Studies in Computational Intelligence   404

Editor-in-Chief

Prof. Janusz Kacprzyk
Systems Research Institute
Polish Academy of Sciences
ul. Newelska 6
01-447 Warsaw
Poland
E-mail: kacprzyk@ibspan.waw.pl

For further volumes:
http://www.springer.com/series/7092

Ahmad Taher Azar (Ed.)

Modeling and Control of Dialysis Systems

Volume 1: Modeling Techniques of Hemodialysis Systems

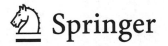 Springer

Editor
Ahmad Taher Azar, PhD, IEEE Member
Assistant Professor, Computer and Software Engineering Department,
Faculty of Engineering,
Misr University for Science & Technology (MUST),
6th of October City, Egypt.
Editor in Chief of International Journal Of System Dynamics Applications (IJSDA),
IGI-Global, USA.

Additional material to this book can be downloaded from http://extra.springer.com

ISSN 1860-949X   e-ISSN 1860-9503
ISBN 978-3-642-27457-2   e-ISBN 978-3-642-27458-9
DOI 10.1007/978-3-642-27458-9
Springer Heidelberg New York Dordrecht London

Library of Congress Control Number: 2011945321

Printed on acid-free paper

Springer is part of Springer Science+Business Media (www.springer.com)

Dedication

I dedicate this book to my wife, her endless prayers through days and nights keep lighting me the way and without her patience, understanding and support the completion of this work would not have been possible. To my dearest, beautiful and extraordinary daughters Hla and Nadine to whose love will always be an inspiration for me. I wish to dedicate this book also, to my mother. She taught me to persevere and prepared me to face challenges with faith and humility. She is a constant source of inspiration to my life. I always feel her presence used to urge me to strive to achieve my goals in life. Also, to my sisters for their endless love, patience, trust and sacrifices for me.

Preface

The primary purpose of the book is to facilitate education in the increasingly important areas of dialysis. It is written as a textbook for a course at the graduate or upper-division undergraduate level for biomedical engineering students. The biomedical engineering is the inter marriage of engineering and medicine. The need to effectively utilize high technology equipment and systems in the dialysis field necessitates the expertise of clinical engineers, hospital physicians and computer scientists. Hardly any patient today would pass through a hospital or even a family physician's chamber without the use of this technology.

Although there is enough material in the text for nephrologists, nurses, technicians and other members of the health care team resolve the myriad of problems confronting the patients undergoing dialysis. The text is also suitable for self study and for short, intensive courses of continuing education. The authors include a senior consultant nephrologist with considerable expertise in all aspects of dialysis. Advanced topics and future challenges are addressed as well, with the researchers in the field in mind. The introductory material, application oriented techniques, and case studies should be particularly useful to practicing professionals.

While several books are available today that address the principles of dialysis, none, unfortunately, provides the practicing knowledge engineer, system analyst, and biomedical researchers with specific, practical information about various modeling and control techniques in the field of dialysis and their applications. The book discusses novel ideas and provides a new insight into the studied topics. The book on this subject will constitute an important contribution in the field of hemodialysis and peritoneal dialysis.

The book is unique for its diversity in contents, clarity and precision of presentation and the overall completeness of its chapters. Each chapter in the book openes with a chapter outline, chapter objectives, key terms list and chapter abstract. Each chapter ends with a conclusion and bibliographic references related to the text. The book is basically broken into two volumes with five parts. The first volume includes the first part of the book from chapters 1–14 which covers overview of dialysis treatment and urea kinetic modeling techniques. There are three treatment modalities available for patients with chronic renal failure: hemodialysis (HD), peritoneal dialysis (PD), and renal transplantation (RT). Although these treatment modalities have proved to be life sustaining, patients with end-stage renal disease (ESRD) continues to grow in the worldwide. The incident population of patients with ESRD is increasing at approximately 6% each year. Kidney transplantation is considered the treatment of choice for many people with severe chronic kidney disease because quality of life and survival are often better than in people who use dialysis. Despite assiduous efforts to utilize renal transplantation as a viable option for potential recipients with ESRD, the donor organ shortage has been one of the major barriers to kidney transplantation. Patients who are not candidates for kidney transplantation or who must wait for a kidney can usually be treated with either hemodialysis or peritoneal dialysis. Dialysis prescription must ensure that an adequate amount of dialysis is delivered to the patient. Numerous studies have shown a correlation between the delivered dose of hemodialysis and patient morbidity and mortality. Therefore, the delivered dose should be measured and monitored routinely to ensure that the patient receives an adequate amount of dialysis. Urea Kinetic Modeling (UKM) is beneficial because it assists clinicians in individualizing dialysis prescriptions and provides the hemodialysis care team with guidance about which specific parameters of the prescription to modify to achieve the target hemodialysis dose. The presentation of these chapters requires only a basic knowledge of linear algebra, differential equations and probability theory.

The second volume of the book includes the remaining parts (from part 2 to part 5). The second part of the book from chapters 15–19 describes online dialysis monitoring devices and continuous therapy. In the past few years, several devices have been developed in the field of dialysis. These devices obviate the need for blood sampling, minimize random measurement errors, and allow a whole range of parameters to be calculated which are likely to be of future clinical value. These new devices also may be coupled on-line to a central database so that measured and calculated values can be recorded without manual intervention, allowing almost instant information of clinical value to the patient.

The third part of the book from Chapters 20–25 covers biofeedback Systems and soft computing Techniques of dialysis. Biofeedback represents the first step towards a 'physiological' HD system incorporating adaptive and logic controls in order to achieve pre-set treatment targets and to ensure delivery of the prescribed dialysis dose. Soft computing approaches in decision making have become increasingly popular in many disciplines. Soft computing concerns the use of theories of fuzzy logic, neural networks, and evolutionary computing to solve real-world problems that cannot be satisfactorily solved using conventional crisp computing techniques. A novel applications of soft computing techniques are discussed in this part of the book. While sufficient theory of each technique is presented, it is offered in a simplified manner for the benefit of the students.

The fourth part of the book from Chapters 26–30 covers the overview of peritoneal dialysis and its modeling techniques.

Finally, the fifth part of the book has two chapters to cove the future challenges and general guidelines of dialysis.

It is hoped that the book will be a very good compendium for almost all readers — from students of undergraduate to postgraduate level and also for researchers, professionals, etc. — who wish to enrich their knowledge on dialysis systems' principles and applications with a single book in the best manner.

Solved Examples, Applications, and Implementation Case Studies

A vast array of illustrative examples, implementation case studies for a variety of applications, end-of-chapter questions and problems are used throughout the text. There are over 1000 questions in this textbook. The basic goals of these case studies, examples and questions are as follows:

- ▶ To help illustrate the theory.
- ▶ To encourage good problem-solving skills.
- ▶ To show how to apply the techniques.
- ▶ To help illustrate design procedures in a concrete way.
- ▶ To show what practical issues are encountered in the development and implementation of dialysis systems.

To the Student

The best way to learn new material is by reading, thinking, and doing. This text is designed to help you along the way by providing an overview and objectives for each section, numerous worked-out examples, exercises and self-test questions. Read each section of the text carefully and think about what you have read. Sometimes you may need to read the section more than once. Work through each example problem step by step before you try the related problem that goes with the example. After the end of each chapter, answer the essay questions and multiple choice questions. The abundance of these questions is very useful for you to check your progress and understanding as they require more systematic and in-depth thinking. If you are able to solve the chapter questions for a given objective, you have mastered that objective.

For Instructors

A. Instructor Solutions Manual

Fully worked-out solutions to end-of chapter questions and problems. So you can check your work.

B. Possible Course Structures

The material in this textbook has been designed for a one-semester, two-semester, or three-quarter sequence depending on the needs and interests of the instructor. The material in the book is suitable for a number of courses at the undergraduate and graduate levels. Some possibilities are given below.

▶ Dialysis principles (senior undergraduate or introductory graduate-level course): Chapters 1, 2, 3, 4, 5, 7, 9, 26, 27, 30, 31 and 32.
▶ Modeling techniques of dialysis (senior undergraduate or graduate-level course): Chapters 6, 8, 10, 11, 12, 13, 14, 19, 25, 28 and 29.
▶ Online dialysis monitoring and continuous therapy (senior undergraduate or introductory graduate-level course): Chapters 15, 16, 17, 18, 19, 25.
▶ Biofeedback Systems and Soft computing applications in dialysis (senior undergraduate or graduate-level course): Chapters 20, 21, 22, 23, 24, and 25.
▶ Principles of peritoneal dialysis and its modeling techniques (senior undergraduate or graduate-level course): Chapters 26, 27, 28, 29, and 30.

Feedback on the Book

We are deeply indebted to the many instructors and students who have offered positive feedback and suggestions for improvement. We are delighted whenever we receive email from instructors and students who use the book, even when they are pointing out an error we failed to catch in the review process. We are also open to your suggestions on how to improve the content, the pedagogy, and the presentation in this text by emailing me at ahmad_t_azar@yahoo.com. We are privileged to have the opportunity to impact the educational experience of the many thousands of future engineers who will turn the pages of this text.

Acknowledgements

My sincere thanks to all contributing authors of this book not only because of their expertise in the science of medicine, but because they are physicians who are able to translate and apply their scientific knowledge in a practical way to allow for a systematic and evidence based plan of therapy and treatment in the best interests of patients.

Special thanks go to our publisher, Springer-Verlag Berlin Heidelberg and data processing team Prabu G., and Shenbagavadivu D. for their valuable review during the publication process. Special thanks for the tireless work of the series editor of Studies in Computational Intelligence, Dr. Thomas Ditzinger.

Ahmad Taher Azar, PhD, IEEE Member
Assistant Professor, Computer and Software Engineering Department,
Faculty of Engineering, Misr University for Science & Technology (MUST),
6th of October City, Egypt.
Editor in Chief of International Journal Of System
Dynamics Applications (IJSDA),
IGI-Global, USA.

About the Editor

Dr. Ahmad Azar has received the M.Sc. degree (2006) in System Dynamics and Ph.D degree (2009) in Adaptive Neuro-Fuzzy Systems from Faculty of Engineering, Cairo University (Egypt). He is currently Assistant Professor, Computer and Software Engineering Department, Faculty of Engineering, Misr University for Science & Technology (MUST), Egypt. Dr. Ahmad Azar has worked in the areas of System Dynamics, Intelligent Control, soft computing and Modelling in Biomedicine and is the author of more than 40 papers in these subjects. He is an editor of four Books in the field of Fuzzy logic systems and biomedical Engineering. Dr. Ahmad Azar is closely associated with several international journals as a reviewer. He serves as international programme committee member in many international and peer-reviewed conferences. He currently serves as the Editor of a lot of international journals. His biography was selected to appear in the 27th and 29th Editions of Who's Who in the World, Marquis Who's Who, USA, 2010 and 2012, respectively. Dr Ahmad Azar is currently the Vice chair of IEEE Computational Intelligence Society (CIS) Egypt Chapter and Vice President Of Egypt System Dynamics Chapter. He is an Academic Member of IEEE Systems, Man, and Cybernetics Society Technical Committee on Computational Collective Intelligence and also a member in KES Focus Group on Agent and Multi-agent Systems. His reserach interests include: Control System Analysis, Systems Engineering, System Dynamics, Medical Robotics, Process Control, Neural network, Fuzzy logic controllers, Neuro-Fuzzy systems, System thinking, Mathematical Modeling and Computer Simulation, Statistical Analysis, Decision Making Analysis, Research Methodology, Biofeedback systems, Monitoring and Controlling of Hemodialysis System.

Contents

Contributing Authors

Ahmad Taher Azar
Assistant Professor, Computer and Software Engineering Department,
Faculty of Engineering, Misr University for Science & Technology
(MUST), 6th of October City, Egypt.
Editor in Chief of International Journal of System Dynamics
Applications (IJSDA), IGI-Global, USA.
e-mail: ahmad_t_azar@ieee.org

Alexandre Granger Vallée
Lapeyronie University Hospital - CHRU Montpellier, France
e-mail: alexandre.granger@videotron.ca

Alicja E. Grzegorzewska
Poznań University of Medical Sciences, Poland
e-mail: alicja_grzegorzewska@yahoo.com

Alfonso Lara
Biomedical Engineering Group, University of Sevilla, ESI, Seville, Spain/
Service of Nephrology, University Hospital Virgen Macarena, Seville,
Spain
e-mail: alararnet@hotmail.com

Alfonso Palma: MD, PhD
Senior Researcher at the Biomedical
Engineering Group of the University of Seville, Spain.
e-mail: apalmaa@senefro.org

Andrea Cavalli
"A. Manzoni" Hospital Departement of Nephrology,
Dialysis and Renal Transplant, Italy
e-mail: a.cavalli@ospedale.lecco.it

Antonio Santoro
Nephrology Dialysis Hypertension Unit;
Policlinico S.Orsola-Malpighi, Italy
e-mail: antonio.santoro@aosp.bo.it

Aron S. Bode
Maastricht University Medical Center, The Netherlands
e-mail: dr.as.bode@gmail.com

Ashita Jiwat Tolwani
University of Alabama at Birmingham, USA
e-mail: atolwani@uab.edu

Bernard Canaud MD, PhD
Professor of Nephrology Montpellier II University School of Medicine;
Head, Nephrology, Dialysis and Intensive Care Unit, Lapeyronie Hospital,
Montpellier, France
e-mail: b-canaud@chu-montpellier.fr

Bertrand L. Jaber
Associate Professor of Medicine St. Elizabeth's Medical Center,
Department of Medicine, USA
e-mail: bertrand.jaber@steward.org

Casper F.M. Franssen
University Medical Center Groningen Department of Internal Medicine,
Division of Nephrology, The Netherlands
e-mail: c.f.m.franssen@int.umcg.nl

Celestina Manzoni
"A. Manzoni" Hospital Departement of Nephrology, Dialysis and
Renal Transplant, Italy
e-mail: c.manzoni@ospedale.lecco.it

Claudio Ronco
San Bortolo Hospital, Italy
e-mail: cronco@goldnet.it

Daniel Schneditz
Medical University of Graz, Institute of Physiology, Austria
e-mail: daniel.schneditz@medunigraz.at

Elena Mancini
Nephrology Dialysis Hypertension Unit; Policlinico S. Orsola-Malpighi,
Italy
e-mail: elena.mancini@aosp.bo.it

Elmer Fernandez
CONICET - School of Engineering, Universidad Católica de Córdoba,
Argentina
e-mail: elmerfer@gmail.com

David Naranjo
Network Center of Biomedical Research in Bioengineering,
Biomaterials and Nanomedicine (CIBER-BBN)/
Biomedical Engineering Group,
University of Sevilla, ESI, Seville, Spain
e-mail: davidazuaga@gmail.com

Declan G. de Freitas
Consultant Nephrologist, Assistant Adjunct Professor, UK
e-mail: declan.defreitas@cmft.nhs.uk

Fredrik Uhlin
Department of Nephrology UHL, County Council of Östergötland and
Department of Medical Health Sciences, Faculty of Health Sciences,
Linköping University, Linköping, Sweden
e-mail: fredrik.uhlin@lio.se

Francesco Locatelli
"A. Manzoni" Hospital Departement of Nephrology,
Dialysis and Renal Transplant, Italy
e-mail: f.locatelli@ospedale.lecco.it

Geoff McDonnell
Centre for Health Informatics, University of News South Wales,
Coogee Campus, Sydney
e-mail: gmcdonne@bigpond.net.au

Giuseppe Pontoriero
"A. Manzoni" Hospital Departement of Nephrology,
Dialysis and Renal Transplant, Italy
e-mail: g.pontoriero@ospedale.lecco.it

Hélène Leray Moraguès
Lapeyronie University Hospital - CHRU Montpellier, France
e-mail: h-leray_moragues@chu-montpellier.fr

Ivo Fridolin
Department of Biomedical Engineering, Technomedicum,
Tallinn University of Technology, Estonia
e-mail: ivo@cb.ttu.ee

Jan H.M. Tordoir
Maastricht University Medical Center, The Netherlands
e-mail: j.tordoir@mumc.nl

Javier Reina-Tosina
Network Center of Biomedical Research in Bioengineering,
Biomaterials and Nanomedicine (CIBER-BBN), Spain
e-mail: jreina@us.es

J. Chris White
ViaSim Solutions, USA
e-mail: jcwhite@viasimsolutions.com

J. Sergio Oliva
Biomedical Engineering Group, University of Sevilla, ESI, Seville, Spain
e-mail: joliva@us.es

John H. Crabtree
Department of Surgery, Southern California Permanente Medical Group,
Kaiser Permanente Downey Medical Center, Downey, California;
Visiting Clinical Faculty, Division of Nephrology and Hypertension,
Harbor- University of California Los Angeles Medical Center, Torrance,
California, USA
e-mail: johncrabtree@sbcglobal.net

Jorge Cerda
Albany Medical College, USA
e-mail: cerdaj@mail.amc.edu

José A. Milán
Biomedical Engineering Group, University of Sevilla, ESI, Seville, Spain /
Network Center of Biomedical Research in Bioengineering,
Biomaterials and Nanomedicine (CIBER-BBN)/ Service of Nephrology,
University Hospital Virgen Macarena, Seville, Spain
e-mail: josea.milan.sspa@juntadeandalucia.es

Judith J. Dasselaar
University Medical Center Groningen Department of Internal Medicine,
Division of Nephrology, The Netherlands
e-mail: judithdasselaar@home.nl

Karen Chia-Ying To
McMaster University, Canada
e-mail: karen.to@medportal.ca

Kenneth Scott Brimble
McMaster University, Canada
e-mail: brimbles@mcmaster.ca

Luciano Alberto Pedrini
Department of Nephrology and Dialysis. Bolognini Hospital – Seriate,
Italy
e-mail: luciano.pedrini@fmc.ag.com

Laura M. Roa
Biomedical Engineering Group, University of Sevilla, ESI, Seville, Spain /
Network Center of Biomedical Research in Bioengineering,
Biomaterials and Nanomedicine (CIBER-BBN), Spain
e-mail: lroa@us.es

Laura M. Rosales
Renal Research Institute, USA
e-mail: lrosales@rriny.com

Laure Patrier
Lapeyronie University Hospital - CHRU Montpellier, France
e-mail: l.patrier@chu-montpellier.fr

Leila Chenine Koualef
Lapeyronie University Hospital - CHRU Montpellier, France
e-mail: l-chenine@chu-montpellier.fr

Leonard M. Ebah
Specialist Registrar in Renal Medicine, UK
e-mail: leonard.ebah@cmft.nhs.uk

Manuel Prado Velasco
M2TB, University of Seville, Spain
e-mail: mpradovelasco@ieee.org

Marion Morena
Lapeyronie University Hospital - CHRU Montpellier & Institut de
Recherche et Formation en Dialyse, France
e-mail: marion.morena@gmail.com

Masatomo Yashiro
Division of Nephrology, Kyoto City Hospital, Japan
e-mail: yashiro@pearl.ocn.ne.jp

Michael Francis Flessner
National Institutes of Health USA
e-mail: flessnermf@niddk.nih.gov

Maurizio Nordio
Nephrology and Dialysis Unit - ULSS 15 "Alta Padovana", Italy
e-mail: maurizio.nordio@gmail.com

Miguel Ángel Estudillo
Network Center of Biomedical Research in Bioengineering,
Biomaterials and Nanomedicine (CIBER-BBN)/ Biomedical Engineering
Group, University of Sevilla, ESI, Seville, Spain
e-mail: m.estudillo@gmail.com

Monica Graciela Balzarini
CONICET - Biometrics Department, School of Agronomy,
Universidad Nacional de Cordoba, Argentina
e-mail: mbalzari@gmail.com

Nathan W. Levin
Renal Research Institite, USA
e-mail: nlevin@rriny.com

Nestor Velasco
Crosshouse Hospital, Kilmarnock, United Kingdom
e-mail: Nestor.Velasco@aaaht.scot.nhs.uk

Orfeas Liangos
Adjunct Assistant Professor of Medicine Tufts University
School of Medicine Klinikum Coburg Coburg, Germany
e-mail: liangos_o@hotmail.com

Philip Alan McFarlane
St. Michael's Hopsital, University of Toronto, Canada
e-mail: phil.mcfarlane@utoronto.ca

Pranay Kathuria
University of Oklahoma School of Medicine, USA
e-mail: pranay-kathuria@ouhsc.edu

Rajnish Mehrotra
Associate Chief, Division of Nephrology and Hypertension,
Department of Medicine, Harbor-UCLA Medical Center, Torrance, CA,
and Professor of Medicine, David Geffen School of Medicine at UCLA,
Los Angeles, CA, USA
e-mail: rmehrotra@labiomed.org

Rodolfo Valtuille
Fresenius Medical Care Argentina, Argentina
e-mail: rvaltuille@gmail.com

Salvatore Di Filippo
"A. Manzoni" Hospital Departement of Nephrology, Dialysis and
Renal Transplant, Italy
e-mail: s.difilippo@ospedale.lecco.it

Shamik Shah
Apollo Hospitals Ahmedabad, India
e-mail: shamik.shah@yahoo.com

Silvio Giove
Department of Economics, University of Venice, Italy
e-mail: sgiove@unive.it

Suhail Ahmad MD
Associate Professor of Medicine University of Washington;
Medical Director, Scribner Kidney Center, Seattle, Washington
e-mail: sahmad@u.washington.edu

Thomas M. Kitzler
McGill University-Divison of Nephrology Lyman Duff Medical Building
Montreal, Quebec, Canada
e-mail: thomas.kitzler@mcgill.ca

Wayne G. Carlson
Minntech Corp. USA
e-mail: wcarlson@minntech.com

Part I

Overview of Dialysis Treatment and Modeling Techniques

Chapter (1)

Initiation of Dialysis

Ahmad Taher Azar, Alicja E. Grzegorzewska

CHAPTER OUTLINES

- Structure of Normal Kidneys
- Function of Normal Kidney
- Kidney Failure (Renal Failure)
- Renal Replacement Therapy (RRT)
- Final remarks and conclusions

CHAPTER OBJECTIVES

- Describe the main functions of the human kidney.
- Describe the main structure of the normal kidney
- Discuss the main types of kidney failure.
- Describe the most common metabolic changes that occur during kidney failure.
- Discuss the methods of performing dialysis.
- Discuss kidney transplantation as a method of renal replacement therapy.

KEY TERMS

- Kidney Function
- Acute Kidney Injury (AKI)
- Chronic Kidney Disease (CKD)
- Hemodialysis (HD)
- Peritoneal Dialysis (PD)
- Continuous Renal Replacement Therapy (CRRT)
- Kidney Transplantation

ABSTRACT

The function of the kidney system is to remove waste products of human metabolism and to eliminate extra fluids. When end-stage renal disease (ESRD) occurs, renal replacement therapy (RRT) - dialysis, transplantation - is required. There are two types of dialysis treatment: extracorporeal blood purification (mainly hemodialysis) and intracorporeal blood purification (peritoneal dialysis). All patients with ESRD should be considered for kidney transplantation. Patients without absolute contraindications should be placed on the transplant waiting list, and receive a kidney, if possible. Patients should be educated about each procedure of RRT.

A.T. Azar (Ed.): Modelling and Control of Dialysis Systems, SCI 404, pp. 3–43.
springerlink.com   © Springer-Verlag Berlin Heidelberg 2013

1.1 STRUCTURE OF NORMAL KIDNEYS

The kidney is an essential organ for the healthy functioning of human beings and is the functional organ in the urinary system. Each person normally has two functioning kidneys which are located in the dorsal abdominal cavity in the retro peritoneal space. They are a bean shaped organ about 11 cm in length, 5 to 6 cm wide, 3 to 4 cm thick. Each kidney weighs 120-160 g. The normal human kidney is pictured in Fig. 1.1. The kidneys are protected and kept in place by a tight fitting capsule (renal capsule) and by layers of fat which cushions them from blunt trauma. The kidneys receive blood from the renal arteries which branch off the abdominal aorta and return blood via the renal vein to the inferior vena cava. The kidney has two layers, the outer layer is called the cortex and the medulla is the inner layer. The kidneys receive from 1000 to 1200 mL of blood every minute which is about 25 % of the cardiac output. Blood enters the kidney via the renal artery and splits into anterior and posterior

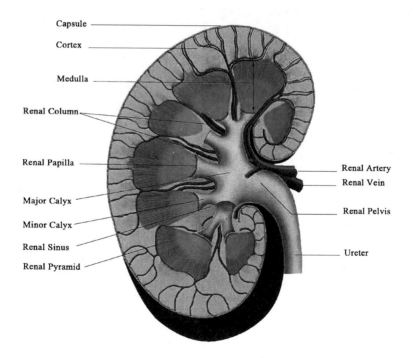

Fig. 1.1 Structure of Kidney

branches and then to lobular arteries which supply the three thirds of the kidney. These arteries split into a large system of capillaries which further break down into tiny vessels called afferent arterioles which enter the glomerulus and form four to eight capillaries in loops which are called the glomerular capillaries. The glomerular capillaries then join again in the efferent arteriole which closely follows the tubular system (for re-absorption and secretion) and then empties into the arcuate vein which joins with other veins and all these small veins exit the kidney via the renal vein (Huether and McCance 2006).

The functional part of the kidney is called the nephron (see Fig. 1.2). Each kidney initially has over one million nephrons: 85% located within the cortex and the other 15% within the juxtamedullary space (Huether and McCance 2006).

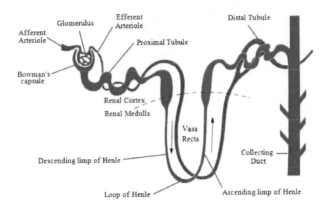

Fig. 1.2 Structure of Nephron-Functional Unit of the Kidney.
Reprinted by permission of Medical Encyclopedia (http://genericlook.com)

Approximately 180 liters of filtrate flow through the nephron system each day. There are two parts of the nephron: the renal corpuscle, and the renal tubule. The renal corpuscle is the initial filtering component of the nephron and is made up of two structures known as the glomerulus and Bowman's capsule (see Fig. 1.3). The Bowman's capsule is a double membrane that cups the glomerulus. The fluid that is filtered into the Bowman's capsule is called the glomerular filtrate.

There are glomerular capillaries inside the glomerulus that are located between the afferent arteriole bringing blood into the glomerulus and the efferent arteriole draining blood away from the glomerulus. The outgoing efferent arteriole has a smaller diameter than the afferent arteriole. The difference in arteriole diameters helps to raise the blood pressure in the glomerulus.

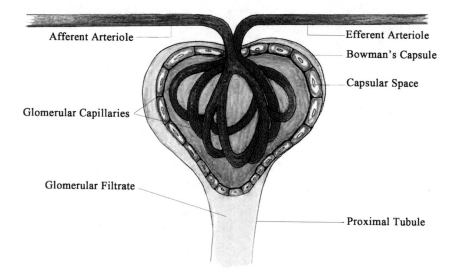

Fig. 1.3 Glomerulus in the Nephron

The renal tubule is the second part of the nephron that receives the filtered plasma from the renal corpuscle. It consists of three parts: the proximal convoluted tubule, the loop of Henle and the distal convoluted tubule. The proximal tubule has a brush border (microvilli) that increases the surface area for absorption. Water and solutes that have passed through the proximal convoluted tubule enter the loop of Henle, which consists of two portions - the descending limb of Henle, then the ascending limb of Henle. The descending limb of Henle is permeable to water, and does not actively transport salt. In the descending limb water diffuses out in response to the high concentration of salt in the interstitium that was created by the ascending loop. This process concentrates the filtrate and reduces its volume, and is known as the countercurrent multiplier system (Fox 2006). The concentrated filtrate then enters the distal convoluted tubule for passage to the collecting duct. Many collecting ducts join together to form several hundred papillary ducts. There are typically about 30 papillary ducts per each renal papilla. The renal papillae are the tips of the renal pyramids, which point towards the centre of the kidney. At each renal papilla the contents of the papillary ducts drain into the minor calyces - the channels through which the fluid passes, via the major calyx, into the centre of the kidney - called the renal pelvis. Because not all of the filtered substances must reach the urinary bladder for elimination, many of the essential substances are absorbed back in the renal tubules through active or passive transport. Water and urea undergo passive transportation whereas glucose, amino acids and some salts go through active transport.

1.2 FUNCTIONS OF NORMAL KIDNEY

The tasks performed by the kidney are summarized in Table 1.1 (Saladin 1999). The kidney has three main functions in the body: the regulation of the volume and composition of extra cellular fluid, the removal of waste products from the body in the form of urine, and the endocrinal functions, which are very important to body homeostasis. These include blood pressure control, erythropoietin production, activation of vitamin D, and acid-base regulation (Huether and McCance 2006). In order to complete their main functions, the kidneys perform complex processes within the nephron (glomerular filtration, tubular secretion and tubular re-absorption of water, electrolytes and metabolic waste products) (Lewis et al. 2004).

Table 1.1 Main Functions of Normal Kidneys

- The kidneys filter blood plasma, separate wastes from the useful chemical, and eliminate the wastes while returning the rest to the blood stream.
- They regulate blood volume and pressure by eliminating or conserving water as necessary.
- They regulate the osmolarity of the body fluids by controlling the relative amounts of water and solutes eliminated.
- They secrete the enzyme renin, which activates hormonal mechanisms (angiotensin, aldosterone) that control blood pressure and electrolyte balance.
- They secrete the hormone erythropoietin, which controls the red blood cell count and oxygen-carrying capacity of the blood.

Table 1.1 (*Continued*)

- They together with the lungs regulate the P_{CO2} and acid base balance of the body fluids.
- They control calcium homeostasis through their role in synthesis of calcitriol (active vitamin D).
- In times of starvation, they deaminate amino acids - remove the–NH_2 group, excrete it as ammonia (NH_3), and make the rest available for glucose synthesis (gluconeogenesis).

1.2.1 Removal of Waste Products from the Body

The kidneys are primarily involved in removing nitrogen-containing wastes to prevent toxic build-up. The metabolic wastes occur during breakdown of nitrogen-containing proteins and purine nitrogenous bases. This metabolism also involves the removal of nitrogen from amino acids, and amino nitrogen is often removed as ammonia, which is extremely toxic to cells and needs to be removed from the blood and body fluids. The liver cells can combine amino nitrogen with carbon dioxide for synthesis of urea, which is much less toxic than ammonia, and is transported in the blood from the liver to the kidneys for excretion with urine. Urea molecule is very small, diffuses easily across cell membranes and requires no specialized transport system. It is osmotically active and can act in regulating osmotic pressure of blood and other body fluids.

Uric acid is a waste product which is also excreted by the kidneys, and while it is a bigger molecule than urea and less soluble, uric acid that appears in urine is mostly secreted by the tubule cells in the kidneys. Uric acid is formed from the metabolism of nucleic acids. Adenosine and guanosine are purine nucleotides, which also contain nitrogen in their ring structure. Purine nitrogenous bases are metabolized to uric acid by the liver cells.

1.2.2 Filtration

Glomerular filtration is the primary process of the nephron and as the name suggests occurs within the glomerulus and Bowman's capsule. The blood passing through the capillaries in the glomerulus is filtered by the capillary membranes which allow the majority of molecules to pass through into the Bowman's capsule. The composition of the filtrate is similar to that of blood however it does not contain larger molecules like blood cells and proteins that are retained in the capillaries (Lewis et al. 2004). The glomerular filtrate is forced across the glomerular membranes by the hydrostatic pressure in the glomerular capillaries (P_{GC}). This pressure is sufficient to overcome the opposing two pressures: the hydrostatic pressure in Bowman's capsule (P_{BC}) and the colloid osmotic (oncotic) pressure in the glomerular capillaries (P_{CO}) (see Fig. 1.4). The hydrostatic pressure is much higher in the glomerulus than in ordinary capillaries. This high hydrostatic pressure enables about 20% of the plasma that flows through the glomerulus to be filtered into the Bowman's capsule. The driving force for filtration is known as the net filtration pressure (NFP). The colloid osmotic pressure in Bowman's capsule is negligible, owing to the virtual exclusion of proteins from the filtrate.

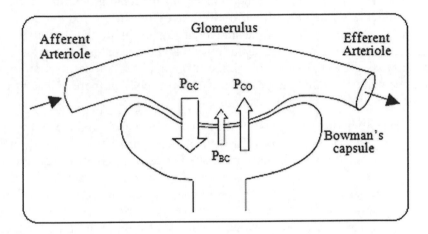

Fig. 1.4 Pressures involved in glomerular filtration (Courtesy of Shirley et al. 2002)

Glomerular filtration rate (GFR) is determined by the product of net filtration pressure (NFP) and the ultrafiltration coefficient (K_f), the latter being a composite of the surface area available for filtration (which is large) and the hydraulic conductance of the glomerular membranes (which is high), and is expressed mathematically:

$$GFR = K_f \times NFP \qquad (1.1)$$

Although direct measurements of P_{GC} and P_{BC} are unavailable in humans, extrapolation from animal studies allows the following estimates of the pressures at the start (afferent end) of the glomerular capillary bed: P_{GC} ~50 mm Hg, P_{BC} ~15 mm Hg, P_{CO} ~25 mm Hg (Shirley et al, 2002). Therefore, NFP is:

$$NFP = P_{GC} - P_{BC} - P_{CO} \qquad (1.2)$$
$$= 50 - 15 - 25 \cong 10 \text{ mm Hg}$$
$$GFR = K_f \times (PGC - PBC - PCO) \qquad (1.3)$$

Since the total GFR for both kidneys is about 125 mL/min and the net filtration pressure is 10 mmHg, so K_f is calculated to be 12.5 ml/min/mmHg of filtration pressure. Changes in K_f probably do not provide a primary mechanism for normal day to day regulation of GFR. Some diseases lower K_f by reducing the number of functional glomerular capillaries (reducing surface area for filtration) or by increasing the thickness of glomerular capillary membrane and reducing its hydraulic conductivity. For e.g. chronic uncontrolled hypertension and diabetes mellitus reduce K_f by increasing the thickness of glomerular capillary basement membrane and eventually by damaging capillaries so severely that there is loss of capillary function (www.similima.com).

Increasing hydrostatic pressure in Bowman's capsule reduces GFR but decreasing this pressure raises GFR. Changes in Bowman's capsule normally do not serve as a primary means for regulating GFR. In certain pathological states associated with obstruction of urinary tract, Bowman's capsule pressure can increase markedly causing serious reduction in GFR. For e.g.: precipitation of calcium or of uric acid may lead to stones that lodge in urinary tract, often in the ureter. Thereby, renal stones obstruct urine outflow from urinary tract, what raises Bowman's capsule pressure and this reduces GFR, and eventually damages or destroys the kidney unless the obstruction is relieved. As blood passes from the afferent arteriole through the glomerular capillaries to efferent arterioles, the plasma protein concentration increases for about 20%, because about one fifth of fluid in capillaries filters into Bowman's capsule, thereby concentrating glomerular plasma proteins that are not filtered. Assuming that the normal colloid osmotic pressure of plasma entering the glomerular capillaries is about 28 mm Hg, this value normally rises to about 36 mm Hg by the time during which blood reaches the efferent end of the capillaries. Average colloid osmotic pressure of the glomerular capillary plasma proteins is midway between 28 and 36 mm Hg or about 32 mm Hg (www.similima.com).

There are two factors that influence the glomerular capillary colloid osmotic pressure: the arterial plasma colloid osmotic pressure and the fraction of plasma filtered by glomerular capillaries (filtration fraction). Therefore, increasing arterial plasma colloid osmotic pressure raises the glomerular capillary colloid osmotic pressure and reduces GFR. Glomerular capillary hydrostatic pressure was estimated to be about 60 mmHg under normal conditions. Changes in glomerular hydrostatic pressure serve as a primary means for physiological regulation of GFR. An increase in hydrostatic pressure raises GFR and a decrease in glomerular hydrostatic pressure lowers GFR. Glomerular hydrostatic pressure is determined by three variables each of which is under physiologic control: (1) Arterial pressure, (2) Afferent arteriolar resistance and (3) Efferent arteriolar resistance. Increased arterial pressure tends to raise glomerular hydrostatic pressure and so increase GFR. Increased resistance of afferent arterioles reduces glomerular hydrostatic pressure and reduces GFR. Dilation of afferent arterioles increases both glomerular hydrostatic pressure and GFR. Constriction of efferent arterioles increases resistance to outflow from glomerular capillaries. This raises glomerular hydrostatic pressure and as long as an increase in efferent arteriolar resistance does not reduce renal blood flow too much, GFR increases slightly (www.similima.com).

Efferent arteriolar constriction also reduces renal blood flow, filtration fraction and glomerular colloid osmotic pressure increase as efferent arteriolar resistance increases. If constriction is severe, rise in colloid osmotic pressure exceeds the increase in glomerular capillary hydrostatic pressure caused by efferent arteriolar constriction. When this occurs the net force for filtration decreases reduction in GFR. Filtrate will constantly drain out of the Bowman's space and into the proximal tubule. When the filtrate enters the proximal tubule, active re-absorption of all the glucose, small proteins and amino acids, and 80% of electrolytes (sodium, chloride, potassium, bicarbonate, phosphate) occurs (Lewis et al, 2004). Some molecules are also secreted into the filtrate: hydrogen ions, foreign substances and creatinine. In the loop of Henle, the concentration process of the filtrate occurs. In the descending loop water is reabsorbed that causes sodium chloride to diffuse back into the blood while urea is being secreted. In the ascending loop chloride ions are reabsorbed via active transport which passively brings across more sodium ions (Huether and McCance, 2006). Thus the filtrate becomes more concentrated.

1.2.3 Regulation of Blood Volume

Volume of fluid in different fluid compartments in human's body depends on the balance between fluid intake and output.

Fluid intake is regulated by thirst. Receptor cells existing in the hypothalamus initiate thirst under hypertonic conditions caused by excessive loss of water or high salt intake. Receptor cells suspend a thirst sense when the hypertonic status is corrected. Specialized receptors in the nervous system correct intake of fluid as well, as they detect the changes in the volume of the blood.

Fluid output as a mechanism of regulation of blood volume takes place by renal excretion of water and sodium. The main hormones involved in this process are the renin-angiotensin-aldosterone system (see 1.2.4 and 1.2.5), anti-diuretic hormone (ADH), and atrial natriuretic peptide (ANP).

ADH, also known as arginine vasopressin, is a potent regulator of blood volume. It is delivered in the posterior pituitary in response to activation of osmoreceptors by increasing plasma osmolarity. The main effect of ADH is increasing the volume of water reabsorbed in the kidneys to limit the fluid lost in urine. ADH binds to receptors on cells in the collecting ducts of the kidneys and causes water reabsorbtion by stimulating insertion of aquaporins ("water channels") into the membranes of kidney tubules. Aquaporins transport solute-free water through tubular cells back into blood. The more free water is absorbed to increase blood volume, the more dilution of the solute concentration occurs. The process of free water reabsorption leads to a decrease in plasma osmolarity and an increase in urine osmolarity. When less urine is formed, more fluid is kept in blood vessels, and the decreased blood volume is regulated. The hypothalamus receptors are not anymore stimulated and ADH secretion is lessened as the osmolarity of the blood and body fluids is reduced. Then the kidneys receive signals to commence water excretion in the urine until the osmolarity of the blood rise for the cycle to commence one more time.

ADH at high concentrations causes constriction of arterioles, which leads to increased arterial pressure. This action explains its name "vasopressin". On the other hand, secretion of ADH is stimulated not only by increasing plasma osmolarity, but also by decreases in blood pressure and volume, conditions sensed by stretch receptors in the heart and large arteries (example hemorrhage).

When blood volume increase, pressure within the atria of the heart increase and atrial dilation occurs. Atrial receptors stretch and transmit a signal for release of ANP, also called atrial natriuretic factor. ANP causes natriuresis, diuresis, and renal vasodilation. It reduces circulating concentrations of renin, aldosterone, and ADH. Thereby ANP secretion is also involved in normalization of circulating blood pressure and volume.

1.2.4 Regulation of Sodium and Potassium

The hormone aldosterone is responsible for regulating the balance of Na^+ and K^+ in the plasma. The renal cortex secretes renin, which triggers the release of aldosterone from the adrenal cortex. When no aldosterone is present, 80% of the sodium and all of the potassium in the filtrate is reabsorbed in the distal convoluted tubule. When aldosterone is present, all of the sodium present in the filtrate is reabsorbed in the distal convoluted tubule. Potassium is actually secreted from the peritubular capillaries into the distal convoluted tubule under the influence of aldosterone.

1.2.5 Regulation of Blood Pressure

The kidneys are involved in the renin-angiotensin-aldosterone system. Renin is the trigger for this system, produced and released from the juxtaglomerular apparatus which is connected to the afferent arteriole next to the glomerulus. The juxtaglomerular apparatus monitors sodium levels in the blood passing through it. Renin acts on angiotensinogen which is constantly present in the blood and converts it to angiotensin I that is converted to angiotensin II by the angiotensin converting enzyme (ACE). Angiotensin II is a powerful vasoconstrictor that acts on the kidney to reabsorb more sodium and water and increases blood flow to the kidney by raising the blood pressure. This system forms an important part of the sodium and water balancing of the body when blood pressure is high or low. Angiotensin II also stimulates the release of aldosterone from the adrenal cortex (Huether and McCance 2006). Aldosterone stimulates more Na reabsorption in the distal tubule, and water gets reabsorbed along with Na. The increased Na and water reabsorption from the distal tubule reduces urine output and increases the circulating blood volume. The increased blood volume helps stretch the heart muscle and causes it to generate more pressure with each beat, thereby increasing the blood pressure. The actions taken by the kidney to regulate blood pressure are especially important during traumatic injury, when they are necessary to maintain blood pressure and conserve the loss of fluids.

1.2.6 Acid-Base Regulation

The kidneys are also responsible for maintenance of acid base balance. This is accomplished by excreting H^+ in the urine and by reabsorbing bicarbonate. Reabsorption of bicarbonate occurs in the proximal convoluted tubule under the direction of the enzyme carbonic anhydrase. Since bicarbonate is almost totally reabsorbed in the nephron, it cannot buffer

H^+ in the urine. Instead, phosphates such as HPO_4^{-2} and ammonia (NH_3) are used.

1.2.7 Erythropoietin Secretion, Vitamin D₃ Production and Glucose Synthesis

The kidneys secrete a substance called erythropoietin that induces red blood cell (RBC) production. Whenever there is hypoxia, or reduced oxygen concentration in the blood, the kidneys secrete erythropoietin in a bid to increase RBC production for elevation the oxygen carrying capacity of the blood. This is why people with severe kidney disease suffer from anemia. The kidneys also convert vitamin D, essential for calcium and bone metabolism, to 1,25-dihydrocholecalciferol or vitamin D_3, the active form of vitamin D. The other amazing function of the kidneys is their ability to produce glucose from amino acids during prolonged periods of fasting in order to sustain the body.

1.3 RENAL FAILURE

Renal failure is the partial or complete reduction of the normal kidney function described above. This is characterized by the inability to remove excess water and metabolic wastes from the body. This subsequently has haemodynamic effects on other systems including blood pressure, blood volume and the blood content (Lewis et al. 2004). Renal failure is classed in two different forms depending on the rate of onset and the cause. The first is Acute Kidney Injury (AKI), the second is Chronic Renal Failure (CRF).

1.3.1 Acute Kidney Injury (AKI)

Up to 2004, the rapid cessation of renal excretory function within a time frame of hours or days, accompanied by a rise in serum urea and creatinine, and accumulation of nitrogenous waste products in a patient whose renal function was previously normal was defined as acute renal failure (ARF). It was usually, but not always, accompanied by a fall in urine output: at least half of all cases with ARF was, however, found to be non-oliguric (Levy et al. 1996; Liano and Pascual 1996; Thadhani et al. 1996; Anderson and Schrier. 1997). Thus, healthy urine output does not ensure normal renal function.

In September 2004, in Vicenza, Italy, the Acute Dialysis Quality Initiative workgroup and representatives from three nephrology societies (ASN,

ISN, and NKF) and the European Society of Intensive Care Medicine used the term acute kidney injury (AKI) to encompass the entire spectrum of the syndrome from minor changes in renal function to requirement for renal replacement therapy. Their definition of AKI is as follows: "An abrupt (within 48 hours) reduction in kidney function currently defined as an absolute increase in serum creatinine of more than or equal to 0.3 mg/dL ($\geq$ 26.4 µmol/L), a percentage increase in serum creatinine of more than or equal to 50% (1.5-fold from baseline), or a reduction in urine output (documented oliguria of less than 0.5 mL/kg per hour for more than six hours)" (Mehta et al. 2007).

AKI is a common complication of critical illness and the predominant reason why patients require continuous renal replacement therapy in the intensive care units (Thakar et al. 2009). Mortality due to AKI requiring dialysis still remains high with over 50% of diagnosed patients dying (Cho et al. 2006, Kellum et al. 2008).

1.3.1.1 Classification of AKI

The first new classification system for AKI is identified by the acronym RIFLE (Risk, Injury, Failure, Loss of kidney function, and End-stage kidney disease) (Bellomo et al. 2004, Kellum et al. 2008). In 2007, a modified version of the RIFLE classification was developed, known as the Acute Kidney Injury Network (AKIN) classification (Mehta et al. 2007).

The Acute Kidney Injury Network (AKIN) offers a staging system for AKI classification which reflects quantitative changes in serum creatinine and urine output (Mehta et al. 2007).

Serum creatinine criteria for AKI stages (Mehta et al. 2007):

- ▸ **Stage 1:** Increase in serum creatinine of more than or equal to 0.3 mg/dL ($\geq$ 26.4 µmol/L) or increase to more than or equal to 150% to 200% (1.5- to 2-fold) from baseline.
- ▸ **Stage 2:** Increase in serum creatinine to more than 200% to 300% (> 2- to 3-fold) from baseline.
- ▸ **Stage 3:** Increase in serum creatinine to more than 300% (> 3-fold) from baseline (or serum creatinine of more than or equal to 4.0 mg/dL [$\geq$ 354 µmol/L] with an acute increase of at least 0.5 mg/dL [44 µmol/L]). Patients who receive dialysis are considered to have met the criteria for stage 3.

Urine output criteria for AKI stages (Mehta et al. 2007):

- ▶ **Stage 1:** Less than 0.5 mL/kg per hour for more than 6 hours.
- ▶ **Stage 2:** Less than 0.5 mL/kg per hour for more than 12 hours.
- ▶ **Stage 3:** Less than 0.3 mL/kg per hour for 24 hours or anuria for 12 hours.

Causes of AKI are the same like those described for acute renal failure: pre-renal, intra-renal and post-renal (Lewis et al. 2004). Pre-renal causes are the most common, forming approximately 55 – 60% of all AKI cases and are also the most readily reversible. They are related to the reduction of blood flow to the kidneys which reduces the glomerular filtration rate due to decreased glomerular perfusion (and decreased glomerular pressure). Failure to recognize and treat pre-renal failure can initiate intra-renal causes such as acute tubular necrosis which is the most common (Huether and McCance 2006). Pre-renal AKI has a number of causes. These are summarized in Table 1.2.

Intra-renal AKI is caused by actual permanent damage occurring to the kidney and kidney structures (Huether and McCance 2006). Acute tubular necrosis is the most common cause which can be started from a number of other causes including ischemic events, nephro-toxic chemicals and drugs, surgery, sepsis, burns and trauma. Once damage has occurred it is generally irreversible. However, human kidneys are able to achieve satisfactory clearance of solutes with decreased numbers of functioning nephrons.

Table 1.2 Causes of acute kidney injury (Lewis et al. 2004)

Pre-renal Causes	Intra-renal Causes	Post-renal Causes
Hypovolaemia Dehydration Haemorrhage Gastro-intestinal fluid losses Excessive diuresis Hypoalbuminaemia Burns	Longstanding Pre-renal ischemia	Prostatic hyperplasia Prostate cancer
Decreased cardiac output Cardiac arrhythmias Cardiogenic shock	Injury to the kidney cells Some antibiotics like gentamycin, amphotericin B Contrast agents	Bladder cancer

Congestive heart failure Myocardial infarction Pericardial tamponade Pulmonary oedema Valvular heart disease	NSAIDS ACE inhibitors Haemolytic blood transfusion reactions Crush injuries Exposure to lead, arsenic or ethylene glycol.	
Decreased peripheral vascular resistance Anaphylaxis Antihypertensive drugs Neurologic injury Septic shock	Acute tubular necrosis (ATN) Acute glomerulonephritis	Bladder calculi formation
Low renal vessel blood flow Renal artery or vein thrombosis Embolism Heparto-renal syndrome	Thrombosis of kidney vessels	Neuromuscular disorders
	Long standing hypertension	Strictures Trauma to the urethra, ureters or bladder
	Allergies to drugs	Spinal cord disease
	Infections	

Post-renal acute renal failure is the least common cause of AKI and occurs when there is urinary tract obstruction affecting both kidneys at the same time. This produces an increased intra-tubular pressure in the kidneys. Backflow from the occlusion causes the glomerulus and the Bowman's capsule to lose their hydrostatic difference and thus filtration, secretion and re-absorption do not occur properly. In this form of AKI, a slow decrease in glomerular filtration rate is shown (Huether and McCance 2006).

1.3.1.2 Common Manifestations of AKI

AKI usually occurs as the result of a sudden interruption in the blood supply to the kidney, or as a result of a toxic overload of the kidneys. Some causes of AKI include accidents, injuries or complications from surgery where the kidneys are deprived of normal blood flow for an extended period of time. Heart-bypass surgery is an example of a situation in which the kidneys receive reduced blood flow. Drug overdoses, whether accidental or from chemical overloads of drugs such as antibiotics or chemotherapy, may also cause the onset of AKI (Feest 1993). Unlike in chronic kidney disease, however, the kidneys can often recover from AKI, allowing the patient to resume a normal life. People suffering from AKI may require supportive treatment until their kidneys recover function, and they often remain at an increased risk of developing kidney failure in the future. Since AKI involves the acute retention of nitrogenous waste products, salt, water, potassium and acids, various physical signs and symptoms may be seen. They are summarized in Table 1.3.

Table 1.3 Common manifestations of AKI

• Nausea and vomiting	• Pleural effusion
• Peripheral oedema	• Weakness
• Breathlessness	• Pericarditis
• Pulmonary oedema	• Depression of consciousness
• Itching	• Oliguria
• Convulsions	• Hypertension

An episode of AKI usually lasts between 7 and 21 days providing the primary insult is corrected in a reasonable time. Irreversible AKI usually occurs either in patients with pre-existing renal disease or in those who experience repeated ischaemic or nephrotoxic insults.

The mortality rate for AKI is variable (Levy et al. 1996). Patients with non-oliguric AKI have a relatively low mortality (10–40%), possibly because they have less severe underlying disease or perhaps because they have been treated more promptly or aggressively. A particularly high mortality rate (80–90%) is found in older patients and in those with serious complications such as preexisting cardiovascular or respiratory disease, severe burns, hepato-renal syndrome, sepsis and multi-organ failure.

1.3.2 Chronic Renal Failure (CRF)

Chronic kidney disease (CKD) is defined by National Kidney Foundation (NKF) as either kidney damage or estimated glomerular filtration rate (eGFR) below 60 mL/min/1.73 m^2 body surface area (BSA) for at least 3 months (NKF-K/DOQI 2002). CKD leads to progressive deterioration of

renal function. At present, according to NKF, five stages of CKD describe
a degree of renal function impairment:

- ▶ Stage 1 describes kidney damage with normal or increased eGFR.
  In stage 1, eGFR is over 90 mL/min/1.73 m^2 BSA. Kidney damage
  is defined by the NKF as "pathologic abnormalities or markers of
  damage, including abnormalities in blood or urine tests or imaging
  studies".
- ▶ Stage 2 means a mild decrease of eGFR (eGFR 60 – 89
  mL/min/1.73 m^2 BSA).
- ▶ Stage 3 means a moderate decrease of eGFR (eGFR 30 – 59
  mL/min/1.73 m^2 BSA).
- ▶ Stage 4 means a severe decrease of eGFR (eGFR 15 – 29
  mL/min/1.73 m^2 BSA).
- ▶ Stage 5 means chronic renal failure (CRF) or end stage renal disease (ESRD). In stage 5, eGFR is below 15 mL/min/1.73 m^2 BSA
  or a patient is treated with dialysis (stage 5D).

Unlike AKI, patients afflicted with CRF do not experience recovery,
and unless treatment is started promptly, their disease will ultimately lead
to death. There are many causes of CRF. The most common cause is diabetes mellitus. The second most common cause is long-standing, uncontrolled, hypertension. Polycystic kidney disease is also a well known cause
of chronic kidney disease. The majority of people afflicted with polycystic
kidney disease have a family history of the disease. Many other genetic
illnesses also affect kidney function. Overuse of some common drugs,
such as aspirin, ibuprofen, and acetaminophen can also cause chronic kidney damage (Perneger et al. 1994). Sometimes people are unaware that
their kidneys are not functioning properly, this is because kidneys are very
adaptable. Even when most of a kidney is not working the remaining portion will increase its activity to compensate for the loss. It is possible to
lead a healthy life with just one kidney instead of the normal two. In fact
patient with kidney failure can stay free of symptoms with just one kidney
working at about 20% of its normal capacity. This is why many patients do
not have any symptoms in the early stages of chronic kidney disease.
People begin to feel ill when their kidney function has dropped to less than
10%, toxic wastes and extra fluids begin to accumulate in the blood. Measuring the level of creatinine in the blood gives an indication of how well
or how poorly the kidneys are working. Kidney failure can cause fluid
overload, producing swelling and high blood pressure; fluid in the lungs
may cause difficulty in breathing and put an added strain on the heart.

Damaged kidneys may not produce enough hormones, which leads to other complications of kidney failure: if the kidneys are not working properly the blood may not have enough red blood cells to carry the oxygen to tissues and patients may become anemic; without the proper amount of hormones and vitamin D, bones begin to lose calcium and become weak.

Many CRF patients develop cardiovascular disease, in fact, heart disease is the main cause of death in CRF patients. Appropriate treatment in the early stages of chronic kidney disease (CKD) may slow or stop the progression of kidney damage. In many patients, CKD does progress to what is known as end stage renal failure (ESRF), end stage renal disease (ESRD) or CKD stage 5. Currently there is no cure for ESRD, the damage done to the kidneys is irreversible and dialysis or a kidney transplantation is needed to replace the lost functions of the kidneys. The amount of time between when patients are first diagnosed with CKD and when they require dialysis or transplantation is different for each patient. It could be a few months or it could be many years depending on the underlying kidney disease, when the kidney disease is first detected, the extent of the damage, and how quickly the remaining kidney function declines.

1.3.2.1 Symptoms of Chronic Kidney Disease (CKD)

Signs and symptoms of CKD depend on the CKD stage. In the early stages (1 – 2), it is possible to detect symptoms related to the underlying kidney disease, like chronic glomerulonephritis, chronic tubulointerstitial nephritis, or diseases causing secondary glomerular involvement, like diabetes mellitus or systemic lupus erythematosus. In more advanced CKD stages, signs and symptoms related to impaired not only renal functions are the greater the higher CKD stage.

Knowing the symptoms of kidney disease can help people detect it early enough to get treatment. These symptoms can include:

- Changes in urination making more or less urine than usual.
- Feeling pain or pressure when urinating.
- Changes in the color of urine, foamy or bubbly urine.
- Swelling of the feet, ankles, hands, or face.
- Arterial hypertension.
- Back or flank pain.

Symptoms related to more advanced CKD stages (3 – 5) are diverse and far-reaching. Since the main function of the kidneys is to cleanse the blood, there is no system that remains unaffected by inadequate removal of waste products. The main clinical changes are seen, when kidney function falls below 25% of normal. They involve not only strict renal symptoms, but also those from other organs, occurring due to their involvement secondary to advanced renal disease. The most commonly observed symptoms include:

- Fatigue or weakness.
- Shortness of breath.
- Having to get up at night to urinate, later decreased or absent urination.
- Swelling of the ankles, feet, and legs.
- Generalized edema (fluid retention).
- Decrease in sensation in the extremities.
- Brushes or bleeding.
- Itching, especially of the legs (pruritus).
- Restless legs.
- Loss of appetite.
- Nausea and vomiting.
- Ammonia breath or an ammonia or metal taste in the mouth, changes in taste, or an aversion to protein foods like meat.
- More hypoglycemic episodes.
- Paleness (anemia).
- Mental disturbances such as agitation, drowsiness, hallucination, or delirium.
- Sleep-disordered breathing.
- Coma.

1.3.2.2 Metabolic Changes Induced by Chronic Kidney Damage

The most common metabolic changes that occur during advanced CKD are elevated levels of serum creatinine and blood urea nitrogen (BUN) due to decreased renal clearance. Clearance is defined as the amount of substance removed from the blood stream in a given time period (clearance is usually expressed in mL/min). Due to the kidney's declining performance, toxins build up in the bloodstream. Three of these molecules, urea, creatinine, and uric acid have already been mentioned. The toxicity of urea has not been established, and indeed many researchers believe that it is not toxic to the body until concentrations are unreasonably high.

Some of the metabolic disturbances associated with decreased kidney function are more difficult to quantify. Patients with advanced CKD also experience a buildup of larger protein fragments and metabolic wastes ("middle molecules") in their blood. There is no definitive answer to the question of what actually causes signs and symptoms seen in CRF patients.

Blood analysis may also indicate that a patient has metabolic acidosis, because bicarbonate ions are used for neutralization of acids, which accumulate in the body due to their low excretion rate with urine. In addition to the buildup of toxins in the blood, water also begins to accumulate in the patient's tissues and spaces (abdominal, pleural, pericardial).

There are also several calcium-related abnormalities that tend to appear as CKD progresses. These include hyperparathyroidism, hypocalcemia, and renal osteodystrophy, all of which result mainly from a loss of production of calcitriol by the kidneys. This loss of calcitriol generally results from an overall decrease in the amount of kidney tissue as decay progresses.

All abnormalities occurring in advanced CKD influence body tissues and organs, resulting in multiple disturbances in their functions.

1.4 RENAL REPLACEMENT THERAPY (RRT)

When the kidneys fail, there are two options for treatment. The most common treatment is dialysis, which shall be described in the following section. The other treatment option is a kidney transplantation, but availability of donor kidneys is limited. Dialysis is often performed as a "bridge to transplant" for stage 5 CKD patients, in order to sustain their life and health until a suitable donor kidney can be found. AKI patients are also given dialysis to substitute for the function of their kidneys until they recover normal renal function.

1.4.1 Dialysis

The most common form of treatment for kidney failure is dialysis. The most renal failure patients spend some time on dialysis while waiting for a donor kidney. Dialysis is a procedure that is performed periodically in order to remove excess water from a patient and to cleanse the blood from metabolic toxins. The procedure is done by placing the patient's blood in contact with a dialysate solution across a semi-permeable membrane. Dialysis was first described by the Scottish chemist Thomas Graham in 1854, who became known as the "Father of Dialysis". Table 1.4 showing the important milestones of dialysis (http://www.edren.org). A History of Hemodialysis is also described in detail in chapter 4.

Table 1.4 Milestones in the development of modern hemodialysis (http://www.edren.org)

1861	The process of dialysis was first described by Thomas Graham (Glasgow)
1913	Artificial kidney developed - John Abel (Baltimore)
1924	First human dialysis - George Haas (Giessen)
1943	Rotating drum dialyzer - Kolff and Berk (Kampen) - the first practical dialyzer
1946	Coil dialyzers - George Murray (Canada), Nils Alwall (Sweden)
1946-7	First dialyses in Britain - Bywaters and Joekes (Hammersmith); Darmady (Portsmouth)
1948	Kolff-Brigham machine - used in the Korean war for acute renal failure
1955	Twin coil dialyzer - Watschinger and Kolff
1956-7	Dialysis recommenced in the UK in Leeds (Parsons), London (Shackman) and RAF Halton (Jackson)
1960	1960 Kiil dialyzer (Oslo)
1960	Scribner shunt (Seattle)
1960	Clyde Shields and Harvey Gentry commenced hemodialysis in Seattle - the first long-term dialysis patients
1961	Dialysis using a domestic washing machine (later leading to the Maytag program in Cleveland; Nose, Japan)
1964	Home dialysis introduced by Shaldon (London), Scribner (Seattle), Merrill (Boston)
1965	Hepatitis outbreaks in the UK
1966	Internal AV fistula developed - Brescia, Cimino (New York)
1972	Aluminium toxicity
1975	Hemofiltration introduced (Henderson, Quellhorst)
1977	Continuous arteriovenous hemofiltration described
1981	Dialysis-related amyloidosis described
1986	Recombinant erythropoietin introduced

There are four main methods of performing dialysis:

- In-Center Intermittent Hemodialysis (IHD)
- Home Hemodialysis (HHD)
- Peritoneal Dialysis (PD)
- Continuous Renal Replacement Therapy (CRRT)

1.4.1.1 In-Center Intermittent Hemodialysis (IHD)

The application of an artificial kidney (an *extracorporeal hemodialysis machine equipped with hemodialyzer)* is sometimes referred to as *hemodialysis*, and the apparatus itself may be called. *Hemo* simply means blood. *Dialysis* is of Greek origin, meaning "to pass through"; the present use implying a filtering (or passing through) process. *Extracorporeal* means "outside the body"; hence an extracorporeal hemodialyzer filters the blood outside the body. Hemodialysis is defined as "any procedure in which impurities and wastes are removed from the blood." It is used in renal failure and other toxic conditions. Standard in-center intermittent hemodialysis (IHD) is performed 3 times a week with each dialysis session lasting 4 hours. IHD is usually managed in specialized units with trained nurses and medical staff. Some patients feel safer getting treatment in a center with doctors, nurses and technicians there to help. They appreciate the chance to meet other people who need dialysis and may make friends at the center. Doing treatments in the center means the home is free of medical supplies. The patient also has days off between treatments and may not think about dialysis. Figure 1.5 presents a diagram of the basic components of hemodialysis system. A hemodialysis machine consists of a set of pumps, mixing chambers, and alarms (not shown) that are designed to pump blood and dialysis fluid into an artificial kidney so that filtration can occur (described in detail in Chapter 3). Once the blood has been filtered and the toxins removed to the dialysis fluid, the used dialysis fluid is sent down the drain, and the cleaned blood is returned to the patient.

In the process of blood purification, the blood, containing high concentrations of waste products such as urea and creatinine, is sent from the patient's body to the dialyzer. The job of the dialyzer is to remove these waste products. This is done by passive diffusion of toxins across the semipermeable membrane. This membrane may be made of cellulose (cuprophane),

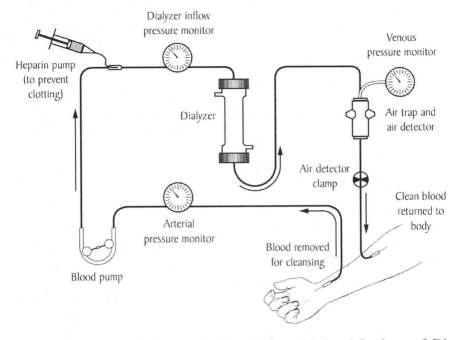

Fig. 1.5 Hemodialysis System. [Adapted from National Institute of Diabetes and Digestive and Kidney Diseases, National Institutes of Health www.kidney.niddk.nih.gov, with permission].

but at present synthetic materials such as polysulphone, polymethylmethacrylate are employed. Urea, creatinine, uric acid, and other small molecules diffuse from the blood through the pores in the membrane into the dialysate driven by a strong concentration gradient. Larger molecules, such as β_2 - microglobulin, cannot pass easily through the conventional dialysis membranes, and are therefore conserved in the patient's blood. Amino acids and vitamins can pass the membrane at a slower rate. For this reason, dialysis patients are often given protein and vitamin supplements to prevent nutritive deficiencies.

Another function of the artificial kidney is known as ultrafiltration. In the process of ultrafiltration, the excess of water is removed from the patient. Inside the dialyzer, there is a certain resistance to the flow of blood. This resistance puts the blood in the dialyzer under a high pressure with respect to the surrounding dialysate bath. As a consequence, water is "squeezed" out of the blood. If the patient has gained more than the recommended amount of fluid since the previous dialysis, negative pressure (suction) can be applied to the dialysate (in the case of a hollow fiber dialyzer) for a removal of a desired water volume. Hemodialysis is not painful, although most patients from time to time experience some discomfort, such as headache, leg cramps, or nausea, particularly during the initial period of adjustment to the treatments. These temporary side effects may respond to the administration of saline solution (infused into the dialyzer's blood lines), or to being placed in a head-lower than- feet position, or to other appropriate medical therapies.

1.4.1.2 Home Hemodialysis (HHD)

Home Hemodialysis is described in detail in Chapter 4. There are three types of hemodialysis that can be performed at home. They are:

1. **Conventional home hemodialysis (CHHD):** This is usually done three times a week for three to four hours or longer each time. Patients are trained to do dialysis safely and to handle any problems that may come up. Training may take from several weeks to a few months.

2. **Short daily home hemodialysis (SDHD):** This is usually done five to seven times a week using new machines designed for short daily home treatment. Dialysis sessions usually last about two hours each. Patients are trained over several weeks. Because patients are doing dialysis more often, less fluid generally needs to be removed each time. This reduces symptoms like headaches, nausea, cramping and feeling "washed out" after the treatment.

3. **Nocturnal home hemodialysis (NHHD):** This term means long (lasting six to eight hours), slow dialysis sessions done at night while sleeping. This is usually done six nights a week or every other night. Some centers monitor the nocturnal sessions by having information from the dialysis machine sent to a staffed location by telephone modem or the Internet. More hours of dialysis each week can increase waste removal.

1.4.1.3 Peritoneal Dialysis (PD)

The other type of dialysis is peritoneal dialysis, in which the patient's own body supplies the dialyzer in the form of the peritoneal membrane. Peritoneal dialysis is described in detail in Chapter 26. The first step toward PD was taken in the 1920s when medical professionals discovered that peritoneal dialysis was effective in treating end stage renal disease (ESRD). Over the years that followed this discovery, developments were made in regard to equipment and materials to ensure safety and cleanliness. In 1968, Henry Tenckhoff created a PD catheter that could remain in a patient's abdomen permanently, instead of being inserted for every treatment. This reduced the risk of infection. Tenckhoff's catheter and the development of continuous cycling peritoneal dialysis (CCPD) in 1981 turned PD into a common form of dialysis treatment. Table 1.5 showing the important milestones of PD dialysis (http://www.edren.org).

The peritoneal cavity contains the various abdominal organs. The organs and the cavity itself are all lined by a highly vascularized layer of peritoneal membrane. This membrane is made of a layer of flattened mesothelial cells that lie over a loose fibrocellular interstitium that contains the blood capillary network. The area covered by this membrane in an adult is 1-2 m^2, and the diffusion distance into the capillaries is short. This membrane is ideal for a natural dialyzer. By introducing fluid into the peritoneal cavity, solutes in the blood are equilibrated with the fluid in a matter of hours (Siroky et al. 2004).

Table 1.5 Milestones in the development of peritoneal dialysis (http://www.edren.org)

1744	Peritoneal lavage undertaken by the Rev. Stephen Hales
1877	Experimental studies of the peritoneum
1923	First human peritoneal dialysis - Ganter
1946	Treatment of acute renal failure by PD - Frank, Seligman, Fine (Boston); Reid (UK); Tanret (Paris); Kop (Netherlands)
1959	Intermittent PD - Ruben and Doolan (Oakland, CA)
1964	Repeated puncture technique introduced - Boen
1965	Stylet catheter (Trocath) introduced
1968	Tenckhoff catheter introduced
1976	CAPD description - Moncrieff and Popovich (Austin, Texas)
1981	CCPD

The peritoneal membrane allows those solutes to pass whose molecular weights are below 30 kDa. The fluid can then be removed and with it the waste materials. The materials that are removed include uremic wastes, excess water, and excess minerals. Since it is not possible to maintain useful hydrostatic pressure across the peritoneal membrane, the dialysate must be hypertonic in order to remove excess water. Glucose is usually used for this purpose. The composition of the dialysate is such that balance of bicarbonate and other biologically important ions is restored. Usually, exchanges of 2 L of fluid are made every 30 – 60 minutes. This can be done by machine, which removes the tediousness of doing it by hand and helps to diminish the possibility of infection by reducing the number of interruptions in the sterile circuit (Siroky et al., 2004). Peritoneal dialysis is commonly administered according to one of the following schedules:

A. Continuous ambulatory peritoneal dialysis (CAPD)
B. Continuous cycling peritoneal dialysis (CCPD)
C. Nocturnal intermittent peritoneal dialysis (NIPD)
D. Tidal peritoneal dialysis (TPD)
E. Intermittent peritoneal dialysis (IPD)

A) Continuous Ambulatory Peritoneal Dialysis (CAPD)

CAPD is the most common type of peritoneal dialysis, it needs no machine, it can be done in any clean, well lit place. CAPD is slow continuous therapy. During CAPD the blood is always being cleaned, the dialysate passes from a plastic bag through the catheter and into the abdomen as shown in Fig. 1.6.

With CAPD, the dialysate stays in the abdomen for 4 to 6 hours; the process of draining the dialysate and replacing fresh solution is performed through the permanent peritoneal catheter and takes 30 to 45 minutes. CAPD requires no external machine, the dialysis is done by connecting the bag of dialysate to the abdominal catheter and allowing the fluid to flow into the abdominal cavity. The empty bag is left attached and rolled up and placed inside clothing around the waist, or in a pocket (or detached). At this point, the patients can return to their normal activity (the patients are free to continue their routine work). After about 4-6 hours, the bag is either removed from the clothing and unrolled or reattached and lowered beneath the abdomen to allow the dialysate to flow back out of the cavity into the bag (via gravity). At this point, the full bag of removed fluid is disconnected and a new bag of dialysate is attached, and the cleaning process begins again. The most CAPD patients perform four exchanges per day, seven days per week. The exchanges are typically done once at wakeup, once at bedtime and two more times during the day (NIDDK 2006).

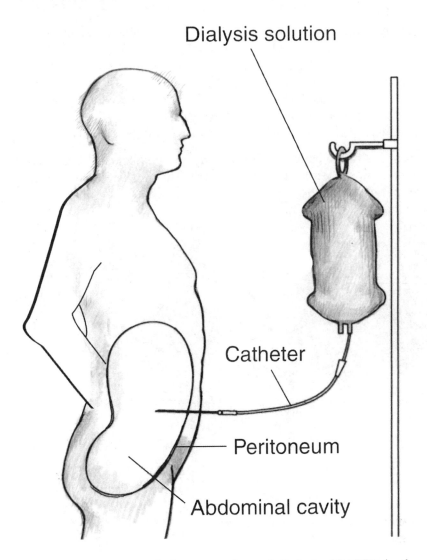

Fig. 1.6 Continuous ambulatory peritoneal dialysis (CAPD) is the most common form of peritoneal dialysis. [Adapted from National Institute of Diabetes and Digestive and Kidney Diseases, National Institutes of Health www.kidney.niddk.nih.gov), with permission]

B) Continuous Cyclic Peritoneal Dialysis (CCPD)

CCPD is similar to CAPD, except that it utilizes a portable cycler machine which is connected to the catheter and automatically warms, fills, drains and weighs the dialysate solution during the night at timed intervals while the patient sleeps as shown in Fig. 1.7. Treatment usually includes 3–5 exchanges during the night over a 10- to 12-hour period. A patient undergoing CCPD typically programs the cycler machine to deliver a dialysate exchange at the end of the nighttime cycler dialysis. In the morning, the patient disconnects from the cycler with a full abdomen and begins a single exchange with a dwell time that lasts the entire day. The patient carries the dialysate in the peritoneal cavity for part or all of the day.

In some cases, the patient performs one or more manual exchanges during the day in addition to the last bag fill exchange. These additional exchanges are usually performed to receive an adequate dose of dialysis and an adequate fluid removal.

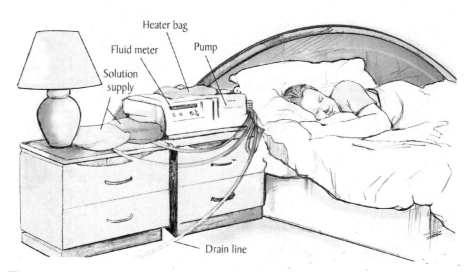

Fig. 1.7 Peritoneal Dialysis Cycler. [Adapted from National Institute of Diabetes and Digestive and Kidney Diseases, National Institutes of Health www.kidney.niddk.nih.gov), with permission]

C) Nocturnal Intermittent Peritoneal Dialysis (NIPD)

NIPD is similar to CCPD, but with more overnight exchanges (at least six) and without the patient performing an exchange during the day. The fluid is drained in the morning, and the abdomen remains empty of dialysis solution the entire day. NIPD patients may be more comfortable without the pressure of dialysate in their abdomens during the day, but they are getting less dialysis than they would with CCPD. For this reason, NIPD is usually reserved for patients whose peritoneums are able to transport waste products very rapidly or who still have substantial remaining kidney function.

D) Tidal Peritoneal Dialysis (TPD)

TPD consists of the repeated instillation of small tidal volumes of dialysis fluid via a cycler machine. The procedure is usually performed nightly. Variables to be set include reserve volume, tidal outflow volume, tidal replacement volume, flow rate, and frequency of exchanges. Theoretically, draining the peritoneal cavity incompletely after each dwell maintains an intraperitoneal reservoir, resulting in more continuous contact of the dialysate with the peritoneal membrane. In addition, the more rapid cycling of dialysis may increase mixing and prevent the formation of stagnant fluid films within the abdomen. It appears that the continual presence of some dialysate in the peritoneal cavity during the cycling procedure of TPD can decrease abdominal discomfort during inflow and outflow. In the most, but not all, studies, however, TPD has not resulted in an increase in urea or creatinine clearance when compared to cycler peritoneal dialysis (Juergensen 2000). The differences in results among these studies stem from differences between the cycler and TPD prescriptions chosen for analysis. A major disadvantage of TPD is the cost of the large volume of fluid needed.

E) Intermittent Peritoneal Dialysis (IPD)

IPD uses the same type of machine as CCPD to add and drain the dialysate. IPD can be done at home, but it is usually done in the hospital. With IPD, treatments are done several times a week, for a total of 36 - 42 hours per week. In practice, IPD is usually performed for 8-12 hours 3 times per week, but sessions may also last up to 24 hours. The automatic dialysis machine has a timer which controls each cycle. The amount of fluid that flows into the abdomen is measured, as well as the amount that flows out. The fluid is left in the abdomen for about 5-10 minutes for equilibration (transperitoneal exchange of solutes between blood and dialysis solution, and water filtration) and then allowed to drain out over about 15 minutes. One inflow, equilibration and outflow is called a cycle. Each cycle takes about 30 minutes to complete and between 16 and 24 cycles complete a treatment. IPD adequacy is measured by calculating how much of the body's waste products carried in the blood is removed during one week.

In many countries, IPD is at present the least popular method of peritoneal dialysis treatment (in-center performance, time-consuming, large volume of dialysis solution used, peritoneal irritation).

1.4.1.4 Advantages and Disadvantages of Dialysis Treatment

Advantages and disadvantages of HD are summarized in Table 1.6.1.

Table 1.6.1 Advantages and disadvantages of hemodialysis

Advantages	Disadvantages
Full medical care during in-center HD sessions	Infections with blood borne viruses (HBV, HCV)
High effectiveness in waste and fluid removal	Muscle cramps
High possibility of individualization of HD schedule	Hypotension episodes
Easy administration of intravenous drugs (erythropoietin stimulating agents, iron)	Dialysis-related amyloidosis
Quick help in sudden situations (pulmonary edema)	Repeated anticoagulation
No anticoagulation for dialysis purposes	Vascular access problems
Most similar to original kidneys	Undernutrition
Self-control over schedule	

Advantages and disadvantages of PD are summarized in Table 1.6.2.

Table 1.6.2 Advantages and disadvantages of peritoneal dialysis

Advantages	Disadvantages
Patient's involvement in self-care	A risk of infection (peritonitis, exit site infection)
If on NIPD, no daytime exchange	Glucose uptake
Less restricted	Placement of permanent abdominal catheter
Clinic visits only once a month	Overhydration in 50% of patients
No needles	Potential weight gain
No anticoagulation for dialysis purposes	Storage space at home for supplies
Most similar to original kidneys	Body image change
Self-control over schedule	A need for a trained helper when a patient is disabled (so called assisted PD)

Differences between HD and PD are summarized in Table 1.7. PD is simple to perform and does not require much training. It is often performed at the patient's home by himself (herself), and the patient can often continue to hold a full time job. The equipment required is much simpler. The removal of fluid and solutes is much gentler on the patient. Neither direct vascular accesses nor anticoagulatory drugs are required.

Table 1.7 Differences between Hemodialysis and PD

	Hemodialysis	**Peritoneal dialysis**
Dialysis characteristics	Hemodialysis is intermittent. Fluid, wastes and chemicals build up between treatments.	CAPD or CCPD is continuous throughout the entire day. Changes in fluid buildup and wastes are not so dramatic and noticeable.
Frequency	Usually three times each week, but may be up to six times a week.	Dialysis solution is exchanged four to five times each day or several times as the patient sleep.
Duration	Usually four hours if the patient has treatment three times a week. About two hours if the patient has treatment six times a week.	Manual exchanges of dialysis solution (inflow and outflow): 30 to 45 minutes for each exchange. During the night using a cycler: 10 to 12 hours.
Type of access	Vascular access, usually in arm.	Peritoneal catheter in the abdomen.
Location	In a dialysis center or home.	Manual exchanges: Many locations, mainly home or at work. During the night using an automated cycler: At home or at the destination if the patient travels.
Supplies needed	Dialysis machine, dialysis solution, treated water and disposable supplies.	Bags of dialysis solution, disposable supplies. A cycler is needed if the patient is treated at home during the night.
Training for home performance	Time-consuming, lot of failure	Simple for an average patient

Some dangers of hemodialysis, such as a rapid drop in blood potassium, do not occur with peritoneal dialysis. The most serious disadvantage associated with peritoneal dialysis is a risk of infection (bacterial, fungal) resulting in peritonitis or in infection of the catheter exit site or tunnel. While usually not life-threatening, it is a painful condition for the patient. Repeated episodes of peritonitis may diminish the permeability of the peritoneal membrane to water and solutes and are the number one cause of drop out in PD programs. Other PD problem is the need for peritoneal access. Once the catheter is surgically implanted, it usually remains clear to get fluid into the cavity, but can often be blocked when trying to remove fluid. This problem is caused by the omentum, a loose sheet of mesothelial tissue that floats freely in the peritoneal cavity. It can wrap around a catheter and block outflow. This problem often must be corrected with surgery, but can occasionally correct itself spontaneously. A fatal PD complication is encapsulating peritoneal sclerosis occurring in long-term PD patients in about 10% of cases.

1.4.1.5 Continuous Renal Replacement Therapy (CRRT)

CRRT is described in detail in Chapter 18. It was initiated due to the restrictions of both peritoneal dialysis (PD) and intermittent hemodialysis (IHD).

PD has been shown to have too low clearance of wastes and insufficient water removal for needs of instable patients with acute kidney injury, a risk of dialysis-related of infections, a limitation of respiratory function as well as difficulties to manage blood glucose levels (Elliot et al. 2007; Cho et l. 2006). Therefore PD is generally not recommended for treating adults in the intensive care units (Ronco et al. 2001).

Standard IHD treatment consists of 4 hour session every second day and needs hemodialysis machines requiring a specialized staff, what means that patients have to be transported to a dialysis unit for treatment, because the intensive care units are usually not prepared for such a treatment. This situation increases risks to the critically ill patient as well as delays the necessary treatment. IHD was also shown to affect the condition of the critically ill patient adversely in a couple of main areas. These included the increased hemodynamic instability, the fluctuations in uraemic and fluid control and decreased metabolic control (Ronco et al. 2001).

1.4.2 Kidney Transplantation

A surgeon places the kidney from a deceased or alive donor inside the lower abdomen of a patient with end-stage renal disease, who is a recipient, and connects the artery and vein of the new kidney to artery and vein of the recipient. The blood flows through the new kidney, which makes urine, just like the original kidneys did when they were healthy. Unless the original kidneys are causing infection or high blood pressure, they are left in place as shown in Fig. 1.8 (www.kidney.niddk.nih.gov).

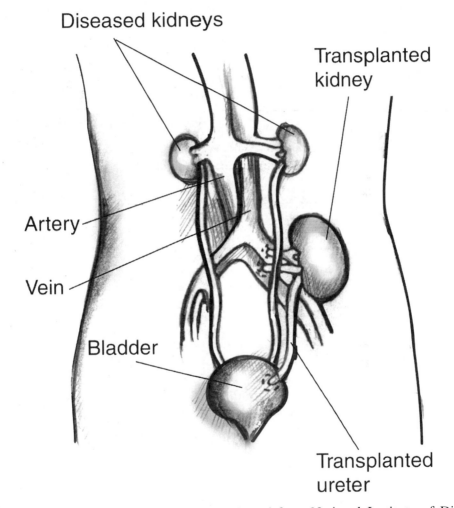

Fig. 1.8 Kidney transplantation. [Adapted from National Institute of Diabetes and Digestive and Kidney Diseases, National Institutes of Health www.kidney.niddk.nih.gov), with permission]

The first successful kidney transplantation was done in 1954 in Boston between identical twins, to eliminate any problems of an immune reaction. It was actually the first successful human organ transplantation in history. Kidney transplants were slow to catch on, for example the first kidney transplantation in the United Kingdom did not occur until 1960 when Michael Woodruff performed one between identical twins in Edinburgh. The important milestones of kidney transplantation are shown in Table 1.8 (http://www.edren.org).

Table 1.8 Milestones in kidney transplantation (http://www.edren.org)

1933	First human renal transplantation (unsuccessful) - Voronoy
1936	Histocompatibility antigens described in mice - Snell
1944	Accelerated rejection of a second transplant described in rabbits - Medawar
1954	First successful human renal transplantation, between identical twins - Murray and Merril (Boston)
1962	First successful cadaver transplantation and the first use of azathioprine - Murray and Calne
1962	Second use of azathioprine - Edinburgh's third renal transplantation
1964	Tissue typing using white blood cells - van Rood and van Leeuwen, Terasaki
1976	UK brain death guidelines facilitate retrieval from heart-beating cadaveric donors
1983	Cyclosporine licensed as new immunosuppressive drug

The most patients receive a renal transplant after having been established on maintenance hemodialysis or peritoneal dialysis. More recently, however, many patients receive a renal transplant before they require dialysis. Indeed, if the supply of kidneys were to increase, this shortcut would become an increasingly common practice. Transplantation before the commencement of dialysis (pre-emptive transplantation) has been convincingly shown to improve posttransplant patient and graft survival. Because of the varied course of advanced chronic kidney disease, it is difficult to provide a precise point when referral for transplantation should be made. However, patients with a glomerular filtration rate (GFR) below 20 mL/min/1.73 m^2 BSA and patients whose course suggests they will be dialysis dependent in 1 to 2 years should be referred. The decision to place a patient on the waiting list for transplantation should be made jointly by the nephrologist and the transplant surgeon. All patients with ESRD should be considered for kidney transplantation, provided no absolute contraindications exist. Patients should receive intermittent re-education about the procedure. Donors require extensive screening to ensure complete health and absence of renal disease. Comorbidity should be regularly re-assessed, especially cardiac disease. The most common problem after transplantation is rejection of the transplanted kidney - the body's immune system sees the transplant as "foreign" and attacks it. To lower the risk of rejection, patients having a kidney transplantation take immunosuppressant drugs to keep the immune system from attacking. These drugs have side effects that may include weight gain, high blood pressure, an increased risk of infection, diabetes mellitus, and certain kinds of cancer. All of these side effects can be managed. Transplant recipients have to follow a special diet, but with many fewer limits than it is indicated for patients on in-center intermittent hemodialysis.

1.5 FINAL REMARKS AND CONCLUSIONS

Healthy kidneys through their excretory, hormonal and regulatory functions maintain homeostasis inside human body. Disturbances in renal function lead to multiorgan consequences. Kidney injury may be acute and reversible or irreversible. Chronic kidney damage due to primary or secondary renal diseases progresses to such a decrease in all kidney functions that further existence is impossible without renal replacement therapy.

Dialysis (peritoneal dialysis, extracorporeal dialysis) is applied for both acute kidney injury and advanced chronic kidney disease (stage 4/5 or 5). Renal transplantation is performed in cases of irreversible kidney damage. The method of renal replacement therapy should be individually chosen for each patient. All these methods are interchangeable: for example peritoneal dialysis complicated with serious peritonitis may be replaced temporarily or permanently with intermittent hemodialysis; renal transplant failed patients may re-start peritoneal or hemodialysis.

Dialysis treatment is not so effective as natural function of healthy kidneys or successful renal transplant function. For this reason a special attention should be paid for adequate dialysis treatment. Currently used methods of estimation of hemodialysis adequacy are described in the next chapters. Adequate hemodialysis is an important integral part of a complex care in end-stage renal disease.

REFERENCES

Anderson, R.J., Schrier, R.W.: Acute renal failure. In: Schrier, R.W., Gott-schalk, C.W. (eds.) Diseases of the Kidney, pp. 1069–1113. Little, Brown, Boston (1997)

Bellomo, R., Ronco, C., Kellum, J.A., et al.: Acute renal failure – definition, outcome measures, animal models, fluid therapy and information technology needs. In: The Second International Consensus Conference of the Acute Dialysis Quality Initiative (ADQI) Group. Crit. Care, vol. 8, pp. R204–R212 (2004)

Cho, K.C., Himmelfarb, J., Paganini, E., et al.: Survival by Dialysis Modality in Critically Ill Patients with Acute Kidney Injury. J. Am. Soc. Nephrol. 17(11), 3132–3138 (2006)

Elliot, D., Aitken, L., Chaboyer, W.: ACCCN's Critical Care Nursing. Elsevier Mosby, Sydney (2007)

Feest, T.G., Round, A., Hamad, S.: Incidence of severe acute renal failure in adults: Results of a community based study. BMJ 306, 481–483 (1993)

Fox, S.I.: Human Physiology, 9th edn. Wm. C. Brown Publishers (2006)

Grzegorzewska, A.E., Kaczmarek-Leki, V., Młot-Michalska, M., Niepolski, L.: Seroconversion rate to positivity for antibodies against core antigen of hepatitis B virus and duration of renal replacement therapy. Nephrol. Dial Transplant 26(3), 970–976 (2011)

Huether, S.E., McCance, K.L.: Pathophysiology: The Biologic Basis for Disease in Adults and Children, 5th edn. Elsevier Mosby, St. Louis (2006)

Juergensen, P.H., Murphy, A.L., Pherson, K.A., et al.: Tidal peritoneal dialysis: comparison of different tidal regimens and automated peritoneal dialysis. Kidney Int. 57(6), 2603–2607 (2000)

Kellum, J.A., Bellomo, R., Ronco, C.: Definition and classification of acute kidney injury. Nephron Clin. Pract. 109(4), c182–c187 (2008)

Kellum, J.A., Mehta, R., Angus, D., Palevskey, P., Ronco, C.: The first international consensus conference on continuous renal replacement therapy. Kidney Int. 62(5), 1855–1863 (2002)

Klahr, S., Miller, S.: Acute oliguria. N. Engl. J. Med. 338(10), 671–675 (1998)

Lewis, S.M., Heitkemper, M.M., Dirksen, S.R.: Medical-Surgical Nursing: Assessment and Management of Clinical Problems, 6th edn. Mosby, St. Louis (2004)

Levy, E.M., Viscoli, C.M., Horwitz, R.I.: The effect of acute renal failure on mortality. JAMA 275(19), 1489–1494 (1996)

Liano, F., Pascual, J.: Epidemiology of acute renal failure: A prospective, multicenter, community-based study. Kidney Int. 50(3), 811–818 (1996)

Mehta, R.L., Kellum, J.A., Shah, S.V., et al.: Acute Kidney Injury Network: report of an initiative to improve outcomes in acute kidney injury. Crit. Care 11(2), 31 (2007)

National Institute of Diabetes and Digestive and Kidney Diseases, NIDDK, Treatment Methods for Kidney Failure: Peritoneal Dialysis (2006), http://www.kidney.niddk.nih.gov

NKF-K/DOQI clinical practice guidelines for chronic kidney disease: evaluation, classification, and stratification. Am. J. Kidney Dis. 39(2 suppl. 1), S1–S266 (2002)

Palevsky, P., Bunchman, T., Tetta, C.: The Acute Dialysis Quality Initiative–part V: Operational Characteristics. Advanced Renal Replacement Therapies 9(4), 268–272 (2002)

Perneger, T.V., Whelton, P.K., Klag, M.J.: Risk of kidney failure associated with the use of acetaminophen, aspirin, and nonsteroidal antiinflammatory drugs. N. Engl. J. Med. 331(25), 1675–1679 (1994)

Ponikvar, R.: Blood purification in the intensive care unit. Nephrol Dial Transplant. 18(suppl. 5), v63–v67 (2003)

Ronco, C., Bellemo, R., Ricci, Z.: Continuous renal replacement therapy in critically ill patients. Nephrol. Dial Transplant 16(suppl. 5), 67–72 (2001)

Saladin, K.S.: Anatomy and Physiology: The Unity of Form and Function. William C Brown McGraw Hill, Boston (1999)

Shirley, D., Capasso, G., Unwin, R.: Renal hemodynamics and glomerular filtration. In: Glynne, P., Allen, A., Pusey, C. (eds.) Acute Renal Failure in Practice, pp. 3–9. Imperial College Press, London (2002)

Siroky, M.B., Oates, R.D., Babayan, R.K.: Handbook of Urology: Diagnosis & Therapy. Williams & Wilkins publisher, Lippincott (2004)

Thadhani, R., Pascual, M., Bonventre, J.V.: Acute renal failure. New Engl. J. Med. 334(22), 1448–1460 (1996)

Thakar, C.V., Christianson, A., Freyberg, R., et al.: Incidence and out-
    comes of acute kidney injury in intensive care units: a Veterans
    Administration study. Crit. Care Med. 37(9), 2552–2558 (2009)
Van Rood, J.J., van Leeuwen, A., Eernisse, J.G., et al.: Relationship of
    leukocyte groups to tissue transplantation compatibility. Ann. N.
    Y. Acad. Sci. 120, 285–298 (1964)

Internet References

- National Kidney Foundation (*http://www.nkf.org*, 2000).
- NKF-DOQI guidelines (*http://www.kidney.org*)
- National Institute of Diabetes and Digestive and Kidney Diseases (NIDDK) (*www.kidney.niddk.nih.gov*)
- www.similima.com

QUESTIONS

1. List the main Functions of Normal Kidney
2. How to make a diagnosis of acute kidney injury?
3. What is the main classification of acute kidney injury?
4. Differentiate between acute kidney injury and chronic renal failure
5. List some of the symptoms of chronic kidney disease
6. What are the clinical manifestations of kidney failure?
7. List the different methods of performing dialysis
8. Compare the main types of home hemodialysis
9. List the main types of peritoneal dialysis
10. Describe the advantages and disadvantages of peritoneal dialysis

SELF-TEST QUESTIONS

Choose the best answer

1. The kidneys produce about....liters of glomerular filtrate per day.
    A. 1,000
    B. 180
    C. 110
    D. 7.5
    E. 1 to 2.

2. The kidneys are located in the....
    A) pelvic cavity
    B) peritoneal cavity
    C) abdominal cavity
    D) retroperitoneal space

3. The cardiac output passing through the kidneys accounts for....
    A) 10%
    B) 25%
    C) 50%
    D) 65%

4. The outermost layer surrounding the kidney is....
    A) cortex
    B) medulla
    C) pelvis
    D) capsule

5. Each kidney contains approximately....nephrons.
    A. 10 million
    B. 1 million
    C. 100,000
    D. 10,000

6. The kidney secretes....for stimulating bone marrow activity.
    A) renin
    B) aldosterone
    C) erythropoietin
    D) somatomedin

7. Decreasing in blood pressure stimulates the kidneys to secrete....
    A) aldosterone
    B) renin
    C) angiotensinogen
    D) angiotensin II

8. A nephron is made up of:
    A. A glomerulus and a tubule
    B. A cortex and a capsule
    C. The loop of Henle and the capillary ball
    D. The bladder and the ureter

9. The functional unit of the kidney is the....
    A. Medulla
    B. Cortex
    C. Calyx
    D. Nephron

10. ....is a hormone that regulates renal excretion of electrolytes.
    A. angiotensin II
    B. aldosterone
    C. angiotensin I
    D. ADH.

11. ....is the last part of the nephron.
    A) collecting duct
    B) renal papilla
    C) distal convoluted tubule
    D) glomerulus

12. The renal medulla is composed of tissue called _____.
    A. Renal pyramids
    B. Nephrons
    C. Renal sinus
    D. Renal pelvis

13. .... directs blood into the glomerulus.
    A)   renal artery
    B)   afferent arteriole
    C)   efferent arteriole
    D)   peritubular capillary

14. Oncotic pressure in the glomerulus....
    A. forces water into the Bowman's capsule
    B. pushes plasma proteins and red blood cells into the Bowman's capsule
    C. pulls water back into the glomerulus

15. Hydrostatic pressure in the Bowman's capsule....
    A. pulls water into the Bowman's capsule
    B. forces water back into the glomerulus
    C. blocks the entry of large plasma proteins

16. If the hydrostatic pressure exerted by the fluid in the capsular space increased, GFR would....
    A) increase
    B) decrease
    C) not change

17. Renin hormone is produced by....
    A) mesangial cells
    B) macula densa
    C) principal cells of the DCT
    D) juxtaglomerular cells

18. If the level of aldosterone hormone increases in the blood....
    A) less sodium is excreted in the urine
    B) less potassium is excreted in the urine
    C) systemic blood pressure decreases
    D) glomerular filtration decreases
    E) both C) and D)

19. With CAPD, the dialysate stays in the abdomen for about....
    A. 5 to 7 hours
    B. 4 to 6 hours
    C. 3 to 5 hours
    D. 4 to 7 hours

20. With IPD, dialysis is done for .... three times per week.
    A. 5-10 hours
    B. 4-6 hours
    C. 3-8 hours
    D. 8-12 hours

Chapter 2

Measurement of Renal Function

Ahmad Taher Azar

CHAPTER OUTLINES

- Stages of chronic kidney disease
- Measurement of residual renal function in adults
- Glomerular Filtration Rate (GFR) in Children with chronic kidney disease
- Conclusion

CHAPTER OBJECTIVES

- Describe the main stages of chronic kidney disease
- Discuss the different methods for calculating Glomerular Filtration Rate in adults.
- Discuss the different methods for calculating Glomerular Filtration Rate in Children.

KEY TERMS

- Chronic kidney disease
- Residual Renal Function
- Glomerular Filtration Rate (GFR)
- Inulin Clearance
- Creatinine Clearance
- Cystatin C
- β-Trace Protein (BTP)
- Iohexol Clearance
- Radioisotopes

ABSTRACT

Chronic kidney disease is a worldwide public health problem with an increasing incidence and prevalence, poor outcomes, and high cost. Outcomes of chronic kidney disease include not only kidney failure but also complications of decreased kidney function and cardiovascular disease. Current evidence suggests that some of these adverse outcomes can be prevented or delayed by early detection and treatment. Residual renal function among patients with end stage renal disease is clinically important as it contributes to adequacy of dialysis, quality of life, morbidity and mortality. The preservation of residual renal function (RRF) is important after initiating dialysis, as well as in the pre-dialysis period. Longer preservation of RRF provides better small and middle molecule removal, improved volemic status and arterial pressure control, diminished risk of vascular and valvular calcification due to better phosphate removal. Deterioration of RRF results in worsening of anemia, inflammation and malnutrition. A direct relationship between RRF value and survival in dialysis patient. is now proved.

A.T. Azar (Ed.): Modelling and Control of Dialysis Systems, SCI 404, pp. 45–98.
springerlink.com   © Springer-Verlag Berlin Heidelberg 2013

2.1 STAGES OF CHRONIC KIDNEY DISEASE

Chronic kidney disease is defined according to the presence or absence of kidney damage and level of kidney function—irrespective of the type of kidney disease (diagnosis). Chronic kidney disease represents a public health threat due to (1) the high burden of the disease; (2) the evidence that the problem is distributed unfairly with regard to ethnicity; (3) the undisputed evidence that upstream preventive strategies could reduce the burden of the condition; and (4) the fact that preventive strategies are not yet in place (Schoolwerth et al. 2006).Among individuals with chronic kidney disease, the stages are defined based on the level of kidney function. In February 2002, the Kidney Disease Outcomes Quality Initiative (K/DOQI) of the National Kidney Foundation (NKF) published 15 clinical practice guidelines on chronic kidney disease (National Kidney Foundation, 2002). The goals of the guidelines are to 1) define chronic kidney disease and classify its stages, regardless of underlying cause; 2) evaluate laboratory measurements for the clinical assessment of kidney disease; 3) associate the level of kidney function with complications of chronic kidney disease; and 4) stratify the risk for loss of kidney function and development of cardiovascular disease (CVD) (Levey et al. 2003). To guide clinicians with the decision-making process, NKFK/ DOQI has developed a classification scheme for stratifying CKD patients based on their level of residual renal function (Table 2.1).

Table 2.1 Stages of Chronic Kidney Disease (NKF-K/DOQI 2002).

Stage	Description	GFR (mL/min/1.73m^2)
1	Kidney damage with normal or increased GFR	$\geq$ 90
2	Kidney damage with mild decreased GFR	60-89
3	Moderately decreased GFR	30–59
4	Severely decreased GFR	15-29
5	Kidney failure	< 15 (or dialysis)

Identifying the presence and stage of chronic kidney disease in an individual is not a substitute for accurate assessment of the cause of kidney disease, extent of kidney damage, level of kidney function, comorbid conditions, complications of decreased kidney function, or risks for loss of kidney function or cardiovascular disease in that patient.

Defining stages of chronic kidney disease requires "categorization" of continuous measures of kidney function, and the "cut-off levels" between stages are inherently arbitrary. Nonetheless, staging of chronic kidney disease will facilitate application of clinical practice guidelines, clinical performance measures and quality improvement efforts to the evaluation, and management of chronic kidney disease (NKF-K/DOQI 2002).

2.2 MEASUREMENT OF RESIDUAL RENAL FUNCTION

In daily clinical practice of urologists and nephrologists the determination of the total renal function as well as the separate renal function (split function) are important tools in the diagnosis and therapy of bilateral and unilateral renal disease. The most important parameter for assessing the renal function is the glomerular filtration rate (GFR). Because GFR varies directly with renal size, which in turn varies with body size, GFR is conventionally factored by body surface area. In normal humans, GFR is approximately 125 mL/min/1.73m^2. The value of 1.73m^2 reflects that GFR is corrected for body surface area represents an average value for normal young men and women. When the GFR is corrected for body surface area, a normal range can be derived to assess renal impairment. Despite adjustment for body surface area, however, the normal GFR for women is approximately 8% lower than for men. GFR is rarely measured clinically except for research when inulin, radioiodinated substance such as iothalamate is used. Estimation of the GFR is used to monitor renal disease, to determine the effectiveness of treatment designed to slow the progression of renal disease, confirm the need for initiating renal replacement therapy (dialysis and transplantation) and to allow for the proper dosing drugs excreted by the glomerular filtration to avoid drug toxicity (NKF-K/DOQI 2002).

2.2.1 The Concept of Renal Clearance

The clearance of a substance from a compartment is defined as the ratio between the elimination rate of the substance (mg/min) from that compartment and the concentration of the substance (mg/mL) in the same compartment. Clearance of a GFR is equivalent to the virtual volume of plasma which contained the amount of the substance removed in unit time and then adjusted for surface area. The GFR can be determined according to two different clearance techniques depending on the samples that are required for the calculation. In clinical practice, renal clearance indicates that urine and plasma samples of the marker are needed, whereas a plasma clearance, also called body clearance, indicates that only plasma samples are needed.

The renal clearance technique was introduces by Rehberg (1926) using exogenous creatinine as a marker. He applied the classic formula:

$$GFR = \frac{U \times V}{P} \qquad (2.1)$$

where U is the urinary concentration of the marker (mg/mL), V is the urine flow rate (mL/min) and P is the average plasma concentration of the marker (mg/mL). The plasma clearance of the marker is calculated by dividing the injected dose with the area under the curve (AUC), which describes the decrease in plasma concentration of the marker from time of injection to infinity. Determination of the GFR requires the utilization of a substance meet the following criteria (Kasiske and Keane 2000): it should be "freely" filtered by the glomerulus and not metabolized, bound to plasma proteins, secreted into or reabsorbed by the renal tubules, not eliminated by extra renal routes, readily diffusible in the extracellular space, safe, convenient and inexpensive. Ideally, the amount of the substance should appear unchanged in urine and be equal to the amount of injected dose. In addition, the marker itself should have no effect on GFR. Another way is to infuse a glomerular substance until equilibration occurs and collect repeated urinary samples while plasma level remains constant. This is the most accurate method but is time consuming.

Various substances (markers) used to measure GFR include exogenous or endogenous substances. Examples of endogenoussubstances are urea, Creatinine, Cystain C). Examples of exogenous substances that may be used as GFR markers are: (a) polysaccharides such as inulin and labeled inulin; (b) water-soluble labeled chelates such as ^{51}Cr-EDTA (ethylenediamine tetraacetic acid), ^{99m}TC-DTPA (technetium-99m-diethylene triamine pentaaceticacid) and non-labeled chelates such as Gd-DTPA; (c) urographic contrast media labeled with a radioactive isotope such as ^{131}I-diatrizoate and ^{131}I-iothalamate; and (d) non-labelled urographic contrast media such as ionic monoers (e.g. metrizoate, diatrizoate, iothalamate), and non-ionic monomers (e.g. iohexol, iopamidol, iopromide). All exogenous marker subtances can be given intravenously either as a constant infusion or as a bolus injection. A bolus injection of the marker is easier to handle for patients and staff than a constant infusion of the marker. Many of these substances do not satisfy the requirement for glomerular substances. The mean of urea and creatinine clearances provides a reasonably accurate GFR.

2.2.2 Exogenous Substances for Measuring GFR

2.2.2.1 Inulin Clearance (C_{In})

The fructose polysaccharide inulin (MW 5200 Dalton) is generally considered the gold standard for GFR measurement. It was proposed by Richards et al (1934); Shannon and smith(1935) as a marker for GFR. The reference ranges for the GFR in normal individuals given by Smith are 88 to 174 mL/min/1.73m^2 for males and 87 to 147 mL/min/1.73m^2 for females (Shannon and smith 1935). Inulin is freely filtered by glomerulus, and is neither reabsorbed nor secreted by the renal tubules. It is metabolically inert and cleared only by the kidney. The amount of inulin filtered at the glomerulus equals the GFR multiplied by the plasma inulin concentration (P_{in}). The amount of excreted inulin equals the urine inulin concentration (U_{in}) multiplied by the urine flow rate (V), (volume excreted per unit time).

$$\underbrace{GFR \times P_{in}}_{\text{Filtered Inulin}} = \underbrace{U_{in} \times V}_{\text{Secreted Inulin}} \qquad (2.2)$$

$$GFR = \frac{U_{in} \times V}{P_{in}} \qquad (2.3)$$

Inulin must be administered intravenously since it is hydrolyzed to fructose in the gas trointestinal tract and is erratically and poorly absorbed from subcutaneous or intramuscular sites. Direct measurement of GFR in routine clinical practice using inulin clearance (C_{In}) is not common because of the complexity, expense and limited availability of testing and overall patient inconvenience. Other inherent difficulties in the use of inulin clearance as a measure of GFR include the necessity for a constant-infusion apparatus and awkward chemical analyses of blood and urine samples. To further compound the problems in clinical practice, shortages of sterile inulin suitable for patient use have recently developed. Because of these factors, other substances have been evaluated as substitutes for inulin.

2.2.2.2 Clearance of Radiolabelled Compounds

A number of radiolabelled chelates have been used to assess the GFR, as very small non-toxic amounts of the compound can be given and can be measured even at very low concentrations using conventional counters. Amongst these are ^{51}Cr-EDTA (ethylenediamine tetraacetic acid), ^{125}I iothalamate, [99]Tcm-DTPA (diethylene triamine pentaaceticacid), ^{131}I-Hippuran (Perrone et al. 1990; Bubeck 1995; Brandstrom et al. 1998).

These compounds are excreted primarily by glomerular filtration but undergo a small degree of tubular secretion. They only overestimate GFR by a few mL/min in patients with underlying renal insufficiency and give comparable results to the standards inulin technique for GFR estimation (Perrone et al. 1990). They require intravenous injection and subsequent blood sampling to measure the rate of loss of isotope from blood. DTPA clearance can be determined by external gamma camera counting over the kidney to estimate the proportion of the isotope taken up by the kidney after a given time. In severe renal failure, isotopic methods are more reliable measures of renal function than serum creatinine or creatinine clearance. The use of these compounds is limited by safety reasons due to exposure to radioactive substances; cost of isotopes and exclusion of certain patients (children and pregnant women) (Gaspari et al. 1998a). Attempt to avoid isotope exposure have led to exploring the plasma clearance of non-radiolablelled compounds like iohexol, a nonionic iodinated contrast agent.

2.2.2.3 Clearance of Non-Radiolabelled Compounds

In addition to inulin, non-radiolabelled contrast media infusion (iothalamate / iohexol) have been used to measure GFR (Nilsson-Ehle and Grubb 1994). One advantage is that urography and an estimation of GFR can be done at a single examination and without exposure to radioactive compounds. Iohexol is a non-ionic compound of low osmolality. Intravenous injection of iohexol is not associated with adverse side effects (Brownand O'Reilly 1991). Once injected, iohexol is not metabolized by the body, bound to plasma proteins, secreted or absorbed by the renal tubules, and is freely filtered at the glomerulus, making it a useful marker for GFR studies. The plasma clearance of iohexol shows excellent correlation with plasma EDTA and inulin clearances (Brandstrom et al. 1998). It has also been shown to be very precise in the group of patients with moderate-severe renal insufficiency (Gaspari et al. 1998b).

A new technique of measuring iohexol clearance using timed dried capillary blood spots was shown by Mafham et al (2007). Blood spot iohexol clearance showed potential in estimating glomerular filtration rate accurately in large-scale epidemiological studies especially among individuals without established chronic kidney disease. Plasma clearance after single injection of iohexol gives a good estimate of glomerular filtration rate and is advantageous for the patients and clinicians (Gowda et al. 2010). In clinical practice, these methods not so simple for quick and repetitive use with patients. They are time consuming, expensive, and often impractical.

2.2.3 Endogenous Substances for Measuring GFR

2.2.3.1 Blood Urea Nitrogen (BUN) Concentration

The blood urea nitrogen (BUN) was one of the first markers for assessing GFR (Kasiske and Keane 2000; Swan and Keane 2001). Urea is the major nitrogenous end product of protein and amino acid catabolism, produced by the liver and distributed throughout the intracellular and extracellular fluid. In the kidneys urea is filtered from blood by glomerulli and is partially being reabsorbed with water (Corbett 2008). The most frequently determined clinical indices for estimating renal function depends upon concentration of urea in the serum. It is useful in differential diagnosis of acute renal failure and pre renal conditions where blood urea nitrogen–creatinine ratio is increased (Mitchell and Kline 2006). Although BUN varies inversely with GFR and it is still widely used, it is however a poor measure of renal function because of its many drawbacks (Swan and Keane 2001). It possesses few of the characteristics of an ideal marker. First its rate of production is not constant; production is determined by protein intake. Urea production is increased with a high protein meal or when there is enhanced tissue breakdown due to corticosteroids or trauma (Kasiske and Keane 2000; Swan and Keane 2001). By comparison, a low protein diet or liver disease can lower BUN without change in GFR (Sherman et al. 2003). Urea is not only filtered at the glomerulus but also is reabsorbed by the tubules. The reabsorption of urea at the proximal and distal tubule parallels tubular fluid reabsorption at these sites. The clearance of urea increases sharply to 2 mL/min and then increases less quickly to a maximal level. Urea is highly diffusible thus when there is hypovolemia or in pre-renal conditions as in congestive cardiac failure, urea concentrate will rise due to increased reabsorption. This accounts for the disproportionate increase seen in pre-renal states. The measurement of urea clearance can be used to assess renal function but it underestimates GFR (Kasiske and Keane 2000). BUN result must be interpreted along with serum creatinine and other electrolyte results to be meaningful.

2.2.3.2 Serum Creatinine (S_{Cr})

The most commonly used measure of overall kidney function in clinical practice is serum creatinine (S_{Cr}) concentration (Walser et al. 1993). Serum creatinine concentration is notoriously insensitive for detecting mild to moderate kidney failure, such that patients must lose 50% or more of their kidney function before the serum creatinine value rises above the upper limit of normal. This situation of a 'normal' creatinine masking a significant decline in kidney function is especially important in elderly patients, in whom the age related decline in kidney function is not reflected by an increase in serum creatinine level because of a concomitant decrease in muscle mass (Baracskay et al. 1997). In cirrhotic patients the additional reasons why Cr is inadequate for renal function assessment are as follows (Cholongitas et al. 2007): (i) decreased hepatic production of creatine (reduction in creatine pool), (ii) the oedematous state that complicates end-stage liver disease, leading to large distribution of Cr in the body and lower serum Cr concentration and (iii) use of drugs such as cephalosporins (used as they are non-nephrotoxic) and calcitriol, which affect the tubular secretion of Cr (Perrone et al. 1992).

The typical human reference ranges for serum creatinine are 0.5 to 1.0 mg/dL (about 45-90 μmol/L) for women and 0.7 to 1.2 mg/dL (60-110 μmol/L) for men. Creatinine (MW 113 daltons) is formed by the nonenzymatic dehydration of muscle creatine. The main determinant (98%) of the creatinine pool therefore is muscle mass. It is produced at a constant rate of about 15-25 mg/kg/day in men and 10-20 mg/kg/day in women. The only other source of creatinine is meat in the diet. Thus the production rate is proportional to muscle mass and dietary meat intake. Like inulin, creatinine is freely filtered across the glomerulus and is not reabsorbed or metabolized by the kidney, however approximately 15% of urinary creatinine is derived from tubular secretion (Shemesh 1985). Creatinine clearance, therefore, usually tends to exceed the GFR by 10 to 15 percent, because of the urinary creatinine that is derived from tubular secretion. Creatinine has been usually measured by the Jaffecolorimetric reaction for more than a century, using alkaline picrate with which it an orange red complex (Rartels and Bohmer 1971).

The measurement of serum creatinine is affected by many factors other than the level of kidney function and varies markedly with age, gender, extra renal excretion, body size, diet and muscle mass (Verhave et al. 2005). Large changes in GFR within the "normal range" are not reflected by concomitant changes in S_{Cr}. The shape of the curve describing serum creatinine to glomerular filtration is a rectangular hyperbola so that large changes in renal function starting from normal kidney function may be reflected by changes within the normal range and small changes in function when the kidneys have failed by large changes in serum creatinine levels. From the age of 20 to 80 years, the GFR declines from about 125 mL/min to about 60 mL/min. However, S_{Cr} may not increase above normal until the GFR is < 50 mL/min (depending on muscle mass). An octogenarian has 50% less renal reserve than a young patient, but the S_{Cr} is still in the normal range. In a cachectic patient with depleted muscle mass, creatinine generation may be so feeble that S_{Cr} remains < 0.9 mg/dL in the face of a GFR < 25 mL/min. Drugs like triamterene, spironolactone, amiloride, probenecid, cimetidine, trimethoprim, high dose salicylates or pyrimethamine inhibit tubular secretion and induce true elevation of plasma creatinine (Weber and Van Zenten 1991). Many substances interfere with Jaffe's colorimetric assay of plasma creatinine and cause falsely high levels i.e. ketones and ketoacids, ascorbic acid, uric acid, glucose, plasma proteins, bilirubin, fatty acids, urea cephalosporins etc. Moreover, there are significant calibration issues associated with the measurement of serum creatinine that lead to inter-laboratory variationof up to 20% (Coresh et al. 2002). Look up universal standardization of creatinine level for eGFR for staging.

Serum creatinine has become a standard laboratory measurement of renal function due to its convenience and low cost, unfortunately it is not a reliable indicator of renal function (Branten et al. 2005). The national kidney foundation (NKF) has recommended that clinicians should not use serum creatinine as the sole means to assess the level of kidney function (NKF-K/DOQI 2002). In clinical practice, the reciprocal of serum creatinine or serial serum creatinine measurements can be used to monitor change in renal function (Levey 1990). A doubling of S_{Cr} implies a halving of the GFR. An increase in S_{Cr} from 0.8 to 1.6 mg/dL may be dismissed, but it indicates a 50% decrease in GFR and the need for early therapeutic intervention. An increase in S_{Cr} from 4 to 8 mg/dL also represents a 50% decrease in GFR, but by this time it is too late for anything other than dialysis. The ratio of the BUN to serum creatinine may be helpful when assessing patients with acute renal failure. The normal ratio is usually around 10:1. An increase > 20:1 implies the existence of a pre-renal syndrome, which includes not only volume depletion but states of increased protein breakdown such as absorption of blood from the GI tract; steroid-induced catabolic activity; major trauma and sepsis.

2.2.3.3 Creatinine Clearance (CrCl)

Creatinine clearance (CrCl) is calculated from the creatinine concentration in the collected urine sample (U_{Cr}), urine flow rate (V), and the plasma concentration (P_{Cr}). Since the product of urine concentration and urine flow rate yields creatinine excretion rate, which is the rate of removal from the blood, creatinine clearance is calculated as removal rate per min ($U_{Cr} \times V$) divided by the plasma creatinine concentration. This is commonly represented mathematically as:

$$CrCl = \frac{U_{Cr} \times V}{P_{Cr}} \qquad (2.4)$$

The CrCl is usually determined from a 24 hour urine collection, since shorter collections tends to give less accurate results. The creatinine clearance can be calculated from a 24 hour urine collection (time, volume, and creatinine concentration), and plasma creatinine as follows:

$$CrCl \ (mL/min) = \frac{U_{Cr} \times U_{Vol}}{S_{Cr} \times T_{hr} \times 60} \qquad (2.5)$$

Where U_{Cr} is the urine creatinine in mg/dL, U_{vol} is the urine volume in mL, S_{CR} is the serum creatinine in mg/dL, T_{hr} is the time in hours. To allow comparison of results between people of different sizes, the CrCl is often corrected for the body surface area (BSA) and expressed compared to the average sized man as mL/min/1.73 m^2. While most adults have a BSA that approaches 1.7 (1.6-1.9), extremely obese or slim patients should have their CrCl corrected for their actual BSA.

$$CrCl_{corrected} = \frac{CrCl \times 1.73}{BSA} \qquad (2.6)$$

Example 2.1

If a person has a plasma creatinine concentration of 0.02 mg/mL and in 1 hour produces 65 mL of urine with a creatinine concentration of 1.35 mg/mL, calculate the creatinine clearance.

Solution

According to Eq. (2.4), CrCl can be calculated as follows:

$$CrCl = \frac{1.35 \ mg/mL \times 65 mL/hr}{0.02 mg/mL} = 4387.5 \ mL/hr = 73.125 \ mL/min$$

There are two major errors that can limit the accuracy of the CrCl, an incomplete urine collection and increasing renal tubular creatinine secretion (Rodrigo et al. 2002). The completeness of urine collection can be estimated from the knowledge of normal creatinine excretion which depends on age, gender and lean body mass. In adults under the age of 50, daily creatinine excretion should be 20-25 mg/kg of lean body weight in men and 15-20 mg/kg of lean body weight in women (Sherman et al. 2003). From ages 50-90 there is a progressive decline in creatinine excretion to about 10 mg/kg in men due to age related fall in muscle mass (Kasiske and Keane 2000). Tubular secretion also increases in progressive renal failure as the GFR and can increase by over 50 %. This leads to gross over estimation of GFR (Walser 1998).

There are two solutions in order to compensate for the tubular secretion of Cr and the overestimation of GFR by the CrCl (Rodrigo et al. 2002): to calculate the Cl as the mean value between the urea and Cr clearances, and to calculate CrCl after reducing the tubular secretion with cimetidine. Because the urea is reabsorbed and the urea clearance underestimates the GFR, it has been suggested that the mean of urea and Cr clearances may be used as the measurement of GFR in patients with CRF. This calculation does not have physiologic support and is subject to greater variability as well as the problems in collecting urine. In order to cancel the tubular secretion of Cr and thus avoid one of the sources of overestimating GFR in pre-dialysis, oral administration of cimetidine, an organic cation like Cr that competitively reduces its secretion, has been proposed (Olsen et al. 1989). With cimetidine, the ratio between CrCland GFR approaches unity (van Acker et al. 1992).

2.2.3.4 β_2-Microglobulin

Beta2-microglobulin has been advocated as a better predictor of GFR (Nolte et al. 1991) but its serum concentration can increase as an acute phase reactant in disorders, such as lupus nephritis, that clearly require adequate assessment of GFR. Beta-2 microglobulin (MW 11815 dalton) is a low molecular weight protein freely filtered through the glomerular capillary wall and almost completely reabsorbed by proximal tubular cells. Subsequently more than 99.9% is reabsorbed and degraded in renal tubule. Because it is filtered so readily, its plasma concentration in health is low (average 1.5mg/ L). The plasma concentration increases as the glomerular filtration rate declines reaching about 40mg/l in terminal uremia. The logarithm of the plasma concentration is linearly related to the logarithm of glomerular filtration rate throughout the whole range so that it provides an excellent marker for renal dysfunction. The plasma concentration of β_2-microglobular is not affected by muscle mass or by sex of individual. As its estimation involves expensive radioimmunoassay it has not yet become more useful in clinical practice. This is a major impediment to its use in kidney disease. Also in patients with some tumors and inflammatory diseases there may be increase in plasma concentration due to increased production rather than reduced clearance (Shardijin and Statius van Epps 1987).

2.2.3.5 Cystatin C

Given the problems with creatinine production and secretion, other endogenous markers have been evaluated in an effort to provide accurate estimation of GFR (Coll et al. 2000). The protease inhibitor Cystatin C is a non-glycosylated low molecular weight protein. Cystatin C has been proposed to be a marker as it is produced by all nucleated cells at a constant rate and is freely filtrated by the glomeruli and completely catabolized in the proximal tubules. The concentration of serum Cystatin C is mainly determined by glomerular filtration, which makes Cystatin C an endogenous marker of glomerular filtration rate (Randers and Erlandsen 1999). Its production is unaffected by inflammatory or malign processes and is not muscular mass- or sex-dependent. The normal plasma level of cystatin C is <1.20 mg/L for patients under 50 years of age and <1.55 mg/L for patients over 50 years of age, while increasing levels are detected in the plasma of patients with reduced GFR. Plasmatic cystatin C correlates well and linearly with the GFR, so that it is more sensitive than Cr for detecting slight alterations in the GFR (Coll et al. 2000; Dharnidharka et al. 2002). Other studies have shown similar results when compared with other markers such as α 1-microglobulin and β_2-microglobulin (Guido et al. 2002). Cystatin C was found to be an effective marker for glomerular filtration rate in patients with cirrhosis following liver transplantation (Gowda et al. 2010; Cholongitas et al. 2007; Gerbes et al. 2002). It has been found more useful for detecting early renal impairment in both type 1 and type 2 diabetic patients (Pucci et al. 2007). Moreover Cystatin C was also found to be associated with mild kidney dysfunction with increased risk for cardiovascular events, peripheral arterial disease and heart failure (Shlipak et al. 2005).

If Cystatin C, which is clearly more expensive, is used, the choice of the cystatin C determination method and an adjusted prediction equation is essential. Therefore, several formulae for estimating GFR based upon serum-cystatin C determination have been proposed. Since there is no international standard for cystatin C these GFR estimates vary with the analytical method and the formula the local laboratory uses to calculate the GFR from the analysis result. A summary of the GFR estimating formulae based on s-cystatin C is shown in Table 2.2 (Le Bricon et al. 2000; Hoek et al. 2003; Filler and Lepage 2003; Larsson et al. 2004; Grubb et al. 2005a; Sjostrom et al. 2005; Flodin et al. 2007). Cystatin C concentrations, determined using reagents from DAKO (DAKO A/S, Glostrup, Denmark), were used for the eGFR formulae of Larsson, Grubb and Orebro-cyst DAKO.

Table 2.2 GFR estimating formulae based upon s-cystatin C
(Tidman et al. 2008)

Reference	Formula	No.	Patient characteristics
Le Bricon et al (2000)	$GFR = \dfrac{78}{s\text{-}SysC} + 4$ $(mL/min/1.73\ m^2)$	25	Adults with renal transplants& GFR was determined by ^{51}Cr-EDTA clearance
Hoek et al (2003)	$GFR = \dfrac{80.35}{s\text{-}SysC} - 4.32$ $(mL/min/1.73\ m^2)$	123	Adults with renal disease& GFR was determined with ^{125}I-iothalamate
Larsson et al (2004)	$GFR = 99.43 \times s\text{-}SysC^{-1.5837}$ using Dade Behring calibration $GFR = 77.24 \times s\text{-}SysC^{-1.2623}$ using DakoCytomation calibration (mL/min)	100	Adults referred for measurement of iohexol clearance
Grubb et al (2005b)	$GFR = 83.93 \times s\text{-}SysC^{-1.676}$ or $GFR = 86.94 \times s\text{-}SysC^{-1.686}$ $\times (0.948\ \text{if female})$	536	adults referred for determination of GFR by iohexol clearance
Orebro-cyst (DAKO) (Sjostrom et al. 2005)	$GFR = \dfrac{119}{s\text{-}SysC} - 33$ $(mL/min/1.73\ m^2)$	393	Adults referred for determination of GFR by iohexol clearance
Orebro-cyst (Gentian) (Sjostrom et al. 2005)	$GFR = \dfrac{100}{s\text{-}SysC} - 14$ $(ml/min/1.73\ m^2)$	393	Adults referred for determination of GFR by iohexol clearance
Rule et al (2006)	$GFR = 76.6 \times s\text{-}SysC^{-1.16}$ $(mL/min/1.73\ m^2)$	460	Adults referred for determination of GFR by iothalamate clearance
MacIsaac et al (2006)	$GFR = \dfrac{84.6}{s\text{-}SysC} - 3.2$ $(mL/min/1.73\ m^2)$	251	Adults with diabetes and GFR determined by ^{99}Tcm-DTPA

s-Cys C:Serum cystatin C in mg/L.

Since the formulae by Hoek and le Bricon were based on the nephelo-metric determination of cystatin C using reagents from Dade-Behring, the cystatin C concentrations obtained with the Gentian (Gentian AS, Moss, Norway) method were used for these formulae (Tidman et al. 2008). Tid-man el al (2008) showed that the concentrations obtained by the Gentian method were approximately 10% lower than the DAKO method within the normal GFR range but were approximately 40% higher within the low GFR range. The linear regression between 1/s-cystatin C and GFR showed a better correlation with the Gentian method compared with the DAKO method (R = 0.9322 and 0.8350, respectively).

Example 2.2

A 29-years old male has a serum cystatin C equal to 1.84 mg/l. Calculate the estimated GFR for this patient using Le Bricon, Hoek, Rule, and MacIsaac then classify this patient according to the Stages of Chronic Kidney Disease.

Solution

GFR can be calculated using Le Bricon, Hoek, Rule, and MacIsaac*formulae as follows:*

Reference Method	GFR (mL/min/1.73 m²)
Le Bricon	$GFR = \dfrac{78}{1.84 \text{ mg/l}} + 4 = 46.4$
Hoek	$GFR = \dfrac{80.35}{1.84 \text{ mg/l}} - 4.32 = 39.34$
Rule	$GFR = 76.6 \times 1.8^{-1.16} = 37.8$
MacIsaac	$GFR = \dfrac{84.6}{1.84 \text{ mg/l}} - 3.2 = 42.8$

It is noted that there are significant differences between cystatin C-based equations for GFR. The patient is classified to be in stage 3 of CKD in each method. An international calibrator for cystatin C would greatly improve its use as a marker for GFR.

2.2.3.6 β-Trace Protein (BTP)

This protein is filtered at glomerulus and then reabsorbed in proximal tubule or excreted in urine and hence have potential to meet the criteria for use as a marker of glomerular filtration rate (Poge et al. 2005). Beta Trace Protein is a low-molecular weight glycoprotein belonging to the lipocalin protein family with 168 amino acids and a molecular weight of 23000–29000, depending on the degree of glycosylation. It has been reported to be a better indicator of reduced glomerular filtration rate than serum creatinine (Priem et al. 1999; Woitas et al. 2001). Serum β -Trace Protein has been found to be elevated in patients with renal diseases (Hoffmann et al. 1997). However, when compared, Cystatin C is still a better indicator than Serum β-Trace Protein (Priem et al. 2001). As a tool for GFR measurement; BTP has been found to have a few distinct advantages.

It has been reported that serum BTP levels do not have a significant relationship with C-reactive protein and that they are unaffected by body composition (Filler and Lepage 2003; Huber and Risch 2005). During the third trimester of pregnancy, BTP, but not CysC, has been shown to adequately reflect the GFR (Akbari et al. 2005). Unlike CysC, thyroid function has not been reported to affect the concentration of BTP (Manetti et al. 2005). Another possible advantage would be the lack of effect of corticosteroid administration on BTP concentrations. However, there is conflicting evidence on this property (Abbink et al. 2008; White et al. 2007). Serum concentrations of BTP have had limited clinical utility owing to the absence of a formula to convert the serum concentration of BTP into an estimate of GFR. Therefore White et al. developed a novel GFR estimation (eGFR) equation on adults based on serum BTP concentration as follows (White et al. 2007):

$$eGFR = 112.1 \times BTP^{-0.662} \times Urea^{-0.280}$$
$$\times (0.880 \text{ if patient is female}) \tag{2.7}$$

where BTP in mg/L, Urea in mmol/L and estimated GFR in mL/min/1.73m^2. If urea is unavailable, the best fit model using creatinine (in μmol/L) would be calculated as follows (White et al. 2007):

$$eGFR = 167.8 \times BTP^{-0.758} \times Creatinine^{-0.204}$$
$$\times (0.871 \text{ if patient is female}) \tag{2.8}$$

where BTP in mg/L, creatinine in μmol/L and estimated GFR in mL/min/1.73m^2. These derived equations require external validation in other populations to determine their accuracy, clinical utility, and generalizability (White et al, 2007).

Poge et al (2008) also developed three BTP-based GFR formulae derived by multiple regression analyses and they validated the diagnostic performance of these BTP-formulae in 102 consecutive renal transplant recipients (RTR), who underwent a technetium diethylenetriamine pentaacetic acid (DTPA) clearance for GFR measurement. The best-performing BTP formula was found to be:

$$eGFR = 89.85 \times BTP^{-0.5541} \times Urea^{-0.3018} \qquad (2.9)$$

Where BTP in mg/L, Urea in mmol/L and estimated GFR in mL/min/1.73m^2. The precision of Poge et al BTP-formula was significantly better than the White equation, but no differences were found between the BTP-formula and MDRD equation (described in the next sections), and none between the MDRD and White equations (Poge et al. 2008). BTP is considerably more expensive than creatinine. Thus, the suggested BTP-based equation for GFR calculation will gain public recognition only when its performance is demonstrated to be clearly superior to the MDRD equation. Further studies are needed to elucidate this issue more clearly.

Example 2.3

A 65-years old female has a serum BTP equal to 1.26 mg/L, serum creatinine equal to 148 μmol/L and a serum urea concentration equal to 10 mmol/L Calculate the estimated GFR for this patient using White and Poge formulae.

Solution

GFR can be calculated based on BTP according to White formula Eq. (2.7) and Poge formula Eq. (2.9) as follows:

White formula using serum urea and BTP concentration:

$$eGFR = 112.1 \times 1.26^{-0.662} \times 10^{-0.280} \times 0.880 = 44.43 \, mL/min/1.73m^2$$

White formula using serum creatinine and BTP concentration:
$$eGFR = 167.8 \times 1.26^{-0.758} \times 10^{-0.204} \times 0.871 = 44.26 \, mL/min/1.73m^2$$

Poge formula: $eGFR = 89.85 \times 1.26^{-0.5541} \times 10^{-0.3018} = 39.46 \, mL/min/1.73m^2$

2.2.4 Prediction Formulae of GFR from Plasma Creatinine

In clinical practice an approximation of bedside GFR is often obtained from plasma creatinine concentration alone albeit with limited accuracy (Perrone et al. 1992). Several formulae have been developed to allow an immediate prediction of GFR from plasma creatinine. Few pitfalls of formula derived GFR need to be kept in mind. Approximation of GFR from plasma creatinine may give unreliable results because plasma creatinine is not only dependent on GFR but also on muscle mass which varies with age, weight and gender. In cirrhosis and diseases with reduced muscle mass, plasma creatinine is low; conversely a high protein intake can lead to 10% increase in plasma creatinine (Cholongitas et al. 2007).

Furthermore a marked reduction in GFR can be present before it is reflected in plasma creatinine concentration above the upper limit of normal range. The value to these formulas for GFR prediction is likely to increase when an accurate plasma creatinine assay is performed along with inhibition of tubular secretion by cimetidine. To improve the estimation of GFR from plasma creatinine concentration, formulas which incorporate variables like age, weight, height and gender can be used. These formulas are based on the idea that the excretion of Cr is constant and equal to its production, which, in turn, is proportional to muscular mass. The calculation of estimated GFR (eGFR) using an empirical mathematical formula has been encouraged as a simple, rapid and reliable means of assessing kidney function (Levey et al. 1999). In most cases, eGFR is at least as accurate as measuring creatinine clearance (NKF-K/DOQI 2002). There are no fewer than 47 different prediction equations currently available (Johnson 2005), although the two most common in use are the Cockcroft-Gault (Cockcroft and Gault 1976) and the abbreviated Modification of Diet in Renal Disease (MDRD) formula (Levey et al. 1999).

2.2.4.1 Cockcroft & Gault (CG) Method

The Cockcroft-Gault equation is probably the most widely used equation to estimate creatinine clearance (Cockcroft and Gault 1976). The Cockcroft-Gault formula is widely available on medical software and specialized semi-automated calculators. This equation can only be used in patients with stable renal function. It takes into account the increased production of creatinine with increasing weight, the decreased production with age and sex related differences in muscle mass as follows (Cockcroft and Gault 1976):

$$\text{CrCl (mL/min)} = \frac{(140 - age) \times (\text{weight in kg}) (\times 0.85 \text{ if female})}{72 \times S_{cr}} \quad (2.10)$$

Where S_{CR} is the serum creatinine in mg/dL. Cockcroft-Gaultequation needs to be normalized to a body surface area (BSA) of 1.73 m² by multiplying Eq. (2.10) by BSA/1.73. GFR can be calculated from Cockcroft and Gault formula as follows (Manjunath et al. 2001):

$$\text{GFR estimate} = 0.84 \times \text{CrCl} \quad (2.11)$$

The formula overestimates GFR in individuals who are obese or edematous and should therefore not be used in such patients. Several authors have reported good correlation between measured GFR and the predicted Ccr from Cockcroft and Gault formula (Bostom et al. 2002).

Example 2.4

A 42-years old, 66 kg, 150 cm in tall female patient has a serum creatinine equal to 1.8 mg/dL. Calculate the estimated creatinine clearance and GFR for this patient using Cockcroft and Gault formula.

Solution

According to Eq. (2.10), the estimated creatinine clearance based on Cockcroft-Gault formula can be calculated as follows:

$$\text{CrCl}_{est} = \frac{(140 - 42) \times (66) \times 0.85}{72 \times 1.8} = 42.42 \text{ mL/min}$$

The body surface area can be calculated according to DuBois and DuBois formula (Dubois and Dubois 1989):

$$BSA = 0.007184 \times 150^{0.725} \times 66^{0.425} = 1.61 \text{ m}^2$$

The corrected creatinine clearance for body surface area is:

$$\text{CrCl}_{est} = 42.42 \text{ mL/min} \times \frac{1.61}{1.73} = 39.5 \text{ mL/min/1.73m}^2$$

According to Eq. (2.12), the estimated GFR is:

$$\text{GFR estimate} = 0.84 \times 39.5 = 33.2 \text{ mL/min/1.73m}^2$$

Table 2.3 describes some of the other equations that have been used to predict creatinine clearance from serum creatinine.

Table 2.3 Equations predicting creatinine clearance

Reference	Formula
Jelliffe (1971)	$C_{Cr}(mL/min/1.73m^2) = \dfrac{100}{S_{Cr}} - 12$ (Male) $C_{Cr}(mL/min/1.73m^2) = \dfrac{80}{S_{Cr}} - 7$ (Female)
Modified Jelliffe, Jelliffe (1973)	$C_{Cr}(mL/min/1.73m^2) =$ $\dfrac{(98 - 0.8 \times (age - 20))}{S_{Cr}} \times$ (0.9 if female)
Mawer et al(1972)	$C_{Cr}(mL/min)$ For male = $\dfrac{weight \times [29.3 - (0.203 \times age)] \times [1 - (0.03 \times S_{Cr})]}{(14.4 \times S_{Cr}) \times (70 / weight)}$ $C_{Cr}(mL/min)$ For Female = $\dfrac{weight \times [25.3 - (0.175 \times age)] \times [1 - (0.03 \times S_{Cr})]}{(14.4 \times S_{Cr}) \times (70 / weight)}$
Bjornsson (1979)	$C_{Cr}(mL/min) = \dfrac{[27 - (0.173 \times age)] \times weight \times 0.07}{S_{Cr}}$ (Male) $C_{Cr}(mL/min) = \dfrac{[25 - (0.175 \times age)] \times weight \times 0.07}{S_{Cr}}$ (Female)
Hull et al (1981)	$C_{Cr}(mL/min) =$ $\left[\dfrac{(145 - age)}{S_{Cr}} - 3\right] \times \dfrac{weight}{70} \times (0.85 \text{ if female})$
Gates(1985)	$C_{Cr}(mL/min)$ For male = $(89.4 \times S_{Cr}^{-1.2}) + (55 - age) \times (0.447 \times S_{Cr}^{-1.1})$ $C_{Cr}(mL/min)$ For Female = $(60 \times S_{Cr}^{-1.1}) + (56 - age) \times (0.3 \times S_{Cr}^{-1.1})$
Effersoe (1957)	$C_{Cr} = 10(-1.09 \times \log S_{Cr} + 1.9)$ (for male) $C_{Cr} = 10(-1.06 \times \log S_{Cr} + 1.78)$ (For Female)

Table 2.3 (*continued*)

Salazar and Corcoran (1988)	C_{Cr} (mL/min) For male = $$\frac{(137 - age) \times \left[(0.285 \times weight) + (12.1 \times height^2) \right]}{(51 \times S_{Cr})}$$ C_{Cr} (mL/min) For Female = $$\frac{(146 - age) \times \left[(0.287 \times weight) + (9.74 \times height^2) \right]}{(60 \times S_{Cr})}$$
Edwards and Whyte (1959)	C_{Cr} (mL/min) $= (94.3/S_{Cr}) - 1.8$ (for male) C_{Cr} (mL/min) $= (69.9/S_{Cr}) + 2.2$ (for Female)
Sanaka et al (1996)	C_{Cr} (mL/min) For Male = $$\frac{\left[(19 \times alb) + 32 \right] \times weight}{100 \times S_{Cr}}$$ C_{Cr} (mL/min) For Female = $$\frac{\left[(13 \times alb) + 29 \right] \times weight}{100 \times S_{Cr}}$$
Mitch et al (1980)	$$CrCl = \left[\frac{27.81}{S_{Cr}} - 0.04 \right] \times 0.69 \times weight \quad \text{For Male}$$ $$CrCl = \left[\frac{23.63}{S_{Cr}} - 0.04 \right] \times 0.69 \times weight \quad \text{For Female}$$
Reciprocal of creatinine	C_{Cr} (mL/min) $= 100/S_{Cr}$
Yukawa et al (1999) (Japanese)	$$C_{Cr} \text{ (mL/min)} = \frac{(470 - age) \times weight}{(3.26 \times S_{Cr}) + 98.7}$$
Wright et al (2001)	C_{Cr} (mL/min) For Male = $$\frac{\left[6580 - (38.8 \times age) \right] \times BSA}{S_{Cr}}$$ C_{Cr} (mL/min) For Female = $$\frac{\left[6580 - (38.8 \times age) \right] \times 0.832 \times BSA}{S_{Cr}}$$

Scr, serum creatinine level (mg/dL); BSA, body surface area; age, in years; weight, in kilograms. GFR measurement (mL/min per 1.73 m^2).

2.2.4.2 Original Six-Variables Modification of Diet in Renal Disease (MDRD) formula

The MDRD formula was created by a stepwise regression analysis of measured GFR ($_m$GFR) by renal clearance of a single-bolus subcutaneous injection of ^{125}Iiothalamate in 1628 participants of the MDRD study, which included only patients with chronic kidney disease (CKD) (Levey et al. 1999). There are two forms of the original MDRD, one with and the other without urine biochemistry variables as follows (Levey et al. 1999):

$$GFR = 170 \times S_{Cr}^{-0.999} \times age^{-0.176} \times (0.762 \text{ if female})$$
$$\times (1.180 \text{ if black}) \times S_{U}^{-0.170} \times Alb^{+0.318} \tag{2.12}$$

$$GFR = 198 \times S_{Cr}^{-0.858} \times age^{-0.167} \times (0.822 \text{ if female})$$
$$\times (1.178 \text{ if black}) \times S_{U}^{-0.293} \times UUN^{+0.249} \tag{2.13}$$

where S_{Cr} is the serum creatinine in mg/dL, S_U is the serum urea nitrogen concentration in mg/dL, Alb is the serum albumin in g/dL and UUN is the urine urea nitrogen in g/dL. The GFR calculated using the MDRD method is already corrected for surface area and requires no measurement of weight or additional normalization. Value obtained must be multiplied by 0.762 for females and by 1.180 for black patients. To assess precision, each of these equations was adjusted to correct for bias. The equation that includes urine biochemistry variables was most accurate. The equation that includes only serum and demographic variables was only slightly less accurate (Levey et al. 1999).

2.2.4.3 Revised Six-variables Modification of Diet in Renal Disease (MDRD) formula

Urinary clearances of ^{125}I-iothalamate after subcutaneous infusion were determined at clinical centers participating in the MDRD Study (Levey et al.1999). Serum and urine ^{125}I-iothalamate were assayed in a central laboratory. All serum creatinine values reported in this study are traceable to primary reference material at the National Institute of Standards and Technology (NIST), with assigned values based on isotope-dilution mass spectrometry (IDMS) (Levey et al. 2006).

The serum creatinine samples from the MDRD Study were originally assayed from 1988 to 1994 in a central laboratory with the Beckman Synchron CX3 (Global Medical Instrumentation, Inc., Ramsey, Minnesota) by using a kinetic alkaline picrate method. Samples were re-assayed in 2004 with the same instrument. The Beckman assay was calibrated to the Roche/Hitachi P module Creatinase Plus enzymatic assay (Roche Diagnostics, Basel, Switzerland), traceable to an isotope-dilution mass spectrometry (IDMS) assay at NIST (Junge et al. 2004; Levey et al. 2005). On the basis of these results, the 6-variable MDRD Study equation is re-expressed for use with standardized serum creatinine assay. The creatinine values were used as IDMS calibrated data and as values converted to the Cleveland Clinical Laboratory using an equation proposed by Levey (2005) to convert the IDMS adapted values to the values of the Cleveland Clinical Laboratory (CCL). The calibration of CCL to IDMS can be expressed as follows (Levey et al. 2005):

$$\text{IDMS calibrated creatinine} = 0.95 \times \text{original MDRD study creatinine} \tag{2.14}$$

Thus, the original equations using revised calibration of serum creatinineare expressed as (Levey et al. 2006):

$$\begin{aligned} \text{GFR} &= 161.5 \times \text{Standardized } S_{Cr}^{-0.999} \times \text{age}^{-0.176} \\ &\times (0.762 \text{ if female}) \times (1.180 \text{ if black}) \times S_{U}^{-0.170} \times \text{Alb}^{+0.318} \end{aligned} \tag{2.15}$$

$$\begin{aligned} \text{GFR} &= 188.1 \times \text{Standardized } S_{Cr}^{-0.858} \times \text{age}^{-0.167} \\ &\times (0.822 \text{ if female}) \times (1.178 \text{ if black}) \times S_{U}^{-0.293} \times \text{UUN}^{+0.249} \end{aligned} \tag{2.16}$$

Where S_{Cr} is the serum creatinine in mg/dL, S_{U} is the serum urea nitrogen concentration in mg/dL, Alb is the serum albumin in g/dL and UUN is the urine urea nitrogen in g/dL.

The Cockcroft–Gault equation was not re-expressed because the original serum creatinine samples were not available for calibration to standardized serum creatinine assay.

Example 2.5

Calculate the estimated GFR using the original MDRD formula for a 38-years old male patient if the measured serum creatinine is 5.5 mg/dL and is recalibrated to be traceable to IDMS, serum urea nitrogen concentration is 95 mg/dL and the serum albumin is 3.4 g/dL.

Solution

a) Since the creatinine is recalibrated to be traceable to IDMS, the estimated GFR using original MDRD formula can be calculated according to Eq. (2.15) as follows:

$$\text{GFR} = 161.5 \times 5.5^{-0.999} \times 38^{-0.176} \times 95^{-0.170} \times 3.4^{+0.318} = 10.6 \text{ mL/min/1.73 m}^2$$

2.2.4.4 Quadratic Mayo Clinic Equation (MC formula) and Rule's Refitted MDRD Formula

Recently, Rule et al (2004) suggested two modified MDRD equations to overcome some of the disadvantages of the original MDRD formula. Their first formula is also known as the new 'Mayo Clinic Equation' and has been used in several recent studies (Maaravi et al. 2005). In contrast to the MDRD study cohort which included only patients with diminished renal function (GFR <60 mL/min), the study of Rule et al (2004) comprised 580 healthy persons and 320 patients with chronic kidney diseases. Covering the whole range of GFR thus the Mayo Clinic (MC) equation potentially could serve as a tool to identify patients with renal insufficiency and may be more accurate than the MDRD equation in estimating GFR when kidney disease status is unknown. The Quadratic Mayo Clinic Equation (MC formula) is expressed as follows (Maaravi et al. 2005):

$$\text{GFR (mL/min/1.73m}^2) = \exp\left(1.911 + \frac{5.249}{S_{Cr}} - \frac{2.114}{S_{Cr}^2} - \right.$$
$$\left(0.00686 \times \text{age}\right) - 0.205 \text{ (if female)}\right) \tag{2.17}$$

If $S_{Cr} < 0.8$ mg/dL, use 0.8 for S_{Cr}

The second formula was proposed to optimize the MDRD formula in patients with known renal disease. This modification was termed as the Rule's refitted MDRD formula (RR-MDRD) (Rule et al. 2004).

This RR-MDRD formula and the MC equation are based on creatinine values which were determined at the Mayo Clinic Laboratory. RR-MDRD formula for chronic kidney diseases is expressed as follows:

$$\text{GFR (mL/min/1.73m}^2) = 297 \times S_{Cr}^{-1.29} \times \text{age}^{-0.290}$$
$$\times (0.767 \text{ if female}) \tag{2.18}$$

Poge et al (2007) evaluated a refit version of the MDRD equation and the Mayo Clinic Quadratic equation to improve estimation of GFR in renal allograft recipients. They revealed that the RR-MDRD can be used as an alternative approach to the MDRD equation in patients after kidney transplantation. The calibration of creatinine to the IDMS method significantly enhances the performance of the MDRD formula. Nonetheless, re-expressed MDRD was outperformed by the MC and the RR-MDRD formula.

Example 2.6

A 52-years old female has a serum creatinine clearance equal to 2.1 mg/dL. Calculate the estimated GFR for this patient using:

a) Quadratic Mayo Clinic formula
b) Rule's refittedMDRD formula

Solution

a) The estimated GFR is calculated using Quadratic Mayo Clinic formula according to Eq. (2.17):

$$GFR = \exp\left[1.911 + \frac{5.249}{2.1} - \frac{2.114}{(2.1)^2} - (0.00686 \times 52) - 0.205\right]$$

$$= 29.1 \text{ mL/min}/1.73 \text{ m}^2$$

b) Using Rule's refitted MDRD formula [Eq. (2.18)], GFR can be estimated as follows:

$$GFR = 297 \times 2.1^{-1.29} \times 52^{-0.290} \times 0.767 = 27.8 \text{ mL/min}/1.73\text{m}^2$$

2.2.4.5 Abbreviated MDRD (4-Variable MDRD)

Another simplified or abbreviated equation to estimate GFR has also been developed using data from MDRD study. The abbreviated MDRD equation is much easier, requires only Scr, age, sex and race and expressed as (Levey et al. 2000):

$$GFR = 186.3 \times S_{Cr}^{-1.154} \times \text{age}^{-0.203} \times (0.742 \text{ if female})$$
$$\times (1.212 \text{ if black}) \tag{2.19}$$

The calculation can be made using available web-based and downloadable medical calculators www.nkdep.nih.gov/GFR-cal.htm. This 4-variable MDRD formula was almost as good as the formula using six variables and provided a better estimate of GFR than the Cockcroft-Gault formula.

2.2.4.6 Abbreviated MDRD using Revised Calibration of Serum Creatinine

The four-variable MDRD Study equation is re-expressed with IDMS traceable serum creatinine as follows (Levey et al. 2006):

$$GFR = 175 \times \text{Standardized } S_{Cr}^{-1.154} \times \text{age}^{-0.203}$$
$$\times (0.742 \text{ if female}) \times (1.212 \text{ if black}) \qquad (2.20)$$

The availability of standard reference materials and accurate assays, such as the Roche enzymatic method, will enable instrument manufacturers and clinical laboratories to calibrate serum creatinine assays to IDMS-traceable values.

Example 2.7

Calculate the estimated GFR using abbreviated MDRD formula for a 53-years old African-American male if the measured serum creatinine is 6.5 mg/dL and is recalibrated to be traceable to IDM.

Solution

The estimated GFR can be calculated according to Eq. (2.20) because the creatinine is recalibrated to be traceable to IDMS as follows:

$$GFR = 175 \times 6.5^{-1.154} \times 52^{-0.203} \times 1.212 = 10.97 \text{ mL/min/1.73m}^2$$

2.2.4.7 Chronic Kidney Disease Epidemiology Collaboration (CKD-EPI) Equation

The Chronic Kidney Disease Epidemiology Collaboration (CKD-EPI) is a research group funded by the National Institute of Diabetes, Digestive and Kidney Disease (NIDDK) to develop and validate improved glomerular filtration rate (GFR) estimating equations by pooling data from research studies and clinical populations. Studies include individuals with diverse clinical characteristics, with and without kidney disease, and across a wide range of GFR. CKD-EPI developed estimating equations to relate measured GFR to predictor variables including serum levels of endogenous filtration markers and clinical characteristics. Equations were developed and internally validated in a database of 10 studies (6 research studies and 4 clinical populations) with a total of 8,254 participants, divided randomly into separate datasets for development (n=5,504) and internal validation (n=2,750). The equations were then externally validated in a database of 16 other studies with a total of 3,896 participants. The CKD-EPI equation, expressed as a single equation, is (Leveyet al. 2009):

$$eGFR = 141 \times \min\left(\frac{S_{Cr}}{k}, 1\right)^{a} \times \max\left(\frac{S_{Cr}}{k}, 1\right)^{-1.209} \times (0.993)^{age}$$
$$\times 1.018 \text{ [if female] } x \text{ 1.159 [if black]}$$
(2.21)

where s_{cr} is serum creatinine, k is 0.7 for females and 0.9 for males, a is -0.329 for females and -0.411 for males, min indicates the minimum of Scr/k or 1, and max indicates the maximum of Scr/k or 1.

The CKD-EPI creatinine equation is more precise and accurate than the MDRD Study equation across various study populations and clinical conditions and could replace it for routine clinical use. Bias is improved, especially at higher estimated GFRs, although precision remains suboptimal. Improved accuracy of the CKD-EPI equation could have important implications for public health and clinical practice. The CKD-EPI equation could replace the MDRD Study equation in general clinical use to estimate GFR (Levey et al. 2009). The greater accuracy of the CKD-EPI equation should improve clinical decision making in patients with decreased kidney function. In particular, lower bias should reduce the rate of false-positive diagnoses of stage 3 chronic kidney disease (estimated GFR <60 mL/min per 1.73 m^2) in patients without chronic kidney disease (measured GFR >60 mL/min per 1.73 m^2 and no markers of kidney damage) (Levey et al, 2009).

Example 2.8

A 55-years old female has a serum creatinine equal to 5.3 mg/dL. Calculate the estimated GFR for this patient using CKD-EPI formula.

Solution

The estimated GFR using CKD-EPI formula can be calculated according to Eq. (2.21) as follows:

$$\text{eGFR} = 141 \times \min\left(\frac{5.3}{0.7},1\right)^{-0.329} \times \max\left(\frac{5.3}{0.7},1\right)^{-1.209} \times (0.993)^{55} \times 1.018$$

$$= 141 \times \min(7.57,1)^{-0.329} \times \max(7.57,1)^{-1.209} \times (0.993)^{55} \times 1.018$$

$$= 8.44 \text{ mL / min / } 1.73\text{m}^2$$

2.2.4.8 Other Formula for estimating GFR

Table 2.4 lists some of the other equations that have been derived to predict GFR. In all equations, GFR is adjusted for body size, age, gender and serum creatinine. Unfortunately, all prediction equations based on serum creatinine concentration are of limited value in patients who are not in a steady state of creatinine balance, for example patients with acute renal failure and patients who are taking drugs or have medical conditions that interfere with the secretion or measurement of creatinine (Levey et al.1990). Other significant limitations include variations in creatinine measurements due to differences in the creatinine assay technique itself. For example, the Jaffe reaction, which provides a colorimetric assay of creatinine, overestimates serum creatinine because it measures non-creatinine chromogens as well. Accurate estimation of GFR at higher levels requires standardization of calibration in creatinine measurements across clinical laboratories.

Table 2.4 Equations predicting glomerular filtration rate

Reference	Formula
Lubowitz et al (1967) and Lavender et al (1969)	$\text{GFR (mL/min)} = \left(\dfrac{C_{urea} + C_{\check{C}r}}{2}\right)$
Mogensen and Heilskov (1980)	$\text{GFR (mL/min)} = \dfrac{\left[\dfrac{113.12}{S_{Cr}} - 14\right]}{0.90}$
Walser et al (1993)	GFR (mL/min/1.73 m²) For Male $= \dfrac{7.57}{S_{Cr}} - (0.103 \times \text{age}) + (0.096 \times \text{weight}) - 6.66$ GFR (mL/min/1.73 m²) For Female $= \dfrac{6.05}{S_{Cr}} - (0.08 \times \text{age}) + (0.08 \times \text{weight}) - 4.81$

Table 2.4 (*continued*)

Davis and Chandler (1996)	$\text{GFR (mL/min)} = \dfrac{140 - age}{S_{Cr}} \times (0.85 \text{ if female})$
Toto et al (1997)	GFR (mL/min/1.73m^2) For male = $-0.30 \times (age - 52) + \dfrac{105}{S_{Cr}} + (weight - 86)$ GFR (mL/min/1.73m^2) For Female = $-0.29 \times (age - 52) + \dfrac{88}{S_{Cr}} - 0.77 \times (BMI - 30)$

Scr, serum creatinine level (mg/dL); age, in years; weight, in kilograms; GFR measurement (mL/min per 1.73 m^2).

The MDRD prediction equation offers several advantages over other equations (Manjunath et al. 2001). First, it appears to be more accurate than other equations developed. Second, it is easily implemented in clinical practice as it can be computed and reported by the clinical laboratory that receives the blood and the patient's demographic data. Furthermore it does not require collection of a timedurine sample, or measurement of height and weight. Third, it predicts GFR rather than creatinine clearance, and does so over a wide range of values, to follow the progression of renal disease and finally to detect the end stage of renal disease. Fourth, it includes a term for ethnicity, which is important because chronic renal disease is more prevalent among black patients. Since the MDRD equations were derived from patients with renal failure, they can be reliably used in those with significant renal dysfunction and have been validated in kidney transplant recipients.

Several studies have compared the accuracy and precision of both Cocroft and Gault formula and the MDRD formula against standard methods of GFR assessment. It has been demonstrated that the Cockcroft-Gault formula can overestimate GFR at low renal function levels (Poggio et al. 2005; Froissart et al. 2005; Kuan et al. 2005) and underestimate high GFR values (Rule et al. 2004). Other GFR overestimation biases have been demonstrated for overweight, young and female individuals (Poggio et al. 2005; Froissart et al. 2005). The MDRD equation clearly underestimates GFR in cases with high renal function levels (Lin et al. 2003; Poggio et al. 2005; Froissart et al. 2005; Kuan et al. 2005; Rule et al. 2004) and Levey et al (1999) emphasized the need for caution in applying the

MDRD formula to individuals with a S_{Cr} within the "normal" range because it has not been validated in people without renal disease. The MDRD underestimates GFR was also recently demonstrated in renal failure, in females (Kuanet al. 2005; Cirillo et al. 2005) and in overweight patients (Kuan et al. 2005), while the opposite is true of lean subjects (Beddhu et al. 2003).

2.3   GLOMERULAR FILTRATION RATE IN CHILDREN WITH CHRONIC KIDNEY DISEASE

In pediatric nephrology a reliable and accurate method for assessment of glomerular filtration rate (GFR) is essential, especially in cases of cytotoxic drug treatment, urinary tract malformation, renal transplantation and reduced renal function.

2.3.1   Exogenous Methods

2.3.1.1   Inulin Clearance

The renal clearance of inulin remains the gold standard for the evaluation of GFR in children and adults. Classic (standard) inulin clearance requires an intravenous priming dose of inulin followed by a constant infusion to establish a steady-state inulin plasma concentration. The process requires the maintenance of a steady-state concentration for about 45 min, followed by serial urine samples collection every 10 to 20 min (Arant et al. 1972). If urine is collected without catheterization, good hydration is requested to maintain a high urine flow rate.

Furthermore, complete voiding at the end of each urine collection is crucial for the precise determination of inulin clearance. The method is time consuming and uncomfortable for the child and is primarily used for research purposes and not for daily routine practice. Moreover, the determination of inulin concentration is problematic, as the assays are imprecise (Rahn et al. 1999). In addition to inulin, Inulin clearance can also be determined by a constant infusion technique measuring plasma clearance, without collecting urine (Cole et al. 1972). After the inulin reaches equilibrium in its distribution space, the excretion rate equals the infusion rate and the clearance of inulin can be calculated as follows (Schwartz and Work 2009):

$$C_{In} = I_{In} \times R / S_{In} \qquad (2.22)$$

where I_{In} is the infusion concentration of inulin, R is the infusion rate (mL/min), S_{In} is the serum concentration of inulin, and C_{In} is the clearance of inulin in milliliters per minute per 1.73 m^2. There is a difficulty associated with this method, because it is difficult to obtain constant inulin plasma or serum concentrations during intravenous infusion (Rahn et al. 1999). In addition, inulin has a high molecular weight, and this takes time to fully equilibrate. If the steady state is not reached, unequilibrated samples will show lower concentrations, and this would lead to an apparent overestimation of GFR (Rahn et al. 1999).

2.3.1.2 Iohexol Clearance

Iohexol is a non-ionic x-ray contrast medium of low osmolality, extensively used in clinical radiology and considered essentially free from side effects (Almen 1983; Schrott et al. 1986; Albrechtsson et al. 1985). It is not secreted, metabolized, or reabsorbed by the kidney (Gaspari et al. 1995). Iohexol diffuses into the extracellular space, but has less than 2% plasma protein binding, and is eliminated exclusively without metabolism by the kidneys (Back et al. 1988).There is close agreement between GFR values obtained with iohexol clearance compared with inulin clearance (Rahn et al. 1999; Gaspari et al. 1995; Erley et al. 2001). There is also a very good correlation between iohexol clearance and ^{51}Cr-EDTA plasma clearance (Krutzen et al. 1990). Iohexol may equilibrate faster than inulin within the various body compartments based on its smaller size. Iohexol has been found to have an extremely low toxicity even when used in radiographic doses which are 10 to 50 times higher than those used for GFR determination (Sterner et al. 1996; Nilsson-Ehle 2001).

Iohexol can be measured in deproteinized serum by high performance liquid chromatography (HPLC), thereby obviating the need for radioactivity. There are two isomers, both of which are handled similarly by the body (Schwartz et al. 2006; Krutzen et al. 1990; Gaspari et al. 1995). In practice, the major peak, eluting at about 5 min, is used for plasma disappearance curves. The single-injection approach is technically less demanding than a constant infusion with urine collection and can be accomplished with less technical assistance.

2.3.1.3 Radioisotopes

In addition to inulin, the plasma clearance of an exogenous tracer that after intravenous injection is exclusively eliminated by renal ultrafiltration is an accurate and precise method for measuring GFR. The most commonly used tracers are ^{51}Cr-EDTA, ^{99}Tc- DTPA, ^{125}I-iothalamate. The total plasma clearance is calculated from the injected dose divided by the total area under the plasma curve obtained on the basis of a number of blood samples drawn from the time of injection and up to 5 h or more. The technique has been simplified to include only a single or a few blood samples, to increase convenience for the child (Ham and Piepsz 1991). However, the simplified techniques are not precise in the case of GFR values below 30 mL/min per 1.73 m^2 body surface area and become inaccurate at GFR values below 10–20 mL/min per 1.73 m^2 (Piepsz et al. 2001). Care should be taken in the case of significant edema or ascites, where tracer will disappear into the expanded extra-cellular volume, leading to GFR overestimation. The plasma clearance of ^{51}Cr-EDTA has been shown to correlate well with the renal clearance of inulin (Rehling et al. 1984). Table 2.5 shows normal values for ^{51}Cr-EDTA clearance in infants and children (Piepsz et al. 2006).^{125}Iothalamate has been used extensively to measure GFR in children, both by standard renal clearance and by constant infusion and plasma disappearance; however, there are problems with this agent (Bajaj et al. 1996). The use of renal iothalamate clearances with the collection of urine result in major inaccuracies, especially in children, because of the inability to assure quantitative emptying of the bladder (Hellerstein et al. 2006). Although accurate and precise, the exogenous methods are relatively cumbersome, invasive, and expensive, and they can exclusively be done at nuclear medicine or biochemistry departments. To avoid serial blood sampling and thereby simplify the procedure for radionuclide GFR measurement, several gamma camera methods have been proposed (Rehling et al. 1985; Itoh et al. 2000). However, as the accuracy of such methods is inferior to that of plasma-sample techniques, the present consensus is restricted to the determination of relative clearance (Prigent et al. 1999).

Table 2.5 Plasma ^{51}Cr-EDTA clearance in normal infants and children (Piepsz et al. 2006)

Age (mo) Mean	GFR ± SD (mL/min/1.73 m^2)
≤ 1.2	52.0 ± 9.0
1.2–3.6	61.7 ± 14.3
3.6–7.9	71.7 ± 13.9
7.9–12	82.6 ± 17.3
12–18	91.5 ± 17.8
18–24	94.5 ± 18.1
> 24	104.4 ± 19.9

2.3.2 Endogenous Methods

2.3.2.1 Plasma Creatinine Concentration

The estimation of GFR from the renal clearance of creatinine has been used frequently in the pediatric patient due to the expense and time needed of using the exogenous markers for the determination of a true GFR. A reduction in GFR is reflected by an increase in plasma creatinine. In children, interpretation of plasma creatinine value is difficult. One reason is the steady and muscle mass-related increase in plasma creatinine level in children above 2 years of age, although mean GFR measured by ^{51}Cr-EDTA remains constant at 104 mL/min per 1.73 m^2 (Schwartz et al. 1987). To obtain a meaningful estimate of renal function from the level of plasma creatinine, therefore narrow age-related reference ranges is needed. To compensate for the increasing muscle mass during childhood, creatinine-based formulas that include height and body composition have been developed. The most widely studied of these are the Schwartz and Counahan-Barratt formulae. Both provide an estimate of GFR based on a constant multiplied by the child's height divided by serum creatinine. Comparison of GFR prediction equations using serum creatinine is shown in Table 2.6.

2.3.2.2 Creatinine Clearance

The creatinine clearance (CrCl) method involves precise urine collection for 24 h, which is hard to obtain in children, time-consuming, and impracticable for routine use. Moreover, urine collection will not eliminate bias introduced by tubular secretion of creatinine. As the endogenous 24-h-creatinine clearance is less precise then the Schwartz estimate (Aufricht et al. 1995), the creatinine clearance is estimated from the plasma level of creatinine by the Schwartz formula.

Table 2.6 Equations predicting glomerular filtration rate in Children based on serum creatinine

Reference	Formula
Schwartz Formula (Schwartz et al. 1976, 1984, 1985, 1987)	$\text{GFR} = \left(\dfrac{k \times L}{S_{Cr}} \right)$ Where k is a constant, L is the height in cm and S_{cr} is the serum creatinine in mg/dL k = 0.33 in preemie infants k = 0.45 in term infants to 1 year of age k = 0.55 in children to 13 years of age k = 0.70 in adolescent males (not females because of the presumed increase in male muscle mass, the constant remains .55 for females).
Counahan-Barratt formula (Counahan et al. 1976)	$\text{GFR} = \left(\dfrac{0.43 \times L}{S_{Cr}} \right)$

Table 2.6(*continued*)

Shull Formula (Shull et al. 1978)	$GFR = \dfrac{[(0.035 \times Age) + 0.236] \times 100}{S_{Cr}}$
Traub Formula (Traub et al. 1980)	$GFR = \left(\dfrac{0.48 \times L}{S_{Cr}} \right)$
Ghazali- Barratt Formula (Ghazali and Barratt 1974)	$GFR = \dfrac{0.12 \times [15.4 + (0.46 \times age)] \times Wt}{S_{Cr} \times BSA}$
Revised Schwartz Formula (Schwartz et al. 2009)	$GFR = \left(\dfrac{0.413 \times L}{S_{Cr}} \right)$
	$GFR = 40.7 \times \left(\dfrac{HT}{S_{Cr}} \right)^{0.640} \times \left(\dfrac{30}{BUN} \right)^{0.202}$
Leger formula (Leger et al. 2002)	$GFR = \dfrac{(0.641 \times Wt) + (0.00161 \times L^2)}{S_{Cr}}$
Morris formula (Morris et al. 1982)	$GFR = \left(\dfrac{0.452 \times L}{S_{Cr}} \right)$

Scr, serum creatinine level (mg/dL); age, in years; Wt: weight, in kilograms; L: height in cm; HT: height in m; BSA, body surface area in m^2, GFR measurement (mL/min per 1.73 m^2).

Example 2.9

Calculate the estimated GFR using Revised Schwartz and Leger formula for a 12-years old male patient if the measured serum creatinine is 9.2 mg/dL. The patient weight and height are 35 Kg and 127 cm respectively.

Solution

The estimated GFR using Revised Schwartz formula can be calculated as follows:

$$GFR = \left(\frac{0.413 \times L}{S_{Cr}} \right) = \frac{0.413 \times 127}{9.2} = 5.7 \text{ mL} / \text{min} / 1.73 \text{m}^2$$

The estimated GFR using Leger formula can be calculated as follows:

$$GFR = \frac{(0.641 \times Wt) + (0.00161 \times L^2)}{S_{Cr}} = \frac{(0.641 \times 35) + (0.00161 \times (127)^2)}{9.2}$$

$$= 5.3 \text{ mL} / \text{min} / 1.73 \text{m}^2$$

2.3.2.3 Cystatin C

Recent studies have suggested that serum or plasma cystatin C (CysC) may be better markers for GFR than serum creatinine (Dharnidharka et al. 2002). CysC offers an advantage over creatinine because of its independence from age and gender (Bokenkamp et al. 1998) but its diagnostic sensitivity for impaired GFR in pediatric patients, particularly in patients with only mildly impaired renal function, has not been better than that of the height/creatinine ratio (Schwartz formula) (Filler et al. 1999). In some studies, the serum concentration of cystatin C may be superior to serum creatinine in distinguishing normal from abnormal GFR (Laterza et al. 2002), and a definitive numerical estimated GFR has been derived from its plasma concentration (Filler et al. 2002, Filler and Lepage 2003). However, cystatin C levels may underestimate GFR in renal transplant patients, which may be a result of inflammation or the use of immunosuppressive therapy (Bokenkamp et al. 1999). Other factors may influence serum cystatin C levels such as high C-reactive protein, smoking status, steroids, diabetes with ketonuria, and thyroid dysfunction (Knight et al. 2004). Therefore, caution must be used when estimating GFR in these situations (Schwartz and Work. 2009).

While there is increasing evidence that CysC is indeed a better marker of GFR, clinicians want an estimation of GFR from cystatin C and not simply a serum concentration. A comparison of GFR prediction equations of children based on CysC is given in Table 2.7.

Table 2.7 Equations predicting glomerular filtration rate in Children based on Cystatin C

Reference	Referred Method	Formula
Bokenkamp (Bokenkamp et al. 1998)	Inulin	$GFR = \dfrac{162}{CysC} - 30$
Filler (Filler and Lepage 2003)	^{99m}Tc- DTPA	$\log(GFR) = 1.962 + \left[1.123 \times \log\left(\dfrac{1}{s\text{-}SysC}\right)\right]$
Grubb (Grubb et al. 2005b)	Iohexol	$GFR = 84.69 \times s\text{-}SysC^{-1.680} \times 1.384 \ (age < 14 \ years)$

Table 2.7(*continued*)

Corrao (Corrao et al. 2006)	^{99m}Tc-DTPA	$\log(\text{GFR}) = 4.03 + \left[0.53 \times \log\left(\text{s-SysC}\right)\right]$
Zappitelli 1 (Zappitelli et al. 2006)	Iothalamate	$\text{GFR} = \left(\dfrac{75.94}{CysC^{1.17}}\right)$ $\left[\times 1.2 \text{ if renal transplant}\right]$

CysC, cystatin C, mg/L; age, in years; Wt: weight, in kilograms; L: height in cm, GFR measurement (mL/min per 1.73 m^2).

Some other equations were developed for predicting glomerular filtration rate in Children based on Cystatin C and serum creatinine as shown in Table 2.8.When using creatinine-based estimating formulas, it is important to know which creatinine assay is being used, because the coefficients of each equation are critically dependent on assay methodology.

Table 2.8 Equations predicting glomerular filtration rate in Children based on Cystatin C and serum creatinine

Reference	Referred Method	Formula
Bouvet (Bouvet et al. 2006)	^{51}Cr-EDTA	$\text{GFR} = 63.2 \times \left[\dfrac{Scr}{96 \times 88.4}\right]^{-0.35}$ $\times \left[\dfrac{CysC}{1.2}\right]^{-0.56} \times \left[\dfrac{Wt}{45}\right]^{0.3} \times \left[\dfrac{age}{14}\right]^{0.4}$
Zappitelli 2 (Zappitelli et al. 2006)	Iothalamate	$\text{GFR} = \dfrac{43.82 \times e^{0.003 \times L}}{CysC^{0.635} \times Scr^{0.547}}$ $\left[\times 1.165 \text{ if renal transplant}\right]$ $\left[\times \dfrac{Scr^{0.925}}{88.4 \times 40.45} \text{ if spina bifida}\right]$
	Iohexol	$\text{GFR} = \dfrac{25.38 \times 1.88^{L}}{CysC^{0.331} \times Scr^{0.602}}$

Table 2.8 (*continued*)

Schwartz (Schwartz et al. 2009)	Iohexol	

$$GFR = 39.1 \times \left[\frac{HT}{Scr}\right]^{0.516}$$

$$\times \left[\frac{1.8}{CysC}\right]^{0.294} \times \left[\frac{30}{BUN}\right]^{0.169}$$

$$\times (1.099)^{if\ male} \times \left[\frac{HT}{1.4}\right]^{0.188}$$

CysC, cystatin C, mg/L; Scr, serum creatinine level (mg/dL); BUN, Blood Urea Concentration (mg/dL); age, in years; Wt: weight, in kilograms; L: height in cm, HT: height in m; GFR measurement (mL/min per 1.73 m^2).

In children, the concentration of serum cystatin C in some studies is better correlated with GFR than is serum creatinine, especially in situations in which there is only a moderate decrease in GFR, suggesting that CysC might be advantageous in 'the creatinine blind area' of initial renal impairment (Dworkin 2001). Moreover, subtle decrements in GFR are more readily detected by changes in serum cystatin C than by serum creatinine, in part because of the shorter half-life of cystatin C (Dworkin 2001).

Thus, although cystatin C is not a conventional marker of GFR, reciprocal values of serum cystatin C levels are reasonably well correlated with GFR in adults (Coll et al. 2000) and in children (Filler et al. 1999). Furthermore, if a CysC-based prediction equation is introduced into a department, derivation of local coefficients has to be performed to overcome problems related to different assays of s-CysC and serum creatinine and different exogenous GFR methods. If this is not possible, a CysC-based equation using the same reference method and s-CysC assay as in the department has to be chosen, to minimize bias. In general, both CysC and creatinine assays have to be improved by international harmonization of methods and calibrators.

Example 2.10

Calculate the estimated GFR using Schwartz formula for a 10-years old female patient if the measured serum cystatin C is 1.9 mg/L, a serum creatinine is 10.2 mg/dL and a blood urea concentration is 55 mg/dL. The patient height is 130 cm.

Solution

The estimated GFR using Schwartz formula can be calculated as follows:

GFR =

$$39.1 \times \left[\frac{HT}{Scr}\right]^{0.516} \times \left[\frac{1.8}{CysC}\right]^{0.294} \times \left[\frac{30}{BUN}\right]^{0.169} \times (1.099)^{\text{if male}} \times \left[\frac{HT}{1.4}\right]^{0.188}$$

$$GFR = 39.1 \times \left[\frac{1.3}{10.2}\right]^{0.516} \times \left[\frac{1.8}{1.9}\right]^{0.294} \times \left[\frac{30}{55}\right]^{0.169} \times \left[\frac{1.3}{1.4}\right]^{0.188}$$

$$= 12.5 \text{ mL/min/1.73 m}^2$$

2.3.2.4 β-Trace Protein (BTP)

A novel formula for the estimation of GFR in children based on BTP was developed by Benlamri et al (2010). A BTP-based formula for estimating GFR was derived using stepwise linear regression analysis as follows:

$$GFR = 10^\wedge \left[1.92 + \left(0.98 \times \log\frac{1}{BTP}\right)\right] \qquad (2.23)$$

$$GFR = 10^\wedge \left[1.90 + \left(0.89 \times \log\frac{1}{BTP}\right)\right] \qquad (2.24)$$

A separate control group of 116 measurements in 99 children was used to validate the novel formula. The validation process revealed that this formula can be used to predict the true GFR with a higher accuracy. The limitation of this study is that it didn't control for corticosteroid use. A recent study suggests that high levels of corticosteroids may influence BTP concentrations (Abbink et al. 2008). In contrast, other studies have not demonstrated any effect of high-dose glucocorticoid therapy on BTP concentrations (Poge et al. 2005; Abbink et al. 2008).

2.4 CONCLUSION

Residual renal function among patients with end stage renal disease is clinically important as it contributes to adequacy of dialysis, quality of life, morbidity and mortality. The glomerular filtration rate (GFR) is considered to be the best overall measurement of renal function in health and disease. Advantages of the GFR as an index of renal function are that it is a direct measure of renal function, it is reduced prior to the onset of symptoms of renal failure and the impairment inGFR is associated with the structural abnormalities observed in CRF. Other tests, such as serum creatinine, creatinine clearance (CrCI), urea clearance, the average of creatinine and urea clearance, and urine volumes (UV) have been used to assess RRF in the CRF population. Urea and creatinine are the simplest measures of GFR but there are many flaws in interpreting their values. Creatinine clearance is best practice measure of GFR but the main limitation is the accuracy of urine collection. Inulin clearance and radioisotopic techniques are the most accurate however cost, non-availability and safety of materials limit their use. A number of different formulae have been developed to estimate CrCl and GFR in patients with CRF without timed urine collections. These formulae were developed and validated on a population with CRF. Cockroft and Gault formula gives a quick estimate of GFR but shouldn't be used below 18 years of age, patients who are obese, cachetic or oedematous. The MDRD formula provided a better estimate of GFR than the Cockcroft-Gault formula and offers several advantages over other equations. It is easily implemented in clinical practice as it can be computed and reported by the clinical laboratory that receives the blood and the patient's demographic data. Measurement of plasma Cystatin C has been proposed as a new and very sensitive endogenous marker of changes in GFR and will soon be available for clinical use

REFERENCES

Abbink, F.C., Laarman, C.A., Braam, K.I., et al.: Beta-trace protein is not superior to cystatin C for the estimation of GFR in patients receiving corticosteroids. Clin. Biochem. 41(4-5), 299–305 (2008)

Akbari, A., Lepage, N., Keely, E., et al.: Cystatin-C and beta trace protein as markers of renal function in pregnancy. Br. J. Obstet Gynaecol. 112(5), 575–578 (2005)

Albrechtsson, U., Hultberg, B., Larusdottir, H., Norgren, L.: Nefrotoxicity of ionic and non-ionic contrast media in aorofemoral angiography. Acta Radiol Diagnosis. 26(5), 615–618 (1985)

Almen, T.: Experimental investigations of iohexol and their clinical relevance. Acta Radiol. 366, 9–19 (1983)

Arant, B.S., Edelmann, C.M., Spitzer, A.: The congruence of creatinine and inulin clearances in children: Use of the Technicon AutoAnalyzer. J. Pediatr. 81(3), 559–561 (1972)

Aufricht, C., Balbisi, A., Gerdov, C., et al.: Formula creatinine clearance as a substitute for 24-hour creatine clearance in children with kidney transplantation. Klin. Padiatr. 207(2), 59–62 (1995)

Back, S.E., Krutzen, E., Nilsson-Ehle, P.: Contrast media as markers for glomerular filtration: a pharmacokinetic comparison of four agents. Scand. J. Clin. Lab Invest. 48(3), 247–253 (1988)

Bajaj, G., Alexander, S.R., Browne, R., et al.: ^{125}Iodine-iothalamate clearance in children. A simple method to measure glomerular filtration. Pediatr. Nephrol. 10(1), 25–28 (1996)

Baracskay, D., Jarjoura, D., Cugino, A., et al.: Geriatric renal function: estimating glomerular filtration in an ambulatory elderly population. Clin. Nephrol. 47(4), 222–228 (1997)

Beddhu, S., Samore, M.H., Roberts, M.S., et al.: Creatinine production, nutrition, and glomerular filtration rate estimation. J. Am. Soc. Nephrol. 14(4), 1000–1005 (2003)

Benlamri, A., Nadarajah, R., Yasin, A., et al.: Development of a beta-trace protein based formula for estimation of glomerular filtration rate. Pediatr. Nephrol. 25(3), 485–490 (2010)

Bjornsson, T.D.: Use of serum creatinine concentrations to determine renal function. Clin. Pharmacokinet. 4(3), 200–222 (1979)

Bokenkamp, A., Domanetzki, M., Zinck, R., et al.: Cystatin C—a new marker of glomerular filtration rate in children independent of age and height. Pediatrics 101(5), 875–881 (1998)

Bokenkamp, A., Domanetzki, M., Zinck, R., et al.: Cystatin C serum concentrations underestimate glomerular filtration rate in renal transplant recipients. Clin. Chem. 45(10), 1866–1868 (1999)

Bostom, A.G., Kronenberg, F., Ritz, E.: Predictive performance of renal function equations for patients with chronic kidney disease and normal serum creatinine levels. J. Am. Soc. Nephrol. 13(8), 2140–2144 (2002)

Bouvet, Y., Bouissou, F., Coulais, Y., et al.: GFR is better estimated by considering both serum cystatin C and creatinine levels. Pediatr. Nephrol. 21(9), 1299–1306 (2006)

Branten, A.J., Vervoort, G., Wetzels, J.F.: Serum creatinine is a poor marker of GFR in nephrotic syndrome. Nephrol. Dial. Transplant. 20(4), 707–711 (2005)

Brandstrom, E., Grzegorczyk, A., Jacobsson, L., et al.: GFR measurements with iohexol and ^{51}Cr-EDTA: A comparison of the two favoured GFR markers in Europe. Nephrol. Dial. Transplant. 13(5), 1176–1182 (1998)

Brown, S.C., O'Reilly, P.H.: Iohexol Clearance for the determination of glomerular filteration rate in clinical practice: evidence for a new gold standard. J. Urol. 146(3), 675–679 (1991)

Bubeck, B.: Radionuclide techniques for the evaluation of renal function: advantages over conventional methodology. Curr. Opin. Nephrol. Hypertens 4(6), 514–519 (1995)

Cholongitas, E., Shusang, V., Marelli, L., et al.: Review article: renal function assessment in cirrhosis - difficulties and alternative measurements. Aliment Pharmacol. Ther. 26(7), 969–978 (2007)

Cirillo, M., Anastasio, P., De Santo, N.G.: Relation of gender, age, and body mass index to errors in predicted kidney function. Nephrol. Dial. Transplant. 20(9), 1791–1798 (2005)

Cockcroft, D.W., Gault, M.H.: Prediction of creatinine clearance from serum creatinine. Nephron 16(1), 31–41 (1976)

Cole, B.R., Giangiacomo, J., Ingelfinger, J.R., Robson, A.M.: Measurement of renal function without urine collection. A critical evaluation of the constant-infusion technic for determination of inulin and para-aminohippurate. N. Engl. J. Med. 287(22), 1109–1114 (1972)

Coll, E., Botey, A., Alvarez, L., Poch, E., et al.: Serum cystatin C as a new marker for noninvasive estimation of glomerular filtration rate and as a marker for early renal impairment. Am. J. Kidney Dis. 36(1), 29–34 (2000)

Corbett, J.V.: Laboratory tests and diagnostic procedures with nursing diagnoses, 7th edn., pp. 90–107 (2008)

Coresh, J., Astor, B.C., McQuillan, G., et al.: Calibration and random variation of the serum creatinine assay as critical elements of using equations to estimate glomerular filtration rate. Am. J. Kidney Dis. 39(5), 920–929 (2002)

Corrao, A.M., Lisi, G., Di Pasqua, G., et al.: Serum cystatin C as a reliable marker of changes in glomerular filtration rate in children with urinary tract malformations. J. Urol. 175(1), 303–309 (2006)

Counahan, R., Chantler, C., Ghazali, S., et al.: Estimation of glomerular filtration rate from plasma creatinine concentration in children. Arch. Intern. Med. 51(11), 875–878 (1976)

Davis, G.A., Chandler, M.H.: Comparison of creatinine clearance estimation methods in patients with trauma. Am. J. Health Syst. Pharm. 53(9), 1028–1032 (1996)

Dharnidharka, V.R., Kwon, C., Stevens, G.: Serum cystatin C is superior to serum creatinine as amarker of kidney function: ameta-analysis. Am. J. Kidney Dis. 40(2), 221–226 (2002)

Dworkin, L.D.: Serum cystatin C as a marker of glomerular filtration rate. Curr. Opin. Nephrol. Hypertension 10(5), 551–553 (2001)

Dubois, D., Dubois, E.F.: A formula to estimate the approximate surface area if height and weight be known. Nutrition 5(5), 303–311 (1989)

Edwards, K.D., Whyte, H.M.: Plasma creatinine level and creatinine clearance as test of renal function. Aust. Ann. Med. 8, 218–224 (1959)

Effersoe, P.: Relationship between endogenous 24-hour creatinine clearance and serum creatinine concentration in patients with chronic renal disease. Acta Med. Scand. 156(6), 429–434 (1957)

Erley, C.M., Bader, B.D., Berger, E.D., et al.: Plasma clearance of iodine contrast media as a measure of glomerular filtration rate in critically ill patients. Crit. Care Med. 29(8), 1544–1550 (2001)

Filler, G., Priem, F., Vollmer, I., et al.: Diagnostic sensitivity of serum cystatin for impaired glomerular filtration rate. Pediatr. Nephrol. 13(6), 501–505 (1999)

Filler, G., Priem, F., Lepage, N., et al.: Beta-Trace protein, cystatin C, β_2-microglobulin, and creatinine compared for detecting impaired glomerular filtration rates in children. Clin. Chem. 48(5), 729–736 (2002)

Filler, G., Lepage, N.: Should the Schwartz formula for estimation of GFR be replaced by cystatin C formula? Pediatr. Nephrol. 18(10), 981–985 (2003)

Flodin, M., Jonsson, A.S., Hansson, L.O., et al.: Evaluation of Gentian cystatin C reagent on Abbot Ci8200 and calculation of glomerular filtrtation rate expressed in mL/min/1.73m^2 from the cystatin C values in mg/l. Scand. J. Clin. Lab Invest. 67(5), 560–567 (2007)

Froissart, M., Rossert, J., Jacquot, C., et al.: Predictive performance of the Modification of Diet in Renal Disease and Cockcroft-Gault equations for estimating renal function. J. Am. Soc. Nephrol. 16(3), 763–773 (2005)

Gaspari, F., Perico, N., Ruggenenti, P., et al.: Plasma clearance of nonradioactive iohexol as a measure of glomerular filtration rate. J. Am. Soc. Nephrol. 6(2), 257–263 (1995)

Gaspari, F., Perico, N., Remuzzi, G.: Application of newer clearance techniques for the determination of glomerular filtration rate. Curr. Opin. Nephrol. Hypertens 7(6), 675–680 (1998a)

Gaspari, F., Perico, N., Matalone, M., et al.: Precision of plasma clearance of iohexol for estimation of GFR in patients with renal disease. J. Am. Soc. Nephrol. 9(2), 310–313 (1998b)

Gates, G.F.: Creatinine clearance estimation from serum creatinine values: an analysis of three mathematical models of glomerular function. Am. J. Kidney Dis. 5(3), 199–205 (1985)

Ghazali, S., Barratt, T.M.: Urinary excretion of calcium and magnesium in children. Arch. Dis. Child 49(2), 97–101 (1974)

Gerbes, A.L., Gülberg, V., Bilzer, M.: Vogeser M Evaluation of serum cystatin C concentration as a marker of renal function in patients with cirrhosis of the liver. Gut. 50(1), 106–110 (2002)

Gowda, S., Desai, P.B., Kulkarni, S.S., et al.: Markers of renal function tests. North Am. J. Med. Sci. 2(4), 170–173 (2010)

Grubb, A., Bjork, J., Lindstrom, V., et al.: A cystatin C-based formula without anthropometric variables estimates glomerular filtration rate better than creatinine clearance using the Cockcroft-Gault formula. Scand. J. Clin. Lab Invest. 65(2), 153–162 (2005a)

Grubb, A., Nyman, U., Bjork, J., et al.: Simple cystatin C-based prediction equations for glomerular filtration rate compared with the modification of diet in renal disease prediction equation for adults and the Schwartz and the Counahan–Barratt prediction equations for children. Clin. Chem. 51(8), 1420–1431 (2005b)

Guido, F., Friedrich, P., Nathalie, L., et al.: β-Trace Protein, Cystatin C, β2-Microglobulin, and Creatinine Compared for Detecting Impaired Glomerular Filtration Rates in Children. Clin. Chem. 48(5), 729–736 (2002)

Ham, H.R., Piepsz, A.: Estimation of glomerular filtration rate in infants and in children using a single-plasma sample method. J. Nucl. Med. 32(6), 1294–1297 (1991)

Hellerstein, S., Berenbom, M., Erwin, P., et al.: Timed-urine collections for renal clearance studies. Pediatr. Nephrol. 21(1), 96–101 (2006)

Hoek, F.J., Kemperman, F.A., Krediet, R.T.: Acomparison between cystatin C, plasma creatinine and the Cockcroft and Gault formula for the estimation of glomerular filtration rate. Nephrol. Dial Transplant. 18(10), 2024–2031 (2003)

Hoffmann, A., Nimtz, M., Conradt, H.: Molecular characterization of ß-trace protein in human serum and urine: a potential diagnostic marker for renal diseases. Glycobiology 7(4), 499–506 (1997)

Huber, A.R., Risch, L.: Recent developments in the evaluation of glomerular filtration rate: is there a place for beta-trace? Clin. Chem. 51(8), 1329–1330 (2005)

Hull, J.H., Hak, L.J., Koch, G.G., et al.: Influence of range of renal function and liver disease on predictability of creatinine clearance. Clin. Pharmacol. Ther. 29(4), 516–521 (1981)

Itoh, K., Tsushima, S., Tsukamoto, E., Tamaki, N.: Reappraisal of single-sample and gamma camera methods for determination of the glomerular filtration rate with 99mTc-DTPA. Ann. Nucl. Med. 14(3), 143–150 (2000)

Jelliffe, R.W.: Estimation of creatinine clearance when urine cannot be collected. Lancet 297(7706), 975–976 (1971)

Jelliffe, R.W.: Creatinine clearance: bedside estimate [letter]. Ann. Intern. Med. 79(4), 604–605 (1973)

Johnson, D.: The CARI guidelines: Evaluation of renal function. Nephrology (Carlton) 10(suppl. 4), 133–176 (2005)

Junge, W., Wilke, B., Halabi, A., Klein, G.: Determination of reference intervals for serum creatinine, creatinine excretion and creatinine clearance with an enzymatic and a modified Jaffe´ method. Clin. Chim. Acta 344(1-2), 137–148 (2004)

Kasiske, B.L., Keane, W.F.: Laboratory assessment of renal disease: clearance, urinalysis and renal biopsy. In: Brenner, B.M. (ed.) Brenner & Rector's The Kidney, 6th edn., pp. 1129–1170. WB Saunders, Philadelphia (2000)

Knight, E.L., Verhave, J.C., Spiegelman, D., et al.: Factors influencing serum cystatin C levels other than renal function and the impact on renal function measurement. Kidney Int. 65(4), 1416–1421 (2004)

Krutzen, E., Back, S.E., Nilsson-Ehle, P.: Determination of glomerular filtration rate using iohexol clearance and capillary sampling. Scand. J. Clin. Lab Invest. 50(3), 279–283 (1990)

Kuan, Y., Hossain, M., Surman, J., et al.: GFR prediction using the MDRD and Cockcroft and Gault equations in patients with end-stage renal disease. Nephrol. Dial. Transplant. 20(11), 2394–2401 (2005)

Larsson, A., Malm, J., Grubb, A., Hansson, L.O.: Calculation of glomerular filtration rate expressed in ml/min from plasma cystatin C values in mg/L. Scand. J. Clin. Lab Invest. 64(1), 25–30 (2004)

Laterza, O.F., Price, C.P., Scott, M.G.: Cystatin C: An improved estimator of glomerular filtration rate? Clin. Chem. 48(5), 699–707 (2002)

Lavender, S., Hilton, P.J., Jones, N.F.: The measurement of glomerular filtration rate in renal disease. Lancet 294(7632), 1216–1218 (1969)

Le Bricon, T., Thervet, E., Froissart, M., et al.: Plasma cystatin C is superior to 24-h creatinine clearance and plasma creatinine for estimation of glomerular filtration rate 3 months after kidney transplantation. Clin. Chem. 46(8 Pt 1), 1206–1207 (2000)

Leger, F., Bouissou, F., Coulais, Y., et al.: Estimation of glomerular filtration rate in children. Pediatr. Nephrol. 17(11), 903–907 (2002)

Levey, A.S.: Measurement of renal function in chronic renal disease. Kidney Int. 38, 167–184 (1990)

Levey, A.S., Bosch, J.P., Lewis, J.B., et al.: A more accurate method to estimate glomerular filtration rate from serum creatinine: a new prediction equation. Modification of Diet in Renal Disease Study Group. Ann. Intern. Med. 130(6), 461–470 (1999)

Levey, A.S., Greene, T., Kusek, J., Beck, G.: A simplified equation to predict glomerular filtration rate from serum creatinine (abstract). J. Am. Soc. Nephrol. 11, 155A (2000)

Levey, A.S., Coresh, J., Balk, E., et al.: National Kidney Foundation. National Kidney Foundation practice guidelines for chronic kidney disease: evaluation, classification, and stratification. Ann. Intern. Med. 15 139(2), 137–147 (2003)

Levey, A.S., Coresh, J., Greene, T., et al.: Expressing the MDRD Study equation for estimating GFR with IDMS traceable (gold standard) serum creatinine values [Abstract]. J. Am. Soc. Nephrol. 16, 69A (2005)

Levey, A.S., Coresh, J., Greene, T., et al.: Chronic Kidney Disease Epidemiology Collaboration. Using standardized serum creatinine values in the modification of diet in renal disease study equation for estimating glomerular filtration rate. Ann. Intern. Med. 15 145(4), 247–254 (2006)

Levey, A.S., Stevens, L.A., Schmid, C.H., et al.: CKD-EPI (Chronic Kidney Disease Epidemiology Collaboration). A new equation to estimate glomerular filtration rate. Ann. Intern. Med. 150(9), 604–612 (2009)

Lin, J., Knight, E.L., Hogan, M.L., et al.: A comparison of prediction equations for estimating glomerular filtration rate in adults without kidney disease. J. Am. Soc. Nephrol. 14(10), 2573–2580 (2003)

Lubowitz, H., Slatopolsky, E., Shankel, S.: Glomerular filtration rate: determination in patients with chronic renal disease. JAMA 199(4), 252–256 (1976)

Maaravi, Y., Bursztyn, M., Stessman, J.: The new Mayo Clinic equation for estimating glomerular filtration rate. Ann. Intern. Med. 142(8), 680–681 (2005)

MacIsaac, R.J., Tsalamandris, C., Thomas, M.C., et al.: Estimating glomerular filtration rate in diabetes: a comparison of cystatin- C- and creatinine-based methods. Diabetologia 49(7), 1686–1689 (2006)

Mafham, M.M., Niculescu-Duvaz, I., Barron, J., et al.: A practical method of measuring glomerular filtration rate by iohexol clearance using dried capillary blood spots. Nephron Clin. Pract. 106(3), 104–112 (2007)

Manetti, L., Pardini, E., Genovesi, M., et al.: Thyroid function differently affects serum cystatin C and creatinine concentrations. J. Endocrinol Invest. 28(4), 346–349 (2005)

Manjunath, G., Sarnak, M.J., Levey, A.S.: Prediction equations to estimate glomerular filtration rate: an update. Curr. Opin. Nephrol. Hypertens 10(6), 785–792 (2001)

Mawer, G.E., Lucas, S.B., Knowles, B.R., et al.: Computer-assisted prescribing of kanamycin for patients with renal insufficiency. Lancet 299(7740), 12–15 (1972)

Mitch, W.E., Collier, V.U., Walser, M.: Creatinine metabolism in chronic renal failure. Clin. Sci. (Lond.) 58(4), 327–335 (1980)

Mitchell, H.R., Kline, W.: Core curriculum in nephrology, Renal Function Testing. Am. J. Kidney Dis. 47, 174–183 (2006)

Mogensen, C.E., Heilskov, N.S.: Prediction of GFR from serum creatinine. Acta Endocrinol Suppl. (Copenh.) 238, 109 (1980)

Morris, M.C., Allanby, C.W., Toseland, P., et al.: Evaluation of a height/plasma creatinine formula in the measurement of glomerular filtration rate. Arch. Dis. Child 57(8), 611–615 (1982)

NKF-K/DOQI, Clinical practice guidelines for chronic kidney disease: evaluation, classification, and stratification. Am. J. Kidney Dis. 39(2 suppl. 1) S1–S266 (2002)

Nilsson-Ehle, P., Grubb, A.: New markers for the determination of GFR: Iohexol clearance and cystatin C concentration. Kidney Int. 46(suppl. 47), S17–S19 (1994)

Nilsson-Ehle, P.: Iohexol clearance for the determination of glomerular filtration rate: 15 years' experience in clinical practice. J. Int. Fed. Clin. Chem. Lab Med. 13(2), 1–5 (2001)

Nolte, S., Mueller, B., Pringsheim, W.: Serum α1-microglobulin and β2-microglobulin for the estimation of fetal glomerular renal function. Pediatr. Nephrol. 5(5), 573–577 (1991)

Olsen, N.V., Ladefoged, S.D., Feldt-Rasmussen, B., et al.: The effects of cimetidine on creatinine excretion, glomerular filtration rate and tubular function in renal transplant recipients. Scand. J. Clin. Lab Invest. 49(2), 155–159 (1989)

Perrone, R.D., Steinman, T.I., Beck, G.J., et al.: Utility of radioisotopic filtration markers in chronic renal insufficiency: Simultaneous comparison of ^{125}I-iothalamate, ^{169}Yb-DTPA, ^{99}Tc-DTPA, and inulin. Am. J. Kidney Dis. 16(3), 224–235 (1990)

Perrone, R.D., Madias, N.E., Levey, A.S.: Serum creatinine as an index of renal function: New insights into old concepts. Clin. Chem. 38(10), 1933–1953 (1992)

Piepsz, A., Colarinha, P., Gordon, I., et al.: Guidelines for glomerular fil-
    tration rate determination in children. Eur. J. Nucl. Med. 28(3),
    BP31– BP36 (2001)
Piepsz, A., Tondeur, M., Ham, H.: Revisiting normal (51) Crethylenedia-
    minetetraacetic acid clearance values in children. Eur. J. Nucl.
    Med. Mol. Imaging 33(12), 1477–1482 (2006)
Poge, U., Gerhardt, T.M., Stoffel-Wagner, B., et al.: β-Trace protein is an
    alternative marker for glomerular filtration rate in renal transplan-
    tation patients. Clin. Chem. 51(8), 1531–1533 (2005)
Poge, U., Gerhardt, T., Stoffel-Wagner, B., et al.: Can modifications of the
    MDRD formula improve the estimation of glomerular filtration
    rate in renal allograft recipients? Nephrol. Dial. Transplant. 22(1),
    3610–3615 (2007)
Poge, U., Gerhardt, T., Stoffel-Wagner, B., et al.: Beta-trace protein-based
    equations for calculation of GFR in renal transplant recipients.
    Am. J. Transplant. 8(3), 608–615 (2008)
Poggio, E.D., Wang, X., Greene, T., et al.: Performance of the Modifica-
    tion of Diet in Renal Disease and Cockcroft-Gault equations in the
    estimation of GFR in health and in chronic kidney disease. J. Am.
    Soc. Nephrol. 16(2), 459–466 (2005)
Prigent, A., Cosgriff, P., Gates, G.F., et al.: Consensus report on quality
    control of quantitative measurements of renal function obtained
    from the renogram: International Consensus Committee from the
    Scientific Committee of Radionuclides in Nephrourology. Semin.
    Nucl. Med. 29(2), 146–159 (1999)
Priem, F., Althaus, H., Birnbaum, M., et al.: ß-trace protein in serum: a
    new marker of glomerular filtration rate in the creatinine-blind
    range. Clin. Chem. 45(4), 567–568 (1999)
Priem, F., Althaus, H., Jung, K., Sinha, P.: ß-Trace protein is not better
    than cystatin C as an indicator of reduced glomerular filtration
    rate. Clin. Chem. 47(12), 2181 (2001)
Pucci, L., Triscornia, S., Lucchesi, D., et al.: Cystatin C and Estimates of
    Renal Function: Searching for a Better Measure of Kidney Func-
    tion in Diabetic Patients. Clin. Chem. 53(3), 480–488 (2007)
Rahn, K.H., Heidenreich, S., Bruckner, D.: How to assess glomerular func-
    tion and damage in humans. J. Hypertens 17(3), 309–317 (1999)
Randers, E., Erlandsen, E.J.: Serum Cystanin C as an endogenous marker
    of the renal function a review. Clin. Chem. Lab Med. 37(4), 389–
    395 (1999)
Rartels, H., Bohmer, M.: Micro-determination of Creatinine. Clinica. Chi-
    mica. Acta 32(1), 81–85 (1971)

Rehberg, P.B.: Studies on kidney function. The rate of filtration and reabsorption in the human kidney. Biochem. J. 20, 447–460 (1926)

Rehling, M., Moller, M.L., Thamdrup, B., et al.: Simultaneous measurement of renal clearance and plasma clearance of ^{99m}Tc-labelled diethylenetriaminepenta-acetate, ^{51}Cr-labelled ethylenediaminetetra-acetate and inulin in man. Clin. Sci. 66(5), 613–619 (1984)

Rehling, M., Moller, M.L., Lund, J.O., et al.: ^{99m}Tc-DTPA gamma-camera renography: normal values and rapid determination of single-kidney glomerular filtration rate. Eur. J. Nucl. Med. 11(1), 1–6 (1985)

Richards, A.N., Westfall, B.B., Borr, P.A.: Renal excretion of inulin, creatinine and xylose in normal dogs. Proc. Soc. Erp. Biol. Med. 32, 73–75 (1934)

Rodrigo, E., de Francisco, A.L., Escallada, R., et al.: Measurement of renal function in pre-ESRD patients. Kidney Int. Suppl. (80), 11–17 (2002)

Rule, A.D., Larson, T.S., Bergstralh, E.J., et al.: Using serum creatinine to estimate glomerular filtration rate: accuracy in good health and in chronic kidney disease. Ann. Intern. Med. 141(12), 929–937 (2004)

Rule, A.D., Bregstraalh, E.J., Slezak, J.M., et al.: Glomerular filtration rate estimated by cystatin C among different clinical presentations. Kidney Int. 69(2), 399–405 (2006)

Salazar, D.E., Corcoran, G.B.: Predicting creatinine clearance and renal drug clearance in obese patients from estimated fat-free body mass. Am. J. Med. 84(6), 1053–1060 (1988)

Sanaka, M., Takano, K., Shimakura, K., et al.: Serum albumin for estimating creatinine clearance in the elderly with muscle atrophy. Nephron 73(2), 137–144 (1996)

Schoolwerth, A.C., Engelgau, M.M., Hostetter, T.H., et al.: Chronic kidney disease: a public health problem that needs a public health action plan. Prev. Chronic. Dis. 3(2), A57 (2006)

Schrott, K.M., Behrends, B., Clauss, W., et al.: Iohexol in excretory urography. Fortschr. Med. 104, 153–156 (1986)

Schwartz, G.J., Haycock, G.B., Edelmann Jr., C.M., Spitzer, A.: A simple estimate of glomerular filtration rate in children derived from body length and plasma creatinine. Pediatrics 58(2), 259–263 (1976)

Schwartz, G.J., Feld, L.G., Langford, D.J.: A simple estimate of glomerular filtration rate in full-term infants during the first year of life. J. Pediatr. 104(6), 849–854 (1984)

Schwartz, G.J., Gauthier, B.: A simple estimate of glomerular filtration rate in adolescent boys. J. Pediatr. 106(3), 522–526 (1985)

Schwartz, G.J., Brion, L.P., Spitzer, A.: The use of plasma creatinine concentration for estimating glomerular filtration rate in infants, children, and adolescents. Pediatr. Clin. North Am. 34(3), 571–590 (1987)

Schwartz, G.J., Furth, S., Cole, S.R., et al.: Glomerular filtration rate via plasma iohexol disappearance: pilot study for chronic kidney disease in children. Kidney Int. 69(11), 2070–2077 (2006)

Schwartz, G.J., Munoz, A., Schneider, M.F., et al.: New equations to estimate GFR in children with CKD. J. Am. Soc. Nephrol. 20(3), 629–637 (2009)

Schwartz, G.J., Work, D.F.: Measurement and Estimation of GFR in Children and Adolescents. Clin. J. Am. Soc. Nephrol. 4(11), 1832–1843 (2009)

Shannon, J.A., Smith, H.W.: The excretion of inulin, xylose and urea by normal and phiorhizinized man. I. Clin. Invest. 14(4), 393–401 (1935)

Shardijin, G., Statius van Epps, L.: ß2-Microglobulin: its significance in the evaluation of renal function. Kidney International 32(5), 635–641 (1987)

Sherman, D.S., Fish, D.N., Teitelbaum, I.: Assessing renal function in cirrhotic patients: problems and pitfalls. Am. J. Kidney Dis. 41(2), 269–278 (2003)

Shlipak, M.G., Katz, R., Fried, L.F., et al.: Cystatin-C and mortality in elderly persons with heart failure. J. Am. Coll. Cardiol. 45(2), 268–271 (2005)

Shull, B.C., Haughley, D., Koup, J.R., et al.: Useful method for predicting creatinine clearance in children. Clin. Chem. 24(7), 1167–1199 (1978)

Sjostrom, P., Tidman, M., Jones, I.: Determination of the production rate and non-renal clearance of cystatin C and estimation of the glomerular filtration rate from the serum concentration of cystatin C in humans. Scand. J. Clin. Lab Invest. 65(2), 111–124 (2005)

Sterner, G., Frennby, B., Hultberg, B., Almen, T.: Iohexol clearance for GFR-determination in renal failure—single or multiple plasma sampling? Nephrol. Dial. Transplant. 11(3), 521–525 (1996)

Swan, S.K., Keane, W.F.: Clinical evaluation of renal function in primer on kidney diseases. In: Greenberg, A. (ed.) 3rd edn., pp. 25–28. Academic press (2001)

Tidman, M., Sjostrom, P., Jones, I.: A Comparison of GFR estimating formulae based upon s-cystatin C and s-creatinine and a combination of the two. Nephrol. Dial. Transplant. 23(1), 154–160 (2008)

Toto, R.D., Kirk, K.A., Coresh, J., et al.: Evaluation of serum creatinine for estimating glomerular filtration rate in African Americans with hypertensive nephrosclerosis: results from the African-American Study of Kidney Disease and Hypertension (AASK) Pilot Study. J. Am. Soc. Nephrol. 8(2), 279–287 (1997)

Traub, S.L., Johnson, C.E.: Comparison of methods of estimating creatinine clearance in children. Am. J. Hosp. Pharm. 37(2), 195–201 (1980)

Van Acker, B.A., Koomen, G.C., Koopman, M.G., et al.: Creatinine clearance during cimetidine administration for measurement of glomerular filtration rate. Lancet 340(8831), 1326–1329 (1992)

Verhave, J.C., Fesler, P., Ribstein, J.: Estimation of renal function in subjects with normal serum creatinine levels: influence of age and body mass index. Am. J. Kidney Dis. 46(2), 233–241 (2005)

Walser, M., Drew, H.H., Guldan, J.L.: Prediction of glomerular filtration rate from serum creatinine concentration in advanced chronic renal failure. Kidney Int. 44(5), 1145–1148 (1993)

Walser, M.: Assessing renal function from creatinine measurernent in adults with chronic renal disease. Am. J. Kidney Dis. 32(1), 23–31 (1998)

Weber, J.A., Van Zenten, A.P.: Interferences in current methods for measurement of creatinine. Clin. Chem. 37(5), 695–700 (1991)

White, C.A., Akbari, A., Doucette, S., et al.: A novel equation to estimate glomerular filtration rate using beta-trace protein. Clin. Chem. 53(11), 1965–1968 (2007)

Woitas, R.P., Stoffel-Wagner, B., Poege, U., et al.: Low-molecular weight proteins as markers for glomerular filtration rate. Clin. Chem. 47(12), 2179–2180 (2001)

Wright, J.G., Boddy, A.V., Highley, M., et al.: Estimation of glomerular filtration rate in cancer patients. Br. J. Cancer 84(4), 452–459 (2001)

Yukawa, E., Hamachi, Y., Higuchi, S., et al.: Predictive performance of equations to estimate creatinine clearance from serum creatinine in Japanese patients with congestive heart failure. Am. J. Ther. 6(2), 71–76 (1999)

Zappitelli, M., Parvex, P., Joseph, L., et al.: Derivation and validation of cystatin C-based prediction equations for GFR in children. Am. J. Kidney Dis. 48(2), 221–230 (2006)

ESSAY QUESTIONS

1. List the main stages of Chronic Kidney Disease.
2. Define the concept of renal clearance.
3. What are the main criteria to select a substance for determination of GFR?
4. List three endogenous substances used to measure GFR.
5. List some exogenous substances used to measure GFR.
6. What are the disadvantages of direct measurement of GFR in routine clinical practice using inulin clearance?
7. What are the disadvantages of using radiolabelled. chelates to assess the GFR?
8. Why BUN is a poor measure of renal function?
9. What are the two major errors that can limit the accuracy of the CrCl?
10. What are the main advantages of the MDRD prediction equation over other equations?

MULTIPLE CHOICE QUESTIONS

Choose the best answer

1. In normal humans, GFR is approximately …

    A. $120 \ mL/min/1.73m^2$
    B. $125 \ mL/min/1.73 \ m^2$
    C. $110 \ mL/min/1.73m^2$
    D. $130 \ mL/min/1.73m^2$

2. The normal GFR for women is approximately …% lower than for men.
    A. 10 %
    B. 15 %
    C. 5 %
    D. 8 %

3. If a patient has a GFR of $65 \ mL/min/1.73m^2$, then he is classified to be in ….of CKD
    A. Stage 4
    B. Stage 3
    C. Stage 2
    D. Stage 1

4. The typical human reference ranges for serum creatinine are ... for women

    A. 0.5 to 1.0 mg/dL
    B. 0.7 to 1.2 mg/dL
    C. 0.5 to 1.2 mg/dL
    D. 0.7 to 1.0 mg/dL

5. The typical human reference ranges for serum creatinine ... for men.

    A. 0.5 to 1.0 mg/dL
    B. 0.7 to 1.2 mg/dL
    C. 0.5 to 1.2 mg/dL
    D. 0.7 to 1.0 mg/dL

6. The following radiolabelled chelates have been used to assess the GFR except ...

    A. ^{51}Cr-EDTA
    B. ^{99}Tc- DTPA
    C. ^{125}I-iothalamate
    D. Iohexol

7. The following exogenous substances are used for measuring GFR except ...

    A. Inulin Clearance (C_{In})
    B. β-Trace Protein (BTP)
    C. Clearance of Radiolabelled Compounds
    D. Clearance of Non-Radiolabelled Compounds

8. The normal plasma level of cystatin C is ... for patients under 50 years of age.

    A. < 1.3 mg/L
    B. < 1.4 mg/L
    C. < 1.2 mg/L
    D. < 1.55 mg/L

9. The normal plasma level of cystatin C is ... for patients over 50 years of age.

   A. < 1.55 mg/L
   B. > 1.55 mg/L
   C. < 1.25 mg/L
   D. < 1.35 mg/L

10. The renal clearance of ... remains the gold standard for the evaluation of GFR in children and adults.

   A. Inulin
   B. Creatinine
   C. Systatin C
   D. Radiolabelled Compounds

11. The most widely methods for estimating GFR in childrens are ...

   A. Leger formula
   B. Schwartz and formulae
   C. Counahan-Barratt
   D. B and C

12. If a creatinine clearance is measured in a 62-year-old man to monitor changes in renal function. The serum creatinine, measured at the midpoint of the 24-hour urine collection, was 2.2 mg/dL. Urine creatinine concentration was 45 mg/dL, and urine volume was 1200 mL. The patient's creatinine clearance is:

   A. 23.2 mL/min
   B. 17.1 mL/min
   C. 20.6 mL/min
   D. 16.5 mL/min

13. A 43-years old male has a serum BTP equal to 1.5 mg/L, serum creatinine equal to 135μmol/L, the estimated GFR for this patient using White-formula is:

   A. 25.6 mL/min/1.73m^2
   B. 50.3 mL/min/1.73m^2
   C. 35.5 mL/min/1.73m^2
   D. 45.4 mL/min/1.73m^2

14. A 57-years old, 64 kg, 166 cm in tall male patient has a serum creatinine equal to 11.21 mg/dL. The corrected estimated creatinine clearance and GFR for this patient using Cockcroft and Gault formula is:

    A. 6.62 mL/min
    B. 7.54 mL/min
    C. 8.55 mL.min
    D. 9.45 mL/min

15. A 38-years old male has a serum creatinine clearance equal to 11.95 mg/dl, the estimated GFR for this patient using Rule's refitted MDRD formula is:

    A. 3.8 mL/min/1.73m^2
    B. 5.6 mL/min/1.73m^2
    C. 4.2 mL/min/1.73m^2
    D. 6.8 mL/min/1.73m^2

16. If a 41-years old African-American female has a serum creatinine of 13.55 mg/dL and is recalibrated to be traceable to IDM, the estimated GFR using abbreviated MDRD formula is:

    A. 3.2 mL/min/1.73m^2
    B. 3.7 mL/min/1.73m^2
    C. 2.8 mL/min/1.73m^2
    D. 4.5 mL/min/1.73m^2

17. A 52-years old male has a serum creatinine equal to 6.6 mg/dL, the estimated GFR for this patient using CKD-EPI formula is:

    A. 8.4 mL/min/1.73m^2
    B. 7.3 mL/min/1.73m^2
    C. 5.8 mL/min/1.73m^2
    D. 6.5 mL/min/1.73m^2

18. For a 14-years old female patient, the measured serum creatinine is 7.1 mg/dL. The patient height is 140 cm. The estimated GFR using Counahan-Barratt formula is:

    A. 8.5 mL/min/1.73m^2
    B. 9.6 mL/min/1.73m^2
    C. 11.3 mL/min/1.73m^2
    D. 6.9 mL/min/1.73m^2

19. If a 13-years old African-American male has serum cystatin C is 2.3 mg/L, the estimated GFR using Filler formula is:

  A. 45.7 mL/min/1.73m^2
  B. 35.95 mL/min/1.73m^2
  C. 32.6 mL/min/1.73m^2
  D. 49.4 mL/min/1.73m^2

20. If the measured serum cystatin C is 1.88 mg/L, a serum creatinine is 6.5 mg/dL and a blood urea concentration is 60 mg/dL for 8 years-old male. If the patient height is 120 cm, the estimated GFR using Schwartz formula is:

  A. 20.43 mL/min/1.73m^2
  B. 22.13 mL/min/1.73m^2
  C. 17.24 mL/min/1.73m^2
  D. 12.35 mL/min/1.73m^2

Chapter (3)

Hemodialysis System

Ahmad Taher Azar and Bernard Canaud

CHAPTER OUTLINES

- Principles Of Dialysis
- Hemodialysis Machine
- Advanced options for hemodialysis machines
- Conclusion

CHAPTER OBJECTIVES

- Describe the principles of dialysis.
- Define the basic principles of diffusion, filtration, ultrafiltration, convection, and osmosis.
- Describe the major components of hemodialysis machines.
- Describe the Extracorporeal Blood Delivery Circuit.
- Describe the Dialysate Delivery Circuit.
- Describe the purpose and chemical composition of dialysate.
- Discuss the various types of dialyzers and their structure.

KEY TERMS

- Hemodialysis
- Diffusion
- Convection
- Extracorporeal Blood Circuit
- Dialysate Delivery Circuit
- Hemodialyzer
- Biocompatibility

ABSTRACT

The function of the dialysis system is to eliminate toxic wastes products, to restore "internal milieu composition" and to correct extracellular fluid overload. When complete renal failure occurs, the use of an artificial kidney is required. An artificial kidney is a machine that provides a means for removing uremic toxins from the blood and adding deficient components to it (e.g., bicarbonate, calcium). This is done using the principle of dialysis. There are two types of dialysis treatment: peritoneal dialysis (PD) and hemodialysis (HD). The peritoneal dialysis (PD) uses the abdominal cavity and its largely perfused serous membrane as a "built-in dialyzer" by creating and renewing periodically an artificial ascites. PD is a simple and safe technique that does not imply an extracorporeal blood circuit and usually performed at home. The hemodialysis and its related techniques are a much more complex and risky procedure that requires an extracorporeal blood circuit. HD is usually performed in hemodialysis facilities (center, self-care) but may be alternatively performed at home after training.

A.T. Azar (Ed.): Modelling and Control of Dialysis Systems, SCI 404, pp. 99–166.
springerlink.com   © Springer-Verlag Berlin Heidelberg 2013

Hemodialysis machines deliver a patient's dialysis prescription by controlling blood and dialysate flows through the dialyzer. In addition, they incorporate monitoring and alarm systems that protect the patient against adverse events that may arise from equipment malfunction during the dialysis treatment. This chapter will focus on essential principles of hemodialysis, the major components of HD machines and their respective monitoring devices.

3.1 PRINCIPLES OF DIALYSIS

Hemodialysis or "dialysis" are generic terms covering all forms of renal replacement therapy that share an extracorporeal blood circulation, a module of exchange (dialyzer) and an electrolytic solution serving as vector to solutes (see Fig. 3.1). This complex interaction between hemodialysis system and chronic kidney disease patient is schematically presented on Fig. 3.2. As illustrated, the clearing capacity of uremic toxins of dialysis patient is restricted by series of factors related to the hemodialyzer performances and to the complexity of body compartments and composition. In other words, the clearance concept that is generally used to define and quantify dialysis efficacy must be splitted in two different aspects: hemodialyzer clearance and body or effective clearance.

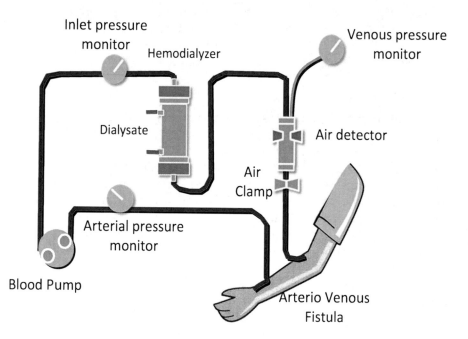

Fig. 3.1 Principle of hemodialysis

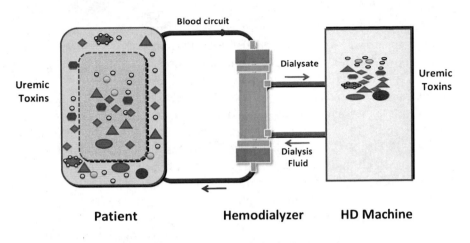

Fig. 3.2 Patient/hemodialysis Interaction

3.1.1 Hemodialyzer Clearance

The process of dialysis occurring in a hemodialyzer unit involves bidirectional movement of molecules across a semi-permeable membrane embedded in a housing unit. Solute movement takes place in and out of blood, across a semi-permeable membrane according to the membrane permeability and operational conditions of use (blood flow, dialysate flow…). Solute removal in dialysis relies on three different basic and physical transmembraneous mechanisms: diffusion, convection, and adsorption. The relative contribution of each of these three mechanisms to the removal of a given solute during dialysis serves to define the renal replacement modality: when diffusion is predominant the method is named "hemodialysis"; when convection is predominant or exclusive the method is named "hemofiltration", when diffusion and large convection occur simultaneously the method is named "hemodiafiltration". Some qualifiers are usually added to the renal replacement modality to qualify solute fluxes (low or high-flux, low or high-efficiency), flow rates (high or low blood rates or dialysate flow rates), substitution site and/or volume in convective therapies (post, predilutional, low or high substitution volume…).

3.1.1.1 Diffusive Transport

If two solutions of different concentrations are separated by a semi-permeable membrane, solute will move from the side of higher to the side of lower solute concentration. This process of solute movement on a concentration gradient is called *diffusion* in water solution and dialysis when a membrane is interposed between two solutions. This phenomenon is caused by the random movement of the solute molecules striking and moving across the membrane (See Fig. 3.3). Several factors influence this random movement and thus the rate of diffusion. The transport of any solute or solvent molecule is dependent on the physical size of the molecule relative to the size of the pores in the membrane (Byrne and Schultz 1994). Any molecules larger than the pores of the membrane cannot pass through. Similarly, the electrical charge, the shape and hydrophilic property of the molecule also determine the rate of transport across the membrane. If the membrane has a negative charge, particles with a like charge will have limited transport as compared with those with a positive or a neutral charge (Ahmad 2009). In dialysis, diffusion occurs across an artificial semipermeable membrane. This is how wastes and fluid are removed from the patient's blood, and electrolytes are balanced. Diffusion of a solute through a solvent is governed by Fick's first law (Sargent and Gotch 1996):

$$J = -DA\frac{dC}{dx} = -DA\frac{\Delta C}{\Delta x} \tag{3.1}$$

Fick's first states that the flux, J, of a material over a short distance, dx, is proportional to its concentration difference, dc, over this distance and the area of the diffusion, A. The constant of proportionality is the diffusivity, D, measured in cm^2/sec. The sign convention is used to indicate that the diffusion in the positive direction; material moves from the region of higher to that of lower activity so that concentration will be decreasing (dc/dx < 0) in the direction of flux (Sargent and Gotch 1996).

If the value of Δx is constant, the major variables that determine the flux of dialyzer will be the concentration difference and area, D being a constant at any particular temperature (Sargent and Gotch 1996). Thus, Equation (1) can be written as follows:

$$J = -K_o A\Delta C \tag{3.2}$$

In Eq. (3.2), K_o is a new proportionality constant, the overall mass transfer coefficient (cm/ min), and is defines as (Sargent and Gotch 1996):

Concentration Gradient

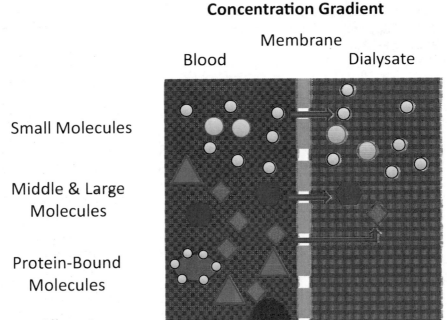

Fig. 3.3 Diffusive Transport, Dialysis

$$K_o = \frac{J/A}{-\Delta C} = \frac{\text{Diffusive flux}}{\text{Driving force}} \qquad (3.3)$$

By comparing Eq. (3.1) and Eq. (3.3), it is noted that K_o is directly proportional to the diffusivity of the solute being transferred and inversely proportional to the diffusion distance characteristics of the dialyzer. By rewriting Eq. (3.3), the diffusive mass transfer during hemodialysis is governed by the following integrated mass balance equation:

$$N = J/A = -K_o \Delta C = \frac{-\Delta C}{1/K_o} = \frac{-\Delta C}{R_o} \qquad (3.4)$$

Where $1/K_o$ is the resistance to transport. The overall resistance to diffuse mass transfer of a particular solute (R_O) is the sum of three resitances in series: blood compartment resistance (R_B), resistance due to the membrane itself (R_M), and dialysate compartment resistance (R_D) (Lysaght 1995; Ward et al. 2001).

$$R_O = R_B + R_M + R_D \qquad (3.5)$$

Thus, the overall resistance to diffusive mass transfer of a particular solute (R_o) by a dialyzer has three components: blood compartment resistance (R_B), resistance due to the membrane itself (R_M), and dialysate compartment resistance (R_D) (Clark et al. 1999). Minimizing the mass transfer resistance in the blood compartment primarily requires the use of relatively high flow rates (that is, shear rates) that decrease unstirred layers. Dialysate-side mass transfer resistance is likewise decreased by increasing the flow rate, but optimal dialysate perfusion of fiber bundles is also a consideration (Clark et al. 1999). The resistance of the three segments can be calculated as follows (Sargent and Gotch 1996):

$$R_B = \frac{\Delta x_B}{D_B}$$

$$R_M = \frac{\Delta x_M}{k D_M} = \frac{\Delta x_M}{D^*_M} \qquad (3.6)$$

$$R_D = \frac{\Delta x_D}{D_D}$$

Where k is the solute distribution coefficient between the membrane material and the solution. This equation indicates that the blood compartment resistance (R_B) and the dialysate compartment resistance (R_D) are governed by the effective diffusion distances from the main stream to and from the membrane (Δx_B and Δx_D, respectively) (Sargent and Gotch 1996). The membrane resistance (R_B) still depends on the thickness of the membrane but in addition, it is sensitive to the effective diffusivity of the membrane (D^*_M) which can vary according to its chemical composition. Therefore, a decrease in membrane resistance can be achieved either by a decrease in membrane thickness or an increase in membrane diffusivity. On the blood side, R_B decreases as the flow rate and the shear rate increase. On the dialysate side, R_D also decreases with increasing flow rate, but is additionally dependent on the distribution of flow through the fiber bundle. The flow distribution in the dialysate compartment may be influenced by the packing density of the fibers in the dialyzer housing and the inclusion of spacer filaments between the membrane fibers or undulations in the membrane fiber in some dialyzers (Ronco et al. 2002).

3.1.1.1.1 Factors Affecting Diffusive Process

The diffusive transport of a solute depends on:

a) The concentration gradient for the solute between the two solutions: Solutes can move through a membrane in either direction, but always toward the area of lesser concentration. A gradient is a difference. As the concentration gradient increases, solute movement increases. Diffusion stops when the concentrations on both sides of the membrane are equal i.e. *Equilibrium* as shown in Fig. 3.4. Concentration gradients allow dialysate to remove wastes from a patient's blood and to balance electrolytes in the blood with electrolytes in the dialysate. The maximum rate of solute transfer occurs initially when the concentration gradient is greatest. The dissipation of the concentration gradient can be minimized and the transfer of solute optimized by increasing the volume of the fluids. In a flowing system (comparable to hemodialysis) this accomplished by increasing the flow rate of parent fluid (blood) or recipient fluid (dialysate).

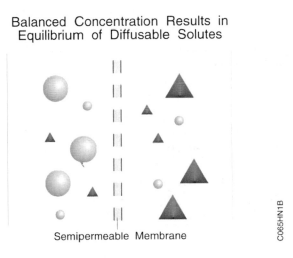

Fig. 3.4 Balanced Concentration Results in Equilibrium of Diffusable Solutes. Reprinted with permission, Copyright 2003, ECRI institute, www.ecri.org, 5200 Butler Pike, Plymond Meeting, PA 19462. 610-825-6000

b) Permeability of the membrane to the solute: membrane with more pores per square centimeters allows faster diffusion. Larger pores allow larger molecules to pass through. Thinner membrane and better designed pore structures (nanotechnology) increase diffusive rate of solutes.

c) Surface area of the membrane: Larger surface areas allow more diffusion.

d) Molecular weight of the solutes: The hydrated size of the solute is highly correlated with its molecular weight. The heavier, larger solute moves more slowly along the concentration gradient than smaller lighter solutes. Thus, dialysis is most effective in removing small solutes and less effective in removing larger solutes, particularly those over 1000 Dalton.

e) Blood protein content affects the diffusive transport of solute across the membrane by two different mechanisms:

1. The binding of the solute to protein (mainly to albumin): Diffusible substance may bind to proteins forming dialysis membrane impermeable complex. Such solutes are no longer available for diffusion (40-50% of measured calcium in patient blood is available for diffusion). The percentage of the total concentration of a diffusible solute (actually free to diffuse) is described as "solute activity". This is also a limiting factor for protein-bind toxins (e.g., paracresyl sulfate, indoxyl sulfate) that are tightly bound to albumin with small removable free-fraction (see Table 3.1)

2. The Gibbs-Donnan effect: Blood proteins are dialysis membrane impermeable, negatively charged and tend to accumulate at the membrane surface during dialysis. Corresponding numbers of membrane permeable cations such as sodium, calcium, magnesium must then retain in the blood to preserve electroneutrality. This results in imbalance in the concentration of ions across the dialysis membrane. The protein-induced ion transport asymmetry is called the *"Gibbs-Donnan effect"*. It indirectly affects the magnitude of the concentration gradients required to drive diffusion across dialysis membrane.

Table 3.1 Uremic toxins (Vanholder et al. 2003)

Small water soluble solutes	Protein-bound solutes	Middle molecules
Asymmetric dimethylarginine	3-Deoxyglucosone	Adrenomedullin
Benzylalcohol	CMPF*	Atrial natriuretic peptide
ß-Guanidinopropionic acid	Fructoselysine	$ß_2$-Microglobulin
ß-Lipotropin	Glyoxal	ß-Endorphin
Creatinine	Hippuric acid	Cholecystokinin
Cytidine	Homocysteine	Clara cell protein
Guanidine	Hydroquinone	Complement factor D
Guanidinoacetic acid	Indole-3-acetic acid	Cystatin C
Guanidinosuccinic acid	Indoxyl sulfate	Degranulation inhibiting protein I
Hypoxanthine	Kinurenine	Delta-sleep-inducing peptide
Malondialdehyde	Kynurenic acid	Endothelin
Methylguanidine	Methylglyoxal	Hyaluronic acid
Myoinositol	N-carboxymethyllysine	Interleukin 1ß
Orotic acid	P-cresol	Interleukin 6
Orotidine	Pentosidine	Kappa-Ig light chain
Oxalate	Phenol	Lambda-Ig light chain
Pseudouridine	P-OHhippuric acid	Leptin
Symmetric dimethylarginine	Quinolinic acid	Methionine-enkepahlin
Urea	Spermidine	Neuropeptide Y
Uric acid	Spermine	Parathyroid hormone
Xanthine		Retinol binding protein
*CMPF is carboxy-methyl-propyl-furanpropionic acid		Tumor necrosis factor alpha

3.1.1.1.2 Role of Blood and Dialysate Flows in Diffusive Clearances

The blood and dialysate flows are critical for optimizing the solute clearances in hemodialysis. As shown on Fig. 3.5, at constant dialysate flow rate of 500 mL/min, increasing the blood flow rate has a positive impact on instantaneous solute clearance. This is particularly marked for small molecular weight substances (urea, creatinine) while this is not hold for middle and large molecular substances (β2-microglobulin). Note that in all cases solute clearances are linked to blood flow rates by a parabolic function. Such relationship underlines the fact that solute clearance is linearly correlated to blood flow in the first part of the curve (less than 300 mL/min), plateaued thereafter and become flow independent afterwards.

In clinical practice, that underlines the fact that blood flow rates are crucial in hemodialysis for optimizing solute clearances. Blood flows over 300 mL/min are required to ensure best solute removal performances of small molecules.

3.1.1.2 Convective Solute Removal

Convective solute removal occurs as a result of water flow, known as solvent drag effect, through the membrane in response to a hydrostatic pressure difference (transmembrane pressure, TMP) applied across the

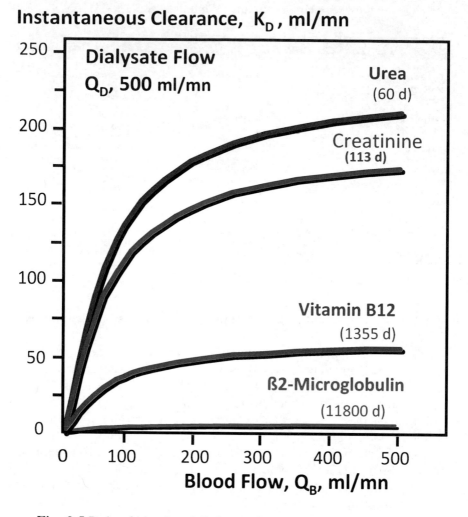

Fig. 3.5 Role of blood and dialysate flows in diffusive clearances

membrane, a process known as ultrafiltration. The fluid removed is the ultrafitrate (UF) that has the solute composition of plasma water of the hemodialysis patient (see Fig. 3.6). Low ultrafiltrate volume (e.g., < 3,0 liters per session) does not need any substitution and is intended to restore the extracellular fluid overload (water and salt removal) without significant effect on uremic toxins removal. Larger ultrafiltrate volumes (e.g., >10 liters per session) require an isovolumetric substitution of infusate and are intended to clear efficiently uremic toxins. In this case the dialysis modality is named hemofiltration and/or hemodiafiltration. Online convective therapies are presented on Fig. 3.7. Note that in all cases, an UF is required during dialysis for removing sodium and water accumulated by ingestion of fluid or by metabolism of food during the interdialytic period. It is essential to prescribe and control the fluid removal rate so that total fluid removed during dialysis will be equal to the total fluid gained since the previous dialysis or from the dry weight. Stable dialysis patients generally can tolerate an ultrafiltration rate of less than 20 ml/kg/hour (Ahmad 2009). It is important to determine which patients are stable and which are not (Mitchell 2002). A more conservative approach is to limit the ultrafiltration rate to 1% of the estimated dry weight per hour (Gutch et al. 1999; Mitchell 2002).

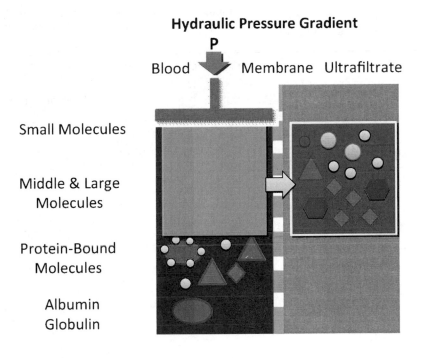

P, Hydraulic Pressure
UF, Ultrafiltrate

Fig. 3.6 Convective Transport, Ultrafiltration

Convective therapies

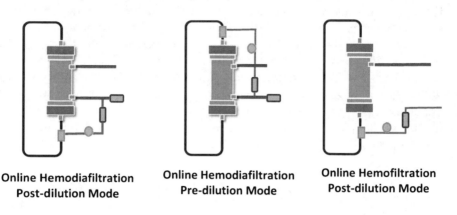

| Online Hemodiafiltration Post-dilution Mode | Online Hemodiafiltration Pre-dilution Mode | Online Hemofiltration Post-dilution Mode |

Fig. 3.7 Online Convective Therapies

The ease with which the solute is dragged along is determined by the size of the solute molecule relative to the size of the membrane pores. Smaller and non-protein-bound solutes are transported easily and the entire solution can sieve across the membrane without any change in concentration. In contrast, larger solutes move more slowly and the rate of convective transport is slower. Thus, the convective transport of a solute depends on how porous (both size and numbers of holes) the membrane is. This measurement of porosity is known as the sieving coefficient (SC) of the membrane (Ahmad 2009). On the opposite, the total solute reflection point known as "cutoff" of the membrane is the molecular size beyond which all solutes are retained. Sieving coefficient of 1.0 means that, barring other clinical factors, the membrane could allow 100% of a given solute to pass. Sieving coefficient of 0.4 means that only 40% of a solute would pass and 60% would be kept in the blood. Darcy's law gives a general equation for ultrafiltration:

$$J_U = h_m \cdot A \cdot \Delta P \tag{3.7}$$

Where J_u is the volumetric flux (m³/s), h_m is the hydraulic permeability (m/s/Pa), A is the area of ultrafiltration (m²), and ΔP is the pressure difference (Pa).

3.1.1.2.1 Factors Governing Ultrafiltration

1. Hydrostatic pressure

The primary driving force for ultrafiltration is the hydrostatic pressure difference across the membrane, which is the Transmembrane Pressure (TMP), expressed in millimeters mercury (mmHg). The TMP is determined by the average or mean pressure in the blood compartment minus the mean dialysate compartment pressure. The relationship of ultrafiltrate to TMP is entirely dependent on the membrane (hemodialysis) properties. The permeability of dialyzer membranes to water is high, varies considerably, and is a function of membrane thickness and pore size. The total capacity of the dialyzer for ultrafiltration is given by the Ultrafiltration Coefficient (K_{UF}). The K_{UF} is defined as the number of milliliters of fluid per hour that will be transferred across the membrane per mmHg pressure gradient across the membrane (described in detail in Chapter 8).

2. Blood flow rate and protein cake formation

During conventional hemodialysis the ultrafiltration rate applied to correct the fluid gain during the interdialytic session, remains relatively low (10-25 mL/min) being not significantly altered by dialysis prescription (blood flow rate, dialysis time duration). In other words, effective blood flow is not critical for preventing TMP increase during the dialysis session.

With high efficient convective therapies (hemofiltration and hemodiafiltration), the blood flow rate become quite critical having a direct effect on the targeted ultrafiltration rate. This phenomenon known as the protein-cake formation onto the surface of the membrane (second protein layer concentration-polarization) reduces the ultrafiltration rate capacity and is enhanced by maintaining too high trans-membrane pressure. To overpass this ultrafiltration threshold limit, increasing blood flow and shear stress are the only means capable of scrubbing protein-cake and restoring hydraulic permeability of the membrane. This is illustrated on Fig. 3.8.

It is of interest noting that higher ultrafiltration rates are associated with a reduced sieving coefficient, a phenomenon that also depends on the protein concentration-polarization effects onto the membrane surface. This is illustrated on Fig. 3.9.

In clinical practice, these phenomenon translates in dialysis prescription that should favor high blood flow rates (>350 mL/min), reduced filtration fraction (20 to 30%) in post-dilutional methods with limited transmembrane pressure (300 mmHg) regimen. If high blood flow cannot be achieved, the ultrafiltration rate should be reduced and predilutional substitution methods should be preferred.

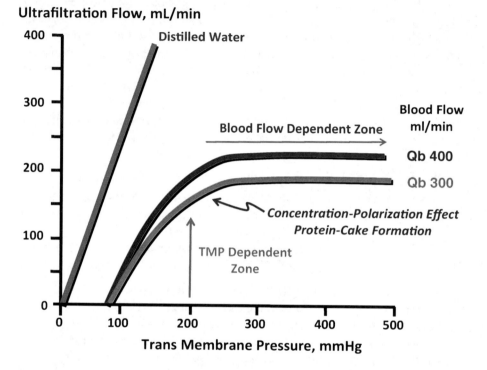

Fig. 3.8 Relationship between Ultrafiltration Rate and Trans-membrane Pressure

3. Patient hemorheologic conditions

Ultrafiltration rate is also limited by patient's characteristics such hematocrit, total protein concentration, fibrinogen and lipid concentrations. High concentrations of these parameters have a negative impact on the ultrafiltration by increasing the viscosity, the oncotic pressure and the blood cells concentration within the hemodialyzer reducing the free plasma water accessible.

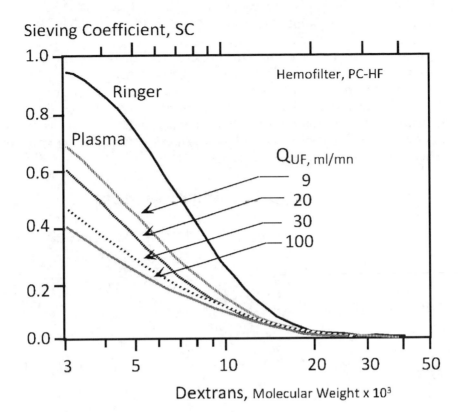

Fig. 3.9 Sieving coefficient of uncharged Dextrans is reduced while increasing ultrafiltration

4. Osmotic Ultrafiltration (this is more relevant to hemodynamic tolerance of dialysis session than dialysis efficacy)

Osmotic ultrafiltration does play an indirect role in total ultrafiltration; water shifts from intracellular to the extracellular compartment which occur during hemodialysis (so-called plasma refilling) can be optimized by introduction of an effective concentration of an osmotic agent into the extracellular space. Sodium is employed in some dialysis practice especially during sodium profiling.

3.1.1.3 Adsorptive Solute Removal

Adsorption occurs when material sticks to the dialyzer membrane as shown in Fig. 3.10. Adsorption to the membrane depends on the physicochemical properties of the membrane surface and the solute being adsorbed (Henrich 2009). Discrepancies between blood-side and dialysate side clearance measurement for some membranes indicated that adsorption can be a factor of considerable clinical relevance in solute removal. In general, adsorption is limited to proteins.

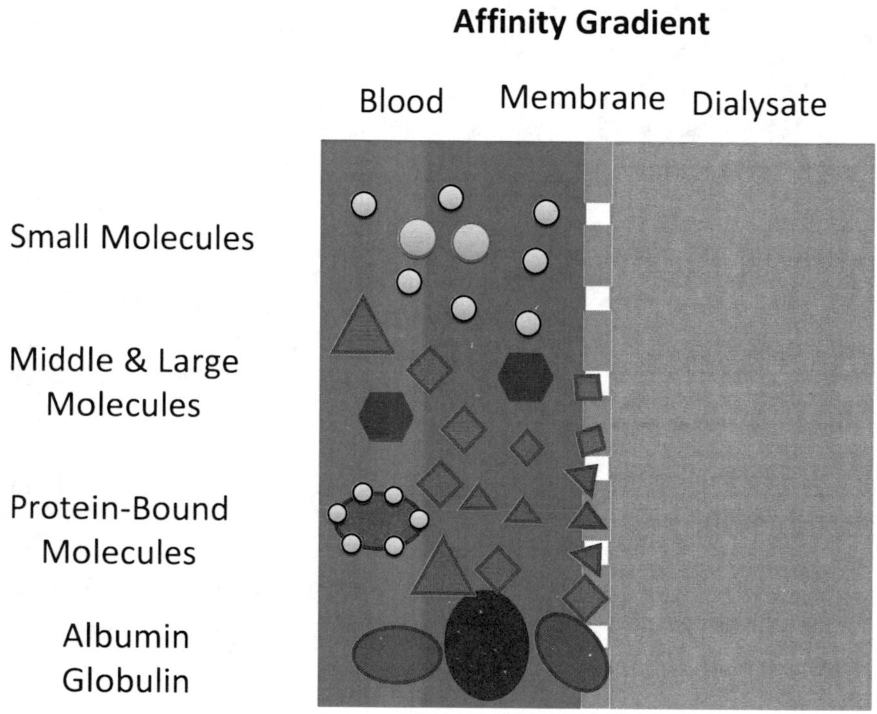

Fig. 3.10 Adsorptive Transport, Adsorption

The contribution of adsorption to removal of low-molecular-weight proteins varies considerably among membranes and among proteins, even for those membranes fabricated from nominally similar polymers but with different physicochemical properties (Ouseph et al. 2008). While the physicochemical interactions that determine protein adsorption to a membrane are incompletely understood, in general more hydrophobic membranes adsorb more protein than more hydrophilic membranes. Manipulation of the surface properties of a membrane may change its adsorptive affinity for protein. For example, the creation of hydrophilic and hydrophobic micro-domains on the surface of Polyflux membranes may impede the formation of the stable hydrophobic protein-surface interactions required for adsorption (Deppisch et al. 1998; Ronco et al. 2003). The adsorption surface of a membrane resides primarily in its pore structure and thickness rather than its nominal surface area, and that adsorption of any middle or low molecular weight protein will depend on it having access to the membrane's internal pore structure (Clark et al. 1999, 1994). This is thought to explain why polyacrylonitrile (PAN) and polymethylmethacrylate (PMMA) membranes can adsorb more β2-microglobulin (MW 11818) than EPO (MW 34000). High-flux membranes, which have a greater number of larger pores, adsorb more protein than low-flux membranes, which have few large pores (Clark et al. 1994. Larger proteins may also become trapped in the pores of the membrane by steric hindrance without actually adsorbing to the surface of the pore. Protein adsorption to a membrane may decrease the diffusive and convective transport of low-molecular-weight proteins through the membrane as dialysis session proceeds, possibly by creating a protein layer that effectively reduces the pore size of the membrane (Morti and Zydney 1998). Because of adsorption to the membrane, the amount of protein retrieved from the dialysate may, under some circumstances, substantially underestimate the net clearance of that protein from the blood. Adsorption of plasma proteins other than β2-microglobulin can have a negative effect on the performances of the individual membranes or dialyzers. Protein adsorption into the membrane during treatment, as well as the eventual retention of such proteins even after reprocessing, leads to so-called "membrane fouling". This term is generally used to describe the deterioration of membrane performance by the presence of a secondary layer of plasma components. This layer increases the diffusive length for blood solutes (thus decreasing diffusion) and blocks pores-whereby membrane hydraulic permeability, adsorption capacity for β2-microglobulin and convective removal properties are negatively affected.

3.1.2 Effective Body Clearance

Effective body clearance is the main target of any form of hemodialysis. It is the end product of a complex interaction between the patient and the hemodialysis system that expresses the real efficacy of the renal replacement treatment. Body clearance integrates major factors affecting hemodialysis efficacy: instantaneous dialyzer clearance, intracorporeal kinetics of solutes defined as their mass transfer coefficient, treatment time and vascular access performances. It is not our intent to review in details all these factors but just to remind that dialysis prescription should consider all these items for tailoring treatment schedule to patient's needs and making sure that dialysis delivery prescribed is achieved.

In clinical practice, dialysis adequacy is a quite complex concept that covers a wide spectrum of metabolic disorders that need to be clearly identified and individually controlled using a series of targeted markers. This is summarized in a recent review (Canaud 2004).

3.2 HEMODIALYSIS MACHINE

The operational system of the HD machine represents a complex array of detectors, controllers, monitors, and safety devices to ensure a safe operation. The system is a totally self-contained machine that provides the necessary control functions for hemodialysis therapy. Basic functions of the unit are: Automatically primes extracorporeal circuit; Prepares dialysate; monitors dialysate and blood; pumps blood and anticoagulant at predetermined rates; controls fluid removal; automatically cleans, disinfects, and rinses dialysate flow path. Single-patient hemodialysis systems can be divided into three major components: (1) the extracorporeal blood-delivery circuit, (2) the dialysate delivery system, and (3) the dialyzer. Blood is taken via the extracorporeal circuit, passed through a dialyzer for solute and fluid removal, and returned to the patient. Each system has its own monitoring and control circuits.

3.2.1 Extracorporeal Blood Delivery Circuit

The extracorporeal blood circuit (see Fig. 3.11) consists of an access device (needles or catheter), blood tubing, blood pump, Heparin pump; Air leak detector; Clamps and dialyzer. The role of the blood circuit is to deliver blood to the dialyzer at the prescribed flow rate and then return the blood to the patient. This goal must be achieved without damaging blood components and without loss of circuit integrity that may lead to blood loss or the entry of air or other harmful substances, such as bacteria, into the blood. Usually, an artery and a vein in the patient's arm are surgically joined for circulatory access; this junction is called an arteriovenous (AV) fistula. Bypassing capillary beds, where arterial blood pressure is markedly decreased, the blood entering the fistula maintains high pressure, causing the diameter of the vein to expand greatly. One or two large-bore needles can then be inserted into the enlarged vessel.

Another technique for vascular access is the external AV shunt, which is made of Teflon and Silastic and connects to both a vein and an artery in the forearm or lower leg. It is less often used because of the risk of infection, thrombosis, and accidental dislodgment. Dialysis vascular access is described in detail in Chapter 5.

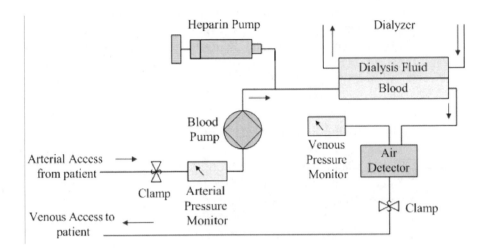

Fig. 3.11 The extracorporeal circuit in hemodialysis

3.2.1.1 Blood Tubing

Blood is drawn from the patient into the blood tubing, either through a central venous catheter or through a needle inserted into the patient's vascular access. Blood tubing is made of biocompatible and nontoxic material. The blood tubing in the pump segment is treated with silicone to minimize blood clotting. Because of its high cost, the use of silicone-treated blood tubing in single-use systems is uncommon (Misra 2005). Leaching of phthalate di-(2-ethylhexyl) phthalate (DEHP) from polyvinyl chloride (PVC), a constituent of the blood tubing, may occur into the blood circulation and lead to liver damage. Phthalate may very rarely lead to anaphylaxis (Misra 2005). Blood tubing can be divided into two major segments. The segment that carries blood from the patient to the dialyzer is traditionally called the "arterial segment," while the segment that carries blood from the dialyzer back to the patient is called the "venous segment." Usually, each of these segments has a drip chamber into which blood flows and any air rises to the top. Blood drains from the drip chamber into the blood tube, continuing its course toward the dialyzer from the arterial and to the patient from the venous drip chamber (Ahmad 2009). Each set of blood tubing has different, specialized parts. The order in which those parts are installed in the delivery system varies with the system's design, prescribed treatment, and the monitoring desired. Parts of blood tubing include (Curtis et al. 2008):

- **Patient connectors**: A tip, or Luer-Lok® connector, at the end of the arterial and venous blood tubing segments connects the tubing to the patient's needles or catheter ports.
- **Dialyzer connectors:** Luer-Lok connectors at the other end of the blood tubing segments connect the tubing to the dialyzer. The arterial blood tubing segment connects to the arterial end of the dialyzer. The venous blood tubing segment connects to the venous end of the dialyzer.
- **Saline infusion line:** This line allows saline to be given to the patient during dialysis. It is most often placed on the arterial blood tubing segment just before the blood pump, so saline can be pulled into the circuit. If the saline infusion line is not clamped correctly, too much fluid or air can enter the extracorporeal circuit.

3.2.1.2 Arterial Pressure Monitor (Pre-Pump)

The arterial pressure is measured by means of a pressure transducer that is connected to the pressure line of the blood tubing system with an intermediate, hydrophobic membrane filter as protection from contamination (see Fig. 3.12). This component monitors the pressure between the blood access and the blood pump, and if it goes beyond the set ranges, the alarm sounds and the blood pump stops. The pressure is negative between the access and the blood pump but achieves a high positive range post-blood pump (see Fig. 3.13). The pressure transducer signal is amplified and converted to an electrical signal. Alarms may indicate patient disconnection, separation of blood tubing, or obstruction/kink in the blood circuit. The normal pressure reading in this segment of the blood circuit is negative (subatmospheric). Negative pressure makes this segment prone to entry of air into the bloodstream. Longer needles with smaller bores increase negative pressure readings in this segment. Likewise, negative-pressure augmentation may be seen when longer catheters with smaller internal diameter bores are used, especially with higher blood flows. Out-of-range pressures trigger the machine to clamp the blood line and activate the appropriate alarms. Some systems have an additional arterial pressure monitor between the blood pump and the dialyzer that enables the reading of pressure between the pump and the dialyzer (Ahmad 2009). Causes of high and low arterial pressure alarms are listed in Table 3.2.

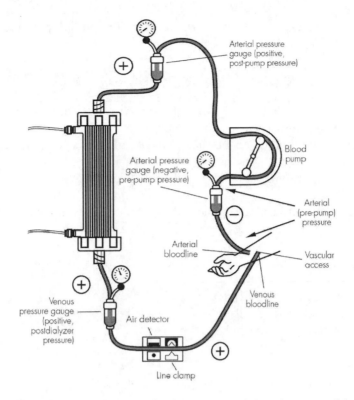

Fig. 3.12 Pressure monitoring devices on arterial and venous bloodlines. Published with permission of Amgen Inc. http://www.amgen.com

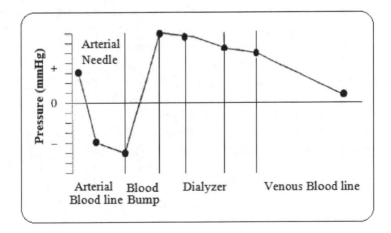

Fig. 3.13 The pressure profile in the blood circuit with an arteriovenous fistula as the blood access. Adapted from From Misra M (2005) The basics of hemodialysis equipment. Hemodial Int; 9: 30-36, with permission.

Table 3.2 Causes of low and high arterial (pre-pump) pressure alarms (Reddy and Cheung 2009)

Low (more negative) arterial pressure alarm	High (less negative) arterial pressure alarm
Blockage of arterial blood flow from the vascular access	Increase in patient's blood pressure
Compression or kinking of the arterial bloodline	Arterial blood line disconnection
Improper positioning of the arterial needle	Blood leak between the patient and the pressure monitoring site
Blood pump set at a rate higher than the vascular access can supply	Infusion of saline and medications into the arterial tubing
Hypotension	A decrease in the blood pump speed
Vasoconstriction (tightening of the patient's blood vessels)	
Poorly working central catheter	

3.2.1.3 Venous Pressure Monitor (Post-dialyzer)

The venous pressure may build up owing to resistance to venous return anywhere between the venous drip chamber and the venous needle (together with the access pressure) (see Fig. 3.12). The venous drip chamber also has a level and air detector. If the blood level drops below the detector level because of too much air, an air alarm sounds, the pump stops, and the tubing segment below the drip chamber is clamped to prevent any air being introduced into the patient (Ahmad 2009). Venous pressure monitors-normally read positive pressures. Out-of-range pressures trigger clamping of the blood line, stopping of the blood pump, and activation of appropriate alarms, with shutting of the venous return. Causes of high and low arterial pressure alarms are listed in Table 3.3. The drop in pressure between post pump pressure and venous pressure represents the effect of ultrafiltration. For the calculation of transmembrane pressure (TMP), either the average of the two pressures (if post pump arterial pressure is measured) or the venous pressure is used (Ahmad 2009).

Table 3.3 Causes of low and high venous (post-pump) pressure alarms (Reddy and Cheung 2009)

Low (less positive) venous pressure alarm	High (more positive) venous pressure alarm
Separation of blood tubing from the venous needle or catheter.	Blood clotting in the venous drip chamber
Low blood pump speed	Kinks in the venous blood tubing
A severely clotted dialyzer	Venous outflow stenosis in vascular access
Blockage in the blood tubing before the monitoring site	Poorly functioning central venous catheter

3.2.1.4 Blood Pump

The most widely used pumps in hemodialysis machines are composed of a rotor with rollers, a stator and tubing compressed between the rollers and the stator, these are called flow regulated pumps or peristaltic pump, since the flow depends mostly on the rotation speed of rollers (see Fig. 3.14). Negative pressure before the pump and positive pressure after the pump have only a small influence on the blood flow. In pressure dependent pumps the pump tubing is stretched upon a vertical rotor without a stator. In this system blood flow is mostly dependent on the pre and post pump pressures and less dependent on the pump speed. The blood pump takes and returns the blood from the patient via the arterial and venous needles. The blood is confined to the disposable plastic tubing and doesn't come in contact with any part of the machine. The pump segment tubing material is silicone rubber and the rest of the blood tubing is usually made of polyvinyl chloride.

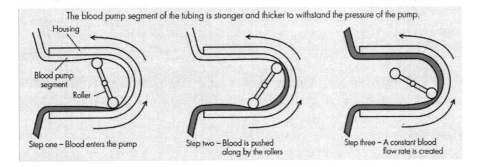

Fig. 3.14 Blood pump. Published with permission of Amgen Inc. http://www.amgen.com

The blood pump is the distinct feature on all dialysis machines. The pumping is done by squeezing the plastic tube inside the pump using a pair of spring loaded rollers. The suction is done by the elasticity of the tube, which expands after released from the rollers and sucks the blood from the arterial needle. The blood coming from the pump flows to the dialyzer and the blood that leaves the dialyzer returns to the patient through the venous needle. The blood pump segment of the blood tubing is threaded between the rollers and the pump head. The rollers turn, blocking the tubing and pushing blood out of the segment (Curtis et al. 2008). After the roller has passed, the segment resumes its shape and blood is drawn in to refill the pump segment. In this way, blood is pulled into and pushed out of the segment at the same time. By changing the roller speed, blood flow through the extracorporeal circuit can be set according to the prescription. Blood flow rates can be varied between 0 mL/min and 600 mL/min (Curtis et al. 2008). If the pump is set at a certain rate but access is unable to provide blood at that rate, the pressure in the arterial chamber drops below the set range and the alarm stops dialysis. Similarly, any excessive resistance to blood being returned to the patient increases pressure in the venous drip chamber and the system will stop if the set range is exceeded. The blood flow rate is calculated based on the pump RPM (revolution per minute), and the stroke volume based on diameter of the tube, entered by a screwdriver driven selector in the pump as follows:

$$BFR = RPM \, (\text{measured directly}) \times$$
$$\text{tubing volume} \, (\pi \times r^2 \times l) \tag{3.8}$$

Where r is the internal radius of the tubing and l is the length of the tubing being compressed between the two rollers. Owing to limited rigidity, the tubing between the two rollers flattens with a high negative pressure and the above formula overestimates the blood flow at high BFR.

3.2.1.5 Heparin Pump

Unfractionated heparin is used to suppress clotting stimulated by the extracorporeal blood circuit. The heparin pump delivers heparin to the blood tubing. The pump is a regular syringe that is pushed by a controlled motor. Heparin is infused downstream into the positive-pressure segment of the blood circuit (post-blood pump, pre-dialyzer) (see Fig. 3.15). If infused pre-pump in the negative-pressure segment, the risk of air embolism is

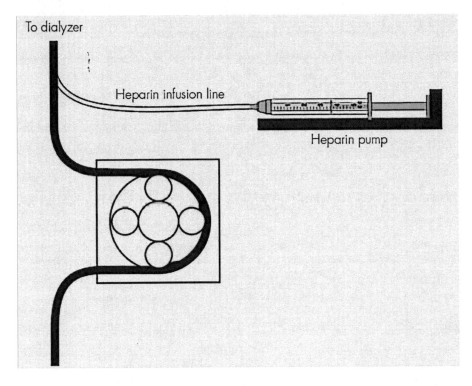

Fig. 3.15 Heparin infusion line. Published with permission of Amgen Inc.
http://www.amgen.com

enhanced. On all machines the rate can be adjusted. On newer machines
the end time can be programmed too. Usually an initial dose of heparin is
given when the treatment begins, then the pump delivers heparin until one
hour before the end. Note that not all patients need continuous heparin. In
case of a patient after surgery or another kind of bleeding, heparin is used
sparingly or not at all. To avoid clotting in the dialyzer it is rinsed with 100
ml saline every hour or so. In spite of that, the blood in the dialyzer may
clot, but unless the patient has a very low blood count no treatment is required (of course the heparin dose should be increased when possible).
Nowadays, prevention of the extracorporeal blood circuit thrombosis may
be easily achieved by using low molecular weight heparin injected IV 2
minutes before launching the blood circuit or regional sodium citrate anticoagulation in high bleeding risk patients (Davenport 2011; Evenepoel et
al. 2007). Several alternatives based on novel anti-anticoagulant agents
(Factor X inhibitors, Direct thrombin inhibitors, Oligosaccharides) are under clinical evaluation.

3.2.1.6 Air Leak Detector

The penetration of air into the patient's extracorporeal blood circuit may cause an air embolism, therefore even a small amount of air or foam stops the machine and starts the alarm. In order to catch limited amounts of air and to separate accompanying air bubbles, the venous blood line is expanded (venous drip chamber). A major task of the air detector is to monitor the presence of air, foam, and microbubbles in the venous drip chamber (see Fig. 3.16). Two types of air-leak detectors are in use: the ultrasonic and the optical detectors. Ultrasonic devices check for changes in a sound wave sent through a cross-section of the blood path. Sound travels faster through air than liquid. Therefore, any air in the blood will raise the speed at which the sound wave passes through the blood, setting off an alarm (see Fig. 3.17). The detector is placed distally in the venous blood line and monitors for and prevents air embolus (incidence of major air embolus is approximately in 1:2000 treatments). The usual volume of air needed to result in this complication is 60 to 125 mL (1 mL/kg/min, may vary), especially if rapidly injected. The air presents as foam with microbubbles. The hemodialysis system should detect the presence of a series of microbubbles that occur within a short period of time and total more than 1.5 mL/30 s. The manufacturer shall disclose the sensitivity of the air detector and the method used for testing. The test method used shall be described in sufficient detail to permit reproducible results and verification of sensitivity by the user. Loss of power to the air detector shall cause the blood pump to be turned off and the venous return line clamp to occlude the venous line. Means shall be provided for manual release of the venous clamp to allow for return of blood in emergency situations. If the air detector has not been activated and the system is being operated when the patient is connected to the dialysis machine, both audible and visual indicators shall alert the operator that the air detector is not activated. The optical detector serves to detect if there is blood or saline solution or air in the venous return line downstream of the bubble catcher.

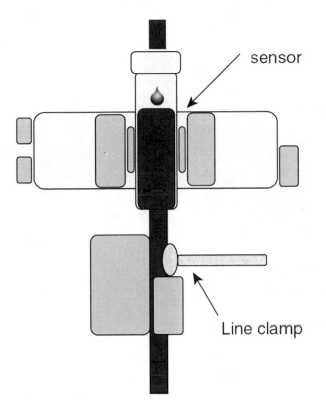

Fig. 3.16 Air-foam detector. Adapted From Pittard JD (2008) Safety monitors in hemodialysis, In: Nissenson AR, Fine RN (eds): Handbook of Dialysis Therapy (4th ed). Philadelphia, PA, Hanley & Belfus, Inc., pp 188-223, with permission of Elsevier.

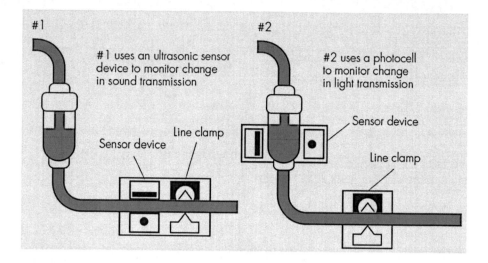

Fig. 3.17 Ultrasound Air detector. Published with permission of Amgen Inc. http://www.amgen.com

3.2.2 Dialysate Delivery Circuit

The term dialysate refers to the fluid and solute that have crossed a membrane i.e. effluent dialysis fluid. Dialysate can also replace needed substances, such as calcium and bicarbonate, which helps keep the body's pH balance. During a treatment, the patient's blood is on one side of the membrane, in the blood compartment. The dialysate is on the other side, in the dialysate compartment. Dialysate and blood never mix, unless the membrane breaks. Dialysis patients' blood has high concentrations of waste products and excess water. Dialysate is prescribed to have desired levels of solutes the patient needs and none of the ones that must be removed completely. The osmolality (solute particle concentration) of dialysate should closely match the blood to keep too much fluid from moving across the membrane (Curtis et al. 2008). The concentration gradients created decide the diffusion rates of each solute across the membrane. Unwanted solutes leave the blood and move into the dialysate; desired solutes stay in the blood (Salai 2007). Some solutes are added to dialysate in amounts that can cause them to enter the patient's blood. Most often, these are sodium, bicarbonate, and chloride. The principal functions of the dialysate circuit are to prepare dialysate from concentrate and water, to deliver it to the dialyzer at the prescribed temperature (generally 35–37°C) and flow rate, and to control fluid removal from the patient. Most current machines allow the composition of the dialysate and the fluid removal rate to be varied during the treatment according to some predetermined profile.

3.2.2.1 Types of Dialysate

Dialysis solutions are usually prepared from concentrates and contain either *acetate* or *bicarbonate* as a buffer.

a) Acetate Dialysate

In the early 1960s acetate became the standard dialysate buffer for correcting uremic acidosis and offsetting the diffusive losses of bicarbonate during hemodialysis. Acetate is physiologically compatible with blood and metabolized to bicarbonate in the liver. It is mixed with water in proportioning system, usually 1 part concentrate and 34 parts of water, to form the dialysate. A typical composition of acetate containing dialysate (after mixing) contains, Sodium 135-145 mmol/L, potassium 0-4 mmol/L, Calcium 1.25-1.75 mmol/L, Magnesium 0.5-1 mmol/L, Acetate 35-38 mmol/L, Chloride 100-119 mmol/L, Dextrose mmol/L, PCO_2 0.5 mmHg. Over the next several years reports began to accumulate that linked routine use of acetate contribute to cardiovascular instability with vasodilatation and hypotension, nausea, vomiting, and post dialysis fatigue (Palmer, 1999). As a result, nowadays dialysate containing bicarbonate has become the principal dialysate buffer worldwide.

b) Bicarbonate Dialysate

Calcium and magnesium will not remain in solution with bicarbonate because of low hydrogen ion content (high pH). To solve this problem, two separate concentrate are used. The proportioning (delivery) system mix and monitor three liquids instead of two.

1. The "A" concentrate
2. The "B" concentrate or powder.
3. Purified water

The "A" -indicating acidified- concentrate contains sodium, calcium, magnesium and potassium, chloride. To maintain low pH enough to keep the calcium and magnesium in solution when mixed into dialysate a small amount of acetic acid is included. The "B" -indicating bicarbonate-concentrate contains the sodium bicarbonate. Sodium chloride may be included in some preparation to raise the total conductivity. Manufacturers utilize a delivery system that accepts a closed container of dry (powder) bicarbonate onto a special holder. Warm water passes through the column producing a saturated solution of bicarbonate that is proportioned with water then with the A concentrate by conductivity controlled feedback system (e.g. Bicart as described in section 3.2.4). The advantage of this technique avoids the problems of bacterial growth in bicarbonate concentrate and reduces the cost of storage.

3.2.2.2 Composition of Dialysate

The composition of dialysate is listed in Table 3.4 (Daugirdas et al. 2007). The composition can be varied substantially in special clinical circumstances.

Table 3.4 The Composition Of Commercial Dialysate For Hemodialysis (Daugirdas et al. 2007)

Solute	Dialysate (mmol/L)
Sodium	135 – 145
Potassium	0 – 4
Chloride	98–124
Calcium	1.25 – 1.75
Magnesium	0.5 – 0.75
Acetate /Citrate	2 – 4
Bicarbonate	30 – 40
Dextrose	11
Glucose (g/L)	0 – 2
P_{CO_2} (mmHg)	40-110
PH	7.1–7.3

a) Sodium

Sodium is removed from the blood primarily by convection instead of diffusion during hemodialysis, so that there is little change in plasma sodium concentration. In the early days of hemodialysis, the dialysate sodium concentration was deliberately set low, usually in the range of 135-145 mmol/L to avoid problems of chronic volume overload such as hypertension and heart failure. As volume removal became more rapid because of shorter dialysis times, symptomatic hypotension emerged as a common and often disabling problem during dialysis. It soon became apparent that changes in the serum sodium concentration-and more specifically changes in serum osmolality-were contributing to the development of this hemodynamic instability. A decline in plasma osmolality during regular hemodialysis favors a fluid shift from the extracellular space to the intracellular space, thus exacerbating the volume-depleting effects of dialysis. With the advent of high-clearance dialyzers and more efficient dialysis techniques, this decline in plasma osmolality becomes more apparent, as solute is removed more rapidly. Use of dialysate of low sodium concentration would tend further to enhance the intracellular shift of fluid, as plasma tends to become even more hyposmolar consequent to the movement of sodium from plasma to dialysate. The use of a higher sodium concentration dialysate (>140 mmol/L) has been among the most efficacious and best tolerated therapies for episodic hypotension (Flanigan 2000). The high sodium concentration prevents a marked decline in the plasma osmolality during dialysis, thus protecting the extracellular volume by minimizing osmotic fluid loss into the cells. The concentration of sodium in the dialysate can be varied during the course of individual treatments in order to actively influence plasma sodium levels, a process called *sodium profiling* or *sodium modeling* (Donauer et al. 2000; Oliver et al. 2001; Stiller et al. 2001; Zhou et al. 2006). Independent of the time course of a profile, an important consideration is its influence on the post-dialysis plasma sodium concentration; this results from diffusive sodium transport during the treatment and represents the respective diffusive sodium balance. A wide variety of sodium profiles (i.e., decreasing, increasing, and alternating) and diverse profiles forms (e.g., linear, stepwise, and exponential) have been used for different clinical situations (Stiller et al. 2001). During this process, the dialysate sodium concentration at the beginning of the dialysis session is set at a higher value (e.g. 160 mEq /L) with subsequent falls to a lower value (e.g. 140 mEq/L) at the end of the session. Sodium profiling is designed to reduce intradialytic intravascular hypovolemia and symptomatic hypotension as well as the post-dialysis washed-out feeling; however, increasing the sodium concentration in the dialysate may also produce post-dialysis hypernatremia and increase interdialytic thirst, intradiaytic fluid weight gain, and hypertension (Meira et al. 2007).

b) Potassium

The dialysate potassium concentration is 4 mmol/L, depending on the patient's pre-dialysis plasma potassium concentration. The commonly used dialysate potassium concentrations are 2-3 mmol/L. Use of low potassium dialysate concentration may contribute to arrhythmias, especially in those patients with underlying coronary artery disease or those taking digoxin. On the other hand, use of dialysate with high potassium concentration may predispose patients to pre-dialysis hyperkalemia. In patients who are at high risk for arrhythmias on dialysis, modeling the dialysate potassium concentration so as to maintain a constant blood to dialysate potassium gradient throughout the procedure may be of clinical benefit.

c) Calcium

The dialysate calcium concentration has implications with regard to metabolic bone disease, hemodynamic stability, and long-term effects on vascular calcification. The calcium concentration in the dialysate can be varied extensively according to the individual needs of the patient. The most common concentrations used are 1.25, 1.5, and 1.75 mmol/L, respectively, corresponding to 2.5, 3.0, 3.5 mmol/L and 5.0, 6.0, 7.0 mg/dL. The most recent National Kidney Foundation's Kidney Disease Outcomes Quality Initiative (NKF-KDOQI) guidelines recommend a dialysate calcium concentration of 1.25 mmol/L as being a useful compromise between optimization of bone health and reductions in cardiovascular risk (Monge et al. 2006). To maintain a neutral calcium balance in hemodialysis patient a dialysate calcium concentration of 1.50 mmol/L is usually the best option for a majority of patients. However, as with the other dialysate constituents, the calcium concentration should be individually tailored to the patient (Palmer 1999). Studies have shown that the dialysate calcium concentration has significant hemodynamic effects and PTH secretion effects when low dialysate calcium concentrations were used (Argiles et al. 1993). In normal individuals, serum calcium concentration can affect blood pressure by two methods: 1) a change in systemic vascular resistance; 2) a change in cardiac output mediated through a change in myocardial contractility. Studies in ESRD patients indicate a direct relationship between dialysate calcium concentration and blood pressure (Van der Sande et al. 1998).

In patients prone to intradialytic hypotension who are at risk for hypercalcemia, dialysate calcium profiling can be used as a strategy to improve hemodynamic stability and yet minimize the potential for hypercalcemia (Kyriazis et al. 2002). Most patients with normal serum calcium do well with a dialysate calcium in the range of 2.5 to 3 mEq/L, and this appears a reasonable choice for starting such a patient on dialysis (NKF-K/DOQI 2003). If serum calcium increases above 2.50 mmol/L, dialysate calcium can be reduced to 1.25 to 1.50 mmol/L. Dialysate concentrations below this range are associated with increased hypotensive episodes. Increases in serum calcium caused by administration of vitamin D in the treatment of hyperparathyroidism can also be treated with a decrease in dialysate calcium. If the serum calcium is low (below 2.20 mmol/L), the dialysate calcium concentration can be increased to 1.5 to 1.75 mEq/L. However, high dialysate calcium concentrations have been reported to be associated with a higher incidence of ventricular arrhythmias (Nishimura et al. 1992). The goal should be to keep the pre-dialysis serum calcium between 2.25 and 2.45 mmol/L and the postdialysis calcium below 2.75 mmol/L. Mild hypercalcemia in this range appears to be fairly well tolerated as long as the serum phosphorus is not excessively high. Patients with low serum albumin have a decrease in the bound fraction of calcium and need to have an adjustment made. Typically, the goal serum calcium should be reduced by 1 mg/dl for every gram that the serum albumin is below 3.5 mg/dL.

d) Magnesium

The usual concentration of magnesium in the dialysate is 0.5 to 0.75 mmol/L and is only rarely manipulated. In an attempt to minimize the development of hypercalcemia associated with the use of calcium-containing phosphate binders and vitamin D, there has been interest in using magnesium-containing compounds as a phosphate binder (Speigel 2007). The use of oral magnesium requires the use of a low magnesium dialysate concentration so as to avoid the development of hypermagnesemia.

e) Chloride

The concentration of chloride in dialysate depends on the contents of chemicals such as sodium chloride, potassium chloride, magnesium chloride, and calcium chloride. Dialysate chloride ranges from 98–124 mmol/L (Curtis et al. 2008). Normal plasma chloride levels are 98–111 mmol/L.

f) Glucose

Glucose may be added to dialysate to prevent loss of serum glucose and to reduce catabolism (muscle breakdown). Adding glucose calories can help patients who are diabetic or malnourished. Dialysate glucose levels may range from 0–2 g/L (0-11mmol/L). The glucose in dialysate can be two to three times higher than in normal blood (0.7–1.05 g/L) (Curtis et al. 2008). This means that dialysate with glucose has an osmotic (water-pulling) effect that aids ultrafiltration.

g) Bicarbonate

Bicarbonate is a buffer—a substance that tends to maintain a constant pH in a solution, even if an acid or base is added (Curtis et al. 2008). Bicarbonate dialysate usage went from essential nonexistence in the middle 1970s to 22% in 1986 and 72% in 1989 (Alter et al. 1991; Van Stone, 1994). Bicarbonate is added to dialysate to help maintain patients' pH. Bicarbonate is used by the body to neutralize acids that are formed when cells metabolize proteins and other foods used for fuel (Curtis et al. 2008). The optimal level of dialysate base concentration varies on a patient to patient basis. The majority of dialysis units dialyze all of their patients with a single base concentration, usually in the range of 35 mEq/L (Van Stone, 1994). Using high bicarbonate dialysate may improve nutrition, bone metabolism, and hemodynamic stability (Graham et al. 1997). With regard to hemodynamics, increasing the bicarbonate concentration to 32 mmol/L is associated with a reduced incidence of both symptomatic and asymptomatic hypotension when compared to a bath bicarbonate concentration of 26 mmol/L (Gabutti et al. 2003).

h) Phosphorus

Although the vast majority of chronic hemodialysis patients have trouble with hyperphosphatemia, a small number of patients have low serum phosphorus concentrations. This hypophosphatemia is further aggravated by hemodialysis using the typical phosphorus- free dialysate (Van Stone 1994). In a typical dialysis session, the rate of phosphorus removal is greatest during the initial stages of the procedure and then progressively declines to a low constant level toward the end of the treatment. This decline is due to the decrease in plasma concentration and the slow efflux of phosphorus from the intracellular space and/or mobilization from bone stores. Although dialysis membranes differ with respect to plasma clearance of phosphate, it is the slow transfer of phosphorus to the extracellular space due to its low intracorporeal mass transfer coefficient (MTC PO4 $\approx$ 35mL/min), where it becomes accessible for dialytic removal, which is the most important factor limiting phosphorus removal (Sam et al. 2006). There are only a few situations in which one might consider adding phosphorus to the dialysate.

Hypophosphatemia can be an occasional finding in the chronic dialysis patient who is malnourished, suffering from some chronic disease state and in patients treated by daily or long nocturnal hemodialysis sessions or in acute setting with continuous renal replacement therapies. In such patients, adding phosphorus to the dialysate may be an effective means to treat hypophosphatemia without having to use a parenteral route of administration. The phosphate must be added to the bicarbonate component of a dual proportioning system to avoid the precipitation of calcium phosphate that would result from addition to the calcium-containing acid concentrate. Another situation in which addition of phosphate to the dialysate may be useful is in the setting of an overdose. In a patient with normal renal function and a normal serum phosphate concentration, use of a phosphate-free dialysate will commonly result in hypophosphatemia. In most circumstances, the hypophosphatemia is of short duration and is of little clinical consequence. However, some intoxications may increase the risk for complications of hypophosphatemia such that addition of phosphate to the dialysate may be warranted. Finally, hypophosphatemia has been noted in patients treated with prolonged daily nocturnal hemodialysis (Pierratos et al. 1998). In this setting, adding phosphate to the dialysate may prove useful as a means to normalize the serum phosphate concentration.

3.2.2.3 Components of the Dialysate Circuit

The major components of the dialysate circuit (see Fig. 3.18) are:
- a) Heating and Deaeration
- b) Proportioning
- c) Monitoring
- d) UF
- e) Disinfection

a) Heating and Deaeration

The purified water is heated to physiologic temperatures (35°C–38°C). This function is monitored downstream by the dialysate temperature control monitor in the dialysate circuit. Deaeration is accomplished by applying a negative pressure (300 to 600 mmHg below atmospheric) to the heated water to remove its air content. Alternatively, deaeration may be accomplished by heating the water to 85°C followed by cooling before proportioning system (Misra 2005). Air in the dialysate can impair flow in the dialyzer and cause the malfunctioning of blood leak and conductivity monitors.

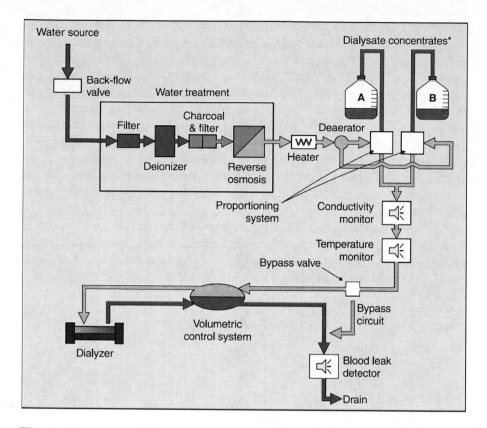

Fig. 3.18 Dialysate circuit. Adapted from From Ahmad S (2009) Manual of Clinical Dialysis. 2nd Ed. Springer: Springer-Verlag GmbH Berlin/Heidelberg, with permission.

b) Dialysate proportioning machine

In a proportioning system, dialysate is made by mixing fresh concentrate with fixed amounts of treated water. The mixing is controlled by the internal mechanical and hydraulic design of the delivery system. The proportioning system ratio depends on the type of dialysate concentrate used and the type of fluid delivery system (Curtis et al. 2008). The exact amount of water and concentrate is set by the center's policies and procedures. Failure to use the correct machine setting or to use the correct concentrates with a given machine can lead to patient injury. There are different types of proportioning systems based on whether dialysate, water, or both are metered. The two basic types of proportioning systems are fixed-ratio mixing and servo-controlled mixing (Pittard 2008).

- **Fixed-ratio mixing**: In the fixed-ratio proportioning systems, cylinders of known volumes are used to proportion dialysate concentrate and treated water in exact amounts, and a series of valves control the cyclic filling and emptying of each cylinder. All available fixed-ratio systems incorporate an electrical conductivity sensor to monitor the mixture and to initiate action (e.g., bypass, alarms) if the conductivity of the dialysate is not within preset limits.
- **Servo-controlled mechanisms** use a control sensor to monitor the conductivity of the dialysate and regulate the flow of the dialysate concentrate within the specified conductivity limits. Flow can be regulated using variable-speed pumps, variable-orifice valves, or other mechanisms. Like fixed-ratio systems, servo systems also employ a second conductivity sensor to monitor the mixture and to initiate action (e.g., bypass, alarms) if conductivity is not within specified limits.

Thus, while fixed-ratio proportioners will mix specific volumes of concentrate and treated water, servo-controlled proportioning systems will attempt to deliver as much or as little concentrate as required to satisfy the conductivity sensor.

c) Monitoring of the dialysate circuit

For safety, several monitors and detectors are used in the dialysate circuit:

i) Conductivity monitor

The dialysate proportioning system checks the total electrolyte level in dialysate by testing conductivity (how much electricity the fluid will conduct). The conductivity of pure water is zero and that of the dialysate depends mainly on the amount of sodium in it. While there are many electrolytes in the dialysate, sodium is the major component. Different amount of potassium or calcium hardly make any noticeable change. Conductivity is checked by placing a pair of electrodes in the dialysate. Voltage is applied to the electrodes, and the current is measured. The measurement gives the estimated total ion concentration of the dialysate (see Fig. 3.19). A sensor cell may be used instead of the electrodes. Most hemodialysis delivery systems have two or more independent conductivity monitors with separate sensors and monitoring circuits. One sensor measures the mixture of the first concentrate (most often acid) with water. The other sensor measures the final dialysate after the second concentrate is added (Curtis et al. 2008). Some machines use conductivity sensors to make the dialysate itself. These have a second set of sensors to check the mixtures, apart from the ones that control the mixing. This multiple monitoring system, called redundant monitoring, is used so two sensors would have to fail before a patient could be harmed (Pittard 2008). The units of conductivity are millisiemens per centimeter. The normal range is 12 to 16 mS/cm; high and low alarm settings should be within ±5% of the sensitivity settings. Because this monitor essentially checks the electrolyte concentrations in the final dialysate, any malfunction that is accompanied by abnormal proportioning can be potentially fatal for the patient. When the dialysate concentration moves outside the preset safe limits, it triggers a conductivity monitoring circuit. The circuit stops the flow of dialysate to the dialyzer and shunts it to the drain. This is called bypass. Bypass keeps the wrong dialysate from reaching the patient. The circuit also sets off audible and visual alarms to alert the staff (Curtis et al. 2008).

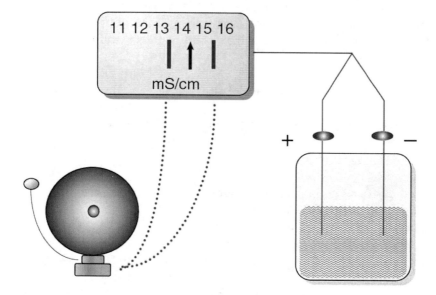

Fig. 3.19 Conductivity monitor. Adapted From Pittard JD (2008) Safety monitors in hemodialysis, in Nissenson AR, Fine RN (eds.): Handbook of Dialysis Therapy (4th ed). Philadelphia, PA, Hanley & Belfus, Inc., pp 188-223, with permission of Elsevier.

ii) pH sensors

The pH is a measure of the acidity or basicity of an aqueous solution. Solutions with a pH less than 7 are said to be acidic and solutions with a pH greater than 7 are basic or alkaline. The pH of a solution is based on the number of acid ions (hydronium ions) or alkali (base) ions (hydroxyl ions) it contains (Curtis et al. 2008). Some machines have a pH electrode as part of the proportioning system which puts out a small voltage when placed in a solution (Ahmad 2009). The voltage is read by a detection circuit that converts the signal into a pH value and displays it. Test strips coated with a chemical that changes color based on pH are another way to measure pH. These are generally used to prevent any mistake in connecting the appropriate concentrates to the machine (e.g., B concentrate not being connected) (Ahmad 2009).

iii) Temperature monitor

The temperature monitor is a heat sensor that monitors the dialysate temperature near the dialyzer; it should have a short feedback loop to the heater element to allow quick adjustment of the temperature. The accuracy of temperature control and monitoring should be ± 1 °C. The usual recommended temperature range is 35 to 42°C. Any increase in temperature beyond the set range triggers an alarm and dialysis is stopped. An alarm condition shall interrupt delivery of dialysate to the hemodialyzer, activate audible and visual alarms, and stop the blood flow in the extracorporeal circuit. The internal high limit should be set at no higher than 41°C. Normal red blood cells (RBCs) begin to hemolyze at 42°C. Overheated dialysate can cause hemolysis and even death (Fortner et al. 1970; Berkes et al. 1975). Cooling dialysate below 36.5°C has been recognized as an important factor contributing to hemodynamic stability of patients during hemodialysis. Many studies show that cool dialysate improves cardiovascular tolerance of hemodialysis and reduces hypotension episodes during hemodialysis (Yu et al. 1995; Ayoub and Finlayson 2004; Azar 2009). If low-temperature dialysate is used, the total dialysis time needs to be increased by about 8% for every 3°C below 37°C because that is the theoretical loss in diffusivity with temperature decrease. With dialysate temperatures below 37°C, patients will complain of being cold and some will actually shiver in an attempt to increase their core body temperature. An increase in cardiac irritability in patients with coronary vessel disease may be observed.

iv) Dialysate Pressure Monitor

Dialysate pressure is monitored similar to monitoring of pressure in the blood circuit. The pressure range is −400 to +350 mmHg with an accuracy ±10%; alarm limits are set at ±10% of the pressure setting. The dialysate pressure monitor monitors ultrafiltration pressures. It is a critical function of dialysis therapy that ensures accurate and safe fluid removal from the patient (Papadimitriou and Kulatilake 1969). One method of regulating the patient's ultrafiltration is by application of the Transmembrane pressure (TMP) (the pressure difference at the blood and dialysate outlets). TMP is adjusted to achieve the desired rate of UF, as low as 50 mL/hr. Newer machine models have ultrafiltration/volumetric control circuits. The dialysis personnel set the goal for the desired fluid removal, set the duration of dialysis, and activate the ultrafiltration control mode. The machine will automatically calculate and apply the required transmembrane pressure to achieve the desired ultrafiltration rate. Volumetric control systems have different design features. A common design uses balancing chambers to precisely measure fluid volume entering and leaving the dialyzer. These machines automatically adjust the TMP. Volumetric control systems use matched pumps, usually diaphragm pumps. The pumps are controlled by valves and are integrated after proportioning of dialysate. Valves located above and below the balancing chambers open and close to direct the flow of fresh and used dialysate. Fresh dialysate is pushed out to dialyzer, whereas used dialysate is pushed out to drain. The two chambers alternate functions, creating a constant flow of fresh dialysate. The system is a closed loop, with both chambers exactly balanced (Petitclerc et al. 1997). Air is removed from the used dialysate, in a separation chamber, to ensure accurate measurement.

v) Blood-Leak Detector

Blood leak sensors are placed on the dialysate outflow line to detect blood leakage and prevention of dialysate contamination by blood downstream of the dialyzer. These are usually flow-through photo-optical or blue frequency spectrum sensors (Ahmad 2009). This sensor functions by transmitting filtered or unfiltered light through a column of effluent dialysate that has exited the dialyzer (see Fig. 3.20). Leaks in the dialyzer membrane cause RBCs to leak into the dialysate, interrupting the light transmission. The machine response to a blood-leak alarm is to effect audible and visual alarms, stop the blood pump, and engage the venous line clamp. The sensitivity of monitor is 0.25 of 0.35 ml of blood per liter of dialysate. False blood-leak alarms can be caused by the presence of air bubbles in the path or by cloudy or dirty optical lenses.

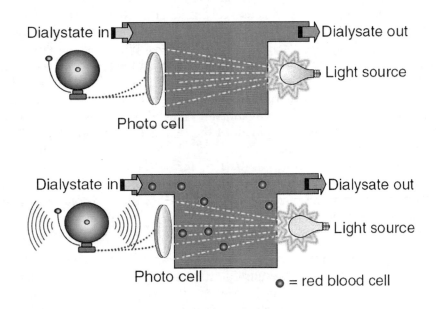

Fig. 3.20 Blood-leak detector. Adapted From Pittard JD (2008) Safety monitors in hemodialysis, in Nissenson AR, Fine RN (eds): Handbook of Dialysis Therapy (4th ed). Philadelphia, PA, Hanley & Belfus, Inc., pp 188-223, with permission of Elsevier.

vi) Dialysate Flow Monitor

The usual dialysate flow rate for conventional dialyzers is a minimum of 500 ml/minute. For high-efficiency and high-flux dialyzers, it is usually 700 to 800 ml/minute. Most machines have a continuous audible alarm for low incoming water pressure to the machine, dialysate pump failure, and obstruction in the flow path and power failure. Dialysis personnel must be diligent in monitoring this aspect. Dialysis personnel must monitor the dialysate effluent line to the drain to ensure that it is not obstructed and that it is properly placed in the drain. An obstruction can cause back-pressure into the dialysate compartment and may decrease the dialysate flow rate.

d) Ultrafiltration Control System

However, intradialytic hypotension remains the most frequent complication occurring in up to 33% of patients (Leunissen et al. 2000; Daugurdas 2001; Schreiber 2001). The causes of intradialytic hypotension are complex and multifactorial. The basic concept, however, is that hypotension during HD only occurs when the normal cardiovascular compensatory mechanisms cannot compensate for the inevitable blood volume reduction that occurs when a large volume of water is removed over a short period of time (Daugirdas 2001; Andrulli et al. 2002). Former studies shown that the first half of the hemodialysis treatment is much less hypotensive episodes in comparison with the second half of the treatment (Schmidt et al. 2001a; Wolkotte et al. 2002; Mancini et al. 2007). In conclusion, it was obviously more beneficial to ultrafilter in the first part of hemodialysis as much as the actual systolic blood pressure allows with the consequence of low ultrafiltration rates at the end of hemodialysis. Ultrafiltration control systems display the ultrafiltration rate or, alternatively, the ultrafiltration time, current volume removed, target ultrafiltration volume, and units of measure.

Ultrafiltration control systems have an automated or manual method of verifying the integrity of the ultrafiltration control or balancing system at the beginning of each dialysis session. Ultrafiltration is controlled by transmembrane pressure (TMP), which is the hydrostatic pressure difference between the blood and dialysate compartments. Older dialysis machines used pressure-controlled ultrafiltration, in which the dialysis personnel calculates the necessary TMP (based on the ultrafiltration coefficient (K_{UF}) of the dialyzer membrane and the desired amount of fluid removed), monitors the filtration, and readjusts the TMP as needed. Modern dialysis machines use a volumetric fluid balancing system. This type of system uses two chambers that fill and drain to control the volume of dialysate going to and coming from the dialyzer. This is known as *volumetric control* (Curtis et al. 2008). Volume-controlled ultrafiltration machines are mandatory for high flux dialyzers in order to prevent excessive fluid removal. Another type of machine uses sensors in the fluid path to and from the dialyzer to control and monitor the flow rate of the dialysate. This is known as *flow control* (Curtis et al. 2008). Testing of the ultrafiltration control system monitor shall be performed to determine accuracy deviations in the presence of a single fault in the control system. The monitor shall either automatically take appropriate control actions to minimize the risk of fluid removal error or clearly signal to the system operator to take appropriate actions to minimize fluid removal error.

i) Volumetric Control System

One of the main components of the volumetric control system is the balancing chambers as shown in Fig. 3.21 (Curtis et al. 2008). One chamber is filling with used dialysate, pushing fresh dialysate to the dialyzer. At the same time, the other chamber is filling with fresh dialysate, pushing the used dialysate to the drain. The balancing system uses matched pumps (usually diaphragm pumps) with appropriate valves to keep the dialysate inflow exactly equal to the dialysate outflow establishing a quasi closed loop. Two diaphragm pumps are used out of phase to establish matched continuous flow of dialysate and keep constant flow through the dialyzer. One pump moves the proportioned dialysate to the balance chambers. A second pump pulls dialysate from the dialyzer and pushes it to the balance chambers (Curtis et al. 2008). A separate ultrafiltration pump is used to remove fluid from the quasi closed loop at the desired rate of ultrafiltration. As the pump removes fluid from the closed loop, the same amount is replaced, moving across the dialyzer membrane into the loop. This allows the machine to precisely remove the right amount of fluid from the patient. Other important component in the system is pressure sensors to control pump speeds, prevent over pressurization, calculate TMP, and detect leaks within the system. Air separation chambers are used to remove any air coming out of the dialyzer. Any air in the system could result in incorrect fluid removal. The air separation chamber maintains a level of fluid while releasing air out the top that is routed to the drain (Curtis et al. 2008). The accuracy of this system depends on two factors, accurate calibration of the pump that removes fluid from the loop and accurate balancing of the dialysate inflow and outflow rates. Accurate balancing requires appropriate design of the matched pumps and appropriate sealing of the valves used in the balancing system.

ii) Ultrafiltration Flow Control System

This system uses flow sensors in the dialysate inflow and outflow streams to measure the rate of dialysate flow to and from the dialyzer as shown in Fig. 3.22 (Curtis et al. 2008). Inlet and outlet flow pumps are set so the flow measured at the inlet and outlet flow sensors is equal (Curtis et al. 2008). The difference between the outflow and inflow rates is the ultrafiltration rate. This difference is measured by digital circuitry and is fed

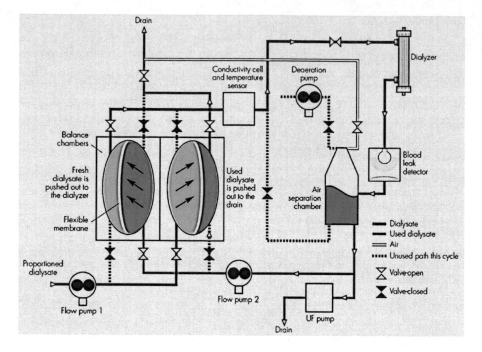

Fig. 3.21 Volumetric UF control system. Published with permission of Amgen Inc. http://www.amgen.com

back to the transmembrane pressure circuit. The transmembrane pressure is varied until the measured and desired rates of ultrafiltration become equal. Post-dialyzer ultrafiltration pump is used to removes fluid at the ultrafiltration rate calculated by the machine. The speed of the pump is equal to the ultrafiltration rate. Two types of sensors have been used. One is a bearingless rotor. The speed of rotation of the bearingless rotor is measured with an optical beam and correlated to flow rate. The other is an electromagnetic flow sensor which measures the voltage developed by the flow of a conductive solution through a magnetic field. The voltage developed is proportional to the flow rate. In electromagnetic type, the inflow and outflow streams flow through a differential flow sensor so that the difference is directly measured rather than measuring each flow rate and then calculating the difference. Both electromagnetic and bearingless rotor systems can develop microbiological contaminants and biofilm that can disrupt the flow sensor paths. Therefore, the flow sensors must be kept clean and free of bacterial slim and particulates for accurate determination of flow rates. Frequent bleaching and routine sterilization procedures of flow sensors are recommended to ensure cleanliness and reliable operation.

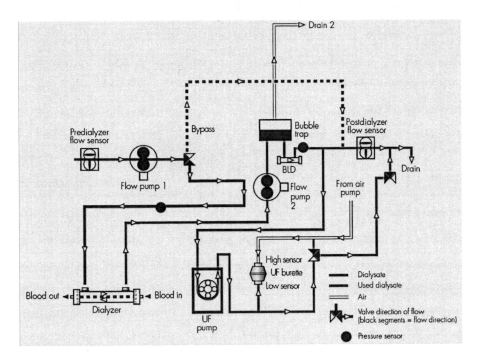

Fig. 3.22 Flow control UF system. Published with permission of Amgen Inc. http://www.amgen.com

e) Cleaning, Disinfection and Rinsing

All fluid pathways in the dialysis machines must be routinely rinsed, cleaned, and disinfected (Lonnemann 2000; Pontoriero et al. 2003). The rinsing and cleaning process keeps the internal environment of the dialysis machine clean and free of cellular debris or deposits for proper operation. The disinfection eliminates bacterial growth and prevents the risk of pyrogen reactions. The same is true for all dialysate concentrate containers that store dialysate concentrate. Some machines also incorporate a hot water disinfection cycle that can be used as an alternative to chemical disinfection. All current machines require the operator to develop a separate cleaning and disinfection protocol for this section of line to prevent its colonization with biofilm that will continually reinfect the fluid pathways of the machine (Koda and Mineshima 2009). Inadequate disinfection can be due to lack of frequent disinfection, too low concentrations of cold chemical disinfectants, and inadequate contact time of the disinfectant. Therefore, single-patient hemodialysis machines must be disinfected at least daily with a chemical disinfectant such as sodium hypochlorite (bleach). The machine should be in bypass mode during disinfection with dialysate alarms overridden. The blood pump power supply should be off as a safeguard. The effluent dialysate line should be isolated from the drain with an air break to prevent backflow and siphoning.

3.2.3 Hemodialyzer

A dialyzer is an artificial kidney designed to provide controllable transfer of solutes and water across a semi permeable membrane separating flowing blood and dialysate streams. Nowadays, only hollow fiber dialyzer are produced by manufacturers and available commercially on the market.

Hollow fiber dialyzer is the only one type used in which approximately 10000 to 20000 thin fibers run longitudinally through the dialyzer as shown in Fig. 3.23. The fibers have an inner diameter of about 0.2 mm, and a length of 150 mm. This dialyzer makes use of countercurrent flow.

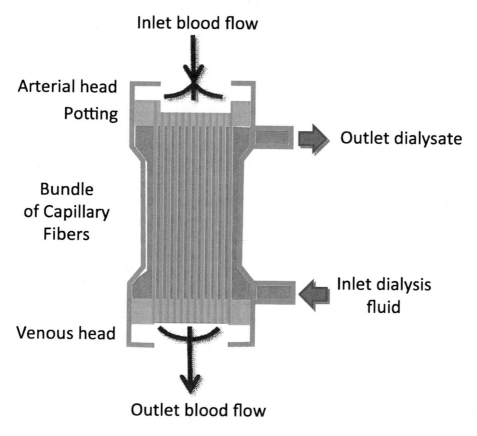

Fig. 3.23 Hollow Fiber Capillary Dialyzer

Countercurrent flow is where the blood is flowing in one direction and the dialysate is flowing in the opposite direction to maintain optimized concentration gradients over the whole length of the dialyzer.

3.2.3.1 Structure of Hollow Fiber Dialyzer

The major components of hollow fiber dialyzer are:

- **Blood ports**: These ports carry blood into (arterial port) and out of (venous port) the dialyzer.
- **Headers:** From the blood port, the blood enters the arterial header space and dialyzed blood enters the venous header space (before entering the venous blood port). Geometry and shape of the header determine the blood distribution within the housing and so influence the priming procedure and thrombosis risk. Therefore, headers were and still are a target for improvement. Removable headers are appreciated in clinics that practice dialyzer reuse because they allow a visible inspection of possibly clotted header regions and fibre ends. Manufacturers prefer sealed caps because high sterility can be guaranteed better with this design.
- **Potting material:** The function of potting material is to ensure a tight seal between the blood and dialysate compartments and to hold the hollow fibers. Potting material belongs to the polyurethane group which has a high affinity for ethylene oxide (ETO) (Lee et al. 1985). The effective surface area is increases when less potting compound is used. Further, the isocyanates used in the potting polymerization are haptens and can theoretically cause immunoallergic reactions. However, this has not been documented clinically.
- **Capillary fibers:** There are about 10,000 to 20000 capillary fibers made of permeable material are contained within the dialyzer casing. The blood flows inside the fibers and the dialysate flows on the outside. The quality of the fibre bundle construction is of considerable importance for performance of a dialyzer. The geometric characteristics of a hollow fiber determine the membrane surface area, which can be varied by changing the number of fibers, their length, and their internal diameter. Fiber diameter of currently available dialyzers varies between 190 and 220 μm, and fiber length between 185 and 270 mm. If fiber length is increased at constant fiber diameter and surface area, the number of fibers can be reduced. The increased length would increase shear rate and

magnify the pressure drop. These two events have opposing effects: the increment in shear rate increases ultrafiltration in the first part of the dialyzer; the fluid volume control of the dialysis machine implies backfiltration of dialysis fluid to maintain a neutral volumetric balance in the second part of the dialyzer. This design has been developed by dialyzer manufacturers to enhance convective clearances (internal hemodiafiltration) and increase middle molecule removal. Now, it should be stressed that such dialyzers require the use of ultrapure dialysis fluid to prevent passage of microbial derived products. A substantial pressure drop occurs if fiber diameter is decreased. This would limit the ultrafiltration profile along the fiber and may also make it more difficult to rinse the dialyzer free of blood at the end of the procedure. A critical minimal inner fiber diameter has been considered to be 180 μm. Fiber wall thickness varies depending on the nature of the membrane. Fibre bundle size and swelling of the membrane determine the priming blood volume. This is an important parameter in the choice of dialyzer for patients with low blood volume, especially children.

- **Housing Material**: Blood comes into contact with the housing material in the inlet and outlet end caps. These are made of amorphous, rigid, and transparent material usually consisting of polystyrene, polycarbonates, or other polymers. They may be gas permeable, and polycarbonates can adsorb ethylene oxide (ETO) during the sterilization process. The coloring of the end caps for inlet/outlet differentiation while useful in practical terms, interferes with the ability to examine the device at the end of the procedure for determination of the proportion of clotted fibers.
- **Dialysate ports:** There are two ports on the side of the casing, one for dialysate inflow and one for the outflow.

3.2.3.2 Hemodialysis Membrane Materials

The type of membrane material used may determine the performance and biocompatibility of the membrane. There are two broad categories of membranes based on the material used for manufacturing: cellulose-based membranes and synthetic membranes (Korwer et al. 2004; Strathmann and Gohl 1990).

1. Cellulose membranes are further classified into unsubstituted cellulose and substituted cellulose membranes

- Unsubstituted cellulose membranes: Cellulose is obtained from processed cotton. Regenerated cellulose and cuprammonium cellulose (or Cuprophan®) are examples of unsubstituted cellulose membranes. There are a large number of free hydroxyl groups on the cellulose polymer that are thought to be responsible for the activation of serum complement proteins and, consequently, the activation of leukocytes, causing bioincompatibility (Schiffl et al. 1998).

- Substituted cellulose membranes: Chemical substitution of free hydroxyl groups on cellulose membranes results in modified cellulose membranes. The free hydroxyl groups can be substituted by acetate (cellulose acetate, cellulose diacetate, or cellulose triacetate), tertiary amino compounds (Hemophan®), and other moieties.

2. Synthetic membranes are manufactured from non-cellulose synthetic polymers and have decreased tensile strength compared to cellulose membranes. Synthetic membranes in clinical use include polyacrylonitrile (PAN), polyamide, polymethylmethacrylate (PMMA), polysulfone, polycarbonate, or a combination of some of these polymers (Lysaght 1995). Synthetic membranes are more biocompatible than unsubstituted cellulose membranes, by most criteria used in the nephrology literature (Lang et al. 1995; Gastaldello et al. 2000; Takemoto et al. 2011).

3. Bioactive synthetic membranes are now available and may offer interesting perspectives in chronic kidney disease patients. Until now, two types of membranes have been developed: the first is a polysulfone vitamin E-coated membrane (Vitabrane, Asahi) associated with a reduction of oxidative stress markers in dialysis patient (Calò et al. 2011); the second is polyacrylonitrile heparingrafted membrane (HeprAN, AN69ST, Evodial, Hospal, Gambro) reducing anticoagulant needs during dialysis session (Lavaud et al. 2003).

In practice, hemodialyzer fitted with synthetic membranes (low flux and high flux) are increasingly used in renal replacement therapy worldwide. Nanotechnology has significantly improved performances and reduced size of dialyzers. Cellulosic unsubstituted membranes are not anymore produced by manufacturers. Bioactive membranes need to prove their superiority in clinic.

3.2.3.3 Biocompatibility of the Membrane

Bioincompatibility refers to a variety of biologic responses that occur in a patient induced by contact of blood with the dialysis membrane and other components of the extracorporeal circuit (Schiffl et al. 1998). The biologic responses elicited by blood–membrane interactions include activation of the complement system, coagulation system, other plasma proteins and lipids, platelets, leukocytes, and erythrocytes. It is generally accepted that unsubstituted cellulose is the most bioincompatible membrane, while modified cellulose membranes and synthetic membranes are considered to be more biocompatible (Lang et al. 1995; Gastaldello et al. 2000). Epidemiologic studies suggest that the chronic use of unmodified low-flux membranes is associated with higher patient mortality, compared to synthetic membranes and modified cellulose membranes. However, many of the dialyzers that are made of more biocompatible membranes are also high flux dialyzers (Takemoto et al. 2011). Therefore, it is difficult to distinguish the effects of biocompatibility from flux on clinical outcomes in these studies. Microbiological purity of dialysis fluid represents an additive factor of confusion in the biocompatibility evaluation. It has been clearly shown that the regular use of ultrapure dialysis fluid prevents microinflammation, reduces morbidity and has several additional benefits in dialysis patients (Masakane 2006).

3.3 Advanced Options for Hemodialysis Machines

3.3.1 Online Clearance Monitor (OCM)

Online Clearance is performed at different times during a dialysis treatment to determine the average effective urea clearance (K) which describes the blood flow volume that is completely cleared, the dialysis dose (Kt/V) and the plasma sodium concentration during dialysis (Kuhlmann et al. 2001). The measurement can be started by the operator on the dialysis machine or can be programmed in the SETUP to start with each dialysis treatment providing a continuous quality control tool.

Sodium dialysance is a convenient method to provide instantaneous online determination of small-solute clearance for the assessment of dialyzer performance (Song et al. 2005). By changing the water proportioning ratio, a momentary change is initiated in the sodium concentration of the dialysis solution flowing into the dialyzer. A conductivity sensor then estimates the overall change in sodium of the dialysis solution leaving the dialyzer. Ionic dialysance is a parameter calculated from the dialysate conductivity at the dialyser inlet and outlet for two steps of inlet dialysate conductivity, and tends to become an on-line monitoring parameter of the effective dialysis dose actually delivered to the patient (Petitclerc 2005; Moret et al. 2006; Pozzoni et al. 2007; Ridel et al. 2007; Maduell et al. 2008). The on-line measurement during hemodialysis of ionic dialysance provides an estimation of urea clearance with a good and already proven correlation (Mercadal et al. 1998, 2002; Moret et al. 2007; Rosa Diez et al. 2010)

3.3.2 Ultrafiltration Profiling

In order to maintain the intravascular volume and prevent symptomatic hypotension, the ultrafiltration rate and dialysate sodium concentration can be changed automatically during dialysis session according to individual patient needs. Most methods attempt to increase the UF rate when the patient is most apt to be able to refill quickly. Some UF profiles are designed to allow periods of high ultrafiltration rate followed with periods of low ultrafiltration (Donauer et al. 2000; Oliver et al. 2001; Stiller et al. 2001; Zhou et al. 2006). The technique of altering ultrafiltration rates during hemodialysis is known as ultrafiltration modeling or ultrafiltration profiling. If dialysate sodium and ultrafiltration profiling are combined, high fluid removal can be matched to high dialysate sodium concentration early in dialysis. The ability to match the appropriate ultrafiltration profile to the rest of the dialysis prescription (i.e. sodium variation) is necessary to optimize fluid removal without morbid events. This technique should effectively reduce intradialytic symptoms but has undergone limited critical evaluation (Levin and Goldstein, 1996; Oliver et al. 2001; Schmidt et al. 2001b).

3.3.3 Blood Temperature Monitor (BTM)

The blood temperature monitor (BTM) is a module built to fit current Fresenius hemodialysis machines (Fresenius Medical Care, Deutschland G.m.b.H., Bad Homburg, Germany). The BTM can be operated in two control modes (Schneditz et al. 2003). The T-control mode requires the prescription of an hourly change in body temperature. The body temperature of the patient corresponds only by the approximation with arterial fistula temperature measured by the BTM. The blood entering the extracorporeal circuit consists of the blood flowing from the heart to the fistula (from the most part) and the recirculation blood. So the arterial blood temperature is determined by the body temperature as well as by temperature of the venous blood flowing back to the patient. Therefore, body temperature can only measured by the BTM if the scope of recirculation is known or both fistula temperatures don't differ much. To control for a constant body temperature throughout a treatment one would have to prescribe a temperature change rate of $\pm 0.00°C/h$. The BTM controller uses the error signal between desired and actual change in temperature to actuate a bounded change in dialysate temperature (T_{dia}) which changes the temperature of the venous (T_{ven}) blood returning to the patient thereby changing the extracorporeal heat flow (Schneditz et al. 2003). The BTM can also be operated in an E-control mode, which controls for the rate of thermal energy removal (dE/dt, in kJ/h). The thermal energy balance control runs as follows: after the control function has been started, the BTM calculates the venous blood temperature by which the thermal energy flow rate prescribed by the used is achieved. Then the dialysate temperature is changed in such a way that the desired venous blood temperature is reached. In regular intervals the BTM examines whether there is a deviation of the actual mean energy flow rate from the setting value. If this is the case, the dialysate temperature is changed so that the deviation is compensated for within a short period of time. With this method the desired thermal energy flow can be met with great accuracy (Schneditz et al. 2003).

3.3.4 Blood Pressure Monitor (BPM)

It is desirable to have periodic blood pressure data and blood pressure parameter monitoring during a hemodialysis treatment (Sankaranarayanan et al. 2004). The wide variations in blood pressure in the course of a hemodialysis treatment are due primarily to reductions in the circulating volume (ultrafiltration) and the physiological reactions to these reductions. It is, therefore, extremely helpful to have a record of the blood pressure variations over the time of each dialysis treatment. It is also helpful to have a system whereby alarm limits can be set, based on the patient's case history, so that safeguards can be provided that are meaningful for each individual patient. The BPM is a fully automatic non-invasive blood pressure instrument utilizing the oscillometric principle. Upon start of a measurement, the pump of the Blood Pressure Monitor builds up a pre-selectable pressure in the cuff. Controlled by the central unit, the relief valve then deflates the cuff pressure. The low-amplitude pulse-depending changes in the cuff pressure are superimposed on the cuff pressure generated by the-pump and controlled by the relief valve. As soon as the amplitude of the superimposed pulse waves starts to increase, the current cuff pressure corresponds to the systolic blood pressure. The moment when the amplitude of the oscillations no longer descends, identifies the diastolic pressure. That cuff pressure, at which the pulse-dependent oscillations reach their peak value, corresponds to the arithmetic mean value (MAP) of the course of the blood pressure. Since each pulsation causes an oscillation in the cuff, the pulse frequency can be determined at the end of measurement, based on the number of pulse waves and the measurement time. With an artefact-free single measurement, the duration of a measurement takes approximately 30 seconds. To be able to determine the measured values, it is necessary to select an inflation pressure which exceeds the patient's systolic blood pressure by approximately 50 mmHg. Otherwise, it would not be possible to determine the point when the oscillation amplitude starts to rise. After the Blood Pressure Monitor has been turned on, an initial inflation pressure of 180 mmHg is preset, since there are no measurement results yet. For all further measurements, the Blood Pressure Monitor adds 50 mmHg to the previous systolic blood pressure value and sets the inflation pressure accordingly. The control system of the Blood Pressure Monitor prevents a cuff pressure of more than 300 mmHg developing during inflation of the cuff or during the measurement. Should this control system fail, an additional independent monitoring system causes an immediate pressure deflation if the cuff pressure exceeds a value of 320 mmHg.

3.3.5 Blood Volume Monitor (BVM)

The continuous surveillance of BV changes may allow for the identification of the critical individual level of hypovolemia in hypotension-prone patients with vascular refilling instability (Mancini et al. 1995; Ronco et al. 2000). The major application of the BVM is the blood volume dependent control of the ultrafiltration. The BVM includes an algorithm which continuously adapts the ultrafiltration rate depending on the measured relative blood volume (RBV) to prevent symptomatic hypotension caused by excessive removal of fluid (Santoro et al. 1998, 2003). This module is described in detail in Chapters 20 and 21. The presently used methods for measuring the blood volume determine the relative blood volume (RBV). This is the ratio of the current blood volume to the blood volume at the start of the dialysis. This means that relative changes of the blood volume are measured; however, this parameter contains the essential information required to prevent blood volume induced drops in blood pressure. RBV monitors differ in the type of blood constituent that they use as a marker. The basis of all methods for measuring RBV is that certain constituents of blood (cells, hemoglobin, plasma protein, total protein) remain confined to the vascular system, whereas the plasma water can pass both the capillary membrane and the dialyzer membrane. Therefore, the blood volume change can be determined from the concentration change of these blood constituents. However, each of these known measuring methods has considerable interference effects which must be compensated by the respective measuring instrument in order to achieve a reliable measuring result. In addition to measuring and controlling the blood volume, the BVM allows to evaluate the hematocrit (HCT), the hemoglobin (HB), the blood water content (BWC) and the blood temperature (T).

3.3.6 Powder Bicarbonate (BiCart (Bi))

By installing the BiCart option on the unit, the clinician has the ability to perform bicarbonate dialysis with on-line production of liquid bicarbonate concentrate instead of connecting bicarbonate jugs. Two components are necessary in order to perform BiCart. Column is a polypropylene column containing sodium bicarbonate powder. This column, fitted into a special holder that is attached to the unit, enables the on-line production of bicarbonate concentrate. BiCart and bicarbonate jug dialysis are not to be performed simultaneously. When the BiCart column is attached to this special holder, fluid will be drawn from the unit through the BiCart column, thus producing a saturated solution of sodium bicarbonate. The bicarbonate proportioning system in the unit proportions this solution. The unit mixes the solution with heated water and acid concentrate to produce a bicarbonate dialysis fluid.

3.3.7 Ultrapure Dialysis Fluid

Apart from the toxic hazards linked to water contaminants (e.g. aluminum), the microbiologic contamination of water has been recognized as a major component of the bioincompatibility hemodialysis network contributing to the complications of the long-term dialysis patients. Water purity has become over the last decade a major concern for nephrologists and microbiologists.

Purified water is the basic form that is suitable for conventional hemodialysis modalities. It is easily obtained from a purification system made of a pretreatment (softener, activated carbon, downsizing microfilters) and a reverse osmosis (RO) module implemented in series in order to prevent mainly aluminum intoxication but also the accumulation of various water pollutants. Microbiological contamination of the delivered water should comply with the recommendations of the European Pharmacopoeia (Bacterial Count < 100 CFU/mL and Endotoxin content < 0.25 EU/mL). Highly purified water (ultrapure water) may be used alternatively on regular basis with all kinds of hemodialysis modalities. Ultrapure water is highly desirable with high flux hemodialysis modalities and is mandatory for dialysis modalities using on-line production of substitution fluid (on-line HF or HDF). Several technical options and arrangements may be used to reach this goal. The most common water treatment system option is based on pretreatment and a double stage RO module in series with a water distribution pipe system allowing a permanent recirculation of purified water. Microbiological contamination of the delivered water should comply with more stringent recommendations (Bacterial Count < 100 CFU/L and Endotoxin content <0.03 EU/mL).

To preserve the microbiologic purity of the dialysis fluid delivered to the patient, very stringent hygienic rules should be adopted for the hemodialysis machine. To ensure delivery of ultrapure dialysis fluid, it is necessary to sterilize the dialysis fluid by a cold sterilization process based on ultrafiltration. Today, quality and purity of the water and the dialysis fluid are of major concern in renal replacement therapy (Canaud et al. 2000).

3.3.8 Single Needle Dialysis (SND)

Another available option is the SN option, which controls on and off cycling of the blood pump to provide blood flow through a single needle access (Y-flow single lumen needle or catheter). In the arterial phase of the cycle, the arterial line is unclamped, the venous line is clamped, and the blood is pumped from the patient until the pressure reaches the venous pressure high trip point. When the pressure reaches this point, the machine switches to the venous phase. The blood pump is stopped, the venous line is unclamped, the arterial line is clamped, and as blood is returned to the patient, the venous pressure falls until it reaches the venous pressure low trip point and the cycle begins again. In addition, the SN set has two pumping chambers (predialyzer and postdialyzer) that provide stroke volume capacity without needing level adjustments.

Single-needle dialysis (SND) was first described by Twiss in 1964 using a time-activated mechanism with a pump and a double clamp for the alternating flow of blood along a caval catheter (Twiss 1964). Kopp et al used blood line clamps controlled by a pressure-activated system (Kopp et al. 1972). Hilderson et al also used a pressure-activated system that controlled a double-headed blood pump (Hilderson et al. 1975). The benefit of SN dialysis is minimizing the risk of fistula damage and destruction since the vascular access will be punctured only once in each session. This will also help to reduce patient discomfort. SN dialysis can also be used in acute dialysis where blood access is made through a single venous catheter. By improving the design of the machine, proper selection of the cannula and setting the

maximum blood flow rate to achieve the target dialysis dose and avoid hemolysis would be of the utmost importance and give the best results to the
patients. Its use, however, has not been widespread and has been confined to
specific situations (Vanholder et al. 1989). The low general utilization of this
technique may be attributed to a number of factors that include poor understanding of the technique, the reluctance to adopt new techniques when established alternatives exist, and the widely held belief that SN dialysis is inferior to conventional double-needle dialysis (DND). This is principally due
to the presence of recirculation, as well as the inability to obtain clinically
acceptable blood flow rates with single-pump tidal flow systems. The potential hazards when using a SN system are principally the same as those for
conventional DN extracorporeal circuits. As example of theses hazards are
the blood loss to the environment due to a rupture or disconnection of the
bloodline, and air embolism (Trakarnvanich et al. 2006). Hemolysis from
shear stresses between red cells and the needle or catheter also is an important complication especially if flows are too high (Polaschegg 2002). The
technique should always be used with needles with a large enough diameter.
The chances for back filtration with the fluctuations in pressure are also
more substantial than for two needle dialysis. Therefore SN dialysis should
be done with ultrapure dialysate. The main disadvantage of SND is the restricted clearance, the maximum achievable clearance in SND is less than
half the maximum DND clearance due to the alternating-flow scheme and
the increased recirculation. Many efforts have been made to improve the efficiency of SND systems, within the inherent limitations just mentioned.
Maximizing the average blood flow is an obvious requirement. Some de-
signers of SND systems have assumed that achieving a continuous or even
constant flow would increase clearance. In consequence, SND is not appropriate for high-efficiency dialysis but is well suited for applications in which
high clearances are not required. Another potential disadvantage is the increased technical complexity of SN systems (and therefore increased treatment cost). The additional technical components required to perform an
SND largely depend on the specific setup used.

3.4 CONCLUSION

Hemodialysis relies on the principles of solute diffusion and convection
across a semipermeable membrane. Movement of metabolic waste
products takes place down a concentration gradient from the circulation into the dialysate. The rate of diffusive transport increases in response to
several factors, including the magnitude of the concentration gradient, the
membrane surface area, and the mass transfer coefficient of the membrane.
The latter is a function of the porosity and thickness of the membrane, the

size of the solute molecule, and the conditions of flow on the two sides of the membrane. According to the laws of diffusion, the larger the molecule, the slower its rate of transfer across the membrane. A small molecule such as urea (60 Da) undergoes substantial clearance, whereas a larger molecule such as creatinine (113 Da) is cleared less efficiently. In addition to diffusive clearance (hemodialysis), movement of toxic materials such as urea from the circulation into the dialysate may occur as a result of convection (hemofiltration and hemodiafiltration). Convective clearance occurs because of solvent drag with solutes getting swept along with water across the semipermeable dialysis membrane and is linearly correlated to volume of substitution and sieving capacity of the membrane. The hemodialysis (HD) machine pumps the dialysate as well as the patient's blood through a dialyzer. The blood and dialysate are separated from each other by a semipermeable membrane. The operational system of the hemodialysis machine represents a complex array of detectors, controllers, monitors, and safety devices to ensure patient safety during the hemodialysis procedure.

REFERENCES

Ahmad, S.: Manual of Clinical Dialysis, 2nd edn. Springer, Heidelberg (2009)

Alter, M.J., Favero, M.S., Moyer, L.A., Bland, L.A.: National surveillance of dialysis-associated diseases in the United States. Trans. ASAIO 37, 97–109 (1991) (1989)

Andrulli, S., Colzani, S., Mascia, F., et al.: The role of blood volume reduction in the genesis of intradialytic hypotension. Am. J. Kidney Dis. 40(6), 1244–1254 (2002)

Azar, A.T.: Effect of dialysate temperature on hemodynamic stability among hemodialysis patients. Saudi J. Kidney Dis. Transpl. 20(4), 596–603 (2009)

Ayoub, A., Finlayson, M.: Effect of cool temperature dialysate on the quality and patients' perception of haemodialysis. Nephrol. Dial. Transplant. 19(1), 190–194 (2004)

Argiles, A., Kerr, P.G., Canaud, B., et al.: Calcium kinetics and the longterm effects of lowering dialysate calcium concentration. Kidney Int. 43(3), 630–640 (1993)

Berkes, S.L., Kahn, S.I., Chazan, J.A., Garella, S.: Prolonged hemolysis from overheated dialysate. Ann. Intern. Med. 83(3), 363–364 (1975)

Byrne, J.H., Schultz, S.G.: An introduction to membrane transport and bioelectricity: foundation of general physiology and electrochemical signalling, 2nd edn. Raven Press, New York (1994)

Calò, L.A., Naso, A., D'Angelo, A., et al.: Molecular biology-based assessment of vitamin E-coated dialyzer effects onoxidative stress, inflammation, and vascular remodeling. Artif. Organs 35(2), E33–
   E39 (2011)
Canaud, B.: Adequacy target in hemodialysis. J. Nephrol. 17(8), S77–S86
   (2004)
Canaud, B., Bosc, J.Y., Leray, H., Morena, M., Stec, F.: Microbiologic
   purity of dialysate: rationale and technical aspects. Blood Pu-
   rif. 18(3), 200–213 (2000)
Clark, W.R., Macias, W.L., Molitoris, B.A., et al.: Membrane adsorption
   of β-2-microglobulin: equilibrium and kinetic characterization.
   Kidney Int. 46(4), 1140–1146 (1994)
Clark, W.R., Hamburger, R.J., Lysaght, M.J.: Effect Of Membrane Com-
   position And Structure On Solute Removal And Biocompatibility
   In Hemodialysis. Kidney Int. 56(6), 2005–2015 (1999)
Curtis, J., Delaney, K., O'Kane, P., et al.: Hemodialysis Devices. In: Core
   Curriculum for the Dialysis Technician: A Comprehensive Review
   of Hemodialysis, 4th edn., pp. 88–112. Medical Education Institute,
   Inc., Madison (2008)
Davenport, A.: What are the anticoagulation options for intermittent he-
   modialysis? Nat. Rev. Nephrol. (2011),
doi:10.1038/nrneph.2011.88; [Epub ahead of print]
Daugirdas, J.T.: Pathophysiology of dialysis hypotension: An update. Am.
   J. Kidney Dis. 38(suppl. 4), S11–S17 (2001)
Daugirdas, J.T., Blake, P.G., Ing, T.S. (eds.): Handbook of Dialysis, 4th
   edn. Lippincott, Williams and Wilkins, Philadelphia (2007)
Deppisch, R., Gohl, H., Smeby, L.: Microdomain structure of polymeric
   surfaces—potential for improving blood treatment procedures.
   Nephrol. Dial. Transplant. 13(6), 1354–1359 (1998)
Donauer, J., Kolblin, D., Bek, M., et al.: Ultrafiltration profiling and measurement of relative blood volume as strategies to reduce hemodialysis-related side effects. Am. J. Kidney Dis. 36(1), 115–123 (2000)
Evenepoel, P., Dejagere, T., Verhamme, P., et al.: Heparin-coated polyacrylonitrile membrane versus regional citrate anticoagulation: a
   prospective randomizedstudy of 2 anticoagulation strategies in patients at risk of bleeding. Am. J. Kidney Dis. 49(5), 642–649 (2007)
Flanigan, M.J.: Role of sodium in hemodialysis. Kidney Int. 76, S72-S78
   (2000)
Fortner, R.W., Nowakowski, A., Carter, C.B., et al.: Death due to overheated dialysate during dialysis. Ann. Intern. Med. 73(3), 443–444
   (1970)

Fresenius Medical Care, Deutschland G.m.b.H., Bad Homburg, Germany, `http://www.fmc-ag.com/`

Gabutti, L., Ferrari, N., Giudici, G., et al.: Unexpected haemodynamic instability associated with standard bicarbonate haemodialysis. Nephrol. Dial. Transplant. 18(11), 2369–2376 (2003)

Gastaldello, K., Melot, C., Kahn, R.J., et al.: Comparison of cellulose diacetate and polysulfone membranes in the outcome of acute renal failure. A prospective randomized study. Nephrol. Dial. Transplant. 15(2), 224–230 (2000)

Graham, K.A., Reaich, D., Channon, S.M., et al.: Correction of acidosis in hemodialysis decreases whole-body protein degradation. J. Am. Soc. Nephrol. 8(4), 632–637 (1997)

Gutch, C.F., Stoner, M.H., Corea, A.L.: Review of hemodialysis for nurses and dialysis personnel, 6th edn. Mosby, St. Louis (1999)

Hilderson, J., Ringoir, S., van Waeleghem, J.P., et al.: Short dialysis with a polyacrylonitrilmembrane (RP 6) without the use of a closed recirculating dialyzate delivery system. Clin. Nephrol. 4(1), 18–22 (1975)

Henrich, W.L.: Principles and Practice of Dialysis, 4th edn. Lippin-cott Williams & Wilkins, USA (2009)

Koda, Y., Mineshima, M.: Advances and advantages in recent central dialysis fluid delivery system. Blood Purif. 27(suppl. 1), 23–27 (2009)

Kopp, K.F., Gutch, C.F., Kolff, W.J.: Single needle dialysis. Trans. Am./ Soc. Artif. Intern. Organs 18, 75–81 (1972)

Korwer, U., Schorn, E.B., Grassmann, A., Vienken, J.: Understanding Membranes and Dialyzers. PABST Science Publishers, Lengerich (2004)

Kuhlmann, U., Goldau, R., Samadi, N., et al.: Accuracy and safety of on-line clearance monitoring based on conductivity variation. Nephrol. Dial. Transplant. 16(5), 1053–1058 (2001)

Kyriazis, J., Glotsos, J., Bilirakis, L., et al.: Dialysate calcium profiling during hemodialysis: use and clinical implications. Kidney Int. 61(1), 276–287 (2002)

Lang, S., Küchle, C., Fricke, H., Schiffl, H.: Biocompatible intermittent hemodialysis. New Horiz. 3(4), 680–687 (1995)

Lavaud, S., Canivet, E., Wuillai, A., et al.: Optimal anticoagulation strategy in haemodialysis with heparin-coated polyacrylonitrile membrane. Nephrol. Dial. Transplant. 18(10), 2097–2104 (2003)

Lee, F.F., Dorning, C.J., Leonard, E.F.: Urethanes as ethylene oxide reservoirs in hollow-fiber Dialyzers. Trans. Am. Soc. Artif. Intern. Organs 31, 526–533 (1985)

Leunissen, K.M., Kooman, J.P., van der Sande, F.M., van Kuijk, W.H.: Hypotension and ultrafiltration physiology in dialysis. Blood Purif. 18(4), 251–254 (2000)

Levin, A., Goldstein, M.B.: The benefits and side effects of ramped hypertonic sodium dialysis. J. Am. Soc. Nephrol. 7(2), 242–246 (1996)

Lonnemann, G.: The quality of dialysate: an integrated approach. Kidney Int. Suppl. 76, S112–S119 (2000)

Lysaght, M.J.: Evolution of hemodialysis membranes. Contrib. Nephrol. 113, 1–10 (1995)

Maduell, F., Vera, M., Arias, M., et al.: Influence of the ionic dialysance monitor on Kt measurement in hemodialysis. Am. J. Kidney Dis. 52(1), 85–92 (2008)

Mancini, E., Mambelli, E., Irpinia, M., et al.: Prevention of dialysis hypotension episodes using fuzzy logic control system. Nephrol. Dial. Transplant. 22(5), 1420–1427 (2007)

Mancini, E., Santoro, A., Spongano, M., et al.: Effects of automatic blood volume control over intradialytic hemodynamic stability. Int. J. Artif. Organs 18(9), 495–498 (1995)

Masakane, I.: Review: Clinical usefulness of ultrapure dialysate - recent evidence and perspectives. Ther. Apher. Dial. 10(4), 348–354 (2006)

Meira, F.S., Poli de Figueiredo, C.E., Figueiredo, A.E.: Influence of sodium profile in preventing complications during hemodialysis. Hemodial. Int. 11(suppl. 3), S29–S32 (2007)

Mercadal, L., Petitclerc, T., Jaudon, M.C., et al.: Is ionic dialysance a valid parameter for quantification of dialysis efficiency? Artif. Organs 22(12), 1005–1009 (1998)

Mercadal, L., Du Montcel, S.T., Jaudon, M.C., et al.: Ionic dialysance vs urea clearance in the absence of cardiopulmonary recirculation. Nephrol. Dial. Transplant. 17(1), 106–111 (2002)

Misra, M.: The basics of hemodialysis equipment. Hemodial. Int. 9(1), 30–36 (2005)

Mitchell, S.: Estimated dry weight (EDW): aiming for accuracy. Nephrol. Nurs. J. 29(5), 421–428 (2002)

Monge, M., Shahapuni, I., Oprisiu, R., et al.: Reappraisal of 2003 NKF-K/DOQI guidelines for management of hyperparathyroidism in chronic kidney disease patients. Nat. Clin. Pract. Nephrol. 2(6), 326–336 (2006)

Moret, K., Beerenhout, C.H., van den Wall Bake, A.W., et al.: Ionic dialysance and the assessment of Kt/V: the influence of different estimates of V on method agreement. Nephrol. Dial. Transplant. 22(8), 2276–2282 (2007)

Moret, K., Aalten, J., van den Wall Bake, W., et al.: The effect of sodium profiling and feedback technologies on plasma conductivity and ionic mass balance: a study in hypotension-prone dialysis patients. Nephrol. Dial. Transplant. 21(1), 138–144 (2006)

Morti, S.M., Zydney, A.: Protein-membrane interactions during hemodialysis. Effects on solute. transport. ASAIO J. 44(4), 319–326 (1998)

NKF-K/DOQI, Clinical practice guidelines for Bone Metabolism and Disease in Chronic Kidney Disease. Am. J. Kidney Dis. 42(4 suppl. 3), S1–S201 (2003)

Nishimura, M., Nakanishi, T., Yasui, A., et al.: Serum calcium increases the incidence of arrhythmias during acetate hemodialysis. Am. J. Kidney Dis. 19(2), 149–155 (1992)

Oliver, M.J., Edwards, L.J., Churchill, D.N.: Impact of sodium and ultrafiltration profiling on hemodialysis-related symptoms. J. Am. Soc. Nephrol. 12(1), 151–156 (2001)

Ouseph, R., Hutchison, C.A., Ward, R.A.: Differences in solute removal by two high-flux membranes of nominally similar synthetic polymers. Nephrol. Dial. Transplant. 23(5), 1704–1712 (2008)

Palmer, B.F.: Dialysate Composition in Hemodialysis and Peritoneal Dialysis. In: Schrier, R.W. (ed.) Atlas of Diseases of the Kidney, ch. 2, vol. 5. Current Medicine, Inc., Philadelphia (1999)

Papadimitriou, M., Kulatilake, A.E.: Relationship between weight loss and venous and dialysate pressures during chronic intermittent haemodialysis. Med. Biol. Eng. 7(3), 317–320 (1969)

Petitclerc, T., Goux, N., Hamani1, A., Béné, B., Jacobs, C.: Biofeed-back technique through the variations of the dialysate sodium concentration. Nefrologia XVII(1), 50–55 (1997)

Petitclerc, T.: Do dialysate conductivity measurements provide conductivity clearance or ionic dialysance? Kidney Int. 70(10), 1682–1686 (2005)

Pierratos, A., Ouwendyk, M., Francoeur, R., et al.: Nocturnal hemodialysis: three-year experience. J. Am. Soc. Nephrol. 9(5), 859–868 (1998)

Pittard, J.D.: Safety monitors in hemodialysis. In: Nissenson, A.R., Fine, R.N. (eds.) Handbook of Dialysis Therapy, 4th edn., Philadelphia, PA, USA, pp. 188–223 (2008)

Polaschegg, H.: Single-needle dialysis. In: Nissenson, A.R., Fine, R.N. (eds.) Handbook of Dialysis Therapy, 4th edn., Philadelphia, PA, USA, pp. 168–187 (2008)

Pontoriero, G., Pozzoni, P., Andrulli, S., Locatelli, F.: The quality of dialysis water. Nephrol. Dial. Transplant. 18(suppl. 7), vii21–vii25 (2003)

Pozzoni, P., Di Filippo, S., Pontoriero, G., Locatelli, F.: Effectiveness of sodium and conductivity kinetic models in predicting end-dialysis plasma water sodium concentration: preliminary results of a single center experience. Hemodial. Int. 11(2), 169–177 (2007)

Reddy, B., Cheung, A.K.H.: Hemodialysis. In: Lai, K.N. (ed.) A Practical Manual of Renal Medicine, 1st edn. World Scientific, Singapore (2009)

Ridel, C., Osman, D., Mercadal, L., et al.: Ionic dialysance: a new valid parameter for quantification of dialysis efficiency in acute renal failure? Intensive Care Med. 33(3), 460–465 (2007)

Ronco, C., Crepaldi, C., Brendolan, A., et al.: Evolution of synthetic membranes for blood purification: the case of the Polyflux family. Nephrol. Dial. Transplant. 18(suppl. 7), vii10–vii20 (2003)

Ronco, C., Brendolan, A., Crepaldi, C., et al.: Blood and dialysate flow distributions in hollow-fiber hemodialyzers analyzed by computerized helical scanning technique. J. Am. Soc. Nephrol. 13(1), S53–S61 (2002)

Ronco, C., Brendolan, A., Milan, M., et al.: Impact of biofeedback-induced cardiovascular stability on hemodialysis tolerance and efficiency. Kidney Int. 58(2), 800–808 (2000)

Rosa Diez, G.J., Bevione, P., Crucelegui, M.S., et al.: Measuring Kt by ionic dialysance is a useful tool for assessing dialysis dose in critical patients. Nefrologia 30(2), 227–231 (2010)

Sankaranarayanan, N., Santos, S.F., Peixoto, A.J.: Blood pressure measurement in dialysis patients. Adv. Chronic. Kidney Dis. 11(2), 134–142 (2004)

Santoro, A., Mambelli, E., Canova, C., et al.: Biofeedback in dialysis. J. Nephrol. 16(suppl. 7), S48–S56 (2003)

Santoro, A., Mancini, E., Paolini, F., et al.: Blood volume regulation during hemodialysis. Am. J. Kidney Dis. 32(5), 739–748 (1998)

Sargent, J., Gotch, F.: Principles and biophysics of dialysis. In: Jacobs, C., Kjellstrand, C., Koch, K., Winchester, J. (eds.) Replacement of Renal Function by Dialysis, 4th edn., pp. 34–102. Kluwer Academic Publishers, Dortdrecht (1996)

Salai, P.B.: Hemodialysis. In: Molzahn, A.E., Butera, E. (eds.) Contemporary Nephrology Nursing: Principles and Practice, pp. 527–574. American Nephrology Nurses' Association, Pitman (2007)

Sam, R., Vaseemuddin, M., Leong, W.H., et al.: Composition and clini-cal use of hemodialysates. Hemodial. Int. 10(1), 15–28 (2006)

Schmidt, R., Roeher, O., Hickstein, H., Korth, S.: Prevention of haemo-dialysis-induced hypotension by biofeedback control of ultrafiltration and infusion. Nephrol. Dial. Transplant. 16(3), 595–603 (2001a)

Schmidt, R., Roeher, O., Hickstein, H., Korth, S.: Blood Pressure Guided Profiling of Ultrafiltration during Hemodialysis. Saudi J. Kidney Dis. Transpl. 12(3), 337–344 (2001b)

Schneditz, D., Ronco, C., Levin, N.: Temperature control by the blood temperature monitor. Semin. Dial. 16(6), 477–482 (2003)

Schreiber Jr., M.J.: Clinical, dilemmas in dialysis: Managing the hypotensive patient. Setting the stage. Am. J. Kidney Dis. 38(suppl. 4), S1–S10 (2001)

Schiffl, H., Lang, S.M., Haider, M.: Bioincompatibility of dialyzer membranes may have a negative impact on outcome of acute renal failure, independent of the dose of dialysis delivered: a retrospective multicenter analysis. ASAIO J. 44(5), M418–M422 (1998)

Song, J.H., Park, G.H., Lee, S.Y., et al.: Effect of sodium balance and the combination of ultrafiltration profile during sodium profiling hemodialysis on the maintenance of the quality of dialysis and sodium and fluid balances. J. Am. Soc. Nephrol. 16(1), 237–246 (2005)

Speigel, D.M.: The role of magnesium binders in chronic kidney dis-ease. Semin. Dial. 20(4), 333–336 (2007)

Stiller, S., Bonnie-Schorn, E., Grassmann, A., et al.: A critical review of sodium profiling for hemodialysis. Semin. Dial. 14(5), 337–347 (2001)

Strathmann, H., Gohl, H.: Membranes for blood purification: state of the art and new developments. Contrib. Nephrol. 78, 119–141 (1990)

Takemoto, Y., Naganuma, T., Yoshimura, R.: Biocompatibility of the dialysis membrane. Contrib. Nephrol. 168, 139–145 (2011)

Trakarnvanich, T., Chirananthavat, T., Ariyakulnimit, S., et al.: The efficacy of single-needle versus double-needle hemodialysis in chronic renal failure. J. Med. Assoc. Thai. 89(suppl. 2), S196–S206 (2006)

Twiss, E.E.: One-cannula haemodialysis. Lancet 284(7369), 1106 (1964)

Yu, A., Ing, T., Zabineh, R., Daugirdas, J.: Effect of dialysate on central hemodynamic and urea kinetics. Kidney Int. 48(1), 237–243 (1995)

Van der Sande, F.M., Cheriex, E.C., van Kuijk, W.H., Leunissen, K.M.: Effect of dialysate calcium concentrations on intradialytic blood pressure course in cardiac-compromised patients. Am. J. Kidney Dis. 32(1), 125–131 (1998)

Vanholder, R., De Smet, R., Glorieux, G., et al.: Review on uremic tox-
    ins: classification, concentration, and interindividual variability.
    Kidney Int. 63(5), 1934–1943 (2003)
Vanholder, R., Hoenich, N., Ringoir, S.: Single needle hemodialysis. In:
    Maher, J.F. (ed.) Replacement of Renal Function by Dialysis, 3rd
    edn., pp. 382–399. Kluwer Academic Publisher, Boston (1989)
Van Stone, J.C.: Individualization of the dialysate prescription in chronic
    hemodialysis. Dial. Transplant. 23(11), 624–635 (1994)
Ward, R.A., Leypoldt, J.K., Clark, W.R., et al.: What clinically important
    advances in understanding and improving dialyzer function have
    occurred recently? Semin. Dial. 14(3), 160–174 (2001)
Wolkotte, C., Hassell, D.R., Moret, K., et al.: Blood volume control by
    biofeedback and dialysis-induced symptomatology. A short term
    clinical study. Nephron. 92(3), 605–609 (2002)
Zhou, Y.L., Liu, H.L., Duan, X.F., et al.: Impact of sodium and ultrafiltra-
    tion profiling on haemodialysis related hypotension. Nephrol. Dial.
    Transplant. 21(11), 3231–3237 (2006)

ESSAY QUESTIONS

1. What are the main different mechanisms of solute removal in di-
    alysis?
2. Define Diffusion Transport Process.
3. List the main factors affecting diffusion process
4. Define the osmosis Process.
5. Compare between the main two mechanisms of ultrafiltration in
    hemodialysis
6. List the major parts of blood tubing
7. What are the major components of the dialysate circuit?
8. List several monitors and detectors used in the dialysate circuit
9. Compare between the main different types of dialyzers.
10. List the major components of hollow fiber dialyzer.

MULTIPLE CHOICE QUESTIONS

Choose the best answer

1. The dominant solute removal mechanism in hemodialysis is…
    A. Diffusion
    B. Convection
    C. Adsorption

2. Membrane with more pores allows…
   A. Lower diffusion
   B. No diffusion
   C. Faster diffusion

3. Hemodialysis relies on diffusion to remove unwanted water from the body.
   A. True
   B. False

4. The measurement of membrane porosity is known as ….
   A. Ultrafiltration coefficient
   B. Permeability coefficient
   C. Sieving coefficient (SC)

5. Osmotic pressure is associated with … membranes.
   A. Semipermeable
   B. Permeable
   C. Permeable and semipermeable

6. The total capacity of the dialyzer for ultrafiltration is given by …
   A. Ultrafiltration coefficient
   B. Sieving coefficient (SC)
   C. Permeability coefficient

7. The maximum rate of solute transfer occurs initially when the concentration gradient is …
   A. Minimum
   B. Maximum
   A) Not-change

8. The primary driving force for ultrafiltration is …
   A. Hydrostatic pressure difference across the membrane
   B. Oncotic pressure difference across the membrane
   C. A and B

9. In hemodialysis units, transmembrane pressure controls …
   A. Dialysate flow rate
   B. Blood flow rate
   C. Ultrafiltration rate

10. Stable dialysis patients generally can tolerate an ultrafiltration rate of less than …
   A. 25 ml/kg/hr
   B. 20 ml/kg/hr
   C. 10 ml/kg/hr
   D. 50 ml/kg/hr

11. The major component of single-patient hemodialysis systems …
   A. Extracorporeal blood-delivery circuit
   B. Dialysate delivery system
   C. Dialyzer
   D. A, B, C

12. The hemodialysis system should detect the presence of a series of microbubbles that occur within a short period of time and total more than …
   A. 2.5 mL/30 s.
   B. 0.5 mL/30 s.
   C. 3.5 mL/30 s.
   D. 1.5 mL/30 s.

13. Arterial pressure monitors normally read ….
   A. Positive pressures
   B. Negative pressures
   C. Zero- pressures

14. Venous pressure monitors normally read …
   A. Zero- pressures
   B. Negative pressures
   C. Positive pressures

15. Deaeration is accomplished by applying … pressure to the heated water to remove its air content.
   A. Negative pressures
   B. Positive pressures
   C. Zero- pressures

16. The dialysate proportioning system checks the total electrolyte level in dialysate by testing …
   A. Dialysate Temperature
   B. Dialysate Conductivity
   C. Dialysate Pressure

17. The dialysate pressure range is …
   A. 200 to -350 mmHg
   B. -300 to 400 mmHg
   C. -350 to 450 mmHg
   D. -400 to +350 mmHg

18. Normal red blood cells (RBCs) begin to hemolyze at …
   A. 40°C
   B. 45°C
   C. 42°C
   D. 39°C

19. If low-temperature dialysate is used, the total dialysis time needs to be increased by about … for every 3°C below 37°C
   A. 8%
   B. 5%
   C. 10%
   D. 3%

20. Dialysate temperature control must keep the temperature within the following tolerance from the set value:
   A. ±0.3°
   B. ±0.5°
   C. ±1°
   D. ±3°

21. The usual concentration of magnesium in the dialysate is …
   A. 0.1 to 0.5 mmol/L
   B. 1 to 3.0 mmol/L
   C. 0.5 to 0.75 mmol/L
   D. 0.2 to 7.0 mmol/L

22. The normal range of dialysate conductivity is …
   A. 10 to 12 mS/cm
   B. 12 to 16 mS/cm
   C. 15 to 18 mS/cm
   D. 11 to 14 mS/cm

23. Artificial kidney filter membrane is … to urea.
   A. Permeable
   B. Semipermeable
   C. Impermeable

24. There are about ... capillary fibers made of permeable material are contained within the dialyzer casing.
  A. 20000 to 25000
  B. 20000 to 30000
  C. 25000 to 30000
  D. 10000 to 20000

25. Countercurrent transport is preferred in hemodialysis because ...
  A. It maintains a concentration difference along the whole path
  B. It maintains a very high concentration difference that decays along the path.
  C. It generates an additional diffusion energy

26. Arterial blood line is ...
  A. The line leading from the patient to the hemodialysis machine
  B. The line returning to the patient from the hemodialysis machine
  C. Any of the above as long as it is connected to an artery in the patient

27. A problem in the dialyzer can be detected using ...
  A. Air bubble detector
  B. Conductivity monitor
  C. Blood leak detector

28. Blood pump is usually selected to be .... type.
  A. Proportioning pump
  B. Peristaltic pump
  C. Flow pump

29. Air bubble detection in hemodialysis is usually done using ...
  A. Ultrasonic sensors
  B. Optical sensors
  C. Electromagnetic sensors
  D. A and B

30. In case of a person weighting e.g. 70 kg, the energy flow rates prescribed should be between ...
  A. 0 kJ/h and −70 kJ/h
  B. 20 kJ/h and −50 kJ/h
  C. 10 kJ/h and −60 kJ/h
  D. 5 kJ/h and −80 kJ/h

Chapter 4

Intensive Hemodialysis in the Clinic and At Home

Philip A. McFarlane, MD, PhD, FRCP (C)

CHAPTER OUTLINES

- Introduction
- The home nocturnal hemodialysis technique
- Rationale for intensive hemodialysis
- Determining adequacy of dialysis in people undergoing intensive hemodialysis
- Economic considerations
- Selecting patients for intensive hemodialysis
- Candidacy and home hemodialysis requirements
- Performing intensive hemodialysis safely
- Conclusions

CHAPTER OBJECTIVES

- To understand the rationale for why conventional hemodialysis may be inadequate in some patients.
- To understand the differing impacts of changes to machine settings or treatment time on small and larger solute clearance.
- To review how a conventional hemodialysis prescription can be intensified by increased the duration or frequency or both of treatments.
- To review some controversies regarding how to measure dialysis adequacy in intensively dialyzed patients.
- To review the existing literature of randomized and non-randomized studies of intensive dialysis, and understand where these techniques may improve patient outcomes.
- To discuss issues that makes hemodialysis in the home environment unique.
- To highlight some issues that need to be addressed in order to ensure that intensive hemodialysis is performed safely.

KEY TERMS

- Conventional hemodialysis
- Hemodialysis adequacy
- Home hemodialysis
- Intensive hemodialysis
- Kt/V
- Nocturnal hemodialysis
- Short daily hemodialysis
- Urea kinetics
- Ultrafiltration
- Urea clearance
- Urea rebound

A.T. Azar (Ed.): Modelling and Control of Dialysis Systems, SCI 404, pp. 167–233.
springerlink.com © Springer-Verlag Berlin Heidelberg 2013

ABSTRACT

Conventional hemodialysis delivered so that urea clearance is adequate may still leave patients with uremic symptoms and unsatisfactory outcomes. This has led to an interest in more intensive hemodialysis prescriptions, where dialysis is delivered with increased frequency, duration or both. Intensive hemodialysis can improve the clearance of small solutes such as urea, but can have an even larger effect on the clearance of larger solutes that tend to maintain a large gradient between blood and dialysate through the course of a dialysis treatment. This is particularly true of intensive hemodialysis prescriptions that increase the total weekly hours of dialysis. Studies have suggested a number of potential benefits for intensive hemodialysis, including improved nutritional markers, easier control of anemia, lower hospitalization rates, improvements in sleep apnea and restoration of fertility. The most convincing studies suggest that intensive hemodialysis can improve blood pressure control, reduce left ventricular mass, improve health related quality of life and improve mineral metabolism parameters. Intensive hemodialysis techniques appear to be associated with an increase in access related difficulties. These techniques also appear to be cost-effective, especially when delivered in the home. The evidence of benefit of intensive hemodialysis generated in these studies has generated increasing interest in these modalities, and their prevalence has been increasing. However, it remains unclear whether intensive hemodialysis should be offered to a wide range of patients with end-stage renal disease, or instead targeted to patients whose clinical status is poor on conventional hemodialysis.

4.1 INTRODUCTION

The purpose of this chapter is not to present an exhaustive review of studies of intensive hemodialysis, but rather to introduce readers to some of the important concepts and principles that form the rationale behind intensive hemodialysis, and provide examples from the literature where intensive hemodialysis has been used successfully. This chapter will also review the five randomized trials comparing intensive to conventional hemodialysis. As intensive hemodialysis is often performed in the home setting, this chapter will also discuss issues unique to performing dialysis safely and successfully in the home setting.

4.1.1 Defining the Terms: Methods of Intensifying a Hemodialysis Prescription

Later, this chapter will explore in detail the benefits and pitfalls of the various intensive hemodialysis prescriptions, but it is important to first outline the different ways that hemodialysis can be prescribed, and the terms associated with these prescriptions (see Fig. 4.1).

Treatment time	3 dialysis sessions per week	4 or more dialysis sessions per week
< 3 to 3.5 hours	Sub-conventional	In-centre or home short daily
3 - 4.5 hours	Conventional	Quotidian conventional
Longer than 4.5 hours	In-centre or home nocturnal, long intermittent (Tassin)	Quotidian home nocturnal

Fig. 4.1 Types of hemodialysis based on treatment duration and frequency

First, most of the discussion in this chapter will focus on comparing various intensive prescriptions to "conventional" hemodialysis. These comparisons are made difficult by the fact that what constitutes conventional hemodialysis varies between countries. For example, From 1996-2001, hemodialysis treatment times were significantly shorter in the United States than in Europe or Japan (US 211 ± 32 minutes, versus 232 ± 41 in Europe and 244 ± 32 in Japan, p<0.05) (Saran et al. 2006). Conventional hemodialysis will refer to dialysis performed three times per week, for about 3.5 hours in the United States and for about 4 hours in most other jurisdictions.

One method for increasing dialysis intensity is to increase the frequency of dialysis treatments to four or more treatments per week. When treatment frequency is increased but the treatment time is kept the same as a conventional schedule, the prescription is referred to as either *daily conventional* or *augmented conventional hemodialysis*. In general, this is an uncommon modality, and typically treatment times are reduced as treatment frequency increases. Short daily hemodialysis refers to treatments that are performed more than three times per week, for less than 3.5 hours per session. Most short daily hemodialysis schedules are performed about five times per week, with treatment times between 2.5 and 3.5 hours. For example, in a randomized controlled study of short daily hemodialysis, treatment frequency in the frequent dialysis group was 5.17 ± 1.11 sessions per week, with an average duration of 154 ± 25 minutes (FHN Trial Group et al. 2010). Other than treatment duration, patients performing short daily hemodialysis usually do not significantly alter the parameters of treatment from a conventional prescription, and so blood and dialysate pump speeds are maintained in a range typical for a conventional prescription.

Another method of increasing dialysis intensity is to lengthen the treatment time. While maintaining the conventional three-times per week frequency, treatment times have been increased in some patients to 6 to 8 hours. With one notable exception, it has been hard to operationalize long treatments during the day in the in-centre environment, and so these long treatments are usually done overnight, and are known as *home nocturnal* or *in-centre nocturnal hemodialysis* depending on location. The notable exception is the group in Tassin, France, which have been using long thrice-weekly treatments as their standard approach to in-centre hemodialysis for over 40 years (Charra et al. 2003). Extended duration treatments performed three times per week in the in-centre unit are referred to as long intermittent hemodialysis. The prescription in this type of dialysis can vary. In some programs, long treatments are executed with blood and dialysate pump speeds similar to conventional treatments (i.e. blood pump speeds 300-450 mL/min, dialysate flows 500-800 mL/min). However, many programs that offer nocturnal hemodialysis perform these treatments with slower pump speeds (i.e. blood pump speeds 250-350 mL/min, dialysate flows 300-500 mL/min or on in some cases even lower) (Bugeja et al. 2009). Lower pump speeds can be justified for a number of reasons. First, a prescription calling for "maximum" blood pump speeds that attempt to deliver the highest possible blood delivery from a dialysis access will tend to produce venous or arterial over-pressure alarms. These can be particularly disruptive and undesirable when a patient is sleeping.

Second, dialysate concentrate containers can run out if high dialysate flows are prescribed for long treatments. This can be mitigated by connecting two dialysate acid and bicarbonate concentrate containers to the machine through a "Y" type connector. While Y-connecting containers can allow for high dialysate flows for long treatments, it adds to the cost of the treatment, as well as making the setup of the machine longer and less convenient. Finally, as will be discussed later, improved clearance of important toxins from the blood in long dialysis treatments does not require high blood or dialysate flows.

The strategies of increasing both dialysis time and frequency can be combined such that dialysis is performed at least every other day for at least 4.5 hours per treatment. Frequent treatments of long duration are hard to operationalize in the in-centre setting, as so such schedules are usually restricted to the home. Originally, the term daily home nocturnal hemodialysis was used to describe this form of dialysis. However, the combination of the terms "daily" and "nocturnal" proved confusing, and so the term quotidian home nocturnal hemodialysis is preferred. Most programs offering quotidian nocturnal hemodialysis use prescriptions with reduced blood and dialysate pumps speeds as described above, although early reports of quotidian nocturnal home hemodialysis used blood pumps speeds between 250-300 mL/min and dialysate flows of only 100 mL/min (Pierratos et al. 1998). Quotidian home nocturnal hemodialysis treatments usually lasting six to eight hours and are usually scheduled five or more times per week.

It is important to note that the categorizations described above overlap, and a patient may meet the common descriptions of more than one intensive dialysis modality at a time. In addition, many home patients will perform a hybrid of these modalities, mixing nocturnal, short daily and conventional treatments depending on medical and social factors. In general, the recommendations for access remain the same for patients receiving intensive hemodialysis as for other hemodialysis patients. Central venous catheters, arteriovenous grafts and fistulae have all been used in intensive hemodialysis (Pierratos 1999). Fistulae can be accessed by standard ladder techniques or by using the buttonhole approach (Twardowski and Kubara 1979). While buttonhole cannulation is usually done as a self-cannulization strategy, it can be operationalized in the in-centre unit as well (Marticorena et al. 2009).

4.1.2 A History of Hemodialysis In-Centre and in the Home

The ability to perform hemodialysis to prevent certain death from renal failure is a recent invention. However, the roots of dialysis stretch back thousands of years. The Romans made extensive use of baths, where hot water and steam were used to cleanse the body. This was purported to have many health benefits and was the first example of dialysis. As they sweated, the skin would act as a semipermeable membrane, allowing salts, waters and toxins to escape the body. In the early 20th century, this technique was the only available treatment for renal failure, and was used up to the 1950's.

In the late 1800s, the Scottish chemist Thomas Graham developed a system for generating hydrous metal oxide colloids by separating them from crystalloids through the use of a membrane, and in the process coined the term "dialysis". His publication "On Osmotic Force" in 1854 outlined his experience with dialysis using a sheep's bladder as the membrane (Graham 1854). In 1889 the Englishman B.W. Richardson, brought Graham's technique to the organic world by describing the selective diffusion properties of colloidon membranes (a film that prevents diffusion of substances with a molecular weight greater than 5000 kDaltons) using animal blood.

The first artificial kidney was developed by Dr. John J. Abel at the Johns Hopkins University in Baltimore.(Abel al. 1990). Their work was first published in 1913, describing their experience in "vividiffusion" of animals. While subsequent research would lead to dialysis membranes that little resemble the current technology, the Abel dialyzer is immediately recognizable by those familiar with today's membranes. Blood would enter and exit the long cylinder at one end, traveling through parallel tubes made of colloidon. Dialysate would flow through the opposite end, bathing the outside of the colloidon tubes. Abel's work recognized some of the fundamental difficulties in the dialysis process. Unless steps are taken, blood will clot outside of the body. Abel used hirudin, an anticoagulant made from the crushed heads of leeches, which lacked the safety and predictability needed for clinical use. The efficiency of dialysis depends on the amount of blood that is exposed to dialysate, a function of the surface area of the membrane. Abel's use of parallel tubes increased the surface area for diffusion within the confines of his cylinder.

In 1915 George Haas of the University Clinic of Giessen, Germany improved upon Abel's designs and performed the first dialysis experiments in humans (Benedum 1986). In tackling the issue of membrane surface area, he connected many dialyzers in parallel. This uncovered other essential issues in dialysis. The volume of the connected dialyzers was large, and the patient's blood pressure was insufficient to pump blood through the system. Haas dealt with this by attaching a blood pump to his system, a standard feature in today's hemodialysis machines. The large dialyzer volume required a significant amount of blood to prime the system, a problem that Haas did not solve. Heparin was vastly superior to hirudin for clinical use at that time, and in 1928 Haas was the first to use heparin as an anticoagulant for dialysis. While previous experiments performed "fractional" dialysis, where small quantities of blood were removed, cleansed and then returned, Haas' design allowed for a continuous flow of blood through the system.

By the 1940's advances in dialysis were continuing, but experiments had been limited to the removal of non-toxic substances. Around this time Willem Kolff from the University of Groningen in the Netherlands suggested that dialysis could be used clinically to remove the toxins from the blood of patients with renal failure (Kolff et al. 1997). Kolff designed his own dialysis machine using sausage skin (made from cellulose acetate) as the membrane. Blood would be passed through 40 meters of sausage skin that Kolff wrapped around a cylindrical drum. The drum was lowered into a tub containing 100 litres of dialysate and then rotated, which would move blood through the sausage casing, diffusing toxins into the dialysate bath along the way. Kolff placed sugar in the dialysate to provide an osmotic pull for ultrafiltration. The process took six hours to perform, but many more hours to prepare. He performed his technique on 15 people before his first patient survived. Sophia Schafstadt, a 68-year-old housewife who developed renal failure secondary to hepatorenal syndrome, became the first human to be successfully treated for renal failure with dialysis. Kolff's techniques were useful for acute renal failure, where it was expected that the patient's own kidney function would return shortly and dialysis was necessary only for a very brief period.

During this time dialysis was spreading from Europe to Canada. In 1940, Gordon Murray performed the first dialysis in North American at the Toronto General Hospital with a machine of his own design. By 1947 dialysis was being performed in Vancouver and the following year in Montreal. 1948 saw the first dialysis treatments in the United States.

Innovations were refining dialysis techniques. Nils Alwall of Sweden placed an external sleeve over the drum and used pumps to generate higher pressures in the blood compartment than in the dialysate. This allowed ultrafiltration by hydrostatic rather than osmotic pressure, an advance still used in modern hemodialysis systems. Alwall also opened the world's first acute hemodialysis clinic in 1950 (Kurkus et al. 2007).

Kolff and others recognized that hand-built machines and lengthy setup procedures would severely limit access to dialysis. George Jernstedt and Westinghouse Corporation in Pittsburg developed the first commercial dialysis machine. They modified the Alwall design to include roller-type blood pumps and monitors for pressures, flow rates and temperatures, all of which are present in every modern-day dialysis machine. Kolff and others developed the Kolff-Brigham Kidney, which expanded on the Westinghouse design to include a dialysate heater and a plastic hood for monitoring of blood leaks. This popular machine continued to be used until the mid-1970's. By standardizing equipment and procedures the Kolff-Brigham Kidney eased setup tremendously. Despite these improvements, starting dialysis remained a time and labour intensive process. First, one had to hand-wind 2 1/2 meters of membrane onto a roller that was then sterilized by boiling for one hour. Next, the membrane was wound onto the drum, the tubing attached, and cannulaes placed into an artery and vein of a patient. Checks were made for blood leaks and repairs to the membrane were made where necessary. The physician had to prepare the 100 L of dialysate by carefully measuring and adding electrolytes to the solution, a process that had to be repeated every two hours during the treatment. Kolff convinced the Singer Sewing Machine Company to develop a machine capable of stitching together a membrane sandwiched between two layers of woven fiberglass screening. By wrapping this membrane around an orange juice concentrate can Kolff developed the first wholly self-contained dialysis membrane. He enrolled the Travenol company to develop this product, and by the mid-1950s the U200A was released. It was the first disposable dialysis membrane, and cost US$59.00. Kolff also modified washing machines to act as the tubs for dialysate. Travenol used this design as the basis for the first complete commercial dialysis system, released on October 30th 1956 for about US$1,200.

Modern commercial dialysis membranes consist of many thousands of capillaries, packed like parallel threads within the dialyzer. Richard D. Stewart at the University of Michigan was the first to develop this type of membrane (Stewart et al. 1966). Initially his design was meant for reverse osmosis water treatment systems. He recognized the potential application for dialysis, and in 1967 the first clinical trial of a hollow-fibre capillary tube dialyzer took place. Instead of cellulose, Stewart's design used cuprammonium for the membrane, improving solute clearance. This design solved two major issues. The array of threads provided a tremendous surface area for diffusion within a compact package, however the internal volume of the capillaries was small, and so large volumes of blood for priming were no longer necessary.

The most vexing problem remaining for performing hemodialysis chronically in patients whose renal function would not recover was the need for routine access to the vascular system. Repeated cannulation of arteries and veins would lead to vessel damage, and the loss of those sites for future treatments. This damage would have to be reduced before long-term dialysis would be viable. Paul Teschan was a U.S. army physician in the Korean war. His interest was in trauma-induced hyperkalemia leading to the death of soldiers on the battlefield. He performed acute dialysis at the 11th evac hospital in Korea (Teschan 1993). Following the war, Teschan developed a cannulae that could be left in a blood vessel. It was made of Tygon tubing and locked with heparin (Teschan et al. 1960). By placing one in an artery and another in a vein, it was possible for the first time to perform multiple dialysis treatments from the same access site. In Seattle, Belding Scribner and associate Wayne Quinton improved upon Teschan's design by connecting the two cannulae externally by a loop made out of PTFE (polytetrafluroethylene, Teflon™). This produced a continuous flow of blood from the artery to the vein through the loop that was positioned outside of the body. PTFE was used commercially to make non-stick cooking pans, and it was felt that the combination of continuous blood flow and a non-stick material would reduce the risk of clotting within the shunt. The shunt could be accessed repeatedly for dialysis, and for the first time allowed for chronic hemodialysis. Despite 50 years of experiments and 20 years of clinical experience with dialysis, the diagnosis of chronic renal failure remained a death sentence. Scribner and Quinton's shunt was the innovation that opened the door to chronic dialysis, allowing patients with irreversible renal damage to survive (Blagg 2011). Clyde Shields was the first patient to receive a Scribner shunt on March 9 1960. Building on this experience, Scribner was able to open the world's first chronic hemodialysis clinic in Seattle. As patients began to be treated longitudinally difficulties with external shunts became apparent, including infections and accidental disconnection with subsequent major blood loss. In response, James Cimino and Kenneth Appel of New York developed the first internal fistulae by connecting the forearm's brachial artery to the cephalic vein. The flow of blood from the high-pressure artery into the lower pressure vein caused the vein to distend and thicken over time, forming a site well suited for the insertion of dialysis needles.

The difficulties facing adoption of dialysis as a practical therapy for renal failure were beginning to fall. Commercial dialysis systems with disposable membranes coupled with training programs for doctors and nurses improved accessibility, while improvements in access techniques opened the possibility for long-term dialysis treatments. Dialysis remained prohibitively expensive for most patients. In American centres that offered dialysis, patient selection committees of health professionals and lay people were struck to decide who would be offered dialysis. These committees were literally charged with deciding who would live and who would not (Alexander 1962). In 1972, public uproar led to the passing of legislation in the US opening funding for dialysis to anyone with kidney failure.

Dialysis remained an expensive undertaking. Resources such as hospital space and staffing remained constrained. Some early nephrologists recognized this, and had begun to look at alternatives to providing dialysis treatments in hospital. If patients could be trained and equipped to perform dialysis at home, many of the resource constraints could be bypassed. Given the complexity of early equipment and techniques, there was little professional support for the concept of home hemodialysis. However, at the 1965 American Society of Artificial Internal Organs meeting reports of small numbers of successes in training patients for home hemodialysis were made. The first home hemodialysis program was in Nose, Japan, followed by the program of Dr. Stanley Shaldon in England. In the US, Boston and Seattle had started home programs. Shaldon trained patients for self-care dialysis, home short daily hemodialysis, and even had patients perform nocturnal hemodialysis three times per week (Shaldon 1968). Spurred by resource pressures and the spread of hepatitis B within hospital-based dialysis programs, home dialysis programs continued to expand. In the US in 1973, as dialysis funding legislation was being implemented, 40% of all dialysis patients performed home hemodialysis. Over the following years, as in-centre dialysis programs expanded the proportion of home hemodialysis declined to a low of about 1% in the 2000s (U.S. Renal Data System 2010).

4.2 THE HOME NOCTURNAL HEMODIALYSIS TECHNIQUE

During the 1970s and into the 1980s, the number and size of centre-based hemodialysis programs expanded rapidly. In addition, peritoneal dialysis was popularized, and become the technique of choice for most people wanted to perform dialysis in the home (Blagg 1996). As a consequence, both the absolute number and relative proportion of people performing hemodialysis in the home began to decline. The standard hemodialysis prescription in an in-centre hemodialysis program was 3 treatments a week, each lasting 4 hours. Interest began to rise in the ability of more intensive forms of hemodialysis to improve patient outcomes. It was identified that the dose of dialysis correlated positively with patient survival (Lowrie et al. 1981; Collins et al. 1994). In Tassin, France, the standard dialysis prescription for their in-centre hemodialysis unit had been 3 times a week, but for 8 to 10 hours per treatment (Laurent et al. 1983). The nephrologists from this area have reported many clinical benefits of longer dialysis treatments, including long-term survival rates higher than reported in any other program (Charra et al. 1983; Laurent et al. 1988; Huting et al. 1989; Charra et al. 1992; Laurent and Charra 1998). In 1993 Dr. Robert Uldall and colleagues from the Wellesley Hospital in Toronto developed a program offering home nocturnal hemodialysis (HNHD). This technique combined prior innovations such as more frequent treatments (Buoncristiani et al. 1988), long treatment times (Laurent and Charra 1998), and treatment in the home setting (Shaldon and Oakley 1966), however, this program was the first to offer quotidian nocturnal hemodialysis as its sole modality to a large number of patients. The HNHD method as practiced in Toronto involved five to seven home-based treatments a week, with the patient dialyzing for 6 to 8 hours overnight as they sleep (Uldall et al. 1994). These individuals placed themselves on dialysis at night and disconnect themselves the following morning. For some patients, remote monitoring during treatments was provided. This service consisted of electronic monitoring of the hemodialysis machine alarms. When an alarm was triggered, this information was relayed to the observation station at the hospital either via the Internet or by a modem over a dedicated phone line. The hospital observers would phone the home if the patient did not respond to the machine alarm, and would dispatch an ambulance if the patient did not respond to the alarm or the phone call.

Selection criteria for this program required that the patient show a capacity for self-care training, functional literacy in English, and a life expectancy of more than one year. In addition, the patient was required to have sufficient manual, visual and auditory abilities unless a spouse or other family member could assist during treatments. Patients received training at the hospital for approximately six weeks. Upon successful completion of training, arrangements were made for the patient to initiate treatments in their home. All equipment and consumables are paid for by the hospital, with the exception of utilities such as water and electricity. The hospital also arranges and pays for any modifications to the home that are necessary, such as routing of plumbing and electrical service to the bedroom.

The combination of longer and more frequent hemodialysis treatments appears to be associated with improved patient outcomes. Quotidian nocturnal hemodialysis has been associated with a number of clinical benefits that will be discussed further later in this chapter.

4.3 RATIONALE FOR INTENSIVE HEMODIALYSIS

As kidney function declines below a critical level, a number of sequelae are seen as a result of loss of renal function. The most obvious is the development of the syndrome of "uremia", which is a poorly defined clinical entity whose onset and manifestations vary significantly between individuals. Common descriptions of uremia would include loss of appetite, malaise, poor energy and exercise tolerance, parageusia, and reduced mental acuity (Almeras and Argilés 2009). Extreme manifestations of uremia would include encephalopathy or pericarditis. Although the original descriptions of uremia date back over 170 years, there continues to be significant debate as to the exact causes of uremia (Piorry 1840; Pierratos 2001). Most clinicians view uremia as a complex interplay between retention products (substances whose concentrations rise beyond physiologic levels in people with kidney disease), intra- and extravascular volume expansion, other sequelae of loss of renal function (ex. metabolic acidosis, disordered mineral metabolism) and the consequences of other comorbid conditions such as diabetes, hypertension and vascular disease. The term "uremia" gained its name from the fact that urea was one of the first identified retention products. However, nearly 100 retention products have been identified, varying widely in their biochemical characteristics (Vanholder et al. 2003). Which of these retention products are important in the generation of uremic symptoms is unclear. However, urea itself is unlikely to be the most significant uremic toxin, as urea loading in hemodialysis patients does not change patient symptomatology (Johnson et al. 1972).

The historical primacy of urea has led to its incorporation into measurements of the adequacy of hemodialysis. The most common measures of hemodialysis adequacy include Kt/V_{urea}, urea reduction ratios and the percent reduction of urea, all of which focus on urea removal during hemodialysis treatments, and declare a patient as being adequately dialyzed once a set proportion of urea has been cleared from the blood. However, an adequately dialyzed patient clears only a fraction of the amount of urea that is normally cleared by healthy kidneys, and measurements of urea clearance tend to overestimate the clearance of other potentially important retention products.

A typical hemodialysis patient whose is achieving a treatment Kt/V_{urea} of 1.4 will remove urea on a weekly basis at a level that is approximately equivalent to 15% of normal kidney function. Patients with progressive kidney failure will typically develop early uremic symptoms at around 25% of normal kidney function (Gotch 1998; McFarlane 2009) (see Fig. 5.2). Most individuals with kidney disease will have at least some symptoms of uremia at 15% of normal kidney function. Even under the best-case scenario assumption that urea clearance by a dialyzer is clinically equivalent to urea clearance by the kidney, it is not surprising that many "adequately" dialyzed patients continue to experience uremic symptoms.

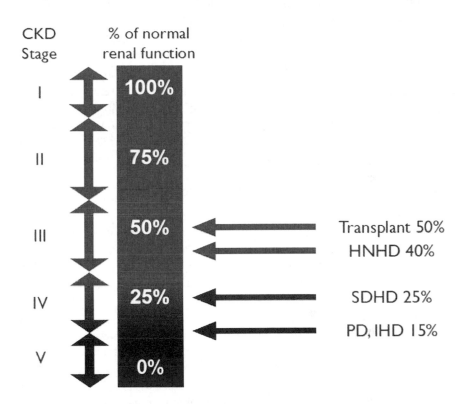

Fig. 4.2 Urea clearance with various forms of renal replacement therapy relative to urea clearance by normal kidney function

Achieving the marginal urea clearance that underlie current hemodialysis adequacy targets would be justifiable if patient outcomes were reasonable, however, it is clear that dialysis patients fare poorly on average. Hemodialysis patients typically report a quality of life that is amongst the worst ever described for a chronic medical condition, with utility scores that are worse on average than those seen in people with significant issues such as paraplegia or untreatable metastatic malignancies (Bell et al. 2001). End stage renal disease is also associated with a significantly accelerated mortality. Older patients on dialysis face a mortality that is 10 times higher than age-matched controls. For younger dialysis patients, the increase in mortality is 1000 times higher than seen in healthy younger individuals (Foley et al. 1998).

In summary, uremia is a common but poorly defined and understood syndrome resulting from kidney failure, and is associated with significant impairments in survival and quality of life. Conventional hemodialysis, even when performed "adequately", is an incomplete replacement of renal function, even when the single parameter of urea clearance is considered. The exciting possibility exists that increasing the dose of dialysis and reducing the uremic toxin load towards a more physiological level could improve the poor outcomes seen in dialysis patients. This chapter will examine the benefits and challenges seen when intensifying the hemodialysis prescription, as well as the advantages and disadvantages of performing hemodialysis in the home.

4.3.1 Principles of Small Molecule Clearance

When considering the process of hemodialysis, it is important to recall that only the blood compartment is being dialyzed, and that toxin removal from the extravascular space (i.e. the majority of the patient) occurs more slowly, as solutes diffuse out of tissues and into the blood where they become available to be dialyzed. In addition, hemodialysis membranes have pores of a particular size that allow passage of smaller molecules but not those that are larger than the pore size. Finally, proteins move across hemodialysis membranes more slowly than smaller molecules, and so retention products that are highly protein bound will be difficult to dialyze (Pierratos 2001). Given these facts, hemodialysis is most efficient at removing solutes that have the following properties; 1) small molecular weight, 2) distribute quickly into the blood compartment, 3) are not highly protein bound. As mentioned, urea has a historical place of primacy in measuring the adequacy of hemodialysis, and coincidentally shares all of the properties of an easily dialyzable molecule, and so can function as an excellent example of small molecule clearance.

During hemodialysis, urea concentration in the blood falls rapidly. By two hours, blood urea levels have fallen about 75% (Kuhlmann 2010) (see Fig. 4.3). During the remainder of the treatment urea levels continue to fall in an asymptotic fashion, with a shrinking concentration gradient between blood and dialysate. Following the discontinuation of dialysis, urea levels rapidly rebound as equilibrium between the intra- and extravascular compartments is restored. For conventional treatments, this rebound is about 15%, but for short high-efficiency treatments the rebound is about 25%, although there is substantial variability in rebound between patients and within patients between treatments (Tattersall et al. 1996). For molecules with similar kinetics to urea, the initial hours of dialysis are the most efficient, with progressively less clearance through the remainder of the treatment. Small molecule clearance can be increased through optimization of the dialysis prescription, including optimizing the blood access, and increasing blood and dialysate flow rates (Gutzwiller et al. 2003).

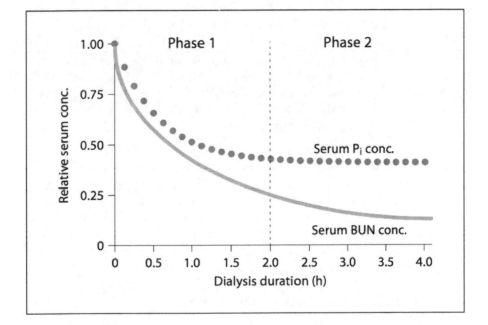

Fig. 4.3 Comparison of intradialytic phosphate and blood urea ni- trogen (BUN) kinetics. Serum Pi concentration sharply drops during the first phase of dialysis (phase 1) and, after reduction of serum Pi to about 40% of predialysis levels, stabilizes throughout the rest of the treatment (phase 2). In contrast, BUN levels steadily decline during dialysis without reaching a plateau. Kuhlmann 2010, reproduced with permission by S. Karger AG, Basel. All rights reserved.

4.3.1.1 Effect of Intensive Hemodialysis on Small Molecule Clearance

As expected, intensive hemodialysis appears to be associated with significant increases in urea removal relative to conventional hemodialysis. One Canadian study involving 39 individuals were examined for 12 months prior to and 12 months following conversion from conventional in-centre hemodialysis (CHD) to three times per week in-centre nocturnal hemodialysis (INHD) (Bugeja et al. 2009). Per-session urea clearance, as expressed by the percentage reduction in urea (PRU) was higher with INHD versus CHD (89% versus 74%, p<0.001). A study from Scotland examining 53 INHD and 53 demographically similar CHD controls found the PRU was higher amongst those with receiving INHD versus conventional controls (77.1% vs. 71.6% respectively, p<0.01) (Powell et al. 2009). In the United States, the Fresenius group reported a higher eKt/V_{urea} amongst 655 INHD patients matched to 15,334 CHD controls (2.21 ± 0.56 and 1.46 ± 0.32 respectively) (Lacson et al. 2009). In one of the only randomized controlled trials in this area, the Frequent Hemodialysis Network (FHN) group demonstrated that short daily hemodialysis also increases total weekly clearance of urea (weekly $stdKt/V_{urea}$ for short daily HD 3.60±0.57 versus 2.57±0.26 for conventional HD, p<0.001) (FHN Trial Group et al. 2010).

Urea removal is dependent on both duration and frequency. In a Canadian study comparing 12 home nocturnal hemodialysis patients (HNHD) to 22 demographically similar IHD patient, the per-session urea clearance was similar, however given the larger number of weekly treatments for those on HNHD (six versus three times per week), the weekly eKt/V was 8.11 ± 0.46 in those performing HNHD, versus 4.26 ± 0.17 in controls (p<0.001) (Suri et al. 2003). Other studies have reported similar findings (McFarlane et al. 2003; Pierratos et al. 2005).

4.3.2 Principles of Middle Molecule Clearance

Larger molecular weight molecules that are still dialyzable are often referred to as "middle molecules". During dialysis, the kinetics of these molecules is quite different from urea. The rate of removal tends to be slower than urea. Larger molecules tend to maintain a significant concentration gradient between blood and dialysate throughout the dialysis treatment, and so removal of these molecules continues through the full treatment duration. The total clearance of these molecules is time dependent, and less dependent on the settings of the dialysis machine (Gutzwiller et al. 2003; Eloot et al. 2007; Tonelli et al. 2009; Kuhlmann 2010) (see Fig. 4.3).

Currently, there are no middle molecules that are routinely measured in hemodialysis patients, nor are there specific adequacy targets for middle molecules. This makes discussions of whether a patient is adequately dialyzed from the perspective of larger solutes difficult. However, phosphate is routinely measured in dialysis patients, and can act as a surrogate for the clearance of middle molecules. Phosphate is a small molecule, but transfers slowly from tissues into the blood, and is extensively hydrated. Due to these characteristics, phosphate kinetics on hemodialysis resembles more closely those of middle rather than small molecules (DeSoi and Umans 1993; Spalding et al. 2002; Gotch et al. 2003).

Phosphate removal on hemodialysis occurs in two phases. During the first phase, serum phosphate levels fall. After approximately 90 minutes, serum phosphate levels stabilize, and can even begin to rise as the treatment continues due to mobilization of phosphate from other pools (Spalding et al. 2002). As a result, a large concentration gradient between blood and dialysate is maintained, even in prolonged treatments. This allows for continued removal of phosphate throughout the dialysis treatment, even when blood urea concentrations have fallen and urea clearance is minimal.

Considering all of these factors, one can conclude that small molecule clearance can be increased through optimization of the dialysis access and the blood and dialysate flow rates, but for larger molecules, increasing clearance will require more hours of dialysis.

4.3.2.1   Effects of Intensive Hemodialysis on Middle Molecule Clearance

Increasing the duration of dialysis from four to eight hours improves clearance of the middle molecule $\beta2$ microglobulin more than that of urea. In a study of 11 anuric patients, eight hour hemodialysis treatments increased removal of $\beta2$ microglobulin by 39.2% ($p<0.0005$) versus an increase of 22.6% ($p<0.003$) for urea removal (Basile et al. 2010). A second study of nine patients confirmed these finding (Eloot et al. 2007). Importantly, these two studies used a hemodialysis system with that created a fixed batch of dialysate, and matched blood and dialysate pump seeds ensuring that the volume of blood and dialysate processed were equal, and the same regardless of the duration of dialysis. These studies were particularly informative as they demonstrate that clearance of uremic retention products is a time dependent phenomenon, and that longer treatments do not increase clearance solely by exposing the blood to more dialysate or processing a greater blood volume.

When considering phosphate removal, one report demonstrated that eight patients converted from conventional to quotidian home nocturnal hemodialysis were able to increase their dietary phosphate intake and stop their phosphate binders but still maintain a phosphate level within the target range. This was attributed to a much higher weekly dialysis phosphate removal (161.6±59.0 vs. 75.8±0.6 mmol/week, p<0.01) (Mucsi et al. 1998). These preliminary results were confirmed in randomized studies which will be discussed below. So far, this discussion has focused on small and middle molecules that are relatively easily dialyzed. Highly protein bound molecules such as homocysteine, in-doxyl sulphate, indole-3-acetic acid and hippuric acid are much more difficult to dialyze, and the impact of more intensive dialysis on these compounds are less clear (Basile et al. 2010).

4.3.3   Principles of Control of Volume Status

Maintenance of a euvolemic state can be difficult in hemodialysis patients, especially those with little or no urine output. Salt and water retention is a common sequelae of end-stage renal disease, and contributes to approximately 80% of cases of hypertension in this population, and can result in episodes of congestive heart failure (Charra and Chazot 2003). While achieving euvolemia is a common goal, it can be difficult to achieve (Charra 1998, 2007). Intradialytic hypotension is a common phenomenon, and can limit the amount of ultrafiltration that is achieved. Although the desire is to return the patient's entire body to a euvolemic state, ultrafiltration is volume removed strictly from the intravascular compartment, which in most people represents about 5 litres. Most conventional dialysis treatments are accompanied by about 2 to 3 litres of ultrafiltration, although some patients can certainly require more in order to reach the desired target weight. Achieving these volumes of ultrafiltration is only possible because of retransfusion of the intravascular space from the extravascular space. However, the rate at which this retransfusion occurs is limited by factors such as the serum albumin, and the weight of the patient (which is correlated with the total capillary cross-sectional area). Hypotension can occur in situations where the dialysis target weight is set too low, leading to an inappropriate contraction of intra- and extravascular volume. It can also occur when the target weight is set correctly, but the rate of ultrafiltration exceeds the rate at which the intravascular space can be retransfused.

Antihypertensive medications that have been prescribed in volume expanded hemodialysis patients can worsen this situation by limiting the ability of the vasculature to contract around a shrinking intravascular volume. Standard procedures for dealing with intradialytic hypotension include intravenous infusion of saline and limiting of further ultrafiltration. These steps can result in a failure to achieve a euvolemic state and perpetuation of the chronic intra- and extravascular volume overload seen in many hemodialysis patients.

4.3.3.1 Effects of Intensive Hemodialysis on Volume Status

All forms of intensive hemodialysis are associated with better control of volume status, and many in turn have also shown positive effects on left ventricular hypertrophy. Long intermittent hemodialysis delivered either during the day or at night has allowed for improvements in blood pressure with fewer or no antihypertensives, as well as less intradialytic hypotension (Charra 1994; Charra et al. 1996). Similarly, the use of short daily hemodialysis has been associated with improved control of hypertension and regression of left ventricular hypertrophy (Ayus et al. 2005; FHN Trial Group et al. 2010). Home nocturnal hemodialysis is the most intensive form of hemodialysis, and is also associated with improved blood pressure control and regression of left ventricular hypertrophy (Pierratos 1999; Chan et al. 2002b, 2003; Culleton et al. 2007).

4.3.4 Principles of Intensification of the Hemodialysis Prescription

The benefits that are expected from an intensive hemodialysis prescription vary depending on whether dialysis frequency, duration or both are increased. When considering short daily hemodialysis, an important question is whether dialyzing more frequently, but maintaining the same total number of dialysis hours per week can gain any incremental benefit. The first potential benefit of more frequent treatments would be a limitation in the interdialytic weight gain. If there is no change in the total weekly fluid consumption, and also no change in the total number of dialysis hours, then the average hourly ultrafiltration rate will be the same in both short daily and conventional hemodialysis. However, the shorter interdialytic period intrinsic to the short daily schedule means that the total weight gain per treatment will be less. Some patients, especially those with ventricular dysfunction, can develop congestive heart failure with large increases in weight between dialysis treatments, in particular during the three day dialysis-free "long stretch" segment of the weekly conventional dialysis schedule. Even those who do not develop heart failure can still find large weight gains to be unpleasant, as this contributes to peripheral edema, can limit exertional capacity, and can make management of hypertension more difficult.

The second potential benefit of short daily hemodialysis lies in the increased number of "first hours" of dialysis. At the start of a hemodialysis treatment, blood concentrations of retention products are at their highest, and then fall as the treatment progresses. In terms of the total amount of a solute that is removed by dialysis, the first hour is the most efficient. For example, as described above urea clearance is highest during the first hour of hemodialysis, and relatively low in the final hour (Spalding et al. 2002). Following the termination of dialysis, the blood concentration of retention products "rebound", as solutes diffuse from the extravascular compartment into the blood. More frequent treatments provide more opportunities for post-treatment rebound and more first hours of dialysis per week. This effect is more prominent for small molecules that are rapidly cleared from the blood, and less dramatic for middle molecules that maintain a large blood-dialysate concentration gradient throughout the treatment (Spalding et al. 2002; Kuhlmann 2010).

Longer treatments increase the total number of dialysis hours per week, which provides the potential for a greater clearance of retention products. Typically, the increased solute clearance seen with longer treatments is facilitated by an exposure of the blood to a greater volume of dialysate. Interestingly, longer treatments are associated with greater solute clearance even when the total volume of blood processed and dialysate used are kept the same (Basile et al. 2010).

Long hemodialysis treatments performed thrice weekly do not help limit interdialytic weight gain, however, as the total weekly ultrafiltration demand is spread over a greater number of hours of dialysis, the average hourly ultrafiltration rate is lower, providing the opportunity for less intradialytic hypotension and treatments that are generally "gentler" and better tolerated.

Home nocturnal hemodialysis prescriptions that increase both dialysis duration and frequency provide the opportunity to gain all of these ultrafiltration and solute removal benefits; lower interdialytic weight gain, lower hourly ultrafiltration rates, and greater solute removal through increased hours of dialysis and a greater number of first hours per week.

4.4   DETERMINING ADEQUACY OF DIALYSIS IN PEOPLE UNDERGOING INTENSIVE HEMODIALYSIS

Much work has been done in modeling urea clearance during hemodialysis and incorporating measures such as the Kt/V_{urea} into assessments of dialysis adequacy. The role of these measures remains controversial, especially in patients undergoing intensive hemodialysis (Gotch 2004; Pierratos et al. 2005). While it is beyond the scope of this chapter to review urea clearance modeling and the optimal method of assessing dialysis adequacy, this section will review some of the most popular methods of assessing adequacy and discuss their role in people receiving intensive hemodialysis.

The Kt/V_{urea} was developed by Gotch and Sargent as a method of estimating urea clearance when analyzing data from the National Cooperative Dialysis Study (Gotch and Sargent 1985). K represents the clearance of urea by the dialyzer in mL/min, and is typically an estimated value based on blood and dialysate flow, as well as clearance information provided by the membrane manufacturer, while t represents the treatment duration, and V represents the volume of distribution of urea. Kt therefor can be thought of as the volume of blood that has been cleared of urea during a dialysis session. When this volume is divided by V to produce the Kt/V_{urea}, the result is a dimensionless ratio of the volume of blood cleared of urea relative to the volume of distribution of urea. On a practical level, calculation of the Kt/V_{urea} requires knowledge of the treatment time, and the pre- and post-dialysis blood urea levels and weight. While the Kt/V_{urea} is widely used as a measure of dialysis adequacy in patients receiving conventional hemodialysis, it has a number of potential flaws. As will be discussed below, urea is a relatively small and easy to dialyze solute compared to the larger middle molecules, and so Kt/V_{urea} overestimates the clearance of these larger molecules. It also models urea distribution using a simplified single compartment approach. For this reason, it is often referred to as the single pool Kt/V_{urea}, or $spKt/V_{urea}$. However, urea rebounds quickly after a hemodialysis session, and follows kinetics that involve more than one compartment. Some have advocated using the equilibrated Kt/V_{urea}, or eKt/V_{urea}, which compensates for the post-dialysis rebound in urea, and therefor may more accurately reflect total body urea removal (Tattersall et al. 1996; Depner et al. 1999). The eKt/V_{urea} is either estimated from the $spKt/V_{urea}$, or measured more directly by having the patient stay for ½ hour after dialysis for an additional blood sample.

The difficulty with these measures is that they have been developed for use in conventionally dialyzed patients, and have not been validated in people receiving a more intensive prescription. The per-session Kt/V can be summed for all of the treatments in a week to produce an estimate of weekly urea clearance, however, these weekly values should not be used to compare different dialysis prescriptions (ex. conventional versus short daily). This is due to the fact that solute removal efficiency increases with treatment frequency, and while Kt/V increases linearly with treatment time, hourly solute clearance tends to decrease as hemodialysis treatment duration increases. For example, when comparing two patients both with a weekly $spKt/V_{urea}$ of 3.6, one whom is dialyzing conventionally and one performing short daily hemodialysis, the patient performing the more frequent dialysis will have higher solute clearance despite the same Kt/V_{urea}. In addition, these models assume that urea generation is constant. This assumption is particularly problematic for patients undergoing nocturnal hemodialysis, as urea generation is significantly lower at night than during the day (Daugirdas et al. 2010).

In response to the need for a measure of dialysis adequacy that could be used across different dialysis techniques, Gotch has also proposed using the standardized Kt/V_{urea} or $stdKt/V_{urea}$ (Gotch 1998). This value is calculated quite differently, and is based on the mid-week pre-dialysis urea level, and so can be used in treatments of different frequency and duration. However, this model is based on a number of assumptions, including that the toxicity of the pre-dialysis urea level in patients undergoing intermittent therapy is the same as for the steady-state urea level in patients undergoing continuous therapy. Related to this is the assumption that urea clearance by various forms of hemodialysis, peritoneal dialysis and native kidney function are all clinically equivalent. Although the idea of a single measure of urea clearance that could be used across modalities is attractive, the $stdKt/V_{urea}$ shares the difficulties listed for the $spKt/V_{urea}$ and the eKt/V_{urea}. The underlying assumptions of the $stdKt/V_{urea}$ have not been confirmed. Indeed, the assumption that urea clearance by dialysis and by native kidney function are clinically equivalent is likely not correct (Bargman et al. 2001; Shemin et al. 2001; Paniagua et al. 2002).

Finally, these measures have not been convincingly validated as predictors of morbidity or mortality in patients undergoing intensive dialysis, and so their utility in these populations are uncertain. As such, the use of the various forms of Kt/V_{urea} is inconsistent across programs that offer intensive hemodialysis, and their role as a driver of clinical decisions is unclear. Many programs simply do not measure urea clearance in intensively dialyzed patients. This raises the question as to how dialysis adequacy should be measured in people receiving intensive hemodialysis?

Although there is no consensus on this subject, it is reasonable to assume that adequacy assessments in this population should not be centered around measures of urea clearance, but rather should be more holistic, integrating the clinical assessment of the patient for signs or symptoms of uremia or volume overload, with an assessment of laboratory measures that correlate with dialysis adequacy such as control of mineral metabolism parameters, dose of erythropoiesis agents and nutritional parameters.

4.4.1 Non-Randomized Trials in Intensive Hemodialysis

A large body of evidence has been developed demonstrating a wide range of benefits for intensive hemodialysis regimens such as short daily or nocturnal hemodialysis when compared to conventional hemodialysis. These studies range from case reports, through case series both cross-sectional and longitudinal and with or without controls, to large-scale epidemiologic studies. Most of these studies were not randomized controlled trials, and as will be discussed below, there are a number of reasons why randomized trials are highly desirable when comparing different dialysis modalities. Because of the potential issues that affect the reliability of these non-randomized studies, they will not be discussed in detail, but rather the focus will be to discuss some general themes that arise from this body of evidence, and present some illustrative examples. Non-randomized studies of patient survival will be examined more closely, as most of the randomized trials in this area were not sufficiently powered to examine mortality.

Short daily hemodialysis has been associated with improved blood pressure control and reductions in left ventricular mass (Fagugli et al. 2001; Ayus et al. 2005). Control of mineral metabolism parameters such as phosphate levels is also better with short daily hemodialysis, although treatment times of at least three hours are most effective (Ayus et al. 2005, 2007). Short daily hemodialysis can improve nutritional status and markers of activation of the malnutrition-inflammation axis (Galland et al. 2001; Ayus et al. 2005). One systematic analysis of the short daily hemodialysis literature summarized the findings of 25 studies (Suri et al. 2006). Improvements were observed in blood pressure in 10 of 11 studies, anemia management in 7 of 11 studies, and serum albumin in 5 of 10 studies.

Long daytime treatments on a three times per week schedule has been a standard approach to dialysis in Tassin, France, and has been associated with improved blood pressure control (Luik et al. 1998), nutrition markers, easier control of anemia, reduced incidence of hyperkalemia and improved markers of mineral metabolism (Charra et al. 2003). Similarly, in-centre nocturnal hemodialysis using six to eight hour treatments three times per week has been shown to improve phosphate control despite using fewer oral phosphate binders, reduce the need for antihypertensives, and maintain hemoglobin levels with lower doses of erythropoiesis stimulating agents (Bugeja et al. 2009). A large report from the US indicated that in-centre nocturnal hemodialysis patients had a lower rate of hospitalization, better serum albumin and lower phosphate levels, and better blood pressure control despite larger interdialytic weight gains than conventional hemodialysis patients dialyzing in a similar geographical area (Lacson et al. 2009).

Patients receiving home nocturnal hemodialysis have experienced improved control of blood pressure (Pierratos 1999), mineral metabolism parameters (Pierratos et al. 2001; Lindsay et al. 2003), sleep apnea (Hanly and Pierratos 2001), as well as improvements in left ventricular hypertrophy (Chan et al. 2002b) and ejection fraction (Chan et al. 2002a). Fertility is rare in women performing conventional hemodialysis, however, fertility can be restored with intensive hemodialysis, and many successful pregnancies have been reported by women performing home nocturnal hemodialysis (Barua et al. 2008).

In terms of markers of quality of life, the use of short daily hemodialysis has been associated with fewer adverse dialysis symptoms and better maintenance of functionality as well as improvements in health-related and global quality of life (Ting et al. 1999; Mohr et al. 2001; Traeger et al. 2001; Heidenheim et al. 2003; Vos et al. 2006). However, improvements in health-related quality of life was an inconsistent finding in a recent systematic review of short daily hemodialysis trials (Suri et al. 2006). Patients performing home nocturnal hemodialysis also report a higher global quality of life (McFarlane et al. 2003). Anecdotally, some patients performing home nocturnal hemodialysis have taken themselves off of the renal transplant waiting list, often as they do not anticipate any further improvements in their global quality of life (McFarlane 2010).

Several studies have examined survival in cohorts of patients receiving intensive hemodialysis through the use of longitudinal data sets and registries. These studies suggest that the use of intensive hemodialysis is associated with better patient survival. For over 40 years, the dialysis program in Tassin, France has been performing eight-hour hemodialysis treatments during the day on a three times per week schedule. As this has been their standard approach to hemodialysis, they have been able to report the results of long treatment times in an unselected cohort (Charra et al. 2003). The mortality rate for their patients appears to be much lower than what is typically reported in other jurisdictions (Laurent and Charra 1998). The Tassin patients have a higher survival than unselected patients receiving conventional hemodialysis in Nottingham, England (Innes et al. 1999). Interestingly, it was not the highest risk patients that benefited the most from long dialysis treatments, but rather the survival differences were most striking in the low and medium risk groups.

Two studies have examined survival in patients receiving home nocturnal hemodialysis. The CAN-SLEEP study examined 247 Canadian patients receiving home nocturnal hemodialysis between 1994 and 2006. One-year adverse event free survival (where adverse events were defined as death or a need to change to a different form of dialysis) was 95.2%, and at 5 years was 80.1% (Pauly et al. 2010). This compared to one- and five-year survival rates of 81% and 38% respectively for unselected contemporaneous Canadian hemodialysis patients (Canadian Institute For Health Information 2008). A more recent study used a propensity score technique to match 94 nocturnal hemodialysis patients to 940 conventional hemodialysis patients identified in the USRDS database (Johansen et al. 2009). The mortality rates differed impressively between these two groups, with patients undergoing nocturnal hemodialysis having a mortality rate that was only one-third of that of the conventional hemodialysis patients (hazard ratio (HR) 0.36, 95% confidence interval (CI) 0.22-0.61, p=0.0001). A large US study of 655 in-centre thrice-weekly nocturnal patients compared with 15,334 patients receiving conventional hemodialysis in a similar geographical area showed a superior survival for those receiving in-centre nocturnal hemodialysis (HR 0.59, 95% CI 0.46 – 0.75, p<..001), however this result was no longer statistically significant after adjusting for case mix and access type (HR .90, p=.4).(Lacson, Wang et al. 2009)

It has been recognized that patients who undergo intensive hemodialysis are highly selected, and their demographics differ significantly from the average hemodialysis patient. For example, Canadian home nocturnal hemodialysis patients are typically younger, less likely to have diabetes, and have been on dialysis for a longer period than the average Canadian hemodialysis patient (McFarlane et al. 2002). However, the direction of bias when comparing intensive dialysis cohorts versus conventional patients is not always easy to predict. While intensive dialysis (especially in the home setting) is often offered to younger, healthier patients, it is also used as rescue therapy for those failing conventional hemodialysis. The studies that have been discussed here have used a variety of methods to minimize confounding and bias and have attempted to generate control groups that are as demographically similar as possible. However, as will be discussed in the next section, residual confounding is almost certain to be present in these studies, making it difficult to conclude with certainty whether these benefits are due to intensive dialysis, or whether they are due to patient factors and residual confounding. Two studies took an interesting approach to finding an appropriate control group to compare to patients undergoing intensive hemodialysis by comparing their survival to another highly selected group – namely patients who have received a renal transplant, who are also known to differ significantly from dialysis patients who are ineligible for transplant, or who are receiving dialysis while on the transplant waiting list (Wolfe et al. 1999). In the first study, 415 patients undergoing short daily hemodialysis either in-centre or at home were found to have a 5-year cumulative survival of $68 \pm 4.1\%$ and a 10-year survival of $42 \pm 9\%$ (Kjellstrand et al. 2008). The standardized mortality ratio again significantly favoured the intensively dialyzed group, with the short daily patients having one third the mortality of conventionally dialyzed patients who were identified in the USRDS database and matched for age, sex, race and primary renal disease (standardized mortality ratio (SMR) 0.34, 95% CI 0.20-0.54, p<0.001). This study also demonstrated that the survival curves for the short daily hemodialysis patients were essentially identical to recipients of a deceased donor kidney transplant who were listed in the USRDS database. In a similar study, 177 Canadian nocturnal hemodialysis patients were compared to 1062 deceased donor renal transplant recipients and 1062 live donor renal transplant recipients identified through the USRDS database (Pauly et al. 2009). Survival was better in the live donor recipients than the nocturnal hemodialysis patients (Hazard Ratio (HR) 0.51, 95% CI 0.28–0.91, p=0.02), but similar between deceased donor recipients and nocturnal hemodialysis patients (HR 0.87, 95% CI 0.50–1.51, p=0.61). These studies suggest that intensive hemodialysis is associated with a significantly higher patient survival rate; however, it remains difficult to determine how much of this benefit is due to patient factors and residual confounding, and how much is attributable to the intensification of the dialysis prescription.

4.4.2 Randomized Trials in Intensive Hemodialysis

Intensive hemodialysis appears to be associated with a number of clinically important benefits in a variety of studies reporting from a large number of jurisdictions from around the world. As discussed above, the vast majority of these reports originate from studies that were not randomized. When possible, conclusions about the risks and benefits of a clinical intervention are best derived from randomized controlled trials. Randomization should lead to study groups that are balanced for parameters that are known to impact on outcome (ex. age, diabetes status, dialysis vintage). More importantly, randomization should also lead to groups that are balanced with respect to variables that correlate with outcome but are either unknown or hard to measure. For studies of intensive hemodialysis, the need for randomization is particularly important. Non-randomized trials are vulnerable to a large range of biases. Of most concern are factors that likely differ between patients who choose intensive hemodialysis versus those who choose conventional hemodialysis, and which are difficult to delineate or measure accurately. For example, two demographically similar patients, one who chooses an intensive hemodialysis prescription versus one who chooses a conventional modality may vary in terms of factors such as motivation, socioeconomic status, quality of care provided by the dialysis team, access to a range of dialysis modalities, etc. These factors and many others known or unknown may differ between patients who opt to perform intensive hemodialysis, and may correlate strongly with outcomes. When considering the impressive body of evidence suggesting that intensive hemodialysis is associated with important clinical benefits, an impartial critique would likely question whether these improvements were due to the "best" dialysis, or because these forms of dialysis were performed on the "best" patients (i.e. those destined to have better outcomes). For these reasons, it is important when critiquing any non-randomized study of intensive hemodialysis to recognize that the study remains particularly vulnerable to important biases that are not evident from a superficial comparison of demographic variables, regardless of the method used to match patients and reduce bias. This places a particular importance for the need for randomized studies in this area. Blinded studies are preferable. Although it would be possible to blind both caregivers and patients to frequency or duration of dialysis through the use of sham dialysis sessions and utilizing periods of hemodialysis where no dialysis occurred by setting the dialysate to bypass the membrane and where no ultrafiltration was performed, such studies would involve obvious practical difficulties, and to date no randomized blinded trials of dialysis dose have been performed.

At the time of the publication of this chapter, there have been five randomized trials of intensive versus conventional hemodialysis. The first was the National Cooperative Dialysis Study (NCDS), which compared a high blood urea target to a conventional target, and short versus longer treatments. The second was the HEMO study, comparing conventional in-centre hemodialysis to a prescription of in-centre hemodialysis that increased and optimized urea clearance. The third was a study from Alberta, Canada, comparing conventional in-centre hemodialysis to home nocturnal hemodialysis. Finally, two trials from the Frequent Hemodialysis Network were reported, comparing conventional in-centre hemodialysis to short daily hemodialysis and home conventional hemodialysis to home nocturnal hemodialysis respectively.

4.4.2.1   The National Cooperative Dialysis Study (NCDS)

The NCDS was the first randomized trial in hemodialysis to examine issues regarding the dose of dialysis (Lowrie et al. 1981). The researchers utilized a two-by-two factorial design where patients were randomized to either a high time averaged concentration of blood urea (TAC_{urea}) or a low TAC_{urea}, and to either short of long dialysis treatment times. The TAC_{urea} represents the mean urea through a hemodialysis treatment, with the high target TAC_{urea} being 40 mmol/L, and the low target being 20 mmol/L. These targets were achieved by manipulating the dialyzer characteristics (membrane type and surface area), and machine settings (blood and dialysate pump speeds, and the relative directions of blood and dialysate flow. The short target treatment time was about 3 hours compared to about 4.5 hours in the long target treatment time. Thus, four study groups were created; I – low TAC_{urea} , long duration, II – high TAC_{urea} , long duration, III – low TAC_{urea} , short duration, and IV – high TAC_{urea} , short duration. One hundred and fifty one hemodialysis patients from 8 US dialysis centres were randomized through a 22-month analysis period in the later part of the 1970s. This study examined prevalent hemodialysis patients, but excluded those with diabetes. The primary outcome was patient morbidity as represented by either patient death or withdrawal from the study for medical reasons. Hospitalization was also studies as an example of patient morbidity.

Removal from study for death or medical reasons occurred in 18%, 45%, 6% and 62% in groups I through IV respectively, indicating a lower removal rate in the low TAC_{urea} groups (p<0.0001). There was no significant effect of time on this outcome. In the analysis of time to first hospitalization it was observed that the first hospitalization occurred earlier in the high TAC_{urea} groups (p<0.0001), with a trend towards similar benefits in the long treatment group (p=0.06). When considering dialysis time, less hospitalization was observed with long dialysis duration regardless of randomized TAC_{urea} assignment. In this analysis, the ratio of observed to expected (O/E) first hospitalizations was examined, so that a ratio less than 1 indicates that fewer hospitalizations occurred in that group than were expected if there were no clinically significant effect of the intervention. For the low TAC_{urea} groups, the O/E for first hospitalization was .31 for the long duration group and 0.54 for the short duration group. Similarly, in the high TAC_{urea} group, the O/E for first hospitalization was 1.62 for those receiving longer dialysis, and 3.09 for those receiving short dialysis. As mentioned, despite the large magnitude of difference, the statistical p value for these differences was 0.06.

The conclusions from this study remain controversial to this day. Despite the small study size and benefits observed in those dialyzed on a longer schedule, the fact that the results came close to but did not achieve statistical significance led to the conclusion that dialysis time was unimportant. The results related to urea clearance ultimately led to the development by Gotch and Sargent of the Kt/V_{urea} parameter, and subsequently the aim to achieve an "adequate" dialysis by reaching a per-treatment single pool Kt/V_{urea} of 1.0 (Gotch and Sargent 1985), As a result, for over 30 years dialysis treatment time has been considered by many nephrologists to be irrelevant, while the dialysis field has remained focused on the primacy of urea clearance.

4.4.2.2 The HEMO Study

The HEMO study aimed to determine whether dialyzing patients more intensively in the in-centre environment would lead to better patient outcomes (Eknoyan et al. 2002). Patients were randomized in a 2-by-2 factorial design to either a conventional hemodialysis prescription or to a prescription that increased urea clearance, and to either a standard or a high flux hemodialysis membrane. The urea clearance goal for the conventional hemodialysis group was an equilibrated Kt/V_{urea} (eKt/V_{urea}) of 1.05, equivalent to a urea reduction ratio (URR) of about 65%, or a single pool Kt/V_{urea} of about 1.25. A low flux dialysis membrane had a mean beta2-microglobulin clearance of less than 10 ml per minute, while a membrane was considered to be high flux if two conditions were met; the membrane ultrafiltration co-efficient had to be more than 14 ml per hour per millimeter of mercury and the mean beta2-microglobulin clearance had to be more than 20 ml per minute. The investigators excluded patients with significant residual renal function, and those who could not achieve an eKt/V_{urea} of 1.3 within 4.5 hours of conventional hemodialysis (i.e., many larger patients were excluded). This study randomized 1846 patients and followed them for an average of 2.8 years. This trial did not demonstrate any statistically significant benefit for either the intensive hemodialysis prescription, or the high flux membrane. With adjustment for baseline factors, there was no difference in death in those with a high versus standard dialysis dose (HR 0.96, 95% CI 0.84-1.10, p=0.53) or in those with a high flux versus low flux dialyzer (HR 0.92, 95% CI 0.81-1.05, p=0.23).

The authors concluded that the study failed to demonstrate any benefit on mortality of either a more intensive dialysis prescription or a high flux membrane. When considering the effect of dialysis intensity, it is important to note that in the HEMO study, the differences in urea clearance between the groups was relatively modest, and urea clearance was intensified through means that involved increasing treatment time as a last resort. As mentioned previously, adjustments of parameters such as blood and dialysate pump speed have a larger effect on the clearance of small solutes such as urea than on middle molecules, which typically require a longer duration of dialysis in order to increase clearance. For these reasons, the HEMO study does not address the question of whether techniques such as short daily or nocturnal hemodialysis have clinically important benefits.

4.4.2.3 The Alberta Study

When the province of Alberta, Canada began offering home nocturnal hemodialysis, they were faced with a large group of patients who were interested in the modality, indeed enough patients that it would take some time to train them all. These patients were offered the opportunity to join a randomized trial. Patients were randomized to either frequent home nocturnal hemodialysis (HNHD) or conventional in-centre hemodialysis (IHD)(Culleton et al. 2007). The training order within the HNHD group was also randomized, and patients who were randomized to the IHD group were offered HNHD at the end of the study period. The primary outcome was change in left ventricular (LV) mass as determined by cardiac magnetic resonance. Between 2004 and 2006, 51 patients were randomized. On average, there was a reduction in left ventricular mass in those receiving HNHD, while LV mass increased in those receiving conventional hemodialysis (HNHD -13.8 g ± 23.0 g, IHD 1.5 g ± 24.0 g, difference of 15.3 g, 95% CI 1.0-29.6 g, p=0.04). In other findings, antihypertensives were reduced or discontinued in 62% of HNHD patients, but only 12% of IHD patients (p<0.001), and HNHD was associated with a 7 mmHg reduction in systolic blood pressure, while systolic blood pressure rose with IHD by 4 mmHg on average. After adjusting for baseline blood pressure, there was a mean difference of 11 mmHg in systolic blood pressure (95% CI 3 to 26 mmHg, p=0.01). Mineral metabolism parameters were better controlled with HNHD. For example, serum phosphate levels at study exit were lower for the HNHD at 1.42 ± .55 mmol/L, versus 1.71 ± 0.61 mmol/L in the IHD group (p<0.01), while parathyroid hormone (PTH) levels fell in the HNHD group but rose in those receiving IHD (-84 ng/L versus +15 ng/L, p=0.05). The improved phosphate occurred despite the reduction or discontinuation of phosphate binders in 19 of the 26 nocturnal patients, versus only 3 of the 25 conventional patients (p<0.001), and was not due to a significant reduction in dietary phosphate intake (Schorr et al. 2011). Unlike in previous non-randomized studies, no difference was found in anemia management parameters and the impact of HNHD on measures of quality of life was less impressive than anticipated from previous studies (Manns et al. 2009). HNHD improved scores in domains of quality of life that were specific to kidney disease (both "effects of kidney disease" and "burden of kidney disease" were improved). The global quality of life score known as the EuroQol 5D (EQ-5D) improved significantly with HNHD when comparing the scores obtained while patients were on HNHD with those at the time of randomization, but not when those scores were compared to the values obtained at baseline as the patients were about to begin HNHD. However, the baseline quality of life scores in this study were much higher than those typically reported for hemodialysis patients, and were in the range typically reported for those with a kidney transplant (Bell et al. 2001).

4.4.2.4 The Frequent Hemodialysis Network (FHN) Trials

The Frequent Hemodialysis Network (FHN) enrolled patients from 2006 to 2009 into two contemporaneous studies involving 65 North American hemodialysis programs (Suri et al. 2007). The first study examined 245 patients who were randomized to receive either conventional three times per week hemodialysis, or six times per week hemodialysis in the in-centre setting (FHN Trial Group et al. 2010). Conventional treatments were of 2.5 to 4 hours duration, with a minimum target equilibrated Kt/V_{urea} of 1.1. Short daily treatments were of 1.5 to 2.75 hours in duration, with a minimum target equilibrated Kt/V_{urea} of 0.9. These studies utilized a somewhat complex analytic plan with two "co-primary" outcomes. The first was a composite of death and change in left ventricular mass, and the second was a composite of death and change in quality of life, as measured by the physical health component score of the Short Form 36 Health Survey (SF-36). As co-primary outcomes, significant improvements would be needed in both of the composites in order for the short daily hemodialysis to be found to be beneficial.

During the study, the short daily group averaged 12.7 hours of dialysis per week, over an average of 5.2 treatments, while the conventional dialysis group averaged 10.4 hours of dialysis over 2.9 treatments per week. The total weekly standard Kt/V_{urea} was 3.60±0.57 in the short daily group versus 2.57±0.26 in those receiving conventional dialysis. After one year of follow-up, significant improvements in both co-primary outcomes were seen with short daily hemodialysis. The hazard ratio for death or increase in left ventricular mass was 0.61 (95% CI 0.46 to 0.82, p<0.001), while the hazard ratio for death or a decrease in the RAND-36 physical-health composite score was 0.70 (95% CI 0.53 to 0.92, p=0.007). There were five deaths in the frequent dialysis group, and 9 in the conventional arm (p=non-signficant (NS)). The left ventricular mass decreased by 16.4±2.9 g in the short daily group, and by 2.6±3.2 g in the conventional group (p<0.001). In contrast to the inconsistent quality of life improvements seen in non-randomized studies of short daily hemodialysis, the physical component of the SF-36 improved by 3.4±0.8 points in the short daily group, and by 0.2±0.8 in those receiving conventional dialysis (p = 0.004) (Suri et al. 2006). The groups started the study with similar blood pressures, but by the end of follow up the systolic blood pressure had fallen by almost 10 mmHg in the short daily group to 137±19 mmHg, but had risen by about 1 mmHg to 147±18 mmHg in the conventional group (p<0.001). This was achieved despite the fact that fewer antihypertensive drugs were needed in the short daily group, and these individuals had a lower rate of intradialytic hypotension 10.9% vs. 13.6% of dialysis sessions, p=0.04). Pre-dialysis phosphorus was also improved by short daily hemodialysis, falling by −0.2 ±.5 mmol/L, while there was essentially no change in the conventional group (p=0.002). Erythropoietin dose fell about 18% in those on short daily, versus a fall of about 5% on conventional, but there was large variability in EPO dose, and this result did not reach statistical significance (p=0.24).

Unfortunately, frequent dialysis came at the cost of an increased number of difficulties with the dialysis access. The time to first access intervention was shorter in the short daily group (HR 1.71, 95% CI, 1.08 to 2.73, p=0.02). Of those receiving short daily hemodialysis, 47% had to undergo at least one access-related intervention, compared to 29% in those on conventional dialysis. In both groups fistulae required the most interventions, followed by grafts then lines.

The FHN group also performed a randomized controlled trial comparing conventional hemodialysis to nocturnal hemodialysis. Both modalities were performed in the home setting. Conventional treatments were of 2.5 to 4 hours duration, with a minimum target equilibrated Kt/V_{urea} of 1.1. Nocturnal treatments were of at least 6 hours duration targeting a standard weekly Kt/V_{urea} of 4.0. At the time of the writing of this chapter, the results of this study have been presented publically, but not yet published, and so only the major themes from this trial will be summarized here. The FHN nocturnal trial shared the identical co-primary endpoints as the short daily hemodialysis trial. The study had major recruiting difficulties, ultimately enrolling only 87 patients, while the power calculation had suggested that enrollment should include 250 patients. There was a trend towards regression of left ventricular hypertrophy in those receiving home nocturnal hemodialysis, but no statistically significant difference in the co-primary outcomes were identified. Like the short daily trial, significant improvements in blood pressure control and control of mineral metabolism parameters were seen in those performing nocturnal hemodialysis, and again there was a trend towards more access interventions is this group.

4.4.2.5 Critique and Synthesis of the Randomized Trials of Intensive Hemodialysis

When considering these trials as a group, some reasonable conclusions can be drawn. First, the advantages of a larger dose of hemodialysis seem to be more striking when conventional dialysis prescriptions are abandoned in favour of either short daily or nocturnal prescriptions. The NCDS suggested no advantage for longer treatment times, however, the trial had a small sample size considering that death or study withdrawal were the components of the primary endpoint. Despite this, strong trends favouring longer treatment times that just missed statistical significance were present but dismissed by the authors. The HEMO study was more adequately powered, but again failed to show a benefit of more intensive hemodialysis. However, the HEMO protocol was not designed to test differences in treatment duration; indeed, treatment time was only increased in the intensive group after all other methods of increasing urea removal had been exhausted. Treatment times in both arms of the HEMO study were relatively short (190 ± 23 and 219 ± 23 minutes for the standard and high dose groups respectively). The Alberta trials and the FHN trials were again quite small and of short duration, but tested significantly more intensive dialysis prescriptions than those examined in the NCDS and HEMO studies. Despite the small size of these studies, clinically and statistically important benefits were demonstrated for short daily and nocturnal hemodialysis. In particular, left ventricular hypertrophy, blood pressure control and control of mineral metabolism parameters consistently appear to improve with hemodialysis prescriptions that significantly increase treatment time, frequency or both. It is important to note that the FHN network nocturnal study showed trends towards improvements in left ventricular hypertrophy, but unlike the Alberta study, these trends did not reach statistical significance despite longer follow-up and a larger sample size (albeit, much smaller than originally called for in the study design). An important difference in these studies is that the FHN group studied incident patients, while the Alberta study examined prevalent patients who had a more significant degree of left ventricular hypertrophy at baseline. It is reasonable to assume that reversal of left ventricular hypertrophy is easier to demonstrate in those with more prominent hypertrophy of the left ventricle. It is also likely that the incident patients in the FHN studies had significantly higher levels of residual renal function, and were less dependent on dialysis to maintain a euvolemic state. It is likely that intensive hemodialysis improves erythropoietin sensitivity and reduces the dose of erythropoietic agents, however, the inter-patient variability of the required dose of erythropoiesis stimulating agents is impressively large, and randomized studies to date have had insufficient statistical power to properly examine this issue. Importantly, these studies demonstrate that quality of life is not adversely affected by a more intensive hemodialysis schedule. Indeed, a number of domains of quality of life appear to improve, in particular those related to the impact of dialysis on quality of life, and those related to physical aspects of quality of life.

The FHN trials provide an important caution; more frequent hemodialysis prescriptions are associated with more access related difficulties. Interestingly central venous lines seem least affected, with fistulae and grafts affected the most. A priority of future research should be to determine the optimal form of access for patients receiving intensive hemodialysis.

Because the average patient on hemodialysis have such profoundly reduced survival and impaired quality of life, these two measures should represent the most important endpoints in trials of dialysis intensity. The Alberta and FHN studies suggest some modest but encouraging improvements in quality of life with nocturnal and short daily hemodialysis. Examining survival amongst hemodialysis patients is more difficult, as studies examining mortality require a very large sample size, even when the effect size is large. For example, between 2000 and 3000 patients would be required in each arm of a study where the effect of intensive hemodialysis reduced mortality by 10%, depending on the assumptions informing the sample size calculation (McFarlane 2008). Of the randomized studies examined here, only the HEMO study approaches the size needed to examine mortality. Although desirable, it is unclear whether a study of the scale required to definitely address whether intensive hemodialysis reduces mortality will ever be performed.

Finally, two intensive hemodialysis techniques remain untested in randomized trials. The group from Tassin, France have reported a number of benefits of long treatment times performed during the day on a three times per week schedule. Similarly, a number of benefits have been reported for in-centre nocturnal hemodialysis performed on a three times per week schedule. These techniques remain untested in randomized trials.

4.5 ECONOMIC CONSIDERATIONS

Hemodialysis is often considered to be the most expensive medical intervention that society will pay for on an ongoing basis (Laupacis et al. 1992). Indeed, hemodialysis is simply too expensive for many jurisdictions, and access to hemodialysis remains highly restricted in many countries (Barton et al. 1996; Cheng 1996; Mittal et al. 1997; Rao et al. 1998; Moosa and Kidd 2006). Intensive hemodialysis regimens are associated with either longer or more frequent treatments, or both. This raises the possibility of increasing the cost of providing hemodialysis, and it is not clear that further increases in dialysis costs would be acceptable to health care payors (McFarlane 2006).

Discussions of the cost-effectiveness of intensive dialysis are often made more confusing when studies compare hospital-based conventional hemodialysis to home-based intensive dialysis, where differences in costs can be driven by both the differences in dialysis modality and the differences in the setting.

There is little published economic data for long in-centre hemodialysis treatments delivered three times per week, such as in-centre nocturnal hemodialysis or long daytime treatments such as in Tassin, France. As the number of treatments is the same, the amount of consumables such as membranes and tubing sets is not increased with these techniques, however, the longer treatments will require more utilities, dialysate and nursing time. Traditionally, utility costs and the cost of producing dialysate are a relatively trivial portion of the overall costs of dialysis, however that may be changing as the cost of electricity and water rise. Staffing, however, is usually a large driver of costs, accounting for about 1/3 of the total costs of in-centre hemodialysis in some studies (McFarlane 2004). Long intermittent dialysis approximately doubles the treatment time, and so have the potential to double staffing costs, in particular those of the nurses supervising the treatment. These additional costs could be mitigated if the patient to nurse ratio is increased, which may be possible, as there tends to be less hemodynamic instability in longer, gentler treatments (Bugeja et al. 2009). These additional costs may be offset if the more intensive treatment improves the patient's condition such that they require less medication or are admitted to hospital less often.

In-centre short daily hemodialysis requires more frequent treatments, and so will incur an increase cost of materials, which typically are a significant driver of dialysis costs, usually accounting for about 10% of the overall cost of conventional in-centre hemodialysis (McFarlane 2004). Depending on the duration of each treatment, the total number of weekly dialysis hours may or may not exceed that of a conventional schedule, and so the impact on staffing costs and the cost of utilities and dialysate may not be substantially impacted. However, the overall efficiency of the dialysis unit may be negatively impacted by short daily hemodialysis. There is time required at the start of a treatment session to assess the patient prior to dialysis, prepare the machine, gain vascular access and initiate dialysis, as well as time needed at the end of the treatment for completing the treatment, achieving hemostasis, and preparing the machine for the next treatment. Because of the time required starting and ending a treatment, three sessions of four hours duration will be more efficient than four sessions of three hours duration, and this may have cost implications to a dialysis program. Again, these costs could be offset as described above.

Finally, moving the treatment location to the home has significant potential cost implications. Staffing and overhead costs are substantially lower in the home. However, capital costs are higher (McFarlane 2004). In the in-centre unit, a single water treatment system typically provides dialysate grade water for all of the dialysis stations, and a single dialysis machine is usually shared amongst six patients. In comparison, each home patient requires their own water treatment system (albeit one substantially less expensive than a whole-unit system), as well as their own dialysis machine. Home patients also require training, which is often relatively staffing intensive. Finally, while in-centre patients typically undergo clinical assessment in the in-centre unit, home patients usually require additional clinical space for their periodic assessments. The costs of utilities increases with more intensive hemodialysis in the home setting, however, that additional cost can be borne by the patient, the dialysis program or the health care payor depending on the jurisdiction, and so whether this is identified as an additional cost will depend on the perspective taken by the study.

Despite the importance of cost in the area of intensive hemodialysis, there have been relatively few publications in this area, and unfortunately, none have been derived from randomized trials to date. It is beyond the scope of this chapter to review all of the studies published in this area, but this section will review briefly four Canadian trials published within 10 years of the writing of this chapter. Costs can vary substantially between jurisdictions, and so trials have been selected from a single country to minimize this effect, and Canada was selected for having example studies across a range of dialysis modalities. Dialysis costs need to be adjusted for the effects of inflation. These techniques may become more imprecise over long time periods, and so the scope has been limited to a ten-year period. All costs presented here are listed in year 2011 Canadian dollars. A study from Alberta, Canada found the costs of conventional home hemodialysis to be substantially less than in-centre conventional hemodialysis ($93,976 vs. $54,936, p<0.001), achieved mainly through savings in nursing and technician costs ($25,590 vs. $5,149) and overhead ($11,288 vs. $4,599). Home patients were hospitalized less frequently, and incurred fewer hospital-related expenses ($11,728 vs. $4,437) (Lee et al. 2002). This study allowed the exploration of the differences in costs between home and in-centre, without contamination based on the number or frequency or duration of treatment. A study from the Canadian city of London examined patients receiving short daily or nocturnal hemodialysis in the home, matched to demographically similar in-centre conventional hemodialysis patients (Kroeker et al. 2003). Home short daily hemodialysis was the least expensive therapy ($82,522), while the costs for home nocturnal hemodialysis was similar to conventional in-centre hemodialysis ($91,218 vs. $89,154 respectively), although the costs of home nocturnal hemodialysis were influenced by a small number of outlier patients with high medication and hospitalization costs. Staffing costs were lower for the home techniques (in-centre conventional HD $32,393, home short daily HD $5,973, home nocturnal HD $5,427) and material costs were higher for daily dialysis (in-centre conventional HD $12,324, home short daily HD $25,037, home nocturnal HD $24,523). A study from Toronto, Canada compared conventional hemodialysis patients who were willing and able to perform home hemodialysis, but were dialyzing at a hospital without a home hemodialysis program to a cohort of home nocturnal hemodialysis patients from another hospital (McFarlane et al. 2002). The cost of home nocturnal hemodialysis was lower despite receiving nearly twice as many dialysis treatments and more than three times the hours of dialysis (in-centre conventional HD $87,172 vs. home nocturnal HD $71,313). As anticipated, nocturnal patients had lower costs for staffing (in-centre conventional HD $27,890 vs. home nocturnal HD $13,846, p<0.001), overhead (in-centre conventional HD $15,692 vs. home nocturnal HD $5,275, p<0.001), as well as trends for lower costs of medications and hospital admissions for those receiving home nocturnal hemodialysis. Nocturnal patients had higher costs for consumables (in-centre conventional HD $8,308 vs. home nocturnal HD $20,967, p<0.001) and capital depreciation (in-centre conventional HD $1,101 vs. home nocturnal HD $7,763, p<0.001). These studies suggest that frequent hemodialysis treatments are associated with higher costs of consumables, and that treatments in the home are associated with lower staffing and overhead costs but higher costs of capital equipment. Most, but not all of these studies suggest lower total costs of these intensive home-based therapies, and none suggest that intensive hemodialysis in the home would be significantly more expensive, despite the greater number of dialysis hours.

The robustness of these conclusions are limited by the fact that none of these trials were randomized, and so it is difficult to be sure that any cost savings are attributable to the modality itself. Both the Alberta and FHN randomized studies included plans for health economic analyses, and so in the future economic data comparing these modalities in a randomized trial setting should be available (Suri et al. 2007).

4.6 SELECTING PATIENTS FOR INTENSIVE HEMODIALYSIS

Intensive hemodialysis has been offered to a wide range of patients. Not surprisingly, it has been used extensively as rescue therapy for patients failing conventional hemodialysis, usually due to ultrafiltration difficulties, persistent uremic symptoms, or persistent disordered mineral metabolism (Bugeja et al. 2009). In one memorable example, a patient had complete resolution of massive tumoral calcinosis with home nocturnal hemodialysis (Kim et al. 2003). However, many patients have chosen to undergo intensive hemodialysis for reasons other than medical failure of conventional dialysis. In-centre nocturnal hemodialysis and all forms of home hemodialysis are attractive to patients who continue to work or have otherwise busy schedules. In the FHN nocturnal trial, greater flexibility and reduced time required to travel to the dialysis centre were the most important incentives that patients perceived when considering switching to home hemodialysis (Pipkin et al. 2010). Anecdotally, patients will also select intensive hemodialysis to allow for more liberal diets and fluid intake, or due to perceptions that more intensive hemodialysis is "better".

However, there is no evidence-based approach to determining who should perform conventional versus intensive hemodialysis. The existing randomized studies examined individuals who met study criteria and were motivated to participate. There have been no randomized studies examining specific patient selection criteria. Should patients with grade 3 or 4 left ventricular systolic function preferentially receive frequent hemodialysis?. Should patients who are unable to reach phosphate control targets despite otherwise adequate dialysis switch to a more intensive hemodialysis schedule?. Should patients who are chronically volume expanded and unable to achieve their blood pressure target despite multiple antihypertensives switch to a more frequent hemodialysis prescription?. These are important questions, and studies would suggest that such patients might benefit from intensive hemodialysis, but at this point there are no trials that have tried to systematically test the value of intensive hemodialysis in specific high-risk populations.

However, the randomized and non-randomized studies of intensive hemodialysis point to a long list of potential benefits. These benefits could apply to a very large proportion of conventionally dialyzed patients. In the absence of rigorous studies identifying clearly which patients should remain on conventional hemodialysis, and which should be converted to a more aggressive prescription, it is this author's opinion that any hemodialysis patient is a candidate for a more aggressive prescription, especially if there are particular medical, social or patient preference issues that are not being addressed by conventional in-centre hemodialysis.

4.7 CANDIDACY AND HOME HEMODIALYSIS REQUIRE-MENTS

Patients performing home hemodialysis need to develop competency in the technical operation of the equipment, the ability to monitor their health status, and perform a number of logistical tasks. The patient's involvement in the performance of hemodialysis is described in more detail in the section in the discussion of the characteristics of an ideal home hemodialysis system, but this section will consider these tasks in the context of patient selection here.

4.7.1 Technical Tasks

The technical aspects of home hemodialysis require patients to learn how to set up their equipment (including both the hemodialysis machine and the water treatment system), how to initiate a hemodialysis session, how to monitor the progress of the treatment, how to terminate a dialysis session and remove themselves from the equipment. Other activities include the "tear-down" phase that follows the end of a hemodialysis session, where used tubing and membranes are removed and disposed, and cleaning and maintenance tasks are completed. If the program allows patients to deliver intravenous medications such as antibiotics or iron, then patients need to be trained to perform this safely. As periodic bloodwork is part of the ongoing monitoring of a home hemodialysis patient, they will also need to be able to draw pre- and post-treatment bloodwork, and centrifuge, store and transport the samples.

Importantly, patients must be able to respond to alarms and errors generated by the equipment. This can be a particularly vexing requirement during training, as the number of potential errors and alarms can be lengthy, and also once the patient is performing dialysis at home, as many errors and alarms occur only rarely, and patients may not recall the procedures required to clear an alarm the further removed from their training they become.

The difficulty of training for home hemodialysis and performing independent hemodialysis can vary widely based on the equipment systems that are selected. Well-designed and simple user manuals and user interfaces can help patients overcome the complexities inherent in performing hemodialysis.

4.7.2 Clinical Tasks

In addition to the technical aspects of performing hemodialysis in the home, the patient must also actively monitor their health status. One of the most important clinical tasks is the ongoing need for an accurate volume status assessment. Patients should measure their weight and blood pressure before and after each treatment, and monitor for signs and symptoms of volume overload (ex. peripheral edema, shortness of breath), or volume contraction (fatigue, poor exercise tolerance, cramping). All of this data must be integrated into an assessment of whether the target weight is set correctly.

Other clinical tasks that patients participate in include monitoring of the adequacy of dialysis by assessing subjective issues like appetite, energy level, and clarity of thought. Patients must be able to recognize dialysis-related complications as they develop, including infectious complications and access-related difficulties. Although patients are dialyzing independently in the home, it is important that they identify clinically important issues as they develop, and relay this information to the home dialysis team so that interventions can be initiated at the earliest possible stage. Finally, patients need to prepare themselves for their routine clinic visits, including all required documentation of their treatments.

4.7.3   Logistical Issues

Performing hemodialysis in the home requires the coordination of a number of visits to the home. Patients need to monitor their stocks of supplies, and order the delivery of consumables in proper quantities and at an appropriate interval. Further home visits are required as hemodialysis equipment requires periodic maintenance, and programs need to monitor water quality on an interval determined by the local water standards. The hemodialysis program may request that their nurses or other members of the multidisciplinary team visit the home to review the physical environment where dialysis is being performed, the state of the dialysis system, and to review issues related to maintenance of competence through testing and retraining. Finally, patients are required to attend their routine clinic visits. All of these tasks require the active participation of the patient, who needs to coordinate the timing of all of these events. Home hemodialysis programs and their associated vendors can ease the burden of these visits by trying to maximize efficiency by performing as many tasks as possible on a single visit.

4.7.4   Patient Selection for Home Hemodialysis

Patients who are being considered for home hemodialysis must be able to perform all of the tasks listed above. Both physical and psychosocial factors impact on a patient's suitability. Physical factors that should be taken into consideration include visual and auditory acuity, manual dexterity, and strength and mobility (ex. sufficient to be able to carry supplies from their storage location to the dialysis machine). Psychosocial factors can often be equally important as physical issues. The patient must have sufficient intelligence and memory to be able to be trained. Motivation and persistence are factors that are difficult to assess but clearly can impact on the likelihood of a patient being able to dialyze successfully in the home.

The patient's home environment also needs to be assessed to ensure sufficient space for the equipment and stores of supplies, proper access to power, water and drainage, and overall cleanliness. Other factors related to the home that the dialysis program should consider relate to distance of the home from the dialysis centre, whether a patient owns or rents their home, how long the patient is expected to stay in their current home, as well as electrical and plumbing issues related to installing the equipment in the desired location in the home. Dialysis programs should consider their ability to support a home hemodialysis patient who lives far from the dialysis centre, including an assessment of how urgent medical issues would be addressed, how supplies would be delivered, and how to address both routine and urgent equipment issues.

While the list of competencies needed for home hemodialysis seems daunting, it is likely that a large portion of patients can perform hemodialysis in their home, and as technology improves, this proportion is likely to increase. As will be discussed below, some jurisdictions have home hemodialysis prevalence rates that are more than an order of magnitude higher than the current rate in the United States. In most jurisdictions there is likely many opportunities to expand the use of home hemodialysis.

4.7.5 Barriers to Recruitment in Home Dialysis Programs

In the United States in the early 1970s, home hemodialysis accounted for nearly 40% of patients on dialysis (Blagg 1996). It has now fallen to 1% (U.S. Renal Data System 2010). A number of factors have contributed to this decline, including changing demographics, improved access to transplantation, the development of peritoneal dialysis as an alternative modality, and the impressive increase in the number of in-centre hemodialysis programs along with the decline in the number of dialysis programs offering home hemodialysis. However, there is substantial variability in the prevalence of home hemodialysis, far more than would be anticipated by differences in socioeconomic and demographic factors, and availability of home hemodialysis. Home hemodialysis is used by 1% of US patients, 2% of Canadian patients, 9% of Australian patients and 16% of patients in New Zealand (U.S. Renal Data System 2010; Briggs et al. 2011; Canadian Institute for Health Information 2011). It is likely that many candidates who would be successful on home hemodialysis are being inappropriately ruled out by their health care team.

However, even in programs that offer home hemodialysis and who approach appropriate candidates, these individuals often do not choose a home-based technique. Over a seven year period, one dialysis program in Toronto, Canada was able to recruit to the home setting (including both peritoneal and home hemodialysis) nearly 40% of the patients who started dialysis after being followed in their pre-dialysis clinic.(Zhang et al. 2010). They did not find any significant differences in demographic or biochemical variables between those who started on home versus centre-based dialysis, with the exception of more males choosing in-centre hemodialysis. The two most important factors that prevented in-centre patients for opting for home–based dialysis was lack of interest by the patient or family (25%) and lack of social support (12%). Interestingly, only 11% of in-centre patients had a medical contraindication to home dialysis. As discussed previously, the FHN nocturnal trial had significant difficulties recruiting the desired sample size. It is important to recall that while this trial compared nocturnal to conventional hemodialysis, all patients in both arms would be performing hemodialysis in their home. The investigators examined the reasons for the lack of willingness to perform home hemodialysis, and again the two most common reasons were lack of patient motivation and unwillingness to leave in-centre hemodialysis (Pipkin et al. 2010). Fear of cannulation was identified as another significant barrier. Surprisingly, education level did not correlate with the length of the training period, suggesting that a lower level of formal education should not exclude a patient from consideration for home hemodialysis.

Ultimately, the barriers to recruiting patients to home dialysis seem to be largely surmountable. Excluding the medically inappropriate still leaves a large pool of eligible candidates. However, it is clear that if home hemodialysis is to increase in prevalence, then dialysis programs are going to have to develop better approaches at overcoming these issues.

4.7.6 A Comparison of In-Centre and Home Hemodialysis from the Patient's Perspective

With the exception of self-care patients, people receiving hemodialysis in a dialysis unit are protected from the bulk of the work related to starting a dialysis treatment through the efforts of the unit's staff. When the patient arrives at the in-centre hemodialysis unit, staff will have already have prepared the equipment for their treatment. The patient is weighed and assessed clinically. Staff prepare their access is prepared and they are connected to the machine. The patient's major contribution to this point has been primarily logistical; they must get themselves to the dialysis centre, and report to the staff any change in their medical condition.

In comparison, a patient performing hemodialysis in the home must perform many additional tasks. To initiate dialysis, supplies must be moved from their storage location, the hemodialysis machine and the water treatment system must be turned on and stepped through their start-up cycle. The patient should ensure that the water and drain lines are properly connected between the water source, the water treatment system, the hemodialysis machine and the drain. The hemodialysis machine must be strung with tubing and a membrane, and acid and bicarbonate concentrates must be connected. Heparin is drawn into a syringe and attached to the machine, as is a bag of saline. The machine must be primed and placed in a state where it is ready to initiate dialysis, and a check is made of the water quality. Patients weigh themselves and check their blood pressure as part of a determination of the volume of ultrafiltration. The parameters of dialysis are programmed into the machine (duration of treatment, ultrafiltration volume and profile, desired blood and dialysate pump speeds, heparin profile, and information about the type of concentrates that have been selected). The patient must then prepare their central line, fistulae or graft, and then connect to themselves to the bloodlines either directly in the case of a central line, or following cannulation in the case of grafts or fistulae. Only now is the patient ready to start their treatment, following a process that typically takes 45 minutes to an hour.

During an in-centre treatment, the patient's primary responsibility is to report any untoward symptoms to the staff. The staff responds to any clinical or equipment related difficulties during the treatment. In the home, the patient also monitors how they feel during the treatment, and must be prepared to adjust or pause treatments if they feel unwell. For example, if the blood pressure falls further than desired, a typical response would be for the patient to reduce the blood pump speed, place the machine in bypass mode, and infuse him or herself with saline. The patient must also respond to any equipment alarms or alerts, and be able to clear these so that the treatment can proceed. In the case of unexpected events, such as a sudden change in medical condition, blood clotting within the system or power or water outages, the patient must be prepared to halt therapy and return their blood. The patient can assist in monitoring the health of their access by noting trends in venous and arterial pressures over time, as well as the frequency of venous or arterial overpressure alarms. The patient is responsible for delivering any medications required during the treatment, and for drawing blood samples before and after dialysis as required.

At the end of a hemodialysis treatment, the patient is disconnected from the machine, the access is cleaned and dressed and hemostasis is ensured. The patient is then weighed, and if clinically well, they can leave the unit. The staff removes and disposes of the lines and the membranes, clean and maintain the equipment and prepare for the arrival of the next patient. A home patient must perform all of these tasks. In particular, the disposal of biohazardous lines and membranes can be a challenge for home patients in some jurisdictions. In addition to being responsible for routine cleaning and maintenance, the home hemodialysis equipment and water treatment system typically require a longer and more involved cleaning and maintenance procedure periodically.

4.7.7   Comparison of Utilization, Maintenance and Turn Over Of In-Centre and Home Hemodialysis Equipment

An in-center hemodialysis machine is used heavily. Typically, such a machine will perform 72 hours of dialysis per week, spread over six days, and shared amongst 6 patients. The typical conventional hemodialysis prescription calls for the maximal blood pump speed that the patient's access will provide, and high dialysate flows. As a consequence of this heavy-duty cycle, most programs purchase more machines than required, to allow for machines to be pulled from usage to allow for regular or unscheduled maintenance. Usually, a team of technicians is available to troubleshoot equipment issues while the dialysis unit is open, and to replace malfunctioning machines on the fly. As each patient arrives for dialysis, the parameters for dialysis, and the acid and bicarbonate solutions are adjusted to their requirements.

In comparison, a home machine typically does not undergo the same duty cycle. It is rare for a home hemodialysis patient to exceed 50 hours of dialysis per week, and most average between 18 and 40 hours. As such, the intensity of usage of home hemodialysis equipment is between about ¼ to ½ of that seen in-centre. While the intensity of usage is less, the home setting also lacks the support infrastructure of the in-centre unit. If the machine is not operational, the home patient is unable to dialyze until the equipment has been repaired, which requires either the swapping of their machine for a functioning unit, or the visit of a technician who is equipped to be able to repair the machine to a functioning state. Some programs have opted to purchase two machines for patients dialyzing in remote locations, as there is no opportunity to rapidly fix or replace equipment for these patients. A home hemodialysis machine is specific to one patient, and so the prescription (other than ultrafiltration target) tends not to vary between treatments.

Centre-based hemodialysis typically utilizes a centralized water treatment system. Each home patient has their own water treatment equipment, typically including one or more charcoal tanks and a reverse osmosis unit. In some homes, a water softener is needed, and some systems utilize an ultrafilter in order to generate ultrapure dialysate.

An important consideration regarding the maintenance of the equipment is that there is usually no redundancy in the home setting. If a hemodialysis machine fails in the in-centre unit, most units have spares that can be used while the machine undergoes repairs. Equipment failure in the home implies that the patient cannot proceed with dialysis until repairs are made or a replacement arrives. In these delays are lengthy enough, then arrangements must be made for the patient to undergo centre-based dialysis. Needless to say, equipment failure in the home is a significant event for the patient, the program and the equipment vendor.

4.7.8 Feature Set of a Home Hemodialysis System

Hemodialysis equipment has evolved significantly over time. This evolution has primarily been driven by the needs of centre-based hemodialysis, and as a result the typical hemodialysis system is not particularly well suited for home hemodialysis. This section will consider the characteristics of an ideal home hemodialysis system by examining the important differences in the patient's perspective between hemodialysis in the centre and the home, and how this equipment is used differently in these environments.

An in-centre hemodialysis machine has to be a multipurpose tool, designed to accommodate the needs of a variety of different patients. As typically the same machine is deployed across a hemodialysis unit, each machine must be able to accommodate the full variety of patients that are cared for in that unit. The requirements for an in-centre program may include the ability to perform across a wide variety of prescriptions, while providing a number of extra features used only occasionally on a subset of patients. Some examples of such features include online monitoring of the hematocrit and urea clearance, complex ultrafiltration ramping protocols, heparin-free dialysis and single needle dialysis (Stiller et al. 2001). The hemodialysis machine may have the ability to identify a patient through a Smart-Card or other identification system, which allows the machine to adjust itself in order to deliver the prescribed dialysis for that patient.

While such features are desirable in the in-centre unit, home based equipment needs to be optimized in other ways. It is difficult to see any value in on-line monitoring of urea clearance, nor is there a need to identify which patient is dialyzing in the home environment. This chapter has already listed many of the tasks that a patient must complete in order to perform a home hemodialysis treatment. Home equipment should be optimized to make these tasks as fast and easy as possible. Time to initiate and time to complete a dialysis session should be important metrics in this area. The use of simple and clear graphical user interfaces can help step patients through their dialysis treatments, as well as provide guidance in how to clear alarms. Such interfaces may also facilitate the successful training of otherwise marginal candidates. Features that improve safety are always desirable. In the case of home hemodialysis, the ability to sense a venous needle disconnection would eliminate a rare but potentially deadly issue. The ability to sense an overly aggressive ultrafiltration rate prior to the patient becoming hypotensive would also be valuable. Some programs would find the ability to perform single needle hemodialysis to be a desirable feature. If a dialysis program wanted to offer many forms of intensive hemodialysis (ex. short daily and quotidian nocturnal), then the equipment should permit both short high-efficiency treatments as well as longer treatments with lower blood and dialysate pump speeds. Such flexibility would also require a short turn-around time between the end of a dialysis session and when the equipment would be ready to perform the next treatment.

The cost of utilities is an increasing concern, particularly the availability of water in some jurisdictions (Agar 2010). Dialysis equipment designed for the home should be as efficient as possible, especially with respect to water consumption. Ideally, the equipment should be designed to operate properly in a wide range of environments such as homes, apartment buildings, and cottages. In some environments, a steady supply of electricity and water is not guaranteed. For example, electrical brownouts are not uncommon is some homes, and in some homes flushing a toilet or running a washing machine can restrict water flow to dialysis equipment. Equipment designed for the home should be forgiving with respect to such utility issues.

There are a number of unique equipment issues that likely don't apply to in the in-centre environment. First, space in the home can be extremely limited, and so equipment needs to be as small as possible. The noises made by the machine are less of a concern in the busy hemodialysis clinic; however, this can be an important issue for both patients and their spouses, particularly when patients are performing nocturnal hemodialysis. A patients perception about the unpleasantness of a noise relates not only to the volume, but the nature of the noise, and so attention should be paid not only to the total volume of noise that the equipment makes, but also the types of sounds that are made during treatments. In the home environment, an important contributor to the total noise during treatment can be the water treatment system, and so this equipment needs to be similarly optimized. Finally, the aesthetics of dialysis equipment is not particularly important in the hospital environment, but many patients object to the medicalization of their home, and so equipment whose appearance and size allows it to blend into the environment as much as possible can help to minimize this issue.

As is evident from this discussion, an ideal home hemodialysis system would be designed from the ground up for the home environment, rather than adapted from a machine designed for the in-centre setting. It is hoped that future hemodialysis systems will allow for a greater number of patients to dialyze safely and successfully in the home.

4.8 PERFORMING INTENSIVE HEMODIALYSIS SAFELY

A number of potential safety issues arise when patients are dialyzing using an intensive prescription. This section will examine safety issues in nocturnal and short daily hemodialysis, as well as suggest some steps to overcome these safety issues.

4.8.1 Excessive Ultrafiltration Rates

High hourly ultrafiltration rates during a hemodialysis session have been associated with excess mortality (Movilli et al. 2007). It is suggested that this increase begins at ultrafiltration rates exceeding 10 mL/h/kg (Flythe et al. 2011) (see Fig. 4.4). There is a sharp increase in risk of mortality between 10 and 13 mL/h/kg, after which the risk continues to rise in a linear fashion. A 75 kg anuric patient performing 5 times-per-week hemodialysis with a modest fluid intake might gain only 1.5 kg a day, which would translate into an ultrafiltration rate of 8 mL/h/kg over a 2.5 hour hemodialysis session. However, a short daily hemodialysis patient who was gaining 3 kg of fluid weight per day would have 6 L to remove after their longest dialysis free interval. Assuming again a 75 kg dry weight, the ultrafiltration rate would now be an impressive 32 mL/h/kg, which is likely to lead to significant intradialytic hypotension as well as being associated with a substantially increased mortality risk. There are many anecdotal reports of patients performing home short daily hemodialysis who became critically hypotensive and were unable to assist themselves or stop the treatment during this very dangerous period. Patients performing short daily hemodialysis should be able to enjoy a less onerous fluid restriction, however, it is still possible for these patients to exceed a safe interdialytic weight gain, especially during periods where they will not be receiving dialysis every day, and especially in the home setting where there may not be someone able to assist if they become critically hypotensive.

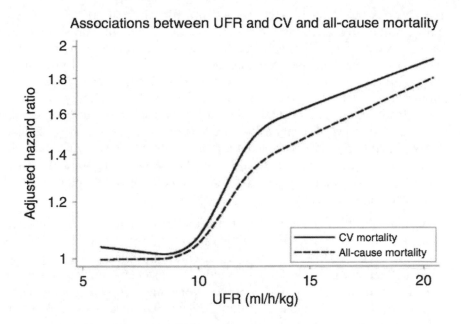

Fig. 4.4 Cubic spline analysis of the associations between ultrafiltration rate (UFR) and cardiovascular (CV) (solid line) and all-cause (dashed line) mortality. Hazard ratios were adjusted for age, sex, interdialytic weight gain, race (black, non- black), smoking status (never, past, current), vintage (<1, 1-2, 2-4, ≥4 years), access type (graft, fistula, catheter), systolic blood pressure (<120, 120-140, 140-160, 160-180, ≥180 mm Hg), residual urine output (p versus 4200 ml/day), diabetes, congestive heart failure, peripheral vascular disease, ischemic heart disease, cerebrovascular disease, serum albumin, creatinine, hematocrit (<30, 30-33, 33-36, ≥36%), and phosphorus, and use of a-adrenergic blocker, angiotensin-converting enzyme inhibitor/ angiotensin receptor blocker, b-blocker, calcium channel blocker, nitrates, and other antihypertensives. Estimates are presented for UFRs between 5.8 ml/h/kg (the 5th percentile of observed UFR in the study sample) and 20.4 ml/h/kg (the 95th percentile). Flythe, Kimmel et al. 2011, Reproduced with permission by Nature Publishing Group. All rights reserved.

In-centre nocturnal patients are vulnerable to the same issue. If an anuric nocturnal patient is gaining 3 kg per day of fluid weight, and dialyzing on a three times-per-week schedule, then they will need to require nine litres of ultrafiltration after the three-day dialysis free interval. Assuming that they weigh 75 kg and are undergoing eight hours of dialysis, this translates into a required ultrafiltration rate of 15 mL/h/kg. While not nearly alarming as the 32 mL/h/kg rate in our short daily hemodialysis example listed above, this may also be a rate of ultrafiltration that is not ideal and not well tolerated in some patients. Under most reasonable assumptions, a patient performing nocturnal hemodialysis on a quotidian schedule (four to seven sessions per week) is unlikely to exceed safe ultrafiltration rates. Patients should be counseled not to exceed safe ultrafiltration rates. When the ultrafiltration target cannot be achieved safely, patients should either increase their treatment time until the hourly ultrafiltration rate is more reasonable, or choose not to remove all of the required fluid during that treatment, and instead remove any retained fluid on subsequent treatments.

A final ultrafiltration difficulty that can arise in intensively dialyzed patients relates to those who gain little or no fluid weight between dialysis treatments. This is most common in patients who retain a large residual urine volume from native kidney function. Most hemodialysis machines have a minimum ultrafiltration rate, and over long treatments in euvolemic patients this obligate amount of ultrafiltration may lead to symptoms of fatigue, cramps or hypotension. In some cases, such patients can overcome these issues by increasing their daily salt and fluid intake, however, some cases patients will require infusion of a volume of normal saline at the beginning of their dialysis session equivalent to the obligate fluid removal dictated by the hemodialysis machine's minimal ultrafiltration rate.

4.8.2 Intradialytic Blood Loss and Water Leaks

Patients performing nocturnal hemodialysis are potentially vulnerable to blood loss during their hemodialysis treatment. For patients performing dialysis with an arteriovenous fistula or graft, the main concern is the inadvertent removal of the venous return needle from the patient's arm. Hemodialysis machines monitor the pressure in the venous side of the hemodialysis circuit, and alarm if the pressure exceeds preset high or low values, or if there is a sudden change in the pressure as would be expected to occur if there were a venous needle disconnect. The pressure in the venous side of the hemodialysis circuit is partly due to resistance in the needle and partly due to factors that contribute resistance of the flow of blood back into patient. The venous pressure correlates directly with the blood pump speed. Patients on nocturnal hemodialysis tend to perform dialysis with low dialysate and blood pump speeds (Pierratos et al. 1998). As a result, the needle provides a large percentage of the total resistance of the venous side of the circuit. If the venous needle is inadvertently disconnected from the patient, then the change in venous pressure may not be enough to trigger an alarm. In a worst-case scenario, the dialysis treatment would proceed with returned blood being released into the environment. These issues are not restricted to those with fistulae and grafts, as inappropriate connections of the patient's central line to the bloodlines can also lead to blood leaks. Similarly, blood leaks can occur from the blood circuit of the dialysis machine, in particular, the connections between the bloodlines and the hemodialysis membrane. To avoid this potentially fatal issue, most dialysis programs recommend the use of a variety of sensors that can detect fluid leaks. Fluid sensitive sensors applied to the access and beneath the hemodialysis machine can assist in increasing the safety in these scenarios. Ideally, such sensors would be incorporated into the dialysis equipment or tubing/dialyzer sets, however off the shelf enuresis or water leak sensors are the most common methods utilized currently to detect such leaks. It is important to recognize that such leaks can occur in in-centre nocturnal hemodialysis programs. Staff working in an environment that is dark and with patients who are asleep should be aware of the importance of periodically checking the access site and local environment for signs of blood leaks. In these settings, it is best if the patient's bedding does not cover their access site during the treatment.

In addition to blood leaks, water or dialysate can leak from the water supply, the water treatment system, the dialysis machine or the hoses connecting these sites. In the home setting, such leaks could do extensive damage. Strategically placed water detectors can detect these leaks so that they can be addressed before damaging the patient's home.

4.8.3 Electrolyte, Acid-Base and Mineral Metabolism Homeostasis

As the total weekly hours of dialysis increases in intensive prescriptions, there is usually an opportunity to reduce or remove the dietary restrictions usually necessary for dialysis patients. Pre- and post-dialysis bloodwork should be performed periodically to monitor levels of potassium, bicarbonate, calcium, phosphate and albumin. Very low dialysate potassium concentrations are usually unnecessary, and as some intensively dialyzed patients will start their dialysis treatment with a potassium level that is in the normal range, it may be necessary to use dialysate potassium concentrations that are much higher than usual, such as a 3.0 or 3.5 mmol/L potassium dialysate. The dialysate potassium level should be progressively raised to ensure a normal pre-dialysis serum potassium level. Similarly, very high dialysate bicarbonate concentrations are usually unnecessary, as some patients will develop a metabolic alkalosis with these solutions. The dialysate bicarbonate concentration should be progressively lowered until a normal pre-dialysis serum bicarbonate level is achieved.

Phosphate clearance increases with intensive dialysis, and many people may be able to reduce or discontinue their oral phosphate binders and eat a diet that is unrestricted in terms of phosphate content (Pierratos 1999). The discontinuation of oral calcium can place patients into a negative calcium balance if they are dialyzed against a standard calcium bath (ex. 1.25 mmol/L). This can result in rising parathyroid hormone and alkaline phosphate levels, and falling bone mineral densities (Pierratos et al. 2001; Lindsay et al. 2003). Because some calcium is removed from the body during ultrafiltration, it may be necessary to ensure that the post-dialysis calcium is higher than the pre-dialysis calcium level in order to maintain parathyroid hormone levels in the target range. As most commercially available have dialysate acid solutions generate a maximum ionized calcium level of 1.5 mmol/L, it may be necessary for patients to add a calcium chloride powder "spike" to the acid solution. For example, in one home nocturnal hemodialysis program, the average dialysate ionized calcium concentration was 1.63 ± 0.10 mmol/L (Pierratos et al. 2001). However, this phenomenon may be more important for nocturnal patients than for those performing short daily dialysis (Al-Hejaili et al. 2003). As total weekly dialysis hours increase, serum phosphate levels fall, leading to a liberalization of the diet. Some patients may become hypophosphatemic despite a fully liberalized diet. At this point, it becomes necessary to add phosphate to the dialysate in order to avoid significant hypophosphatemia. Typically, this is done by adding sodium phosphate to the acid concentrate. Many programs use the Fleet Rectal Solution or an equivalent. Some sodium phosphate solutions contain mineral oil (ex. Fleet Enema), and such solutions should not be added to the dialysate. For example, in one home nocturnal hemodialysis program, the average dialysate phosphate concentration was 0.53 ± 0.29 mmol/L (Pierratos et al. 2001).

4.9 CONCLUSIONS

Conventional hemodialysis can be insufficient in some patients, leaving them chronically uremic or volume expanded. Intensification of the hemodialysis prescription by increasing the treatment frequency, duration or both can help address these issues in some patients. Although hemodialysis is already highly burdensome, studies to date do not show any systematic negative effects on quality of life, although most programs do report a patients dropping back to conventional prescriptions for a variety of non-medical reasons. While currently most hemodialysis programs only offer conventional hemodialysis, it is likely that in the future more programs will also offer some of these intensive techniques, in order to provide a more flexible approach to dialysis with an aim to meet the needs of patients.

REFERENCES

Abel, J.J., Rowntree, L.G., Turner, B.B.: On the removal of diffusable substances from the circulating blood by means of dialysis. Transactions of the Association of American Physicians (1913) (1990); Transfus. Sci. 11(2), 164–165

Agar, J.W.: Conserving water in and applying solar power to haemodialysis: 'green dialysis' through wiser resource utilization. Nephrology 15(4), 448–453 (2010)

Al-Hejaili, F., Kortas, C., Leitch, R., et al.: Nocturnal but not short hours quotidian hemodialysis requires an elevated dialysate calcium concentration. J. Am. Soc. Nephrol. 14(9), 2322–2328 (2003)

Alexander, S.: They decide who lives, who dies: Medical miracle and a moral burden of a small committee. Life Magazine, 102–125 (1962)

Almeras, C., Argilés, A.: The General Picture of Uremia. Semin. Dial. 22(4), 329–333 (2009)

Ayus, J.C., Achinger, S.G., Mizani, M.R., et al.: Phosphorus balance and mineral metabolism with 3 h daily hemodialysis. Kidney Int. 71(4), 336–342 (2007)

Ayus, J.C., Mizani, M.R., Achinger, S.G., et al.: Effects of short daily versus conventional hemodialysis on left ventricular hypertrophy and inflammatory markers: a prospective, controlled study. J. Am. Soc. Nephrol. 16(9), 2778–2788 (2005)

Bargman, J.M., Thorpe, K.E., Churchill, D.N., et al.: Relative contribution of residual renal function and peritoneal clearance to adequacy of dialysis: a reanalysis of the CANUSA study. J. Am. Soc. Nephrol. 12(10), 2158–2162 (2001)

Barton, E.N., Williams, W., Morgan, A.G., Burden, R.P.: A prospective study of ward referrals for renal disease at a Jamaican and a United Kingdom hospital. West Indian Med. J. 45(4), 110–112 (1996)

Barua, M., Hladunewich, M., Keunen, J., et al.: Successful pregnancies on nocturnal home hemodialysis. Clin. J. Am. Soc. Nephrol. 3(2), 392–396 (2008)

Basile, C., Libutti, P., Di Turo, A.L., et al.: Removal of uraemic retention solutes in standard bicarbonate haemodialysis and long-hour slow-flow bicarbonate haemodialysis. Nephrol. Dial. Transplant. 26(4), 1296–1303 (2010)

Bell, C.M., Chapman, R.H., Stone, P.W., et al.: An off-the-shelf help list: a comprehensive catalog of preference scores from published cost-utility analyses. Med. Decis. Making 21(4), 288–294 (2001)

Benedum, J.: Georg Haas (1886-1971), pioneer in hemodialysis. Schweiz Rundsch. Med. Prax. 75(14), 390–394 (1986)

Blagg, C.R.: A brief history of home hemodialysis. Adv. Ren. Replace Ther. 3(2), 99–105 (1996)

Blagg, C.R.: The 50th anniversary of long-term hemodialysis: University of Washington Hospital. J. Nephrol. 24(suppl. 17), S84–S88 (March 9, 1960) (2011)

Briggs, N., Excell, L., Mcdonald, S.: Method And Location of Dialysis. In: Mcdonald, S., Excell, L., Livingston, B. (eds.) Australia and New Zealand Dialysis and Transplant Registry. The Thirty Third Report, pp. 4-2–4-4 (2011)

Bugeja, A., Dacouris, N., Thomas, A., et al.: In-center nocturnal hemodialysis: another option in the management of chronic kidney disease. Clin J. Am. Soc. Nephrol. 4(4), 778–783 (2009)

Buoncristiani, U., Quintaliani, G., Cozzari, M., et al.: Daily dialysis: long-term clinical metabolic results. Kidney Int. Suppl. 24, S137–S140 (1988)

Canadian Institute For Health Information. 2007 Annual Report—Treatment of End-Stage Organ Failure in Canada, 1996 to 2005. Ottawa, Canada, Canadian Institute for Health Information (CIHI) (2008)

Canadian Institute for Health Information. Canadian Organ Replacement Register Annual Report: Treatment of End-Stage Organ Failure in Canada, 2000 to 2009. Ottawa, ON, Canada, Canadian Institute for Health Information (CIHI) (2011)

Chan, C., Floras, J.S., Miller, J.A., Pierratos, A.: Improvement in ejection fraction by nocturnal haemodialysis in end-stage renal failure patients with coexisting heart failure. Nephrol. Dial. Transplant. 17(8), 1518–1521 (2002a)

Chan, C.T., Floras, J.S., Miller, J.A., et al.: Regression of left ventricular hypertrophy after conversion to nocturnal hemodialysis. Kidney Int. 61(6), 2235–2239 (2002b)

Chan, C.T., Harvey, P.J., Picton, P., et al.: Short-term blood pressure, noradrenergic, and vascular effects of nocturnal home hemodialysis. Hypertension 42(5), 925–931 (2003)

Charra, B.: Control of blood pressure in long slow hemodialysis. Blood Purif. 12(4-5), 252–258 (1994)

Charra, B.: 'Dry weight' in dialysis: the history of a concept. Nephrol. Dial. Transplant. 13(7), 1882–1885 (1998)

Charra, B.: Fluid balance, dry weight, and blood pressure in dialysis. Hemodial Int. 11(1), 21–31 (2007)

Charra, B., Calemard, E., Cuche, M., Laurent, G.: Control of hypertension and prolonged survival on maintenance hemodialysis. Nephron 33(2), 96–99 (1983)

Charra, B., Calemard, E., Ruffet, M., et al.: Survival as an index of adequacy of dialysis. Kidney Int. 41(5), 1286–1291 (1992)

Charra, B., Calemard, M., Laurent, G.: Importance of treatment time and blood pressure control in achieving long-term survival on dialysis. Am. J. Nephrol. 16(1), 35–44 (1996)

Charra, B., Chazot, C.: Volume control, blood pressure and cardiovascular function. Lessons from hemodialysis treatment. Nephron Physiol. 93(4), 94–101 (2003)

Charra, B., Chazot, C., Jean, G., et al.: Long 3 x 8 hr dialysis: a three-decade summary. J. Nephrol. 16(suppl. 7), S64–S69 (2003)

Cheng, I.K.: Peritoneal dialysis in Asia. Perit. Dial. Int. 16(suppl. 1), S381–S385 (1996)

Collins, A.J., Ma, J.Z., Umen, A., Keshaviah, P.: Urea index and other predictors of hemodialysis patient survival. Am. J. Kidney Dis. 23(2), 272–282 (1994)

Culleton, B.F., Walsh, M., Klarenbach, S.W., et al.: Effect of frequent nocturnal hemodialysis vs conventional hemodialysis on left ventricular mass and quality of life: a randomized controlled trial. JAMA 298(11), 1291–1299 (2007)

Daugirdas, J.T., Depner, T.A., Greene, T., et al.: Effects of Reduced Intradialytic Urea Generation Rate and Residual Renal Clearance on Modeled Urea Distribution Volume andKt/Vin Conventional, Daily, and Nocturnal Dialysis. Semin. Dial. 23(1), 19–24 (2010)

Depner, T., Beck, G., Daugirdas, J., et al.: Lessons from the hemodialysis (HEMO) Study: An improved measure of the actual hemodialysis dose. Am. J. Kidney Dis. 33(1), 142–149 (1999)

DeSoi, C.A., Umans, J.G.: Phosphate kinetics during high-flux hemodialysis. J. Am. Soc. Nephrol. 4(5), 1214–1218 (1993)

Eknoyan, G., Beck, G.J., Cheung, A.K., et al.: Effect of dialysis dose and membrane flux in maintenance hemodialysis. N. Engl. J. Med. 347(25), 2010–2019 (2002)

Eloot, S., Van Biesen, W., Dhondt, A., et al.: Impact of hemodialysis duration on the removal of uremic retention solutes. Kidney Int. 73(6), 765–770 (2007)

Fagugli, R.M., Reboldi, G., Quintaliani, G., et al.: Short daily hemodialysis: blood pressure control and left ventricular mass reduction in hypertensive hemodialysis patients. Am. J. Kidney Dis. 38(2), 371–376 (2001)

Chertow, G.M., Levin, N.W., et al.: In-Center Hemodialysis Six Times per Week versus Three Times per Week. N. Engl. J. Med. 364(1), 93–107 (2010); FHN Trial Group

Flythe, J.E., Kimmel, S.E., Brunelli, S.M.: Rapid fluid removal during dialysis is associated with cardiovascular morbidity and mortality. Kidney Int. 79(2), 250–257 (2011)

Foley, R.N., Parfrey, P.S., Sarnak, M.J.: Clinical epidemiology of cardiovascular disease in chronic renal disease. Am. J. Kidney Dis. 32(5 suppl. 3), S112–S119 (1998)

Galland, R., Traeger, J., Arkouche, W., et al.: Short daily hemodialysis rapidly improves nutritional status in hemodialysis patients. Kidney Int. 60(4), 1555–1560 (2001)

Gotch, F.A.: The current place of urea kinetic modelling with respect to different dialysis modalities. Nephrology Dialysis Transplant. 13(suppl. 6), 10–14 (1998)

Gotch, F.A.: Definitions of dialysis dose suitable for comparison of daily hemodialysis and continuous ambulatory peritoneal dialysis to conventional thrice weekly dialysis therapy. Hemodial Int. 8(2), 172–182 (2004)

Gotch, F.A., Panlilio, F., Sergeyeva, O., et al.: A kinetic model of inorganic phosphorus mass balance in hemodialysis therapy. Blood Purif. 21(1), 51–57 (2003)

Gotch, F.A., Sargent, J.A.: A mechanistic analysis of the National Cooperative Dialysis Study (NCDS). Kidney Int. 28(3), 526–534 (1985)

Graham, T.: The Bakerian lecture - On osmotic force. Philos. Trans. R. Soc. Lond. 144, 177–228 (1854)

Gutzwiller, J.P., Schneditz, D., Huber, A.R., et al.: Increasing blood flow increases kt/V(urea) and potassium removal but fails to improve phosphate removal. Clin. Nephrol. 59(2), 130–136 (2003)

Hanly, P.J., Pierratos, A.: Improvement of sleep apnea in patients with chronic renal failure who undergo nocturnal hemodialysis. N. Engl. J. Med. 344(2), 102–107 (2001)

Heidenheim, A.P., Muirhead, N., Moist, L., Lindsay, R.M.: Patient quality of life on quotidian hemodialysis. Am. J. Kidney Dis. 42(1 suppl.), 36–41 (2003)

Huting, J., Kramer, W., Charra, B., et al.: Asymmetric septal hypertrophy and left atrial dilatation in patients with end-stage renal disease on long-term hemodialysis. Clin. Nephrol. 32(6), 276–283 (1989)

Innes, A., Charra, B., Burden, R.P., et al.: The effect of long, slow haemodialysis on patient survival. Nephrol. Dial. Transplant. 14(4), 919–922 (1999)

Johansen, K.L., Zhang, R., Huang, Y., et al.: Survival and hospitalization among patients using nocturnal and short daily compared to conventional hemodialysis: a USRDS study. Kidney Int. 76(9), 984–990 (2009)

Johnson, W.J., Hagge, W.W., Wagoner, R.D., et al.: Effects of urea loading in patients with far-advanced renal failure. Mayo. Clin. Proc. 47(1), 21–29 (1972)

Kim, S.J., Goldstein, M., Szabo, T., Pierratos, A.: Resolution of massive uremic tumoral calcinosis with daily nocturnal home hemodialysis. Am. J. Kidney Dis. 41(3), E12 (2003)

Kjellstrand, C.M., Buoncristiani, U., Ting, G., et al.: Short daily haemodialysis: survival in 415 patients treated for 1006 patient-years. Nephrol. Dial. Transplant. 23(10), 3283–3289 (2008)

Kolff, W.J., Berk, H.T., ter Welle, M., et al.: The artificial kidney: a dialyser with a great area. J. Am. Soc. Nephrol. 8(12), 1959–1965 (1944) (1997)

Kroeker, A., Clark, W.F., Heidenheim, A.P., et al.: An operating cost comparison between conventional and home quotidian hemodialysis. Am. J. Kidney Dis. 42(1 suppl.), 49–55 (2003)

Kuhlmann, M.K.: Phosphate Elimination in Modalities of Hemodialysis and Peritoneal Dialysis. Blood Purif. 29(2), 137–144 (2010)

Kurkus, J., Nykvist, M., Lindergård, B., Segelmark, M.: Thirty-five years of hemodialysis: two case reports as a tribute to Nils Alwall. Am. J. Kidney Dis. 49(3), 471–476 (2007)

Lacson Jr., E., Wang, W., Lester, K., et al.: Outcomes Associated with In-Center Nocturnal Hemodialysis from a Large Multicenter Program. Clin. J. Am. Soc. Nephrol. 5(2), 220–226 (2009)

Laupacis, A., Feeny, D., Detsky, A.S., Tugwell, P.X.: How attractive does a new technology have to be to warrant adoption and utilization? Tentative guidelines for using clinical and economic evaluations. CMAJ 146(4), 473–481 (1992)

Laurent, G., Calemard, E., Charra, B.: Long dialysis: a review of fifteen years experience in one centre 1968-1983. Proc. Eur. Dial Transplant. Assoc. 20, 122–135 (1983)

Laurent, G., Calemard, E., Charra, B.: Dialysis related amyloidosis. Kidney Int. Suppl. 24, S32– S34 (1988)

Laurent, G., Charra, B.: The results of an 8 h thrice weekly haemodialysis schedule. Nephrol. Dial. Transplant. 13(suppl. 6), 125–131 (1998)

Lee, H., Manns, B., Taub, K., et al.: Cost analysis of ongoing care of patients with end-stage renal disease: the impact of dialysis modality and dialysis access. Am. J. Kidney Dis. 40(3), 611–622 (2002)

Lindsay, R.M., Alhejaili, F., Nesrallah, G., et al.: Calcium and phosphate balance with quotidian hemodialysis. Am. J. Kidney Dis. 42(1 suppl.), 24–29 (2003)

Lowrie, E.G., Laird, N.M., Parker, T.F., Sargent, J.A.: Effect of the hemodialysis prescription of patient morbidity: report from the National Cooperative Dialysis Study. N. Engl. J. Med. 305(20), 1176–1181 (1981)

Luik, A.J., Charra, B., Katzarski, K., et al.: Blood pressure control and hemodynamic changes in patients on long time dialysis treatment. Blood Purif. 16(4), 197–209 (1998)

Manns, B.J., Walsh, M.W., Culleton, B.F., et al.: Nocturnal hemodialysis does not improve overall measures of quality of life compared to conventional hemodialysis. Kidney Int. 75(5), 542–549 (2009)

Marticorena, R.M., Hunter, J., Cook, R., et al.: A simple method to create buttonhole cannulation tracks in a busy hemodialysis unit. Hemodial Int. 13(3), 316–321 (2009)

McFarlane, P.A.: Reducing hemodialysis costs: conventional and quotidian home hemodialysis in Canada. Semin. Dial. 17(2), 118–124 (2004)

McFarlane, P.A.: Interpreting cost-effectiveness in dialysis: can the most expensive be more expensive? Kidney Int. 69(12), 2120–2121 (2006)

McFarlane, P.A.: Lessons for dialysis investigators from the Steno-2 Study. J. Nephrol. 21(1), 6–13 (2008)

McFarlane, P.A.: More of the same: improving outcomes through intensive hemodialysis. Semin. Dial. 22(6), 598–602 (2009)

McFarlane, P.A.: Should Patients Remain on Intensive Hemodialysis Rather than Choosing to Receive a Kidney Transplant? Semin. Dial. 23(5), 516–519 (2010)

McFarlane, P.A., Bayoumi, A.M., Pierratos, A., Redelmeier, D.A.: The quality of life and cost utility of home nocturnal and conventional in-center hemodialysis. Kidney Int. 64(3), 1004–1011 (2003)

McFarlane, P.A., Pierratos, A., Redelmeier, D.A.: Cost savings of home nocturnal versus conventional in-center hemodialysis. Kidney Int. 62(6), 2216–2222 (2002)

Mittal, S., Kher, V., Gulati, S., et al.: Chronic renal failure in India. Ren. Fail. 19(6), 763–770 (1997)

Mohr, P.E., Neumann, P.J., Franco, S.J., et al.: The case for daily dialysis: its impact on costs and quality of life. Am. J. Kidney Dis. 37(4), 777–789 (2001)

Moosa, M.R., Kidd, M.: The dangers of rationing dialysis treatment: the dilemma facing a developing country. Kidney Int. 70(6), 1107–1114 (2006)

Movilli, E., Gaggia, P., Zubani, R., et al.: Association between high ultrafiltration rates and mortality in uraemic patients on regular haemodialysis. A 5-year prospective observational multicentre study. Nephrol. Dial. Transplant. 22(12), 3547–3552 (2007)

Mucsi, I., Hercz, G., Uldall, R., et al.: Control of serum phosphate without any phosphate binders in patients treated with nocturnal hemodialysis. Kidney Int. 53(5), 1399–1404 (1998)

Paniagua, R., Amato, D., Vonesh, E., et al.: Effects of increased peritoneal clearances on mortality rates in peritoneal dialysis: ADEMEX, a prospective, randomized, controlled trial. J. Am. Soc. Nephrol. 13(5), 1307–1320 (2002)

Pauly, R.P., Gill, J.S., Rose, C.L., et al.: Survival among nocturnal home haemodialysis patients compared to kidney transplant recipients. Nephrol. Dial. Transplant. 24(9), 2915–2919 (2009)

Pauly, R.P., Maximova, K., Coppens, et al.: Patient and Technique Survival among a Canadian Multicenter Nocturnal Home Hemodialysis Cohort. Clin. J. Am. Soc. Nephrol. 5(10), 1815–1820 (2010)

Pierratos, A.: Nocturnal home haemodialysis: an update on a 5-year experience. Nephrol. Dial. Transplant. 14(12), 2835–2840 (1999)

Pierratos, A.: Effect of therapy time and frequency on effective solute removal. Semin. Dial. 14(4), 284–288 (2001)

Pierratos, A., Hercz, G., Sherrard, D.J., et al.: Calcium, Phosphorus Metabolism and Bone Pathology on Long Term Nocturnal Hemodialysis. J. Am. Soc. Nephrol. 12, 274A (2001)

Pierratos, A., McFarlane, P., Chan, C.T.: Quotidian dialysis–update 2005. Curr. Opin. Nephrol. Hypertens 14(2), 119–124 (2005)

Pierratos, A., Ouwendyk, M., Francoeur, R., et al.: Nocturnal hemodialysis: three-year experience. J. Am. Soc. Nephrol. 9(5), 859–868 (1998)

Piorry, P.: Traité d'Alterations du Sang, Paris, France (1840)

Pipkin, M., Eggers, P.W., Larive, B., et al.: Recruitment and training for home hemodialysis: experience and lessons from the Nocturnal Dialysis Trial. Clin. J. Am. Soc. Nephrol. 5(9), 1614–1620 (2010)

Powell, J.R., Oluwaseun, O., Woo, Y.M., et al.: Ten Years Experience of In-Center Thrice Weekly Long Overnight Hemodialysis. Clin. J. Am. Soc. Nephrol. 4(6), 1097–1101 (2009)

Rao, M., Juneja, R., Shirly, R.B., Jacob, C.K.: Haemodialysis for end-stage renal disease in Southern India–a perspective from a tertiary referral care centre. Nephrol. Dial. Transplant. 13(10), 2494–2500 (1998)

Saran, R., Bragg-Gresham, J.L., Levin, N.W., et al.: Longer treatment time and slower ultrafiltration in hemodialysis: associations with reduced mortality in the DOPPS. Kidney Int. 69(7), 1222–1228 (2006)

Schorr, M., Manns, B.J., Culleton, B., et al.: The Effect of Nocturnal and Conventional Hemodialysis on Markers of Nutritional Status: Results From a Randomized Trial. J. Ren. Nutr. 21(3), 271–276 (2011)

Shaldon, S.: Independence in maintenance haemodialysis. Lancet 1(7541), 520 (1968)

Shaldon, S., Oakley, J.J.: Experience with regular haemodialysis in the home. Br. J. Urol. 38(6), 616–620 (1966)

Shemin, D., Bostom, A.G., Laliberty, P., Dworkin, L.D.: Residual renal function and mortality risk in hemodialysis patients. Am. J. Kidney Dis. 38(1), 85–90 (2001)

Spalding, E.M., Chamney, P.W., Farrington, K.: Phosphate kinetics during hemodialysis: Evidence for biphasic regulation. Kidney Int. 61(2), 655–667 (2002)

Stewart, R.D., Baretta, E.D., Cerny, J.C., Mahon, H.I.: An artificial kidney made from capillary fibres. Inv. Urology 3, 614 (1966)

Stiller, S., Al-Bashir, A., Mann, H.: On-line Urea Monitoring during Hemodialysis: A Review. Saudi J. Kidney Dis. Transpl. 12(3), 364–374 (2001)

Suri, R., Depner, T.A., Blake, P.G., et al.: Adequacy of quotidian hemodialysis. Am. J. Kidney Dis. 42(1 suppl.), 42–48 (2003)

Suri, R.S., Garg, A.X., Chertow, G.M., et al.: Frequent Hemodialysis Network (FHN) randomized trials: study design. Kidney Int. 71(4), 349–359 (2007)

Suri, R.S., Nesrallah, G.E., Mainra, R., et al.: Daily hemodialysis: a systematic review. Clin. J. Am. Soc. Nephrol. 1(1), 33–42 (2006)

Tattersall, J.E., DeTakats, D., Chamney, P., et al.: The post-hemodialysis rebound: predicting and quantifying its effect on Kt/V. Kidney Int. 50(6), 2094–2102 (1996)

Teschan, P.E.: Building an acute dialysis machine in Korea. ASAIO J. 39(4), 957–961 (1993)

Teschan, P.E., Baxter, C.R., O'Brien, T.F., et al.: Prophylactic hemodialysis in the treatment of acute renal failure. Ann. Intern. Med. 53, 992–1016 (1960)

Ting, G., Freitas, T., Carrie, B., et al.: Short daily hemodialysis - Clinical outcomes and quality of life. J. Am. Soc. Nephrol. 9, 228A (1999)

Tonelli, M., Wang, W., Hemmelgarn, B., et al.: Phosphate Removal With Several Thrice-Weekly Dialysis Methods in Overweight Hemodialysis Patients. Am. J. Kidney Dis. 54(6), 1108–1115 (2009)

Traeger, J.R., Galland, R., Arkouche, W., et al.: Short daily hemodialysis: A four-year experience. Dial. Transplant. 30(2), 76–86 (2001)

Twardowski, Z., Kubara, H.: Different sites versus constant sites of needle insertion into arteriovenous fistulas for treatment by repeated dialysis. Dial. Transplant. 8, 978–980 (1979)

U.S. Renal Data System, Annual Data Report: Atlas of End-Stage Renal Disease in the United States. Bethesda, MD, National Institute of Health, National Institute of Diabetes and Digestive and Kidney Diseases (2010)

Uldall, P.R., Francoeur, R., Ouwendyk, M.: Simplified nocturnal home hemodialysis (SNHHD): A new approach to renal replacement therapy. J. Am. Soc. Nephrol. 5, 428 (1994)

Vanholder, R., De Smet, R., Glorieux, G., et al.: Review on uremic toxins: classification, concentration, and interindividual variability. Kidney Int. 63(5), 1934–1943 (2003)

Vos, P.F., Zilch, O., Jennekens-Schinkel, A., et al.: Effect of short daily home haemodialysis on quality of life, cognitive functioning and the electroencephalogram. Nephrol. Dial. Transplant. 21(9), 2529–2535 (2006)

Wolfe, R.A., Ashby, V.B., Milford, E.L., et al.: Comparison of Mortality in All Patients on Dialysis, Patients on Dialysis Awaiting Transplantation, and Recipients of a First Cadaveric Transplant. N N Engl. J. Med. 341(23), 1725–1730 (1999)

Zhang, A.H., Bargman, J.M., Lok, C.E., et al.: Dialysis modality choices among chronic kidney disease patients: identifying the gaps to support patients on home-based therapies. Int. Urol. Nephrol. 42(3), 759–764 (2010)

ESSAY QUESTIONS

1. Changing the settings of the hemodialysis machine such as blood and dialysate pumps speeds can affect solute clearance. The degree of impact depends on the solute and the frequency and duration of dialysis. Explain how to optimize the blood and dialysate pump speeds for someone on conventional hemodialysis versus home nocturnal hemodialysis, and explain the reasoning for how these settings will be selected.

2. Discuss how to decide whether a patient receiving hemodialysis is "adequately" dialyzed. Would the approach to assessing dialysis adequacy be different for a patient being dialyzed conventionally versus a patient receiving an intensive form of hemodialysis?

3. Patient safety is an important priority for a dialysis program. Discuss some policies and procedures that you would put in place to maximize patient safety in a home hemodialysis program if you were the program's medical director.

4. You would like to start a home hemodialysis program in order to offer home short daily and quotidian home nocturnal hemodialysis. However, the hospital-based dialysis program where you work is reluctant to support this initiative. They are concerned about the economic viability of a home hemodialysis program. Discuss the potential economic advantages of intensive hemodialysis that would be used to try to convince your administration to support this initiative, and discuss where there might be economic risks to this undertaking.

5. Increasing the duration of a hemodialysis session can increase the clearance of retention products. Discuss the important characteristics of a retention product that determine how its clearance would change with a longer treatment time.

6. Discuss what you would consider to be the imprtant elements of a system for delivering hemodialysis in the home that would allow more people to perform hemodialysis independently than what is possible currently.

7. While the term "uremia" is commonly used in nephrology, it is a difficult term to define. Discuss the important elements of the uremic syndrome, and how one might try to determine if a patient was uremic.

8. There are few randomized trials comparing different doses of hemodialysis, and of those that are available, most are small in size and had a short duration of follow-up. Discuss why randomized trials are important in general, and why randomized trials are so desirable when comparing different methods of providing dialysis. Discuss some of the barriers that exist that make randomized trials difficult to perform in this area, and how these barriers might be overcome.

9. When considering a patient receiving quotidian home nocturnal hemodialysis, what would need to be done to avoid "over-dialysis".

10. Discuss which patients could be considered to be good candidates for an intensive hemodialysis prescription.

MULTIPLE CHOICE QUESTIONS

Choose the best answer

1. In the United States, the typical conventional hemodialysis session lasts for:
   A. 2 hours
   B. 2.5 hours
   C. 3 hours
   D. 3.5 hours
   E. 4 hours

2. In Europe, the typical conventional hemodialysis session lasts for:
   A. 2 hours
   B. 2.5 hours
   C. 3 hours
   D. 3.5 hours
   E. 4 hours

3. Which of the following safety concerns is of the greatest danger to a home short daily hemodialysis patient?
   A. venous needle disconnection
   B. excessively high ultrafiltration rate
   C. air embolism
   D. heparin overdose
   E. membrane rupture leading to blood in the dialysate

4. Which of the following safety concerns is of the greatest danger to a home nocturnal daily hemodialysis patient?
    A. venous needle disconnection
    B. excessively high ultrafiltration rate
    C. air embolism
    D. heparin overdose
    E. membrane rupture leading to blood in the dialysate

5. Mortality amongst older conventional hemodialysis patients is how much higher than age-matched healthy individuals?
    A. It is the same
    B. 2x higher
    C. 10x higher
    D. 100x higher
    E. 1000x higher

6. Mortality amongst young conventional hemodialysis patients is how much higher than age-matched healthy individuals?
    A. It is the same
    B. 2x higher
    C. 10x higher
    D. 100x higher
    E. 1000x higher

7. Excessively high ultrafiltration rates are associated with increased mortality. Exceed what ultrafiltration rate has been associated with increasing mortality?
    A. 10 mL/h/kg
    B. 15 mL/h/kg
    C. 20 mL/h/kg
    D. 25 mL/h/kg
    E. 30 mL/h/kg

8. Quotidian is another terms for:
    A. intensive
    B. of long duration
    C. of short duration
    D. performed in the home
    E. daily

9. Clearance by hemodialysis of which of the following solutes best reflects the clearance of middle molecules?
 A. potassium
 B. urea
 C. creatinine
 D. sodium
 E. phosphate

10. When compared to conventional hemodialysis treatments (3 times per week for 4 hours), long intermittent hemodialysis treatments (3 times per week for 6 – 8 hours) are expected to be associated with:
 A. less fluid gain between treatments and a lower hourly ultrafiltration rate
 B. more fluid gain between treatments, but a lower hourly ultrafiltration rate
 C. the same fluid gain between treatments, but a lower hourly ultrafiltration rate
 D. more fluid gain between treatments and a higher hourly ultrafiltration rate
 E. none of the above

11. Which of the following measures of small solute clearance was developed to improve the accuracy of the single pool Kt/V_{urea} by adjusting for post-dialysis rebound in levels of retention products?
 A. urea reduction ratio (URR)
 B. equilibrated Kt/V_{urea} (eKt/V_{urea})
 C. standardized Kt/V_{urea} ($stdKt/V_{urea}$)
 D. post-dialysis blood urea level
 E. post-dialysis serum creatinine level

12. Which of the following measures of small solute clearance was developed to allow for comparison of solute clearances between different types of dialysis?
 A. urea reduction ratio (URR)
 B. equilibrated Kt/V_{urea} (eKt/V_{urea})
 C. standardized Kt/V_{urea} ($stdKt/V_{urea}$)
 D. post-dialysis blood urea level
 E. post-dialysis serum creatinine level

13. Database studies would suggest that patients receiving nocturnal hemodialysis have survival rates that are:
   A. better than all forms of transplantation
   B. worse than all forms of transplantation
   C. the same as for all forms of transplantation
   D. similar to deceased donor transplantation, but worse than live donor transplantation
   E. similar to live donor transplantation, but worse than deceased donor transplantation

14. Which of the following is NOT commonly needed in quotidian nocturnal hemodialysis patients to prevent "overdialysis"
   a) increased dialysate potassium
   b) addition of sodium phosphate to the dialysate
   c) a lower dialysate calcium
   d) a lower dialysate bicarbonate
   e) none of the above

15. Which of the following is true regarding urea?
   A. it is a large molecule that it likely to be the major cause of uremia
   B. it is a small molecule that is not likely to be the major cause of uremia
   C. it is a small molecule that is likely to be the major cause of uremia
   D. it is a large molecule that is not likely to be the major cause of uremia
   E. none of the above

16. The most significant adverse effect of intensive hemodialysis seen in randomized trials to date is:
   A. reduced bone density
   B. higher blood pressure
   C. lower quality of life
   D. increased hospitalization
   E. more frequent access-related complications

17. What is the typical blood volume for an average sized man?
   A. 5 litres
   B. 7.5 litres
   C. 10 litres
   D. 12.5 litres
   E. 15 litres

18. The HEMO study main results demonstrated:
   A. both higher dialysis dose and high flux membranes reduced mortality
   B. higher dialysis dose reduced mortality, but high flux membranes did not
   C. high flux membranes reduced mortality, but higher dialysis dose did not
   D. neither higher dialysis dose, nor high flux membranes reduced mortality
   E. both higher dialysis dose and high flux membranes increased mortality

19. The group from Tassin, France has used which form of hemodialysis as their standard form of in-centre dialysis:
   A. short daily hemodialysis
   B. quotidian nocturnal hemodialysis
   C. intermittent nocturnal hemodialysis
   D. long intermittent hemodialysis
   E. conventional hemodialysis

20. Which of the following are important contributors to the uremic syndrome?
   A. high levels of retention products
   B. chronic volume overload
   C. effects of comorbid conditions
   D. other sequelae of kidney failure (ex. anemia, acidosis)
   E. all of the above

Chapter (5)

Vascular Access For Hemodialysis Therapy

A.S. Bode, J.H.M. Tordoir

CHAPTER OUTLINES

- End-stage renal disease
- History of vascular access
- Options for vascular access
- Pre-operative work-up
- Using the arteriovenous fistula
- Vascular access complications and their treatment
- Hemodynamic aspects of arteriovenous fistula
- Conclusion and future directions for vascular access

CHAPTER OBJECTIVES

- Elaborate on the different options for vascular access creation
- Elaborate on pre-operative imaging and clinical decision making
- Elaborate on vascular access complications and their treatment
- Elaborate on the hemodynamic changes associated with vascular access creation

KEY TERMS

- End-stage renal disease
- Vascular access
- Arteriovenous fistula
- Arteriovenous graft
- Central venous catheter
- Duplex ultrasonography
- Digital subtraction angiography
- Magnetic resonance angiography
- Cannulation
- Non-maturation
- Stenosis / Thrombosis
- Aneurysm
- Distal ischemia
- Cardiac failure
- Central venous obstruction
- Hemodynamics

ABSTRACT

Therapeutic options for patients suffering from end-stage renal disease have improved tremendously over the last decades and can be divided into three categories: hemodialysis, peritoneal dialysis and kidney transplantation. Transplantation remains the treatment of choice, however, lack of donor organs results in the necessity of performing -temporary-dialysis therapies of which hemodialysis is carried out in the majority of patients.

A.T. Azar (Ed.): Modelling and Control of Dialysis Systems, SCI 404, pp. 235–303.
springerlink.com   © Springer-Verlag Berlin Heidelberg 2013

To facilitate adequate hemodialysis therapy a reliable vascular access is mandatory and can be provided by either surgically connecting an artery with a vein (arteriovenous fistula), surgically connecting an artery with a vein using an interposition of prosthetic graft material (arteriovenous graft) or a central venous catheter. This chapter shortly reviews the condition of end-stage renal disease after which history of vascular access, different options to create a vascular access, pre-operative work-up, surgical procedure, monitoring and usage, post-operative complications and the role of hemodynamics will be discussed. Finally, some future directions for vascular access creation and management will be identified.

5.1 END-STAGE RENAL DISEASE

The kidneys play an important role in maintaining homeostasis inside the human body by their ability to remove metabolic waste products, electrolytes and water from the circulating blood. When the kidneys are no longer able to function at a level needed for daily life, end-stage renal disease (ESRD) occurs. In most patients ESRD is the result of chronic kidney disease (CKD), characterized by a gradual decline in renal function until the capacity of the kidneys is decreased to 5-10% of their original function. Among others, diabetes and high blood pressure are the most common causes for CKD (NKF-K/DOQI 2002). On the other hand acute renal failure (ARF), which comprises a rapid loss of kidney function (in less than 48 hours) induced by either pre-renal, intrinsic or post-renal causes, may also result in -temporary- kidney failure. In both scenarios, the decline in renal function is quantified by the reduction in glomerular filtration rate (GFR), and decreased creatinine clearance rate.

Over the last decades, ESRD has been more and more recognized as a global public health problem with an increasing incidence and prevalence. Based on previous reports (Moeller et al. 2002; Grassmann et al. 2005) and current developments in global registries, Meichelboeck (2010) estimated that the total number of patients with ESRD requiring treatment increased from 1.479.000 in 2001 to 2.310.000 in 2008 (+56%). For these patients, the only treatment option consists of renal replacement therapy (RRT) by modalities such as hemodialysis (HD), peritoneal dialysis (PD) or renal transplantation (NTx). Despite the latter one being the treatment of choice, the number of available donor kidneys is not sufficient to treat all ESRD patients and results in an average time of 4 – 5 years on a surgical waiting list. Therefore, alternative treatment modalities (HD + PD) have to be temporarily exploited before transplantation can take place.

A population analysis by Fresenius Medical Care reveals that the burden on these modalities will continue to increase: approximately 5.5 million patients will be depending on RRT in 2030 (see Fig. 5.1).

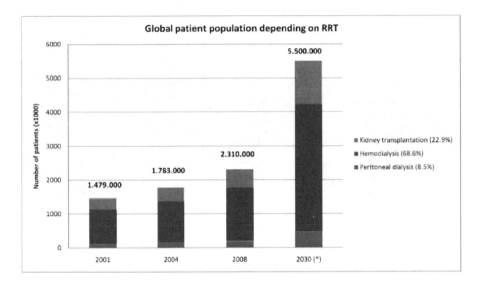

Fig. 5.1 Development of the global ESRD patient population in need of renal replacement therapy over the years 2001, 2004 and 2008 regarding the 3 different treatment modalities (Moeller et al. 2002; Grassmann et al. 2005). Based on the observed growth rates the burden on renal replacement therapy will increase tremendously to a total of approximately 5.5 million by the year 2030 (* extrapolation of global registries based on current growth rates).

Both HD and PD are based on removing waste products from the body by diffusion over a semi-permeable membrane (see Fig.5.2). PD uses the peritoneum (layer of cells covering the abdominal cavity) as a membrane where diffusion takes place between blood vessels and dialysate. This dialysate is inserted in the abdominal cavity by a trans-abdominal catheter which is evacuated and replaced by fresh dialysate after a few hours. In HD blood is extracted from the circulatory system and purified in an artificial kidney where dialysate is flowing in opposite direction to blood. This counter-current flow maximizes the concentration gradient across the membrane to increase the efficiency of HD. The most important requirement for efficient HD therapy is a reliable access to the circulation where blood can be extracted for purification and returned afterwards (see Fig. 5.3).

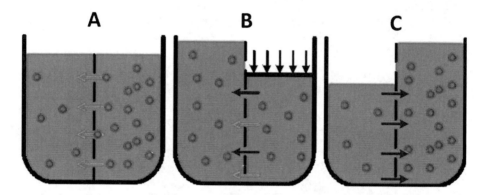

Fig. 5.2 A) Process of diffusion: the exchange of molecules dissolved in a solute over a semi-permeable membrane due to a concentration gradient. By adjusting the concentration of chemicals in the dialysate, the dialysis prescription can be changed to the individual need of a patient. **B)** Process of ultrafiltration: fluid flow over the semi-permeable membrane, forced by a pressure gradient. Consequently, the volume of fluid removed from the patient can be adjusted directly in order to achieve the prescribed weight loss. **C)** The process of osmosis: movement of water over a semi-permeable membrane induced by a difference in solutes.

5.2 HISTORY OF VASCULAR ACCESS

In 1924, Georg Haas performed the first HD treatment as an effort to sustain life and to relieve the features of uremia. Until 1929 he performed 11 treatments in uremic patients whereby he used glass cannulas inserted in the radial artery and a cubital vein for withdrawal and returning of blood. His efforts were continued in 1943 by Willem Kolff who initiated

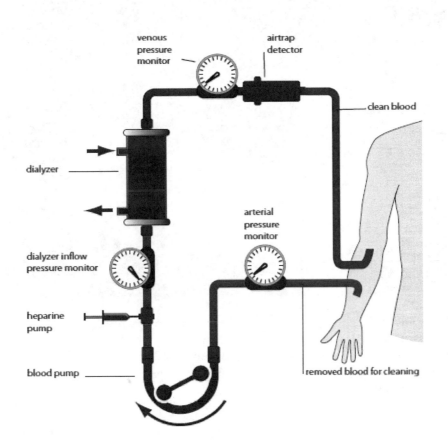

Fig. 5.3 Schematic visualization of a hemodialysis circuit

the development of HD treatment as we know it today. He used a rotating drum kidney (see Fig. 5.4) for extracorporeal purification of blood. Cannulation of the femoral or radial artery was performed for extraction of blood together with cannulation of a large caliber vein for reinfusion. However, severe bleeding after surgical cut down on the one hand and clotting of the extracorporeal circuit due to mismanagement in anticoagulation on the other hand resulted in a major limitation for HD treatment. In short: routine HD therapy was hampered by the lack of a reliable access to the circulation.

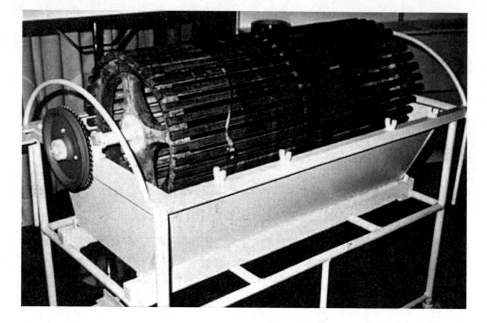

Fig. 5.4 Photograph of the rotating-drum kidney introduced by Willem Kolff in 1943. Blood ran around cellulose tubing which was wound round a drum made of wooden slats, dipping into the 'bath' of dialysate at the bottom of its turn. The movement of blood was powered by the rotation of the drum rather than a blood pump.

The development of the Quinton/Scribner shunt in 1960 resulted in a major breakthrough and represents a landmark in the history of HD: it initiated the possibility of repeated, chronic HD therapy by means of inserting two teflon cannulas: one in the radial artery and one in the adjacent cephalic vein near the wrist (see Fig. 5.5) (Scribner et al. 1960; Quinton et al. 1960). Connecting these cannulas by a silicon rubber bypass tube resulted in a low resistance high flow rate conduit which was suitable for repetitive cannulation. Nevertheless, frequent infections and thrombosis initiated the search for better alternatives.

Only a few years later, Brescia, Cimino and Appel created an internal arteriovenous fistula (AVF) by subcutaneously connecting the radial artery in the wrist to the adjacent cephalic vein using a side-to-side anastomosis (Brescia et al. 1966). Beside the fact that the change in approach resulted in less infectious and thrombotic complications, minimal post-operative problems were encountered using their technique: only two out of 15 operations failed.

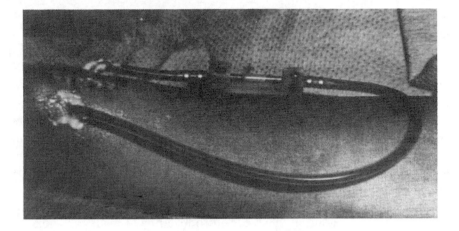

Fig. 5.5 Quinton/Scribner shunt

In the following years, several variations regarding fistula location and anastomotic technique were investigated and minor adjustments were implemented. For example, Gracz and co-workers investigated the possibility of creating a autologous AVF in the proximal forearm by connecting the perforating vein in the elbow to the brachial, radial or ulnar artery which got wide-spread acceptance (Gracz et al. 1977). After these developments, the only hurdle which had to be taken was to come up with a solution in patients with no suitable peripheral veins for autologous AVF creation.

A proposal from James May and Gilberto Flores-Izquierdo in 1969 resulted in creation of a fistula in which a segment of the saphenous vein was implanted between the brachial artery and a proper vein in the elbow (May et al. 1969; Flores Izquierdo et al. 1969). Subsequent steps focused on the development of prosthetic graft material in order not to be dependent on autologous veins. Expanded polytetrafluorethylene (ePTFE) was introduced in vascular surgery in 1972 and was investigated by Baker and co-workers for the creation of a VA. Their first publication in 1976 reported on the results of the use of ePTFE as a VA in 72 HD patients (Baker et al. 1976). Until today, numerous publications established the value of this prosthetic graft material and identified its pro's and con's in the dialysis population. Despite the aforementioned improvements in VA surgery, AVF and AVG functioning was hampered by complications. In particular the development of stenosis within the VA conduit resulted in poor patency rates.

In 1967 Charles Dotter and co-workers performed a transluminal reca-
nalization of an atherosclerotic obstruction and preluded the development
of modern percutaneous angioplasty, which is able to deal with luminal
narrowing within the VA conduit by endovascular dilatation of stenoses
with the use of a balloon (Dotter et al. 1967). Identification of these stenotic lesions became easy with the introduction of digital subtraction angiography (DSA) in 1979 (Ergun et al. 1979). In DSA, images are acquired by
exposing an area of interest with time-controlled x-rays while injecting
contrast medium into the blood vessels. The era of the percutaneous transluminal angioplasty of VA started with a publication by Gordon et al
(1982): "treatment of stenotic lesions in dialysis access fistulae and shunts
by transluminal angioplasty". Another important development in VA creation came from Shaldon in 1961. He introduced hand-made catheters for
insertion in the femoral artery and vein using the percuteneous Seldinger
technique (Seldinger 1953; Shaldon et al. 1961). In the following years,
other vessels proved to be suitable as well: cannulation of the subclavian
vein became the preferred method of temporary VA creation. The current
opinion regarding central venous catheters (CVC) as a VA will be discussed further on.

5.3 OPTIONS FOR VASCULAR ACCESS

For a VA to be suitable for HD, certain criteria need to be met.
Firstly, the VA needs to provide a high flow (usually in excess of 400
ml/min) to allow efficient withdrawal of blood from the circulation as
well as to prevent the VA from clotting. Secondly, the VA needs to be
suitable for repetitive cannulation: a superficial cannulation traject with
a sufficient length and diameter are mandatory to protect the patient
from complications following miscannulation. Furthermore, the VA
should have a good primary patency, have a low risk of complications
and side effects, and leave opportunities for future procedures in the
event of failure. Although the ideal VA conduit does not exist, there are
multiple options for access creation each having specific advantages and
disadvantages. Nowadays, decision-making in clinical practice takes
place according to pre-operative vascular imaging combined with knowledge regarding post-operative complications and patency rates for each
configuration. Vascular imaging is performed to determine arterial and

venous diameters and their continuity within the upper extremity. Several observational studies investigated the relation between minimal arterial and venous diameters and the risk of early failure and nonmaturation (Wong et al. 1996; Silva et al. 1998; Malovrh 2002; NKF-K/DOQI 2001; Tordoir et al. 2007) (see Table 5.1) and thereby importantly influence the strategy in VA creation.

Table 5.1 Minimal vascular diameters for successful creation of a radiocephalic fistula

Study	Radial artery diameter (mm)	Cephalic vein diameter (mm)
Wong et al (1996)	1.6	1.6
Silva et al (1998)	2.0	2.5
Malovrh (2002)	1.5	1.6
KDOQI Guideline (National Kidney Foundation 2001)	2.0	2.5
European Guideline (Tordoir et al. 2007)	2.0	2.0

Regarding post-operative VA patency, the following definitions are applied (Sidawy et al. 2002):

Primary patency: Primary patency (intervention-free access survival) is defined as the interval from time of access placement to any intervention designed to maintain or reestablish patency or to access thrombosis or the time of measurement of patency.

Assisted primary patency: Assisted primary patency (thrombosis-free access survival) is defined as the interval from time of access placement to access thrombosis or time of measurement of patency, including intervening manipulations (surgical or endovascular interventions) designed to *maintain* the functionality of a patent access

Secondary patency: Secondary patency (access survival until abandonment) is defined as the interval from time of access placement to access abandonment or time of measurement of patency, including intervening manipulations (surgical or endovascular interventions) designed to *reestablish* the functionality of thrombosed access

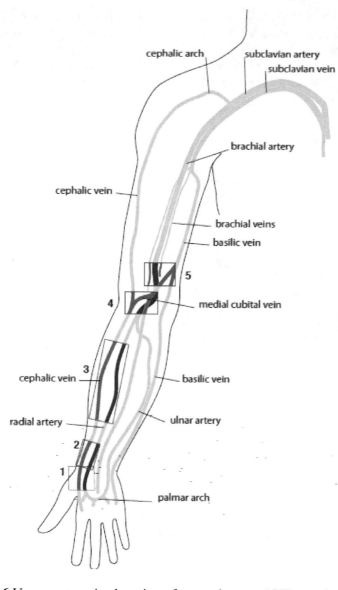

Fig. 5.6 Upper extremity locations for autologous AVF creation. **1)** Arteriovenous fistula at the anatomic snuffbox between the radial artery and the cephalic vein. **2)** Arteriovenous fistula at the level of the wrist between the radial artery and the cephalic vein. **3)** Location for proximalization of an arteriovenous anastomosis after failure at wrist level. **4)** Arteriovenous fistula at the level of the elbow between the brachial artery and the cephalic vein / medial cubital vein. **5)** Arteriovenous fistula at the level of the elbow between the brachial artery and the basilic vein.

According to the NKF-K/DOQI guidelines (NKF-K/DOQI 2001), a direct surgical connection between an artery and a vein as distal as possible in the upper extremity on the non-dominant side is preferred in patients requiring long-term HD. In case distal vascular diameters are not suitable for creation of an AVF, more proximal vessels are utilized (see Fig. 5.6). When proximal vascular diameters are still not suitable or in case autologous vessels are no longer available, the second option is the creation of an AVG, where prosthetic material is used to make the connection. When HD therapy needs to be initiated before either an AVF or AVG is created, a CVC can be used as a temporary VA. However, CVC use should be minimized because of increased risk of sepsis, increased mortality, and development of central venous stenosis or thrombosis which comprises future VA procedures in the ipsilateral upper limb. Unfortunately, many patients require a CVC either to start dialysis or as a bridge between AVF failure and the creation of a new VA.

5.3.1 Primary Vascular Access

A distal radiocephalic arteriovenous fistula (RC-AVF) is considered the best option for initial VA in the vast majority of patients. Although creation of a RC-AVF may be compromised by insufficient vascular diameters or a diseased cephalic vein, post-operative flow enhancement and dilatation of the venous cannulation traject are usually sufficient to meet the demands for dialysis prescription. Furthermore, it leaves more proximal sites for future procedures in the event of failure. To preserve the possibility of distal RC-AVF creation, it is crucial to avoid cannulation of the cephalic vein after the diagnosis ESRD has been established.

After successful creation of a RC-AVF it may function for years with a minimum of complications, revisions and interventions. On the long term, RC-AVFs have a low incidence of thrombosis (0.2 events per patient per year) and infection (2%) compared to more proximal AVFs and the use of grafts. However, relatively high numbers of early thrombosis and nonmaturation are important disadvantages of this fistula configuration. Observational studies report early failure rates varying from 5% to 46% and secondary patency rates from 42% to 83% after one year of follow-up (Silva et al. 1998; Golledge et al. 1999; Wolowczyk et al. 2000; Gibson et al. 2001; Allon et al. 2001; Dixon et al. 2002; Ravani et al. 2002; Rooijens et al. 2004; Biuckians et al. 2008; Huijbregts et al. 2008) (see Table 5.2).

Table 5.2 Failure rates and secundary patency rates of radiocephalic fistulas

Study	Number of AVFs	Early failure (%)	1-year patency (%)
Silva et al (1998)	108	26	83
Golledge et al (1999)	107	18	69
Wolowczyk et al (2000)	208	20	65
Gibson et al (2001)	130	23	56
Allon et al (2001)	139	46	42
Dixon et al (2002)	205	30	53
Ravani et al (2002)	197	5	71
Rooijens et al (2004)	86	41	52
Biuckians et al (2008)	80	37	63
Huijbregts et al (2008)	649	30	70

Older studies incorporated in the meta-analysis performed by Rooijens et al (2004) identified lower primary failure rates (17%), which might be explained by the increase in comorbidities in the ESRD patient population nowadays. Compared to men, women have poorer patency rates which might advocate more proximal AVF creation if the cephalic vein or radial artery is small. When a wrist RC-AVF has failed or is impossible to create, a more proximally located anastomosis from the mid-forearm to the elbow between the radial artery and cephalic vein may be employed before resorting to secondary autologous VA.

Surgical Technique

The patient is positioned on the operating table with the arm in 90 degrees of abduction. Subsequently, venous congestion pressure is applied after which the radial artery and the cephalic vein together with their first order side branches are marked on the skin: the preferred location for the incision is identified. After release of the tourniquet disinfection of the arm can take place. Ideally this procedure is carried out under local or regional anesthesia instead of general anesthesia which is associated with decreased blood pressures during surgery. This procedural drop in blood pressure restricts post-operative flow enhancement and increases the risk of immediate post-operative thrombosis. A local subcutaneous injection of lidocaine 1% (without epinephrine) is usually sufficient to create this type of VA. Some studies have described a beneficiary effect of regional anesthesia: peripheral vasodilatation which potentially results a larger post-operative flow enhancement (Malinzak and Gan 2009; Yildirim et al. 2006).

After a longitudinal or transverse incision near the wrist, the cephalic vein and radial artery are dissected from their surrounding tissue. Next, the cephalic vein is mobilized towards the radial artery where the anastomosis will be created (see Fig. 5.7).

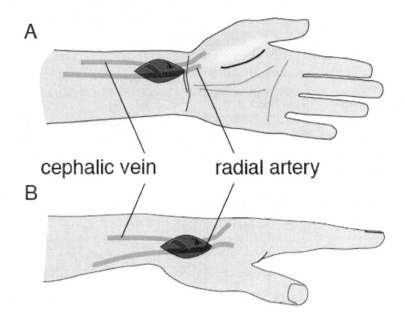

Fig. 5.7 Surgical creation of a radiocephalic fistula **A)** at the level of the wrist, and **B)** at the level of the anatomic snuffbox.

For the RC-AVF, four types of anastomosis can be employed (see Fig. 5.8).

- *End-to-side anastomosis:* Connecting the end of the cephalic vein to the side of the radial artery. This is the most common technique for creating a RC-AVF because it reduces the risk of venous hypertension distally of the anastomosis. Also, by connecting the end of the vein to the side of the artery, retrograde flow from the distal radial artery can enter the fistula conduit. This retrograde flow originates from the ulnar artery and enters the distal radial artery through the palmar arch. Approximately 30% of total fistula flow is generated by retrograde flow which in some patients may induce hemodialysis access induced distal ischemia (HAIDI). These symptoms can be treated by ligating the radial artery distally of the anastomosis, and results in a functional end-to-end fistula configuration.

- *Side-to-side anastomosis:* Connecting the side of the cephalic vein to the side of the radial artery. This anastomosis configuration results in the largest increase in post-operative flow but may result in venous congestion of the hand. Post-operatively, the venous valves distally of the anastomosis are destroyed by the increase of pressure in the vein, resulting in retrograde flow towards the hand.

- *End-to-end anastomosis:* Connecting the end of the cephalic vein to the end of the radial artery: This technique yields the lowest incidence of post-operative HAIDI and venous hypertension but also results in the lowest post-operative flow by excluding retrograde flow from the distal radial artery.

- *Side-to-end anastomosis:* Connecting the side of the cephalic vein to the end of the radial artery. This is not being performed in RC-AVF surgery anymore.
  Its advantages are similar to an end-to-end anastomosis, however it still carries a risk for the development of venous congestion of the hand.

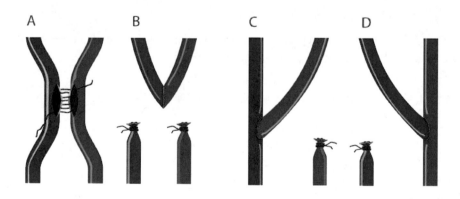

Fig. 5.8 Four different types anastomotic configurations: **A)** Side-to-side anastomosis, **B)** End-to-end anastomosis, **C)** End-to-side anastomosis, and **D)** Side-to-end anastomosis

After appropriate dissection according to the anastomosis technique, coronary dilators are inserted in the radial artery and cephalic vein to measure the actual diameter and to treat any form of vascular spasm by forced dilatation. Before suturing the artery to the vein, heparinized water is used to flush the conduit to prevent the development of clots. A 6-0 or 7-0 polypropylene suture is used for the anastomosis. After completing the anastomosis, the proximal and distal vascular clamps are removed. A soft thrill is felt over the anastomosis, continuing in the venous outflow vein for a moderate distance. Auscultation reveals a soft bruit over the anastomosis. Further exploration should be performed in case pulsation instead of thrill is objectivated which can be caused by obstruction in the venous outflow, e.g. torsion or thrombosis. Intra-operative control by DSA can identify potential problems within the conduit. The incision can be closed using absorbable or non-absorbable sutures.

5.3.2 Secondary Vascular Access

Although the RC-AVF is preferred over any other type of fistula, the first VA procedure in the majority of ESRD patients more and more comprises the upper arm, especially in the dialysis population with associated co-morbidities such as diabetes mellitus, coronary artery disease, and peripheral arterial occlusive disease (Pisoni et al. 2002). In case no more viable options for upper extremity VA are available, one may consider residing to the lower extremity.

5.3.2.1 Forearm Cephalic and Basilic Vein Transposition and Elevation

Forearm vein transposition or elevation results in more possibilities to create a forearm VA. In obese patients it might be necessary to elevate the cephalic vein in order to create a superficial cannulation traject. When the cephalic vein is not suitable due to its size or previous events of thrombophlebitis, the basilic vein can be transposed from the ulnar side to the radial side through a straight subcutaneous tunnel from the elbow to the radial artery.

Alternatively, the basilic vein can also be anastomosed to the ulnar artery, though an additional volar transposition might be necessary to facilitate needling and to improve patient comfort during HD.

Surgical Technique

Positioning and anesthesia are essentially the same as for RC-AVF creation. A longitudinal incision is made from the elbow to the wrist over the course of the vein. After dissection, mobilization, and ligation of side branches a superficial subcutaneous tunnel is created from the elbow to the target artery at the wrist which is already dissected through a separate incision. Subsequently, the vein is passed through the tunnel with special care being taken to avoid torsion. Anastomotic techniques are similar to RC-AVF surgery.

5.3.2.2 Elbow and Upper Arm Cephalic Vein Arteriovenous Fistulas

When forearm fistulas are no longer considered to be an option, more proximal vessel can be utilized for the creation of a autologous AVF. The large caliber brachial artery and the cephalic vein can be anastomosed in the elbow, either directly or by involvement of the perforating vein from the median cubital vein. By ligating the basilic vein proximal to the anastomosis, venous return is directed through the cephalic vein, which results in sufficient dilatation. Brachiocephalic fistulas (BC-AVFs) usually have a high primary function rate and a good 1 year patency (Murphy et al. 2002; Zeebregts et al. 2005; Lok et al. 2005; Woo et al. 2007; Koksoy et al. 2009) (see Table 5.3). The most important disadvantages of upper arm fistulas between the brachial artery and the cephalic vein are the higher incidence of HAIDI and high-output cardiac failure due to relative large flow enhancement.

Table 5.3 Failure rates and secundary patency rates of brachiocephalic fistulas

Study	Number of AVFs	Early failure (%)	1-year patency (%)
Murphy et al (2002)	208	16	75
Zeebregts et al (2005)	100	11	79
Lok et al (2005)	186	9	78
Woo et al (2007)	71	12	66
Koksoy et al (2009)	50	8	87

Surgical Technique

After correct positioning and adequate anesthesia, the superficial antecubital venous system is exposed by a transverse incision in the elbow. Subsequently, the median cubital vein and cephalic vein are dissected and assessed for their continuity with the proximal cephalic vein and the central venous vessels.

In case of large caliber vessels, the perforating branch of the median cubital vein (vena median cubiti profunda) can be identified and used for the anastomosis to limit post-operative flow enhancement. After selection of the most suitable location for the anastomosis, the proximal outflow to the basilic vein is interrupted to ensure maximal dilatation of the cephalic vein. Also the distal cephalic vein is ligated to prevent venous backflow to the hand. Within the selected vein, coronary dilators are used to gently dilate the venous outflow tract and to verify the actual diameters. Next, the brachial artery is exposed by dividing the bicipital aponeurosis after which it is clamped. The arteriotomy should be no more than 5-7 mm to prevent steal syndrome and high output cardiac failure. After flushing the inflow and outflow vessels with heparinized saline, the selected vein is anastomosed to the brachial artery in an end-to-side fashion (see Fig. 5.9). In case the cephalic vein is located too deep in the upper arm, a second stage elevation procedure has to be performed. Post-operatively, 4-6 weeks of maturation have to be taken into account before cannulation can take place.

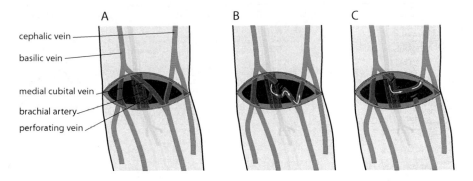

Fig. 5.9 Surgical creation of a brachiocephalic fistula. **A)** vascular anatomy prior to vascular access creation, **B)** Creation of a Gracz fistula by anastomosing the perforating vein of the cubital medial vein to the brachial artery, and **C)** Creation of a brachiocephalic fistula by anastomosing the cephalic vein directly to the brachial artery.

5.3.2.3 Upper Arm Basilic Vein Arteriovenous Fistulas

In case the cephalic vein cannot be used for the creation of an AVF due to previous VA, insufficient diameters or (partial) thrombosis, the more deeply located basilic vein can be utilized. Due to its deep and medial position in the upper arm a superficialization and transposition procedure has

to be performed in order to render the VA suitable for repetitive cannulation. The deep position of the vein also accounts for the absence fibrotic
deformation due to repetitive needling in the past. Patency rates after one
year are reported between 47% to 89%, with primary failure rates of 2% to
23% (Murphy et al. 2002; Koksoy et al. 2009; Segal et al. 2003; Wolford
et al. 2005; Keuter et al. 2008; Harper et al. 2008) (see Table 5.4). Compared with BC-AVFs, brachiobasilic AVFs (BB-AVFs) are more likely to
mature, although they are more susceptible to late thrombosis (Koksoy et
al. 2009). Moreover, the creation of a BB-AVF is preferred over lower
limb VA or the use of prosthetic graft material as evidenced by lower infection and thrombosis rates as well as superior primary and secondary
patency rates (Lazarides et al. 2008).

Table 5.4 Failure rates and secundary patency rates of brachiobasilic
fistulas

Study	Number of AVFs	Early failure (%)	1-year patency (%)
Murphy et al (2002)	74	3	75
Segal et al (2003)	99	23	64
Wolford et al (2005)	100	20	47
Harper et al (2008)	168	23	66
Keuter et al (2008)	52	2	89
Koksoy et al (2009)	50	4	86

Surgical Technique

Although an axillary block eases the procedure significantly, local anesthesia can be used. As described for the BC-AVF, the brachial artery is exposed by dividing the bicipital aponeurosis. Subsequently, a longitudinal
incision on the medial aspect of the upper arm is placed after which the
subfascial basilic vein is mobilized. Special care is taken to preserve the
medial cutaneous nerve of the forearm. During mobilization, venous side
branches are ligated. The vein is ligated distally and a longitudinal mark-
ing on the anterior side is applied to avoid torsion. After creation of a subcutaneous tunnel over the anterior side of the arm, the vein is passed
through and anastomosed to the brachial artery in an end-to-side fashion
(see Fig. 5.10)

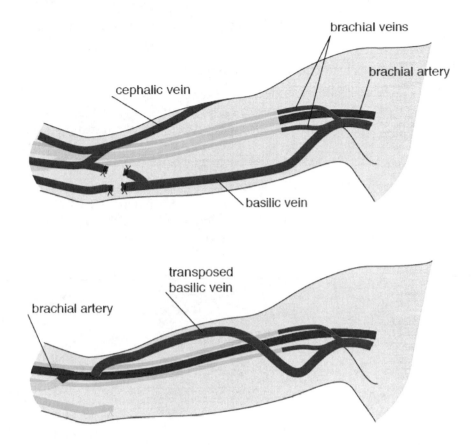

Fig. 5.10 Autologous brachiobasilic arteriovenous fistula. **A)** The basilic vein is completely mobilized from underneath the fascia in continuity with a section of the medial cubital vein through a longitudinal incision. **B)** Then the vein is transposed in a subcutaneous tunnel on the anterior surface of the arm and anastomosed to the brachial artery in an end-to-side fashion.

Alternatively, this procedure can be carried out in two stages. Hereby, the first procedure consists of a small dissection in the elbow in order to anastomose the basilic vein to the brachial artery. After 4-6 weeks of maturation, elevation and transposition are performed in a second procedure. The rationale behind the two-stage procedure is that dissection of the arterialized thick-walled vein is easier after a few weeks of maturation and that size and flow rate of the fistula can be assessed before carrying out the second stage. In case of nonmaturation, the second stage can be abandoned.

5.3.2.4 Nonautologous Prosthetic Vascular Access

When autologous AVF creation in the upper extremity is impossible due to insufficient diameters or when previous fistulas have failed, implantation of prosthetic graft material should be considered the next option. Xenografts such as the ovine sheep (Omniflow) and bovine cow ureter graft (SynerGraft) are popular materials to create an access conduit.

However, the most frequently used grafts are prosthetic ones made of either polyurethane (Vectra) or polytetrafluoroethylene (PTFE). These prosthetic grafts can be implanted on several locations in the upper extremity in either a straight or looped configuration (see Fig. 5.11).

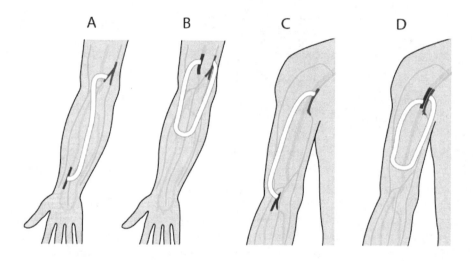

Fig. 5.11 Prosthetic graft configurations in the upper extremity. **A)** Straight forearm arteriovenous graft from the radial artery at the wrist to the antecubital fossa in the elbow, **B)** Looped forearm arteriovenous graft from the brachial or radial artery to the antecubital fossa in the elbow, **C)** Straight upper arm arteriovenous graft from the brachial or radial artery to the axillary vein, **D)** Looped upper arm arteriovenous graft from the axillary artery to the axillary vein.

Short term functional patency is usually good. However, the development of neo-intimal hyperplasia (NIH) with subsequent stenosis increase the risk of thrombotic occlusions. Primary patency rates for prosthetic

AVGs vary from 60% to 80% after 1 year of follow-up and 30% to 40% after 2 years. Secondary patency rates are between 70% to 90% after 1 year and 50% to 70% after 2 years (Glickman et al. 2001; Kaufman et al. 1997; Lenz et al. 1998; Garcia-Pajares et al. 2003). These patency rates can only be obtained with a strict follow-up protocol to diagnose flow decrease at an early stage with subsequent pre-emptive (endovascular) treatment. Measures to improve AVG patency rates have been widely investigated. Changing AVG configuration to create an optimal post-operative hemodynamic profile may have a beneficial effect on the development of NIH as will be argued later on. Improvement of the compliance mismatch between prosthetic graft and both artery and vein was also not proven to delay stenotic obstructions (Hofstra et al. 1994). Also, pharmacological treatment with dipyridamole and apririne showed a significant but modest effect in reducing the risk of stenosis and improved the duration of primary unassisted patency of newly created AVGs (Dixon et al. 2009). Given the available evidence, anti-coagulant agents should be used routinely in patients with AVGs but not in patients with AVFs (Dember et al. 2008).

Surgical Technique

Local, regional and general anesthesia are considered to be an option during placement of an interposition graft between an artery and a vein. Furthermore, a single dose of antibiotics needs to be administered during surgery to reduce the risk of post-procedural infection. Depending on the intended graft configuration, the artery and vein are exposed by either one or two incisions.

Next, a superficial tunnel is created by using a bi-directional tunneling device after which the graft is sewn in an end-to-side fashion. AVG material has the advantage of early cannulation after creation: no period of maturation needs to be taken into account.

5.3.2.5 Lower Limb Vascular Access

In difficult cases, VA surgery can also focus on the thorax or lower extremity (see Fig. 5.12). Probably the only indication for AVF creation in the lower extremity is bilateral central venous obstruction. These obstructions compromise the venous return to the heart and often result in venous hypertension and edema in case an upper extremity fistula is present. The VA conduit in the lower extremity can either be a straight or a looped traject. Initially, the saphenous vein or superficial femoral vein is exploited to create the fistula and result in good patency rates (Antoniou et al. 2009). Pre-operatively, the ankle/ brachial index should be measured to rule out the possibility of peripheral arterial occlusive disease (PAOD) which could be responsible for decreased arterial inflow after VA creation. Post-operatively, a strict follow-up protocol is advocated to monitor for distal hypo-perfusion and infection, in particular when prosthetic graft material is used to create the VA.

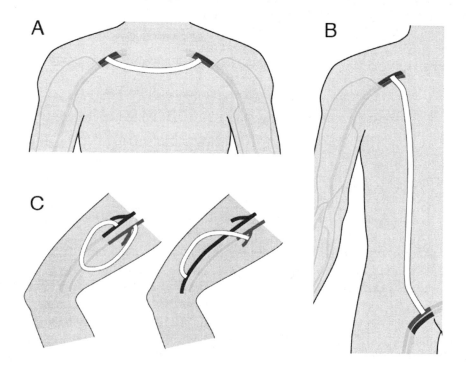

Fig. 5.12 Prosthetic graft configurations for the thorax and lower extremity. **A)** Necklace graft from the subclavian artery on one side to the subclavian vein on the other side, **B)** Straight graft from the axillary artery to the femoral vein, and **C)** Straight and looped prosthetic graft configuration in the lower extremity. Please note that saphenous and superficial femoral vein transposition are the primary options for thigh AV fistulas

A meta-analysis reporting on the outcome of AVFs in the lower extremity distinguishes three different types of VA in the leg: the AVG in the groin, the AVG in the proximal part of the leg and the femoral vein transposition. Mean primary patency after 12 months was 48%, 43% an 83% resp. Mean secondary patency after 12 months was 69%, 67% and 93% resp. Abandonment of the VA occurred more often when a prosthetic graft was used compared to the femoral vein transposition (18% vs. 1.6%; P<0.05). Ischemic complaints manifested more frequently in autologous fistulas when compared to AVGs (21% vs. 7.1%; P<0.05) (Antoniou et al. 2009).

5.3.3 Central Venous Catheters

Temporary CVCs are useful to gain immediate access to the circulation and facilitate HD treatment on short notice. However, the use of this type of VA has some important disadvantages: a shorter usability compared to AVFs, a significant risk of infection and the development of central venous stenosis (Allon 2007). Therefore, placement of a CVC should only be performed in patients with acute renal failure who need immediate dialysis therapy or in patients with chronic renal failure in whom a permanent VA by means of a fistula or graft is not a viable option or has not matured yet. Also, patients with limited life expectancy, severe HAIDI or cardiac failure may be better off using a CVC. The last indication for temporary dialysis by means of a CVC is in patients with a renal transplantation in the near future. Two types of catheters are used in clinical practice: non-tunneled catheters with a limited use and high morbidity; and tunneled catheters, which can be used for several months or even years (see Fig. 5.13).

5.3.3.1 Non-tunneled Catheters

Non-tunneled catheters enable simple and direct cannulation of the internal jugular vein, the subclavian vein or the femoral vein. Preferably, the subclavian vein should not be used for indwelling CVCs because of the very high risk of subsequent venous stenosis (Schillinger et al.1991). Procedural fluoroscopic guidance is advised to rule out the possibility of pneumothorax and to establish correct intravenous positioning (Hameeteman et al. 2010). It is recommended that the use of non-tunneled catheters does not exceed 7 days.

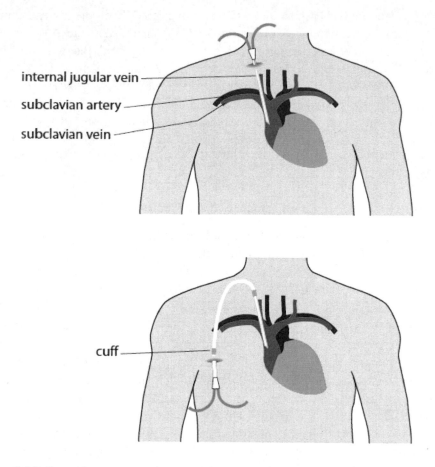

internal jugular vein

subclavian artery

subclavian vein

cuff

Fig. 5.13 Central venous catheters: **A)** Non-tunneled central venous catheter, and **B)** Tunneled central venous catheter

5.3.3.2 Tunneled Catheters

Tunneled CVCs are associated with reduced morbidity rates as well as better performance compared to non-tunneled CVCs (Weijmer and ter Wee 2004). Therefore, tunneled CVCs are preferred in patients with an expected need for HD longer than 3 weeks or in whom a VA is maturing but who require immediate HD. After insertion of the catheter in the internal jugular or femoral vein, a subcutaneous tunnel is created to divert the exit site of the catheter. At the exit point, a Dacron cuff is present which will adhese to the subcutis and prevents the catheter for dislocation and reduces infection rates.

5.3.3.3 Catheter Infection

Compared to patients with an AVF, patients with CVCs have an increased relative mortality risk, most likely because of higher infection rates (Allon et al. 2006). These catheter related infections can be divided into three categories: exit site infections, tunnel infections and generalized bacteremia. Although treatment options are feasible in tunneled catheters, non-tunneled catheters should always be removed. There is no role for trying to salvage temporary catheters. In tunneled catheters, exit site infections usually present as a mild cellulitis around the exit site. These infections respond well to systemic antibiotic therapy and therefore catheter removal is not required. When this infection is not recognized, it might progress to a tunnel infection, characterized by erythema over an area more than 2 cm from the exit site. Purulent discharge may be noticed in these patients, who also complain about fever, pain, swelling, fluctuance, and erythema along the track of the catheter. Untreated tunnel infections potentially result in generalized bacteremia. Opposite to exit site infections, tunnel infections do not respond well to systemic antibiotic therapy due to limited vascular supply in the involved area in combination with the presence of a foreign body: catheter removal is inevitable (NKF-K/DOQI 2001).

Generalized bacteremia should always be considered if a patient with a CVC presents with a fever without a clear focus. Blood specimens taken from peripheral vessels as well as from the CVC are examined for pathogens. Both gram-positive and gram negative organisms have been reported to be responsible for catheter related bacteremia, yet, the Staphylococcus is the most common one (Weijmer et al. 2005). Awaiting the results of the culture, systemic broad-spectrum antibiotic therapy should be initiated which is later on adjusted to the culture results and the local microbiologic epidemiology. The treatment plan in generalized bacteremia asks for catheter removal. Although, before catheter removal is considered it is recommended to wait for the initial response to antibiotic treatment (30% response rate). Furthermore, the presence of metastatic complications, the responsible pathogen, and the availability of other VA sites must be taken in to account in this decision. In case of catheter removal, a new VA needs to be established by placement of a new temporary catheter at another location.

5.3.3.4 Catheter Obstruction

Besides infection, catheter function may be hampered by catheter obstruction caused by endoluminal fibrin deposits and results in insufficient
flows and pressure alarms during the dialysis session. It is of utmost importance to prevent formation of these clots during the interdialytic period
by installing an antithrombotic lock solution within the lumen of the catheter (Allon 2007). Leakage of this solution in the circulation may increase
the risk of hemorrhage. Dysfunctional catheters may be corrected by administration of a fibrinolytic agent (urokinase / tPA) as a lock solution or
by using a mechanical approach (brush). As a final option, the catheter can
be replaced over a guide wire.

5.4 PRE-OPERATIVE WORK-UP

Patients diagnosed with ESRD should be instructed to abstain from ve-
nipunctures in the upper extremity (except the dorsum of the hand) in order to prevent formation of scar tissue: fibrotic changes in the venous wall
hamper dilatation after AVF surgery. When patients approach initiation of
dialysis therapy, referral to a VA surgeon is mandatory. Following pre-
operative examinations, the surgical procedure is performed after which a
period of maturation has to be taken into account before repetitive cannulation can take place. Here, the possibilities of pre-operative work-up are
discussed.

5.4.1 Medical History and Physical Examination

A thorough medical history allows the surgeon to identify patients with
an increased risk for post-operative complications at an early stage. Studies
showed that the chance of successful creation and utilization of a VA is
decreased in women, negroid patients, as well as in patients with diabetes,
peripheral arterial disease and multiple attempts for VA creation in the past
(Allon et al. 2000; Tordoir et al. 2003). When medical history is combined
with physical examination, a first impression regarding the quality of the
vessels can be obtained. For the veins, diameters and distension are estimated after application of a venous congestion pressure. Also, the length
of the future cannulation segment and its corresponding depth are recorded. The arteries are examined by palpation to evaluate the quality of arterial pulsations. Additionally, blood pressure measurements on both arms are
performed to rule out a significant arterial inflow stenosis.

Finally, inspection of the neck should take place to identify collateral veins and skin lesions due to previous indwelling CVCs: previous CVCs might hamper successful creation of an AVF due to central venous stenosis. Besides that interpretation of the physical examination depends on the experience of the physician, less straightforward results may be obtained in obese patients due to a deeper location of the vessels (Mihmanli et al. 2001). When solely depending on results of physical examination, proximal vessels and prosthetic material might be used despite sufficient quality of vessels in the distal forearm. Therefore, objective imaging of arterial and venous structures in the upper extremity is necessary which can be provided by duplex ultrasonography (DUS).

5.4.2 Duplex Ultrasonography

Due to its non-invasive character, clinical availability and low costs, DUS is an important technique to objectively evaluate the vasculature prior to AVF creation. Several studies show that routine DUS examination is responsible for a change in surgical approach: Allon et al (2001) registered an increase in autologous fistula creation when DUS examination was performed instead of only physical examination (64% vs. 34%). The same study showed that the patient population with successful HD on an AVF could be doubled (16% vs. 34%) when a pre-operative DUS examination is performed. Research by Silva et al (1998) reports an increase in the construction of AVFs (from 14% to 63%), a reduction of the use of prosthetic graft material (from 62% to 30%), and a reduction of primary catheter use (from 24% to 7%) when pre-operative mapping of arteries and veins is performed using DUS. However, despite the positive influence of pre-operative DUS, there is still no consensus on the parameters of the examination and how the results should be interpreted.

According to the European Best Practice Guidelines (EBPG) (Tordoir et al. 2007), the complete upper extremity vascular tree should be visualized; from the subclavian artery to the arteries in the wrist and from the distal cephalic and basilic vein to the subclavian vein. Over these vessels diameter, course, continuity, side branches and possible stenotic segments need to be identified. During the examination it is important to apply a venous congestion pressure to induce dilation of the veins, which results in reliable and reproducible measurements (Planken et al. 2006). Examples of arterial and venous DUS acquisitions are visualized in (see Fig. 5.14).

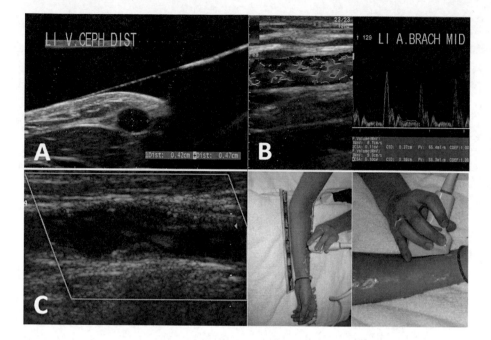

Fig. 5.14 Pre-operative duplex ultrasound examination. **A)** Axial venous diameter measurements are performed on multiple locations over the cephalic and basilic vein together with **B)** longitudinal diameter and flow measurments over the radial, ulnar, brachial and subclavian artery. Furthermore, the detection of pre-existing stenoses (**C**) may influence clinical decision making.

To determine the most optimal location for AVF creation and which vessels should be utilized depends on arterial and venous diameter measurements (Wong et al. 1996; Silva et al. 1998; Malovrh 2002). The guidelines from the Vascular Access Society advocate AVF creation at the most distal location where both artery and vein have a diameter >2.0 mm. American guidelines are more conservative with a venous diameter >2.5 mm (see Table 5.1). Despite the duplex induced increase in autologous AVF creation, DUS has an important limitation: central vessels cannot be visualized adequately due to the location behind the clavicula. As a result, central venous stenoses and arterial inflow stenoses are difficult to identify. For sufficient depiction of these vessels, other imaging techniques have to be employed, particularly in patients with an increased risk for central venous stenoses (multiple CVCs in the past) or when a difference in blood pressure between both arms is registered.

5.4.3 Digital Subtraction Angiography

Additional pre-operative imaging can be performed by means of digital subtraction angiography (DSA). Depending on the position of an intravenous catheter, arterial and venous structures can be visualized separately by injecting a contrast agent during x-ray examination. Although the acquired images are two-dimensional, detailed information regarding the *complete* arterial and venous vascular tree can be obtained. Moreover, stenoses, occlusions, side branches and collateral pathways can be identified easily (see Fig. 5.15).

Although a more thorough vascular evaluation can be performed, DSA has a very important limitation which prevents routine implementation in clinical practice: administration of a contrast agent. Most commonly, nephrotoxic iodined contrast is used which potentially results in a temporary or permanent loss of residual renal function. This happens in approximately 20% of the pre-dialysis patients in whom a DSA is performed (Geoffroy et al. 2001). Therefore, careful selection of patients is required given that residual renal function is strongly correlated to overall patient survival (Jansen et al. 2002). In an attempt to overcome the limitation of administering iodine in patients with ESRD who need a DSA, alternative contrast agents have been investigated: both gadolinium and CO_2 proved to be usefull (Geoffroy et al. 2001; Heye et al. 2006; Heye et al. 2010). However, also the utilization of these contrast agents is not free of risk.

The use of gadolinium in patients with ESRD has been associated with the development of nephrogenic systemic fibrosis (NSF) (Sadowski et al. 2007), a condition characterized by accumulation of gadolinium in the skin and joints due to the inability to remove gadolinium from the body and can result in severe disability or even be lethal (Penfield and Reilly 2007). CO_2 has the disadvantage of requiring large dose administration for diagnostic images, thereby increasing the risk for pulmonary, cardiac an cerebral embolism. Given the associated risks, angiographic techniques should not be used as a first choice for pre-operative imaging. However, in patients who are at risk for central vascular pathology or in patients with an inconclusive DUS examination, DSA is recommended when appropriate precautions have been taken into account: decent pre-hydration, use of the lowest possible dose of contrast, and post-procedural HD in case a CVC is already in use.

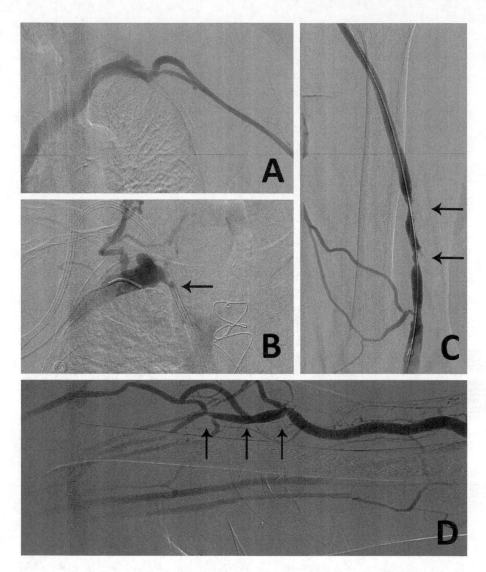

Fig. 5.15 Examples of digital subtraction angiography where **A)** no pathology is detected in the central venous system, **B)** a significant central venous obstruction is depected due to multiple previous indwelling CVSs (note: CVC in place during examination), **C)** two stenoses are detected in the cephalic vein which may compromise post-operative functioning, and **D)** an occluded cephalic vein with multiple venous side branches is visualized.

5.4.4 Magnetic Resonance Angiography

Another possibility to obtain structural and functional data of the upper extremity is magnetic resonance angiography (MRA) which allows the radiologist to visualize both central and peripheral vessels. Prior to the introduction of contrast-enhanced MRA (CE-MRA), non contrast-enhanced MRA (NCE-MRA) was the only option but suffered from many artifacts, limited fields of view and long acquisition times. With the introduction of gadolinium-based contrast agents (GBCA) these limitations were solved and CE-MRA became the standard of reference for diagnostic vessel imaging.

Also in VA surgery, this new method proved to be of additional value: a prospective study of Planken et al (2008b) showed that MRA examination prior to VA creation potentially results in a 30% decrease of non-maturing fistulas because of improved depiction of the most suitable site for VA creation. Figure 5.16 shows a typical example of an upper extremity CE-MRA.

However, several years after the introduction of GBCA a relation seemed to exist between the administration of linear GBCA in patients with ESRD and the development of NSF (Sadowski et al. 2007). Although this condition only occurs in a small percentage of the examined population, GBCA exposure in the ESRD population needs to be restricted. Therefore, the MRI community has shown interest in alternative MRA sequences and contrast agents: novel non contrast-enhanced techniques are focus of current research to abstain from contrast administration in the future, and more stable (macrocyclic) gadolinium contrast agents have been introduced for which no unconfounded cases of NSF have been reported until now. Nevertheless, guidelines advocate to minimize contrast exposure in the ESRD patient population. In case diagnostic vessel imaging is indicated by means of CE-MRA, post-procedural HD should be performed when patients already have a functional fistula or CVC (Penfield and Reilly 2007). The commercial availability of acceptable non contrast-enhanced MRA techniques for imaging the upper extremity vasculature is just a matter of time.

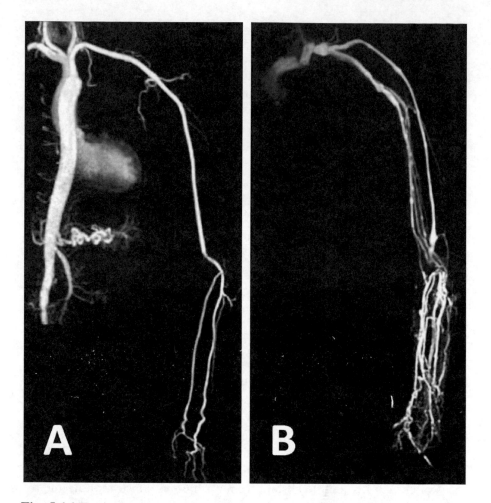

Fig. 5.16 Typical example of a CE-MRA examination of the upper extremity where all arterial (**A**) and venous (**B**) stations are depicted. (With courtesy of Planken et al. 2008a)

5.5 USING ARTERIOVENOUS FISTULA

To facilitate HD, a VA should be easily accessible and suitable for long-term use with minimal risk of complication. It is reasonable to assume that complications caused by cannulation, such as hematoma, infection, and aneurysm formation, lead to morbidity, hospitalization, access revision, and an increased use of CVCs. Besides this, cannulation can be painful and burdensome for the patient.

5.5.1 Pre-Cannulation Assessment

No consensus has been reached on when the VA is suitable for first time cannulation post-operatively. Exploration of the DOPPS-database revealed that 42-62% of the newly created AVGs is cannulated within 2-4 weeks after surgery while 36-98% of the autologous AVFs is cannulated within 2 months (Saran et al. 2004). Early cannulation of autologous AVFs has a negative effect on fistula survival and should therefore be discouraged. Only fistulas with a sufficient flow (>500 ml/min) and diameter (>4.0 mm) are suitable for a first cannulation attempt (Basile et al. 2005; Brunori et al. 2005). These parameters can be investigated by a routine duplex ultrasound evaluation 6 weeks after surgery.

5.5.2 Needling

For repetitive fistula cannulation, three different techniques have been described: the rope-ladder technique, the area puncture technique, and the button-hole technique (see Fig. 5.17). The rope-ladder technique uses the entire length of the cannulation segment for puncturing: every dialysis session, two puncture sites approximately 5 centimeters apart are chosen which avoid the previous cannulation site. As a result, gradual remodeling of the entire cannulation segment will occur. However, in daily clinical practice, often the same area of the fistula or graft is cannulated for reasons of comfort and ease. This may lead to aneurysmatic dilatations of the puncture areas and stenoses in adjacent regions. The button-hole technique centers around cannulating the AVF at exactly the same location, at exactly the same angle for every dialysis session. The first 8-12 times the fistula is cannulated, a sharp needle is used to create a traject which is kept open by inserting a plug after the dialysis session. After formation of the canals, dull needles can be used for cannulation of the AVF after removing the crust on top of the canal.

Which technique should be used in a particular VA is still matter of debate. Studies suggest that AVGs should be cannulated by the rope-ladder technique in order to prevent disintegration of graft material with subsequent aneurysm formation (Hartigan 1994). In AVFs, more and more evidence exists that the button-hole technique is a valuable alternative with a reduced complication rate: less hematomas, less aneurysms, and less pain during cannulation. On the other hand, significantly more attempts are necessary for successful cannulation.

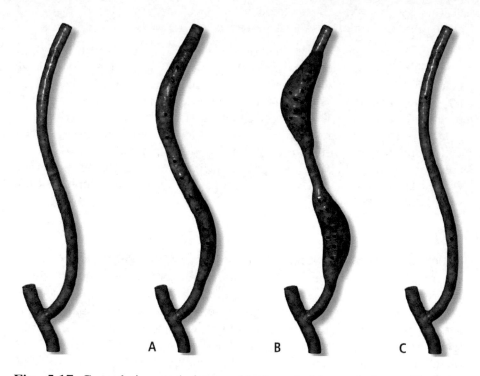

Fig. 5.17 Cannulation techniques. **A)** Rope-ladder technique, **B)** Area technique, and **C)** Button-hole technique

Also a higher infection rate was present in the patients cannulated with the button-hole technique (van Loon et al. 2010). Particularly in patients with a short cannulation segment, the button-hole technique is preferred over other techniques.

5.5.3 Monitoring for Complications

In order to detect VA dysfunction at an early stage and prevent complications, a well-structured monitoring program needs to be implemented on the dialysis ward. Monitoring should consist of a full physical examination of the VA prior to every dialysis session: inspection, palpation, auscultation. Additional measurements include volume flow, recirculation, and static and dynamic arterial and venous pressures which can be performed during the dialysis session. Observed changes over time or abnormalities should be documented and further investigated by means of vascular imaging techniques like duplex, DSA or MRA. Subsequently, preemptive correction of the underlying pathology results in prolonged patency rates of the VA.

5.6 VASCULAR ACCESS COMPLICATIONS AND THEIR TREATMENT

Over the past decades, creation and maintenance of VA has become challenging due to an increase in cardiovascular co-morbidities in the ESRD patient population. These conditions influence the quality of vessels involved in VA creation which makes the patient population more susceptible to post-operative complications, both on the short- and long term. Several studies have revealed that patient variables influence the choice and outcome of VA creation. Lin et al (1998) identified age as an important factor for post-operative flow enhancement. In elderly patients 18.9% of the newly created fistulas failed to mature while in younger patients this was only 13.6%. Moreover, high age in combination with diabetes mellitus resulted in even higher failure rates (28.6%). The influence of gender is controversial in the literature. A study from Caplin et al (2003) showed comparable pre-operative diameters of arteries and veins in both male and female patients which resulted in the successful creation of an AVF in 72% of the female and 77% of the male patients. On the other hand, multiple studies suggest higher rates of nonmaturation and primary failure in the female population with subsequently a higher percentage of AVGs and more endovascular and surgical revisions (Gibson et al. 2001; Enzler et al. 1996; Fisher and Neale 2003; Hirth et al. 1996; Kalman et al. 1999; Polkinghorne et al. 2004).

The meta-analysis of Rooijens et al (2004) illustrated comparable maturation and patency rates for RC-AVFs in male and female patients. Other determinants involved in the decision to create an autologous AVF are peripheral arterial disease, race and obesity (Allon et al. 2000). Elevated homocysteine levela do not induce VA failure (Sirrs et al. 1999), while elevated lipoprotein levels in negroide dialysis patients are believed to be a risk factor for fistula complications (Astor et al. 2001). A retrospective study revealed C-reactive protein (CRP) as an independent predictor for VA thrombosis (Chou et al. 2006). Patients using calcium antagonists, aspirin and angio-converting-enzyme inhibitors prior to AVF creation show a better post-operative patency of AVFs and AVGs.

5.6.1 Nonmaturation of Arteriovenous Fistulas

5.6.1.1 Definition

Although no well-established criteria have been defined for maturation, fistulas are considered mature when they can be routinely cannulated with two large-bore needles and deliver an adequate blood flow (typically 350-450 ml/min) for the total duration of dialysis. Depending on the fistula configuration, a mature forearm AVF will have a blood flow of 400-1200 ml/min while an upper arm AVF will have a flow between 500-2000 ml/min. Therefore, nonmaturation of autologous fistulas is characterized by either insufficient flow enhancement, insufficient venous dilatation or by cannulation difficulties due to a deep location of the cannulation segment which is the consequence of either poor selection of vessels, poor technique, or post-operative hemodynamic instability. Hemodynamical aspects of AVF nonmaturation will be discussed elsewhere.

5.6.1.2 Diagnosis and Treatment

Physical examination combined with DUS or DSA should identify the underlying cause. In the majority of cases nonmaturation is caused by vascular abnormalities in the juxta-anastomotic region (see Fig. 5.18). Using angiography, Beathard et al (2003) identified venous stenoses and accessory veins in 78% of the non-maturing fistulas and 43% of these cases showed abnormalities around the anastomosis. Another study described 61% of the stenoses in non-maturing fistulas to be present in the juxta-anastomotic region while 39% existed in the venous outflow (Turmel-Rodrigues et al. 2001). Proximal arterial inflow stenosis was identified in 25% of the non-maturing fistulas when the complete upper extremity vascular tree was imaged (Duijm et al. 2009).

Therefore, in non-maturing fistulas, the complete arterial inflow and venous outflow should be evaluated for identification of arterial inflow stenosis, venous outflow stenosis, or accessory veins which hamper proper fistula maturation.

Treatment of non-maturing fistulas comprises percutaneous transluminal angioplasty (PTA) of stenoses, thrombectomy, thrombosuction, thrombolysis, ligation or embolisation of accessory veins, main stream banding, and superficialisation of the outflow vein in case the depth of the cannulation segment results in cannulation difficulties. A systematic review by Voormolen et al (2009) revealed an 86% success rate after surgical or endovascular intervention in non-maturing fistulas with primary and secondary patency rates of 51% and 76%, resp. When interventional procedures do not result in successful maturation, surgical revision of the anastomosis can be performed using local anesthesia. When the involved vessels are severely diseased for AVF creation, more proximal vessels can be utilized for AVF creation before residing to implantation of graft material.

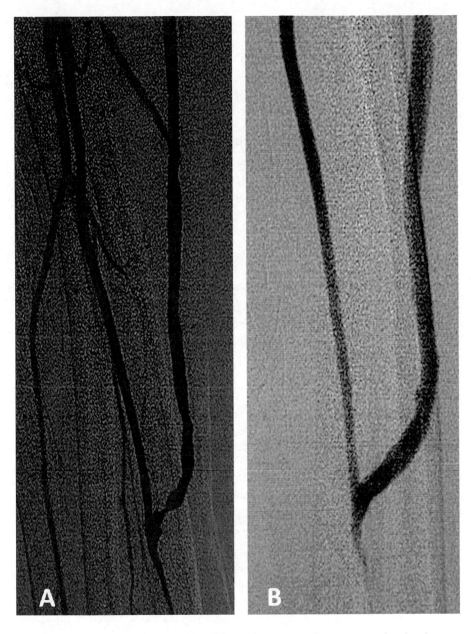

Fig. 5.18 Nonmaturing fistula with a clear stenotic segment in the juxta-anastomotic region. After diagnostic angiography, a balloon is inflated in order to dilate the narrowed vessel segment. Post-procedural angiography reveals no residual stenosis.

5.6.2 Stenosis and Thrombosis

5.6.2.1 Autologous Fistula Stenosis and Thrombosis

After VA creation, stenotic lesions tend to develop around the arteriovenous anastomosis and further on in the venous outflow traject. The timeframe in which they develop varies between fistula configurations and depends on hemodynamic disturbances in flow. The process is usually initiated by neointimal hyperplasia (NIH) due to migrating and proliferating smooth muscle cells, initiated by damage of the endothelial cell layer. As a consequence, luminal narrowing will occur. Progressive stenosis leads to a reduction of access flow which may result in thrombotic occlusion. Reduction of the vessel lumen by more than 50% together with a reduction of access flow (AVF < 500 ml/min; AVG <600 ml/min or >25% decrease with a total flow <1000 ml/min) allow for vascular imaging and preemptive treatment in order to avoid VA failure (NKF-K/DOQI 2002).

Other conditions suspicious for the presence of stenosis are difficulties with cannulation, upper extremity edema, prolonged bleeding time induced by venous hypertension, or ischemic complaints by insufficient arterial inflow. In RC-AVFs, 55-75% of the stenotic lesions occurs around the anastomosis, while 25% is localized in the venous outflow traject. In patients with BC-AVFs stenotic lesions are also often localized where the cephalic vein enters the subclavian vein (cephalic arch), while BB-AVF stenosis frequently occurs where the basilic vein enters the brachial vein (Turmel-Rodrigues et al. 1993, 2000). Endovascular treatment by percutaneous transluminal angioplasty (PTA) is the first option for arterial and venous stenoses and results in good salvage rates (Cohen et al. 2009; Greenberg et al. 2008). During this procedure, a balloon is inflated over the stenosis resulting in luminal widening. Some stenoses may not be sufficiently dilated using conventional balloons, however, cutting balloons or ultra-high pressure balloons may give better results (Trerotola et al. 2004). In case of frequent re-stenosis surgical revision may be performed by proximalisation of the anastomosis or by inserting a patch or graft interposition. AVF thrombosis has an incidence of approximately 0.2 events per patient/year. When present, thrombectomy, thrombosuction or thrombolysis should be performed as soon as possible (<24 hours) in order to prevent thrombus adhesion to the vascular wall. Timely correction might result in the avoidance of CVCs. In order to avoid these stenotic VA complications, regular monitoring of AVFs should be implemented in dialysis care. Early detection of VA dysfunction with subsequent vascular imaging and prophylactic treatment reduces the actual number of complications and results in higher patency rates. Dedicated DUS examination should be performed regularly in order to detect structural and functional abnormalities in the in- and outflow traject of the VA.

5.6.2.2 Arteriovenous Graft Stenosis and Thrombosis

Patients in which prosthetic graft material is used for creation of a VA are also at risk for graft dysfunction and graft thrombosis: on average 0.8 thrombotic complications per patient per year (Tordoir et al. 2004). Graft monitoring by access flow measurements or DUS is recommended; with preemptive endovascular treatment, this may reduce graft thrombosis but does not extend graft patency. Stenoses in AVGs are particularly common near the venous anastomosis due to turbulence and compliance mismatch. Also in the cannulation segment excessive ingrowth of fibrous tissue through the puncture holes results in luminal narrowing. Treatment is indicated by PTA, graft curettage, or partial graft replacement. Initial success rates of 73% and primary patency rates of 32% and 26% at 1 and 3 months have been reported (Marston et al. 1997; Beathard 1995; Beathard et al. 1996). When endovascular treatment fails or is not possible, surgical thrombectomy may be performed with a Fogarty catheter. On-table DSA should be performed after completion of thrombectomy of both arterial and venous limbs of the graft.

5.6.3 Aneurysms

Aneurysm formation within the VA conduit can be induced by elevated intraluminal pressures in combination with a weakened venous wall (Haage and Gunther 2006). Both AVFs and AVGs are subject to aneurysm formation because of repetitive large bore cannulation which negatively influence quality of the cannulation segment. Stenotic deformations in the venous outflow traject are often responsible for the increase in luminal pressure (Vesely and Siegel 2005). Therefore, after aneurysm formation, vascular imaging techniques should be employed to identify these lesions (see Fig. 5.19).

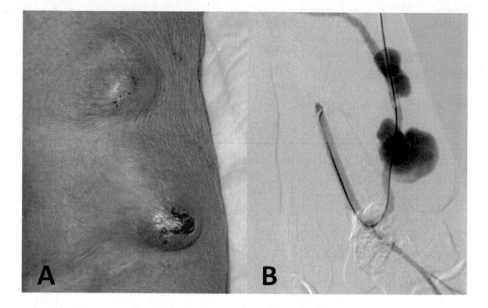

Fig. 5.19 Aneurysmatic dilatation of an arteriovenous fistula due to repetitive cannulation in the same segment (area-technique): **A)** photograph, and **B)** corresponding angiography

Treatment of the stenosis might stop aneurysm expansion: a single study reports that in 73% of the patients, development of venous outflow stenoses is in line with development of aneurysms (Vesely and Siegel 2005). Aneurysms in VA are at risk for thrombosis due to high residence time of blood and accordingly higher risk of platelet aggregation. Aneurysms are detected by inspection of the VA and confirmed by either a DUS examination or DSA. Treatment of these aneurysms is indicated when the diameter of the aneurysm is 2 times the diameter of the graft, a very superficial location of the aneurysm due to skin erosion results in an increased chance of rupture, infectious parameters are present, the aneurysm is painfull or increases in size, or when thrombus is present within the aneurysm with subsequent obstruction of the VA conduit. Treatment of VA aneurysms depends on the type of aneurysm (true or false), the type of VA (AVG or AVF), and the location of the aneurysm. Aneurysm formation near the arteriovenous anastomosis often is a true aneurysm for which surgical correction is the treatment of choice (Yasim et al. 2006). When possible, the anastomosis should be proximalized in order to save the VA conduit, instead of creating a new access. Aneurysmatic dilatation of a longer segment is usually a true aneurysm as well. When treatment is indicated, the diseased segment needs to be excised and replaced by an interposition graft. Recent literature also reports the possibility of endovascular exclusion of the aneurysm by means of a covered stent (Keeling et al. 2008; Barshes et al. 2008; Silas and Bettmann 2003). However, no studies have been performed to identify superiority of one technique over the other.

5.6.4   Hemodialysis Access Induced Distal Ischemia

Although the distal RC-AVF remains the primary option for VA, demographical changes in the ESRD population result in the creation of more upper arm fistulas. These fistulas deliver a higher flow compared to forearm fistulas but also carry a greater risk for impeded perfusion of tissue distally of the anastomosis (Padberg et al. 2008): hemodialysis access induced distal ischemia (HAIDI) or steal syndrome (see Fig. 5.20). The locoregional drop in blood pressure near the anastomosis in combination with progressive atherosclerosis and vascular calcification are believed to play an important role in the development of this complication (Wixon et al. 2000).

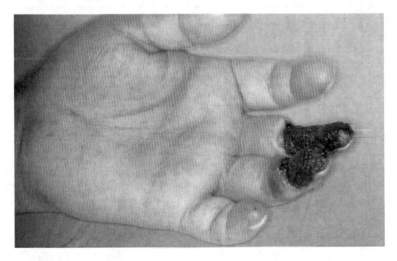

Fig. 5.20 Digital necrosis due to impeded perfusion of the tissue distally of the anastomosis: the most severe clinical manifestation of hemodialysis access induced distal ischemia (HAIDI).

Severe chronic steal syndrome after VA creation is a serious complication with an incidence between 2% and 8% in the HD population (Morsy et al. 1998). However, more than 75% of the dialysis patients report one or more complaints associated with ischemia: coldness, pain, weakness, pallor, and paresthesia (van Hoek et al. 2006). These ischemic complaints can be objectivated by measuring digital blood pressure or transcutaneous oxygen pressure. Digital pressure can be interpreted as an absolute value or in relation to the brachial artery pressure: digital to brachial index (DBI). Healthy individuals and asymptomatic patients with a VA have a DBI (P_{dig} / P_{syst}) > 0.8 while symptomatic patients often have a DBI <0.6 which increases during compression of the fistula (Schanzer et al. 2006; Papasavas et al. 2003; Goff et al. 2000). When complaints, physical examination and finger pressure measurements indicate distal ischemia, classification should be performed; like the Fontaine classification for peripheral arterial occlusive disease, four separate stages have been defined (Tordoir et al. 2007) (see Table 5.5).

Table 5.5 Classification of hemodialysis access induced distal ischemia.

HAIDI	Symptoms
Stage 1	Pale or blue hand without pain; no complaints
Stage 2	Complaints during HD or exercise: a) acceptable b) unacceptable
Stage 3	Ischemic complaints during rest
Stage 4	Ulceration, necrosis and gangrene

The treatment strategy depends on the etiology of the ischemia. Conservative treatment is indicated in patients with stage I and IIa distal ischemia which consists of heat application, adjustments in medication and exercise for improvement of collateral circulation (Scheltinga et al. 2009). In patients with more advanced stages of distal ischemia, diagnostic vessel imaging is needed to rule out any arterial inflow stenoses (DeCaprio et al. 1997). Therefore, angiography is used after which hemodynamic significant arterial stenoses can be treated by angioplasty (Duijm et al. 2009; Guerra et al. 2002). Patients with stage IIb or higher, not responding to conservative and endovascular treatment need to be evaluated for surgical intervention. Flow reduction can be performed by either surgical ligation of the fistula, surgical ligation of side branches and banding of the AVF (see Figure 5.21).

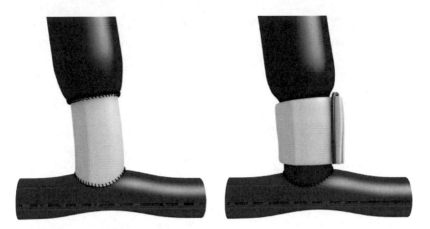

Fig. 5.21 Minimal-invasive Procedures performed to increase the resistance in the venous outflow traject in order to reduce fistula flow and / or increase distal perfusion pressures: **A)** Interposition of graft material with a smaller diameter than the venous outflow traject. **B)** Banding procedure; a non-elastic, non-resorbable prosthetic band is wrapped around the venous outflow near the anastomosis. Fine-tuning of luminal narrowing can be performed by using surgical clips to tighten the band. Afterwards, these clips can be fixed or replaced by multiple sutures. These procedures should be performed under real-time monitoring of fistula flow and finger pressures in order to achieve the desired effect: decrease in flow and increase in peripheral perfusion pressures without putting the fistula at risk for thrombosis.

Also, several bypass procedures are available to the surgeon which improve distal perfusion of the upper extremity. The DRIL-procedure (distal revascularization-interval ligation) consists of a venous bypass from the proximal artery to the distal ischemic forearm (Schanzer et al. 1992) (see Fig. 5.22). Subsequently, the artery distally of the AVF is ligated to prevent steal. Alternatively, a PAI-procedure (proximalization of arteriovenous inflow) can be performed in which the anastomosis in the elbow is disconnected and anastomosed more proximal to the brachial artery by means of an interposition graft (Gradman and Pozrikidis 2004). The RUDI-procedure (revision using distal inflow) is based on extending the inflow traject to a more distal artery (proximal radial artery) by means of a venous interposition.

Intra-operative digital pressure and flow measurements are mandatory to guarantee an adequate surgical intervention with acceptable outcome. The results of these procedures are usually good, however, in some patients, AVF ligation and transition to chronic CVC dialysis or PD may be the only solution.

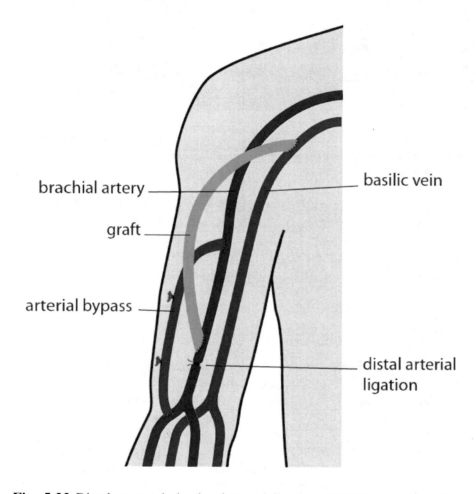

Fig. 5.22 Distal revascularization-interval ligation (DRIL) procedure: the artery is ligated distally of the prosthetic or autologous vascular access. Subsequently, an arterial bypass is created, starting 5-10 cm proximal of the fistula to a point just distal of the ligation (brachial artery / proximal radial artery)

5.6.5 Cardiac Failure

The increase in co-morbidity in the ESRD patient population requires the construction of relatively more upper arm AVFs compared to forearm AVFs. Although upper arm fistulas have good patency rates, the development of high flow over these conduits is a clinical problem which is illustrated by heart failure being the primary cause of death in ESRD patients (Schou et al. 2008; Tian et al. 2008). Creation of an AVF results in a decrease of the peripheral vascular resistance with a subsequent acute and prolonged increase of cardiac output (Warren et al. 1951; Holman 1965). Studies have confirmed that functional AVFs potentially contribute to the development of cardiac failure by provoking a disbalance between oxygen requirement and oxygen delivery to the myocardium (Savage et al. 2002). Besides the presence of a patent fistula, also volume flow is a strong predictor for the development of cardiac failure: the higher the flow, the more cardiac activity is required. A recent study indicated that patients with a fistula flow >2 L/min have a significant higher risk for the development of cardiac failure (Basile et al. 2008). Based on literature, the incidence of these high flow AVFs, is estimated around 4% of which the majority (95%) consists of autologous elbow fistulas. Regular access flow measurements are necessary to identify patients at risk for the development of cardiac failure. In case repetitive access flows >2 L/min are measured and patients complain of dyspnea, additional examinations need to be performed: a thorough physical examination, ECG registration and echocardiography are mandatory. In patients with severe cardiac failure, compression of the fistula may result in bradycardia provoked by the sudden increase of blood pressure (Chemla et al. 2007). Treatment of AVF-induced cardiac failure depends on life expectancy and co-morbidity of the patient.

Conservative treatment can be attempted in patients with minor complaints and consists of correction of anemia, hypertension and electrolytes. Furthermore, blood supply to the heart may be improved by performing endovascular procedures to the coronary arteries. Surgery is performed in patients not responding to conservative treatment with an access flow >2 L/min or in patients with lower access flows but with significant symptomatology of cardiac failure. Basically, to decrease the cardiac burden, fistula flow needs to be reduced (to a level where it still delivers an adequate flow for HD). In order to achieve this, the clinician has the availability over the same procedures as in patients with HAIDI: ligation of the AVF, ligation of hemodynamic important side branches, narrowing of the arteriovenous anastomosis, the RUDI-procedure or the banding procedure.

5.6.6 Central Venous Obstruction

Central venous obstruction is a complication which often results from previous indwelling CVCs or pacemaker leads. 40% of the patients who have had a CVC in the subclavian vein develops a significant stenosis while CVCs through the internal jugular vein result in a stenosis in 20% of the patients (Schillinger et al. 1991). Usually, a central venous obstruction is asymptomatic, however, when an AVF is created in the ipsi-lateral upper extremity symptoms may develop as a result of flow increase and consist of prolonged bleeding time, local swelling, edema or even venous ulcera. Patients with mild complaints benefit from conservative treatment. In case local swelling, venous ulcera or infection hamper fistula cannulation, additional vascular imaging needs to be performed: conventional phlebography visualizing the veins from the upper arm into the superior caval vein (see Fig. 5.15b). Symptomatic central venous obstructions can be treated by endovascular procedures (Dammers et al. 2003), with an initial success rate of 95%. Primary patency however is relatively low (10-20% after 1 year): multiple re-interventions due to re-stenosis are necessary to maintain central vein patency (Sprouse et al. 2004). Some studies suggest better patency rates with additional stent placement over the stenotic segment (Mickley et al. 1997; Haage et al. 1999). If endovascular therapy has failed, a surgical intervention can be attempted and is performed according to patient condition, life expectancy and vascular pathology. Initially, a surgical bypass over the stenosed or occluded segment is indicated and can be directed to the contra-lateral side or even the lower extremity. When surgical bypass fails, ligation of the upper limb VA can be considered to relieve symptoms but requires an alternative VA for dialysis therapy.

5.7 HEMODYNAMIC ASPECTS OF ARTERIOVENOUS FISTULAS

5.7.1 Physiological Setting

Both heart and vascular tree are responsible for efficient transport of blood through the body and are controlled by the nervous system. This neural innervation is dedicated to maintaining optimum hemodynamic parameters by acting on cardiac output, circulating volume, peripheral vascular resistance, and blood viscosity. Within the arterial vascular tree two separate forces can be distinguished which influence local hemodynamics: one acting perpendicularly on the arterial wall which influences all layers of the artery, and one acting parallel on the arterial wall (see Fig. 5.23). The latter one, wall shear stress (WSS), represents the effect of friction of blood flow on the endothelium and is quantified by Pascal (Pa) or dynes per square centimeter.

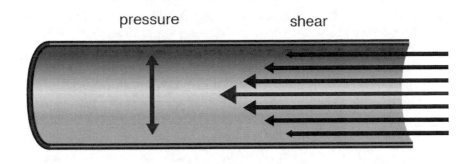

Fig. 5.23 Schematic visualization of forces acting on the arterial wall: Axial pressure (blood pressure) influences all layers over the arterial wall and acts perpendicular in all directions. Wall shear stress acts longitudinal over the inside of the arterial wall and is caused by friction of blood with the endothelial cells. As a result, blood velocity near the vascular wall is lower when compared to the center of the vessel.

5.7.2 Vascular Access Creation

In order to be suitable for HD, flow over the AVF needs to be at least 500 ml/min. For this, the feeding artery needs to dilate. Based on Pouseuille's law, where volume flow (Q) is proportional to the product of the pressure gradient (ΔP) and vessel radius (r) to the fourth power, divided by the viscosity (η) of blood, the brachial artery lumen would need to dilate by nearly 80% to achieve the required flow increase (Dixon 2006). Clinical studies have revealed smaller increases (40-50%) (Dammers et al. 2005; Girerd et al. 1996) but identified other factors influencing postoperative flow enhancement: increase in end diastolic velocity (EDV) and the contribution of retrograde flow on total fistula flow. Therefore, the

surgical connection of an artery with a vein results in a changed hemodynamic profile within the involved arterial inflow and venous outflow
traject. Clinically, three different effects can be distinguished: local, peripheral, and systemic.

5.7.2.1 Local Effects

Local effects are directly provoked by the bypass of the peripheral arterioles: the sudden decrease in peripheral vascular resistance results in
an increased blood flow over the VA conduit. The endothelial cells of
the feeding artery are subject to increased WSS and respond by increasing the production of nitric oxide (NO) (Ben Driss et al. 1997; Tronc et
al. 2000). Initially, NO facilitates relaxation of the smooth muscle cells
but on the long term, also matrix metalloproteinases (MMP's) are activated which break down the fibrous tissue supporting the media layer of
the artery (Tronc 2000). The NO mediated arterial dilatation is initiated
in order to attempt restoring WSS levels to physiological values (Zakrzewicz et al. 2002; Kamiya et al. 1984). The gradual increase in arterial
diameter results in a gradual flow increase to a maximum value within
4-12 weeks after AVF creation (Wong et al. 1996; Corpataux et al.
2002; Remuzzi et al. 2003; Lomonte et al. 2005). Post-operative venous
dilatation ultimately determines fistula suitability. Venous dilatation occurs rapidly after fistula creation and continues for several weeks. Wong
et al (1996) presented a venous diameter increase of 51% one day after
surgery which further increased to 123% after twelve weeks. These findings were confirmed by Corpataux et al (2002) who found that the
venous lumen increased by 86% at 1 week and 179% at 12 weeks. Besides an increase in venous diameter, the vessel wall will also thicken as
a result of elevated pressures and micro trauma following repetitive
cannulation.

Another local hemodynamic consequence of AVF surgery is turbulence.
At the arteriovenous anastomosis, flow is directed from the arterial system
into the venous system over a pressure gradient. The magnitude of this
pressure gradient depends on total vascular resistance of the AVF itself,
and is determined by the location and size of the anastomosis. As discussed above, flow velocity and volume flow increase and become turbulent, which can be felt at the site of the anastomosis and over venous side
branches as a thrill (see Fig. 5.24).

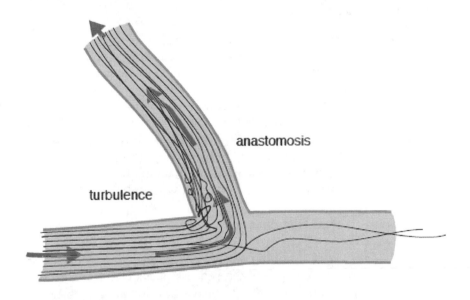

Fig. 5.24 Schematic visualization of turbulence over the anastomotic complex. Due to the pressure drop over the arteriovenous fistula blood is directed into the venous system where it becomes turbulent. This turbulence can be felt over the anastomosis and further on in the venous outflow tract (thrill). In case of a venous outflow stenosis / obstruction, the thrill can become pulsatile.

5.7.2.2 Systemic Effects

All stages of chronic kidney disease are characterized by a gradual decrease in cardiac function. At initiation of dialysis therapy, almost 75% of the patients is diagnosed with left ventricular hypertrophy (LVH), left ventricular dilatation or systolic dysfunction (Foley et al. 1995; Parfrey et al. 1996), and is considered to be the consequence of adaptive remodeling in response to pre-existing pressure- or volume overload (London 2001). Directly upon fistula creation cardiac output increases by means of a reduction in peripheral vascular resistance, increased sympathetic nervous system activity and an increase in stroke volume and heart rate. The lower systemic vascular resistance induces an increase in cardiac output in effort to maintain blood pressure. Iwashima et al (2002) published a significant increase in left ventricular end-diastolic diameter (+4%) and cardiac output (+15%) 14 days after surgery.

5.7.2.3 Peripheral Effects

Depending on the size and location of the anastomosis, peripheral perfusion decreases. Following the creation of an AVF, blood is flowing through the VA conduit, rather than continuing to the distal extremity. Moreover, the anastomotic pressure drop may induce a retrograde flow in the artery distally of the anastomotic complex. This retrograde flow from the distal artery occurs in about 75% of the forearm fistulas and accounts for an average of 25% of the blood flow into the venous limb of the fistula (Sivanesan et al. 1998). Nonetheless, blood supply to the distal extremity may remain adequate because of peripheral dilatation of the arterioles and the development / adaptation of collateral inflow vessels.

5.7.3 Vascular Access Complications

When the process of maturation has been completed and the fistula is suitable for repetitive cannulation, the process of adaptation and remodeling continues. This ultimately results in the development of VA related complications with subsequent dysfunction. The development of stenotic lesions is the most common complication after VA surgery and is most likely induced by vascular injury. According to the traditional theory of neointimal hyperplasia, endothelial and smooth muscle injury (hemodynamic stress, surgical injury, dialysis needles, PTA) result in the migration of smooth muscle cells and myofibroblasts from the media to the intima, where they proliferate and form the lesion of venous neointimal hyperplasia, which narrows the vessel lumen (Roy-Chaudhury et al. 2007).

These lesions can be indentified in the complete venous outflow tract but are more common in certain areas, particularly around the arteriovenous anastomosis where arterial blood runs along the venous wall. Depending on the anastomotic configuration, distribution of WSS differs over the various locations: some sites are exposed to high and others to low WSS. High levels of WSS are associated with appropriate vascular dilatation and a relative lack of neointimal hyperplasia. Most likely this is the result of endothelial quiescence, high levels of NO and low levels of inflammatory cytokines. On the other hand, low or oscillatory shear stress tends to be involved in limited vascular dilatation and an increase in neointimal hyperplasia: endothelial deactivation, low levels of NO and increased inflammatory mediators predispose to the development of vascular stenoses (Roy-Chaudhury et al. 2007) (see Fig. 5.25). While hemodynamic shear stress is the most important factor for stenotic AVF failure, other factors like surgical injury, and repetitive cannulation also play a role. Also, the treatment of AVF stenosis, PTA, can result in significant endothelial and smooth muscle cell injury and potentially result in an exacerbation of the re-stenotic lesion (Chang et al. 2004).

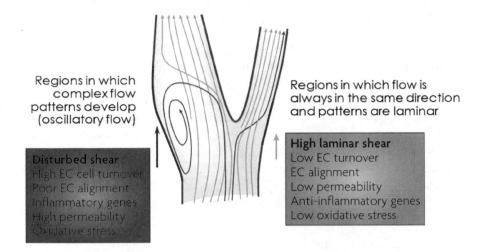

Fig. 5.25 Schematic visualization of the processes involved in the development of stenoses which are influenced by wall shear stress.

The development of steal syndrome and cardiac failure is more straightforward. Both complications arise from insufficient endogenous cardiovascular adaptation mechanisms following the creation of an AVF. In patients with symptomatic steal, pre-existing vascular lesions (e.g. arterial inflow stenosis) or insufficient vascular remodeling (e.g. lack of peripheral arterial dilatation or development of collateral inflow) result in a reduced perfusion pressure of the hand and fingers which can become symptomatic. Cardiac failure on the other hand results from incapability of the myocardium to adapt to the new situation where besides the normal circulation, also a fistula circulation must be provided while maintaining blood pressure. A study performed by Basile et al (2008) reports that patients with a fistula flow >2.2 l/min have a significantly higher mean cardiac output than patients with a fistula flow <2.2 l/min. In the same study, the ROC curve analysis identified that flow values >2.0 l/min predicts the occurrence of cardiac failure accurately with a sensitivity of 89%, a specificity of 100% and a curve area of 99%. Furthermore, they established that upper arm AVFs are associated with an increased risk for high output cardiac failure. In case the heart has difficulty to comply, patients can experience symptoms of cardiac failure as classified by the American Heart Association (Hunt 2005).

5.8 CONCLUSION AND FUTURE DIRECTIONS FOR VASCULAR ACCESS

Although great progress has been achieved over the last decades, VA creation and maintenance remains the Achilles heel of chronic HD treatment. Bearing in mind that the ESRD patient population will increase tremendously over the next years, will be older when the first VA procedure needs to be performed and suffers from co-morbidities which affect the quality of the cardiovascular system, alternative strategies need to be explored to tailor VA management to the individual patient and thereby reducing short- and long-term AVF dysfunction. Recent studies have showed that a multi-disciplinary approach according to national and international guidelines reduce VA related complications (Vassalotti et al. 2004).

Essential in these guidelines is a shift from management of complications to prevention of complications: by detecting VA dysfunction at an early stage, preemptive treatment results in improved patency rates. Within the multidisciplinary team the nephrologist, the vascular surgeon, the interventional radiologist and the dialysis nurse play an important role. This team is involved from the pre-dialysis traject until renal replacement therapy is no longer necessary and plays a crucial role in providing pre-dialysis information and education, timely referral to the vascular surgeon for creation of the AVF, pre-operative screening, observation of fistula maturation, repetitive cannulation of the AVF, post-operative monitoring of the AVF and management and treatment of complications. Another very promising strategy is the development of computational tools for the prediction of post-operative AVF function. This approach requires patient-specific pre-operative modeling of the cardiovascular system and simulation of the effect of VA creation. The more factors (anatomical, physiological, mechanical and demographical) are taken in to consideration, the more reliable the computational tool predicts. Ultimately, the predictive tool should be able to identify the AVF configuration with the most optimal post-operative hemodynamic profile resulting in the lowest post-operative complication rate.

REFERENCES

Allon, M.: Current management of vascular access. Clin. J. Am. Soc. Nephrol. 2(4), 786–800 (2007)

Allon, M., Daugirdas, J., Depner, T.A., et al.: Effect of change in vascular access on patient mortality in hemodialysis patients. Am. J. Kidney Dis. 47(3), 469–477 (2006)

Allon, M., Lockhart, M.E., Lilly, R.Z., et al.: Effect of preoperative sonographic mapping on vascular access outcomes in hemodialysis patients. Kidney International 60(5), 2013–2020 (2001)

Allon, M., Ornt, D.B., Schwab, S.J., et al.: Factors associated with the prevalence of arteriovenous fistulas in hemodialysis patients in the HEMO study. Hemodialysis (HEMO) Study Group. Kidney International 58(5), 2178–2185 (2000)

Antoniou, G.A., Lazarides, M.K., Georgiadis, G.S., et al.: Lower-extremity arteriovenous access for haemodialysis: a systematic review. Eur. J. Vasc. Endovasc. Surg. 38(3), 365–372 (2009)

Astor, B.C., Eustace, J.A., Powe, N.R., et al.: Timing of nephrologist referral and arteriovenous access use: the CHOICE Study. Am. J. Kidney Dis. 38(3), 494–501 (2001)

Baker Jr., L.D., Johnson, J.M., Goldfarb, D.: Expanded polytetrafluoroethylene (PTFE) subcutaneous arteriovenous conduit: an improved vascular access for chronic hemodialysis. Trans. Am. Soc. Artif Intern. Organs 22, 382–387 (1976)

Barshes, N.R., Annambhotla, S., Bechara, C., et al.: Endovascular repair of hemodialysis graft-related pseudoaneurysm: an alternative treatment strategy in salvaging failing dialysis access. Vascular and Endovascular Surgery 42(3), 228–234 (2008)

Basile, C., Lomonte, C., Vernaglione, L., et al.: The relationship between the flow of arteriovenous fistula and cardiac output in haemodialysis patients. Nephrol. Dial. Transplant. 23(1), 282–287 (2008)

Basile, C., Casucci, F., Lomonte, C.: Timing of first cannulation of arteriovenous fistula: time matters, but there is also something else. Nephrol. Dial. Transplant. 20(7), 1519–1520 (2005)

Beathard, G.A., Arnold, P., Jackson, J., Litchfield, T.: Aggressive treatment of early fistula failure. Kidney International 64(4), 1487–1494 (2003)

Beathard, G.A., Welch, B.R., Maidment, H.J.: Mechanical thrombolysis for the treatment of thrombosed hemodialysis access grafts. Radiology 200(3), 711–716 (1996)

Beathard, G.A.: Thrombolysis versus surgery for the treatment of thrombosed dialysis access grafts. J. Am. Soc. Nephrol. 6(6), 1619–1624 (1995)

Ben Driss, A., Benessiano, J., Poitevin, P., et al.: Arterial expansive remodeling induced by high flow rates. Am. J. Physiol. 272(2 Pt 2), H851–H858 (1997)

Biuckians, A., Scott, E.C., Meier, G.H., et al.: The natural history of autologous fistulas as first-time dialysis access in the KDOQI era. J. Vasc. Surg. 47(2), 415–421 (2008); discussion 420-411

Brescia, M.J., Cimino, J.E., Appel, K., Hurwich, B.J.: Chronic hemodialysis using venipuncture and a surgically created arteriovenous fistula. N. Engl. J. Med. 275(20), 1089–1092 (1966)

Brunori, G., Ravani, P., Mandolfo, S., et al.: Fistula maturation: doesn't time matter at all? Nephrol. Dial. Transplant. 20(4), 684–687 (2005)

Caplin, N., Sedlacek, M., Teodorescu, V., et al.: Venous access: women are equal. Am. J. Kidney Dis. 41, 429–432 (2003)

Chang, C.J., Ko, P.J., Hsu, L.A., et al.: Highly increased cell proliferation activity in the restenotic hemodialysis vascular access after percutaneous transluminal angioplasty: implication in prevention of restenosis. Am. J. Kidney Dis. 43(1), 74–84 (2004)

Chemla, E.S., Morsy, M., Anderson, L., Whitemore, A.: Inflow reduction by distalization of anastomosis treats efficiently high-inflow high-cardiac output vascular access for hemodialysis. Seminars in Dialysis 20(1), 68–72 (2007)

Chou, C.Y., Kuo, H.L., Yung, Y.F., et al.: C-reactive protein predicts vascular access thrombosis in hemodialysis patients. Blood Purification 24(4), 342–346 (2006)

Cohen, A., Korzets, A., Neyman, H., et al.: Endovascular interventions of juxtaanastomotic stenoses and thromboses of hemodialysis arteriovenous fistulas. J. Vasc. Interv. Radiol. 20(1), 66–70 (2009)

Corpataux, J.M., Haesler, E., Silacci, P., et al.: Low-pressure environ-ment and remodelling of the forearm vein in Brescia-Cimino haemodialysis access. Nephrol. Dial. Transplant. 17(6), 1057–1062 (2002)

Dammers, R., Tordoir, J.H., Kooman, J.P., et al.: The effect of flow changes on the arterial system proximal to an arteriovenous fistula for hemodialysis. Ultrasound in Medicine & Biology 31(10), 1327–1333 (2005)

Dammers, R., de Haan, M.W., Planken, N.R., et al.: Central vein obstruction in hemodialysis patients: results of radiological and surgical intervention. Eur. J. Vasc. Endovasc. Surg. 26(3), 317–321 (2003)

DeCaprio, J.D., Valentine, R.J., Kakish, H.B., et al.: Steal syndrome complicating hemodialysis access. Cardiovasc. Surg. 5(6), 648–653 (1997)

Dember, L.M., Beck, G.J., Allon, M., et al.: Effect of clopidogrel on early failure of arteriovenous fistulas for hemodialysis: a randomized controlled trial. Jama 299(18), 2164–2171 (2008)

Dixon, B.S., Beck, G.J., Vazquez, M.A., et al.: Effect of dipyridamole plus aspirin on hemodialysis graft patency. N. Engl. J. Med. 360(21), 2191–2201 (2009)

Dixon, B.S.: Why don't fistulas mature? Kidney International 70(8), 1413–1422 (2006)

Dixon, B.S., Novak, L., Fangman, J.: Hemodialysis vascular access survival: upper-arm native arteriovenous fistula. Am. J. Kidney Dis. 39(1), 92–101 (2002)

Dotter, C.T., Judkins, M.P., Rosch, J.: Nonoperative treatment of arterial occlusive disease: a radiologically facilitated technique. Radiol. Clin. North Am. 5(3), 531–542 (1967)

Duijm, L.E., Overbosch, E.H., Liem, Y.S., et al.: Retrograde catheterization of haemodialysis fistulae and grafts: angiographic depiction of the entire vascular access tree and stenosis treatment. Nephrol. Dial. Transplant. 24(2), 539–547 (2009)

Enzler, M.A., Rajmon, T., Lachat, M., Largiader, F.: Long-term function of vascular access for hemodialysis. Clin. Transplant. 10(6 Pt 1), 511–515 (1996)

Ergun, D.L., Mistretta, C.A., Kruger, R.A., et al.: A hybrid computerized fluoroscopy technique for noninvasive cardiovascular imaging. Radiology 132(3), 739–742 (1979)

Fisher, C.M., Neale, M.L.: Outcome of surgery for vascular access in patients commencing haemodialysis. Eur. J. Vasc. Endovasc. Surg. 25(4), 342–349 (2003)

Flores Izquierdo, G., Ronces Vivero, R., Exaire, E., et al.: Venous autologous graft for hemodialysis (original technic). Preliminary report. Arch. Inst. Cardiol. Mex. 39(2), 259–266 (1969)

Foley, R.N., Parfrey, P.S., Harnett, J.D., et al.: Clinical and echocardiographic disease in patients starting end-stage renal disease therapy. Kidney International 47(1), 186–192 (1995)

Garcia-Pajares, R., Polo, J.R., Flores, A., et al.: Upper arm polytetrafluoroethylene grafts for dialysis access. Analysis of two different graft sizes: 6 mm and 6-8 mm. Vascular and Endovascular Surgery 37(5), 335–343 (2003)

Geoffroy, O., Tassart, M., Le Blanche, A.F., et al.: Upper extremity digital subtraction venography with gadoterate meglumine before fistula creation for hemodialysis. Kidney International 59(4), 1491–1497 (2001)

Gibson, K.D., Gillen, D.L., Caps, M.T., et al.: Vascular access survival and incidence of revisions: a comparison of prosthetic grafts, simple autogenous fistulas, and venous transposition fistulas from the United States Renal Data System Dialysis Morbidity and Mortality Study. J. Vasc. Surg. 34(4), 694–700 (2001)

Girerd, X., London, G., Boutouyrie, P., et al.: Remodeling of the radial artery in response to a chronic increase in shear stress. Hypertension 27(3 Pt 2), 799–803 (1996)

Glickman, M.H., Stokes, G.K., Ross, J.R., et al.: Multicenter evaluation of a polytetrafluoroethylene vascular access graft as compared with the expanded polytetrafluoroethylene vascular access graft in hemodialysis applications. J. Vasc. Surg. 34(3), 465–472 (2001); discussion 472-463

Goff, C.D., Sato, D.T., Bloch, P.H., et al.: Steal syndrome complicating hemodialysis access procedures: can it be predicted? Ann. Vasc. Surg. 14(2), 138–144 (2000)

Golledge, J., Smith, C.J., Emery, J., et al.: Outcome of primary radiocephalic fistula for haemodialysis. Br. J. Surg. 86(2), 211–216 (1999)

Gordon, D.H., Glanz, S., Butt, K.M., et al.: Treatment of stenotic lesions in dialysis access fistulas and shunts by transluminal angioplasty. Radiology 143(1), 53–58 (1982)

Gracz, K.C., Ing, T.S., Soung, L.S., et al.: Proximal forearm fistula for maintenance hemodialysis. Kidney International 11(1), 71–75 (1977)

Gradman, W.S., Pozrikidis, C.: Analysis of options for mitigating hemodialysis access-related ischemic steal phenomena. Ann. Vasc. Surg. 18(1), 59–65 (2004)

Grassmann, A., Gioberge, S., Moeller, S., Brown, G.: ESRD patients in 2004: global overview of patient numbers, treatment modalities and associated trends. Nephrol. Dial. Transplant. 20(12), 2587–2593 (2005)

Greenberg, J.I., Suliman, A., Angle, N.: Endovascular dialysis interventions in the era of DOQI. Ann. Vasc. Surg. 22(5), 657–662 (2008)

Guerra, A., Raynaud, A., Beyssen, B., et al.: Arterial percutaneous angioplasty in upper limbs with vascular access devices for haemodialysis. Nephrol. Dial. Transplant. 17(5), 843–851 (2002)

Haage, P., Gunther, R.W.: Radiological intervention to maintain vascular access. Eur. J. Vasc. Endovasc. Surg. 32(1), 84–89 (2006)

Haage, P., Vorwerk, D., Piroth, W., et al.: Treatment of hemodialysis-related central venous stenosis or occlusion: results of primary Wallstent placement and follow up in 50 patients. Radiology 212(1), 175–180 (1999)

Hameeteman, M., Bode, A.S., Peppelenbosch, A.G., et al.: Ultrasound-guided central venous catheter placement by surgical trainees: A safe procedure? J. Vasc. Access 11(4), 288–292 (2010)

Harper, S.J., Goncalves, I., Doughman, T., Nicholson, M.L.: Arteriovenous fistula formation using transposed basilic vein: extensive single centre experience. Eur. J. Vasc. Endovasc. Surg. 36(2), 237–241 (2008)

Hartigan, M.F.: Vascular access and nephrology nursing practice: existing views and rationales for change. Adv. Ren. Replace Ther. 1(2), 155–162 (1994)

Heye, S., Maleux, G., Marchal, G.J.: Upper-extremity venography: CO2 versus iodinated contrast material. Radiology 241(1), 291–297 (2006)

Heye, S., Fourneau, I., Maleux, G., et al.: Preoperative mapping for haemodialysis access surgery with CO(2) venography of the upper limb. Eur. J. Vasc. Endovasc. Surg. 39(3), 340–345 (2010)

Hirth, R.A., Turenne, M.N., Woods, J.D., et al.: Predictors of type of vascular access in hemodialysis patients. JAMA 276(16), 1303–1308 (1996)

Hofstra, L., Bergmans, D.C., Hoeks, A.P., et al.: Mismatch in elastic properties around anastomoses of interposition grafts for hemodialysis access. J. Am. Soc. Nephrol. 5(5), 1243–1250 (1994)

Holman, E.: Abnormal arteriovenous communications. Great variability of effects with particular reference to delayed development of cardiac failure. Circulation 32(6), 1001–1009 (1965)

Huijbregts, H.J., Bots, M.L., Wittens, C.H., et al.: Hemodialysis arteriovenous fistula patency revisited: results of a prospective, multicenter initiative. Clin. J. Am. Soc. Nephrol. 3(3), 714–719 (2008)

Hunt, S.A.: ACC/AHA 2005 guideline update for the diagnosis and management of chronic heart failure in the adult: a report of the American College of Cardiology/American Heart Association Task Force on Practice Guidelines (Writing Committee to Update the 2001 Guidelines for the Evaluation and Management of Heart Failure). J. Am. Coll. Cardiol. 46(6), e1–e82 (2005)

Iwashima, Y., Horio, T., Takami, Y., et al.: Effects of the creation of arteriovenous fistula for hemodialysis on cardiac function and natriuretic peptide levels in CRF. Am. J. Kidney Dis. 40(5), 974–982 (2002)

Jansen, M.A., Hart, A.A., Korevaar, J.C., et al.: Predictors of the rate of decline of residual renal function in incident dialysis patients. Kidney International 62(3), 1046–1053 (2002)

Kalman, P.G., Pope, M., Bhola, C., et al.: A practical approach to vascular access for hemodialysis and predictors of success. J. Vasc. Surg. 30(4), 727–733 (1999)

Kamiya, A., Bukhari, R., Togawa, T.: Adaptive regulation of wall shear stress optimizing vascular tree function. Bull. Math. Biol. 46(1), 127–137 (1984)

Kaufman, J.L., Garb, J.L., Berman, J.A., et al.: A prospective comparison of two expanded polytetrafluoroethylene grafts for linear forearm hemodialysis access: does the manufacturer matter? J. Am. Coll. Surg. 185(1), 74–79 (1997)

Keeling, A.N., Naughton, P.A., McGrath, F.P., et al.: Successful endovascular treatment of a hemodialysis graft pseudoaneurysm by covered stent and direct percutaneous thrombin injection. Seminars in Dialysis 21(6), 553–556 (2008)

Keuter, X.H., De Smet, A.A., Kessels, A.G., et al.: A randomized multicenter study of the outcome of brachial basilic arteriovenous fistula and prosthetic brachial-antecubital forearm loop as vascular access for hemodialysis. J. Vasc. Surg. 47(2), 395–401 (2008)

Koksoy, C., Demirci, R.K., Balci, D., et al.: Brachiobasilic versus brachiocephalic arteriovenous fistula: a prospective randomized study. J. Vasc. Surg. 49(1), 171–177 (2009)

Lazarides, M.K., Georgiadis, G.S., Papasideris, C.P., et al.: Transposed brachial basilic arteriovenous fistulas versus prosthetic upper limb grafts: a meta analysis. Eur. J. Vasc. Endovasc. Surg. 36(5), 597–601 (2008)

Lenz, B.J., Veldenz, H.C., Dennis, J.W., et al.: A three-year follow-up on standard versus thin wall ePTFE grafts for hemodialysis. J. Vasc. Surg. 28(3), 464–470 (1998); discussion 470

Lin, S.L., Huang, C.H., Chen, H.S., et al.: Effects of age and diabetes on blood flow rate and primary outcome of newly created hemodialysis arteriovenous fistulas. American Journal of Nephrology 18(2), 96–100 (1998)

Lok, C.E., Oliver, M.J., Su, J., et al.: Arteriovenous fistula outcomes in the era of the elderly dialysis population. Kidney International 67(6), 2462–2469 (2005)

Lomonte, C., Casucci, F., Antonelli, M., et al.: Is there a place for duplex screening of the brachial artery in the maturation of arteriovenous fistulas? Seminars in Dialysis 18(3), 243–246 (2005)

London, G.: Pathophysiology of cardiovascular damage in the early renal population. Nephrol. Dial. Transplant. 16(suppl. 2), 3–6 (2001)

Malinzak, E.B., Gan, T.J.: Regional anesthesia for vascular access surgery. Anesth. Analg. 109(3), 976–980 (2009)

Malovrh, M.: Native arteriovenous fistula: preoperative evaluation. Am. J. Kidney Dis. 39(6), 1218–1225 (2002)

Marston, W.A., Criado, E., Jaques, P.F., et al.: Prospective randomized comparison of surgical versus endovascular management of thrombosed dialysis access grafts. J. Vasc. Surg. 26(3), 373–380 (1997); discussion 380-371

May, J., Tiller, D., Johnson, J., et al.: Saphenous vein arteriovenous fistula in regular dialysis treatment. N. Engl. J. Med. 280(14), 770 (1969)

Meichelboeck: Trends in ESRD epidemiology and vascular access. in: Angio Access for Hemodialysis, Tours, France, June 14-16 (2010)

Mihmanli, I., Besirli, K., Kurugoglu, S., et al.: Cephalic vein and hemodialysis fistula: surgeon's observation versus color Doppler ultra sonographic findings. J. Ultrasound Med. 20(3), 217–222 (2001)

Mickley, V., Gorich, J., Rilinger, N., et al.: Stenting of central venous stenoses in hemodialysis patients: long-term results. Kidney International 51(1), 277–280 (1997)

Moeller, S., Gioberge, S., Brown, G.: ESRD patients in 2001: global overview of patients, treatment modalities and development trends. Nephrol. Dial. Transplant. 17(12), 2071–2076 (2002)

Morsy, A.H., Kulbaski, M., Chen, C., et al.: Incidence and characteristics of patients with hand ischemia after a hemodialysis access procedure. J. Surg. Res. 74(1), 8–10 (1998)

Murphy, G.J., Saunders, R., Metcalfe, M., Nicholson, M.L.: Elbow fistulas using autogeneous vein: patency rates and results of revision. Postgrad. Med. J. 78(922), 483–486 (2002)

NKF-K/DOQI, clinical practice guidelines for chronic kidney dis-ease: evaluation, classification, and stratification. Am. J. Kidney 39(2 suppl. 1), S1–S266 (2002)

NKF-K/DOQI, Clinical Practice Guidelines for Vascular Access: update 2000. Am. J. Kidney Dis. 37(1 suppl. 1), S137–S181 (2001)

Padberg Jr., F.T., Calligaro, K.D., Sidawy, A.N.: Complications of arteriovenous hemodialysis access: recognition and management. J. Vasc. Surg. 48(5 suppl.), S55–S80 (2008)

Papasavas, P.K., Reifsnyder, T., Birdas, T.J., et al.: Prediction of arteriovenous access steal syndrome utilizing digital pressure measurements. Vascular and Endovascular Surgery 37(3), 179–184 (2003)

Parfrey, P.S., Foley, R.N., Harnett, J.D., et al.: Outcome and risk factors for left ventricular disorders in chronic uraemia. Nephrol. Dial. Transplant. 11(7), 1277–1285 (1996)

Penfield, J.G., Reilly Jr., R.F.: What nephrologists need to know about gadolinium. Nature Clinical Practice 3(12), 654–668 (2007)

Pisoni, R.L., Young, E.W., Dykstra, D.M., et al.: Vascular access use in Europe and the United States: results from the DOPPS. Kidney International 61(1), 305–316 (2002)

Planken, N.R., Tordoir, J.H., Duijm, L.E., et al.: Magnetic resonance angiographic assessment of upper extremity vessels prior to vascular access surgery: feasibility and accuracy. Eur. Radiol. 18(1), 158–167 (2008a)

Planken, R.N., Leiner, T., Nijenhuis, R.J., et al.: Contrast-enhanced magnetic resonance angiography findings prior to hemodialysis vascular access creation: a prospective analysis. The Journal of Vascular Access 9(4), 269–277 (2008b)

Planken, R.N., Keuter, X.H., Kessels, A.G., et al.: Forearm cephalic vein cross-sectional area changes at incremental congestion pressures: towards a standardized and reproducible vein mapping protocol. J. Vasc. Surg. 44(2), 353–358 (2006)

Polkinghorne, K.R., Atkins, R.C., Kerr, P.G.: Determinants of native arteriovenous fistula blood flow. Nephrology (Carlton) 9(4), 205–211 (2004)

Quinton, W., Dillard, D., Scribner, B.H.: Cannulation of blood vessels for prolonged hemodialysis. Trans. Am. Soc. Artif. Intern. Organs 6, 104–113 (1960)

Ravani, P., Marcelli, D., Malberti, F.: Vascular access surgery managed by renal physicians: the choice of native arteriovenous fistulas for hemodialysis. Am. J. Kidney Dis. 40(6), 1264–1276 (2002)

Remuzzi, A., Ene-Iordache, B., Mosconi, L., et al.: Radial artery wall shear stress evaluation in patients with arteriovenous fistula for hemodialysis access. Biorheology 40(1-3), 423–430 (2003)

Rooijens, P.P., Tordoir, J.H., Stijnen, T., et al.: Radiocephalic wrist arteriovenous fistula for hemodialysis: meta-analysis indicates a high primary failure rate. Eur. J. Vasc. Endovasc. Surg. 28(6), 583–589 (2004)

Roy-Chaudhury, P., Spergel, L.M., Besarab, A., et al.: Biology of arteriovenous fistula failure. Journal of Nephrology 20(2), 150–163 (2007)

Sadowski, E.A., Bennett, L.K., Chan, M.R., et al.: Nephrogenic systemic fibrosis: risk factors and incidence estimation. Radiology 243(1), 148–157 (2007)

Saran, R., Dykstra, D.M., Pisoni, R.L., et al.: Timing of first cannulation and vascular access failure in haemodialysis: an analysis of practice patterns at dialysis facilities in the DOPPS. Nephrol. Dial. Transplant. 19(9), 2334–2340 (2004)

Savage, M.T., Ferro, C.J., Sassano, A., Tomson, C.R.: The impact of arteriovenous fistula formation on central hemodynamic pressures in chronic renal failure patients: a prospective study. Am. J. Kidney Dis. 40(4), 753–759 (2002)

Schanzer, A., Nguyen, L.L., Owens, C.D., Schanzer, H.: Use of digital pressure measurements for the diagnosis of AV access induced hand ischemia. Vasc. Med. 11(4), 227–231 (2006)

Schanzer, H., Skladany, M., Haimov, M.: Treatment of angioaccess induced ischemia by revascularization. J. Vasc. Surg. 16(6), 861–864 (1992); discussion 864-866

Scheltinga, M.R., van Hoek, F., Bruijninckx, C.M.: Time of onset in haemodialysis access-induced distal ischaemia (HAIDI) is related to the access type. Nephrol. Dial. Transplant. 24(10), 3198–3204 (2009)

Schillinger, F., Schillinger, D., Montagnac, R., Milcent, T.: Post catheterisation vein stenosis in haemodialysis: comparative angiographic study of 50 subclavian and 50 internal jugular accesses. Nephrol. Dial. Transplant. 6(10), 722–724 (1991)

Schou, M., Torp-Pedersen, C., Gustafsson, F., et al.: Wall motion index, estimated glomerular filtration rate and mortality risk in patients with heart failure or myocardial infarction: a pooled analysis of 18,010 patients. Eur. J. Heart Fail. 10(7), 682–688 (2008)

Scribner, B.H., Buri, R., Caner, J.E., et al.: The treatment of chronic uremia by means of intermittent hemodialysis: a preliminary report. Trans. Am. Soc. Artif. Intern. Organs 6, 114–122 (1960)

Seldinger, S.I.: Catheter replacement of the needle in percutaneous arteriography; a new technique. Acta Radiol. 39(5), 368–376 (1953)

Segal, J.H., Kayler, L.K., Henke, P., et al.: Vascular access outcomes using the transposed basilic vein arteriovenous fistula. Am. J. Kidney Dis. 42(1), 151–157 (2003)

Shaldon, S., Chiandussi, L., Higgs, B.: Haemodialysis by percutaneous catheterization of the femoral artery and vein with regional heparinisation. Lancet 2, 857–859 (1961)

Sidawy, A.N., Gray, R., Besarab, A., et al.: Recommended standards for reports dealing with arteriovenous hemodialysis accesses. J. Vasc. Surg. 35(3), 603–610 (2002)

Silas, A.M., Bettmann, M.A.: Utility of covered stents for revision of aging failing synthetic hemodialysis grafts: a report of three cases. Cardiovasc. Intervent. Radiol. 26(6), 550–553 (2003)

Silva Jr., M.B., Hobson, R.W., Pappas, P.J., et al.: A strategy for increasing use of autogenous hemodialysis access procedures: impact of preoperative noninvasive evaluation. J. Vasc. Surg. 27(2), 302–307 (1998)

Sirrs, S., Duncan, L., Djurdjev, O., et al.: Homocyst(e)ine and vascular access complications in haemodialysis patients: insights into a complex metabolic relationship. Nephrol. Dial. Transplant. 14(3), 738–743 (1999)

Sivanesan, S., How, T.V., Bakran, A.: Characterizing flow distributions in AV fistulae for haemodialysis access. Nephrol. Dial. Transplant. 13(12), 3108–3110 (1998)

Sprouse, L.R., Lesar, C.J., Meier, G.H., et al.: Percutaneous treatment of symptomatic central venous stenosis [corrected]. J. Vasc. Surg. 39(3), 578–582 (2004)

Tian, J.P., Wang, T., Wang, H., et al.: The prevalence of left ventricular hypertrophy in Chinese hemodialysis patients is higher than that in peritoneal dialysis patients. Ren. Fail. 30(4), 391–400 (2008)

Tordoir, J.H., Van Der Sande, F.M., De Haan, M.W.: Current topics on vascular access for hemodialysis. Minerva Urologica e Nefrologica = The Italian Journal of Urology and Nephrology 56(3), 223–235 (2004)

Tordoir, J., Canaud, B., Haage, P., et al.: EBPG on Vascular Access. Nephrol. Dial. Transplant. 22(suppl. 2), ii88–ii117 (2007)

Tordoir, J.H., Rooyens, P., Dammers, R., et al.: Prospective evaluation of failure modes in autogenous radiocephalic wrist access for haemodialysis. Nephrol. Dial. Transplant. 18(2), 378–383 (2003)

Trerotola, S.O., Stavropoulos, S.W., Shlansky-Goldberg, R., et al.: Hemodialysis-related venous stenosis: treatment with ultrahigh-pressure angioplasty balloons. Radiology 231(1), 259–262 (2004)

Tronc, F., Mallat, Z., Lehoux, S., et al.: Role of matrix metallopro-teinases in blood flow induced arterial enlargement: Interaction with NO. Arterioscler Thromb. Vasc. Biol. 20(12), E120–E126 (2000)

Turmel-Rodrigues, L., Mouton, A., Birmele, B., et al.: Salvage of immature forearm fistulas for haemodialysis by interventional radiology. Nephrol. Dial. Transplant. 16(12), 2365–2371 (2001)

Turmel-Rodrigues, L., Pengloan, J., Blanchier, D., et al.: Insufficient dialysis shunts: improved long-term patency rates with close hemodynamic monitoring, repeated percutaneous balloon angioplasty, and stent placement. Radiology 187(1), 273–278 (1993)

Turmel-Rodrigues, L., Pengloan, J., Baudin, S., et al.: Treatment of stenosis and thrombosis in haemodialysis fistulas and grafts by interventional radiology. Nephrol. Dial. Transplant. 15(12), 2029–2036 (2000)

Van Hoek, F., Scheltinga, M.R., Kouwenberg, I., et al.: Steal in hemodialysis patients depends on type of vascular access. Eur. J. Vasc. Endovasc. Surg. 32(6), 710–717 (2006)

Van Loon, M.M., Goovaerts, T., Kessels, A.G., et al.: Buttonhole needling of haemodialysis arteriovenous fistulae results in less complications and interventions compared to the rope-ladder technique. Nephrol. Dial. Transplant. 25(1), 225–230 (2010)

Vassalotti, J.A., Falk, A., Teodorescu, V., Uribarri, J.: The multidisciplinary approach to hemodialysis vascular access at the Mount Sinai Hospital. Mt. Sinai. J. Med. 71(2), 94–102 (2004)

Vesely, T.M., Siegel, J.B.: Use of the peripheral cutting balloon to treat hemodialysis related stenoses. J. Vasc. Interv. Radiol. 16(12), 1593–1603 (2005)

Voormolen, E.H., Jahrome, A.K., Bartels, L.W., et al.: Nonmaturation of arm arteriovenous fistulas for hemodialysis access: A systematic review of risk factors and results of early treatment. J. Vasc. Surg. 49(5), 1325–1336 (2009)

Warren, J.V., Nickerson, J.L., Elkin, D.C.: The cardiac output in patients with arteriovenous fistulas. J. Clin. Invest. 30(2), 210–214 (1951)

Weijmer, M.C., van den Dorpel, M.A., Van de Ven, P.J., et al.: Randomized, clinical trial comparison of trisodium citrate 30% and heparin as catheterlocking solution in hemodialysis patients. J. Am. Soc. Nephrol. 16(9), 2769–2777 (2005)

Weijmer, M.C., ter Wee, P.M.: Temporary vascular access for hemodialysis treatment. Current Guidelines and Future Directions. Contrib. Nephrol. 142, 94–111 (2004)

Wixon, C.L., Hughes, J.D., Mills, J.L.: Understanding strategies for the treatment of ischemic steal syndrome after hemodialysis access. J. Am. Coll. Surg. 191(3), 301–310 (2000)

Wolowczyk, L., Williams, A.J., Donovan, K.L., Gibbons, C.P.: The snuffbox arteriovenous fistula for vascular access. Eur. J. Vasc. Endovasc. Surg. 19(1), 70–76 (2000)

Wolford, H.Y., Hsu, J., Rhodes, J.M., et al.: Outcome after autogenous brachial basilic upper arm transpositions in the post-National Kidney Foundation Dialysis Outcomes Quality Initiative era. J. Vasc. Surg. 42(5), 951–956 (2005)

Wong, V., Ward, R., Taylor, J., et al.: Factors associated with early failure
    of arteriovenous fistulae for haemodialysis access. Eur. J. Vasc.
    Endovasc. Surg. 12(2), 207–213 (1996)
Woo, K., Farber, A., Doros, G., et al.: Evaluation of the efficacy of the
    transposed upper arm arteriovenous fistula: a single institutional
    review of 190 basilic and cephalic vein transposition procedures. J.
    Vasc. Surg. 46(1), 94–99 (2007)
Yasim, A., Kabalci, M., Eroglu, E., Zencirci, B.: Complication of hemo-
    dialysis graft: anastomotic pseudoaneurysm: a case report. Trans-
    plant. Proc. 38(9), 2816–2818 (2006)
Yildirim, V., Doganci, S., Yanarates, O., et al.: Does preemptive stellate
    ganglion blockage increase the patency of radiocephalic arteri-
    ovenous fistula? Scand. Cardiovasc. J. 40(6), 380–384 (2006)
Zakrzewicz, A., Secomb, T.W., Pries, A.R.: Angioadaptation: keeping the
    vascular system in shape. News Physiol. Sci. 17, 197–201 (2002)
Zeebregts, C.J., Tielliu, I.F., Hulsebos, R.G., et al.: Determinants of failure
    of brachiocephalic elbow fistulas for haemodialysis. Eur. J. Vasc.
    Endovasc. Surg. 30(2), 209–214 (2005)

ESSAY QUESTIONS

1. Describe the difference between diffusion and ultrafiltration in hemodialysis therapy
2. Describe the difference between primary and secondary patency of a vascular access.
3. In 1960, Quinton and Scribner proposed a novel way to create a vascular access. What was the principle of this access and what were its shortcomings?
4. Nowadays, clinical decision-making is based on pre-operative vascular imaging and knowledge regarding post-operative complications and patency rated for each configuration. Which vascular parameters are objectivated during the duplex ultrasound examination?
5. Venous congestion of the hand can occur after the creation of a side-to-side anastomosis. How can this be avoided?
6. Describe the rationale of performing a transposition procedure when creating a brachiobasilic fistula
7. The creation of a brachiobasilic fistula can be performed in a one or two-stage procedure. Describe the rational of both procedures.
8. Describe the rationale of a banding procedure in a patient with ischemic complaints

9. Prosthetic graft material can be used for vascular access creation when autologous veins are no longer available / suitable. What are the main disadvantages of using graft material?

10. Identify the arteries and veins in the image below.

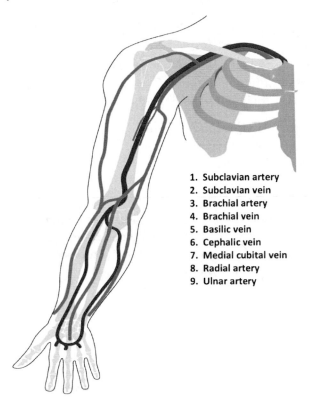

1. Subclavian artery
2. Subclavian vein
3. Brachial artery
4. Brachial vein
5. Basilic vein
6. Cephalic vein
7. Medial cubital vein
8. Radial artery
9. Ulnar artery

MULTIPLE CHOICE QUESTIONS

Choose the best answer

1. After creation of a radiocephalic fistula, retrograde flow in the distal radial artery occurs in a certain percentage of cases. This percentage is…

A. 10%
B. 30%
C. 75%
D. 90%

2. In order to perform adequate hemodialysis, a minimum flow through the vascular access is necessary. This flow is...

   A. 100 ml/min
   B. 300 ml/min
   C. 500 ml/min
   D. 1000 ml/min

3. Central venous catheters may induce the development of central venous stenosis. After insertion of a catheter in the subclavian vein, the chance for development of such a stenosis is...

   A. 10%
   B. 20%
   C. 40%
   D. 80%

4. After creation of a radiocephalic fistula, early failure might occur due to poor selection of vessels. Below a certain venous diameter there is an increased chance of early failure and non-maturation. According to European guidelines, this diameter is...

   A. 1.0 mm
   B. 1.6 mm
   C. 2.0 mm
   D. 2.5 mm

5. A Gracz-fistula is a vascular access at the level of the elbow. It consists of an anastomosis between the...

   A. Brachial artery and cephalic vein
   B. Brachial artery and cubital medial vein
   C. Brachial artery and perforant vein of the cubital medial vein
   D. Proximal radial artery and perforant vein of the cubital medial vein

6. Ischemic complaints of the hand after vascular access surgery are reported in a certain percentage of patients: This percentage is...

   A. 5%
   B. 10%
   C. 50%
   D. 75%

7. Only a certain amount of patients requires treatment for hemodialysis access induced distal ischemia. This percentage is...

    A. Approximately 5%
    B. Approximately 10%
    C. Approximately 15%
    D. Approximately 20%

8. According to clinical practice guidelines certain autologous vascular access conduits are preferred over others. From first choice to least favorite...

    A. Snuffbox fistula, BC-AVF, BB-AVF
    B. Proximal RC-AVF, Distal RC-AVF, BB-AVF, BC-AVF
    C. Lower extremity AVF, BB-AVF, BC-AVF, RC-AVF
    D. Snuffbox fistula, Distal RC-AVF, Proximal RC-AVF, BC-AVF, BB-AVF

9. What is the preferred vascular access in the dialysis population?

    A. A central venous catheter
    B. An arteriovenous graft
    C. An arteriovenous fistula

10 Prior to vascular access surgery vascular imaging needs to be performed to determine the most suitable site for vascular access creation. What examination is recommended in patients with previous indwelling central venous catheters?

    A. Physical examination
    B. Duplex ultrasound examination
    C. Digital subtraction angiography
    D. Magnetic resonance angiography

11. Which cannulation technique is associated with the highest incidence of aneurysm formation?

    A. Rope-ladder technique
    B. Area-technique
    C. Button-hole technique
    D. There is no difference between these techniques

12. What determines the suitability of a vascular access to perform hemodialysis?

   A. Vascular access flow
   B. The diameter of the venous outflow tract
   C. The depth of the cannulation segment
   D. All of the above

13. What is the most common location for the development stenoses in a
native arteriovenous fistula?

   A. The arterial inflow
   B. The juxta-anastomotic region
   C. The venous outflow traject
   D. The central venous system

14. After vascular access creation, peripheral vascular resistance is bypassed. To maintain blood pressure over the cardiovascular system, an increase in cardiac output is required. Cardiac failure is more likely to occur
in patients with a vascular access flow over...

   A. 1000 ml/min
   B. 1500 ml/min
   C. 2000 ml/min
   D. 3000 ml/min

15. Intimal hyperplasia is the result of proliferation and migration of certain cells. These are...

   A. Endothelial cells
   B. Smooth muscle cells
   C. Red blood cells
   D. White blood cells

16. The chance for development of hemodialysis access induced distal
ischemia is the largest in...
   A. RC-AVF
   B. BC-AVF
   C. BB-AVF
   D. Arteriovenous grafts

17. Monitoring of the vascular access by means of frequent physical examination and duplex examination improves survival when preemptive interventional procedures are performed

  A. Yes
  B. No

18. For the creation of a vascular access different types anesthesia exist. Which of the following techniques is the least recommended?

  A. Local anesthesia
  B. Regional anesthesia
  C. General anesthesia

19. Why is regional anesthesia preferred over local anesthesia?

  A. Induction of peripheral venous dilatation
  B. Most adequate treatment of pain
  C. Supervision of a anesthesiologist is necessary
  D. All of the above

20. In order to avoid temporary hemodialysis by a central venous catheter, referral to the department of vascular surgery needs to be well in advance to allow time for sufficient maturation and interventional procedures in case of vascular access dysfunction. The recommended time for referral is...

  A. 3 months prior to the expected start of HD
  B. 6 months prior to the expected start of HD
  C. 9 months prior to the expected start of HD
  D. 12 months prior to the expected start of HD

Chapter 6

Access Flow Monitoring Methods

Daniel Schneditz, Laura M. Rosales, Ahmad Taher Azar

CHAPTER OUTLINES

- Introduction
- Peripheral Access
- Flow Measurement
- Extracorporeal Applications
- Access Flow
- Bolus Approach
- Continuous Infusion Approach
- Line Switches
- Arterio-Venous Gradients
- Conclusion

CHAPTER OBJECTIVES

- To acknowledge the importance of indicator dilution for the measurement of physiologic flows
- To recognize that the connection of the extracorporeal system to the circulation is not as efficient as desired because of recirculation
- To realize that recirculation is related to blood flows and that blood flows can be determined from recirculation measurements
- To understand that the process of hemodialysis itself with material exchanged in the extracorporeal system can be used as indicator
- To realize the potential of extracorporeal applications for automatic flow measurements

KEY TERMS

- Cardiac output
- Systemic blood flow
- Access blood flow
- Access resistance
- Access stenosis
- Blood pressure
- Resistance
- Recirculation
- Access recirculation
- Forced recirculation
- Cardiopulmonary recirculation
- Indicator dilution
- Constant infusion techniques
- Bolus techniques
- Area under the curve
- Double recirculation techniques
- Gradient techniques
- Thermodilution
- Saline dilution
- On-line clearance
- Extracorporeal gradients
- Line switches

A.T. Azar (Ed.): Modelling and Control of Dialysis Systems, SCI 404, pp. 305–345.
springerlink.com   © Springer-Verlag Berlin Heidelberg 2013

ABSTRACT

Low access blood flow has been recognized as the most important cause for access thrombosis and subsequent access failure so that some form of access flow surveillance is recommended in everyday practice. The classic technique to measure flow in physiology is based on indicator dilution as most flow rates are inaccessible to direct measurement. However, extracorporeal blood purification techniques have been designed for the controlled removal and/or delivery of solutes, all of which can be used as indicators to measure selected transport characteristics throughout the intra- and extracorporeal system. It is therefore not surprising that extracorporeal techniques are extremely well suited for access flow monitoring methods based on indicator dilution, also because these techniques can be integrated into the extracorporeal system as part of the purification process and as these procedures have the potential to be fully automated. In this chapter the physiological basis of indicator dilution is briefly summarized with regard to application in hemodialysis considering the limitations as well as the possibilities for integration and automation.

6.1 INTRODUCTION

Chronic extracorporeal therapy relies on high extracorporeal blood flows. With intermittent therapy the elimination rate of solutes removed during short periods of time must be much higher than their continuous generation rate. Therefore, for adequate hemodialysis delivering a Kt/V dose of 1.4 thrice a week, and for the average treatment duration t of 4 h (240 min) in an average 70 kg patient with a total body water volume V in the range of 35 L, the clearance K delivered must be larger than 200 mL/min ($=1.4*V/240$). Thus, in this mode of therapy where efficiency is importantly flow limited an uncomplicated and steady extracorporeal blood flow Q_b of 250 mL/min or more is required. Temporary delivery of sufficient blood flow is possible with venous catheters placed centrally or in femoral veins, but due to the risk of infection and patient discomfort, the extended use of such accesses is not recommended.

Therefore, the peripheral arterio-venous access has been created with the aim to provide sufficient blood flow during extracorporeal treatment while the skin provides the natural barrier to reduce the risk of infection. The pain and discomfort of frequent needle punctures can be reduced by special methods such as the buttonhole technique (Marticorena et al. 2011). However, the vascular access remains a vulnerable interface between the extracorporeal and the cardiovascular system. Adequate flow assures access longevity (Kim et al. 2010) and access blood flow monitoring in combination with physical exam by the nephrologists is likely to reduce access morbidity and costs (Lomonte and Basile 2011, McCarley et al. 2001).

There are several techniques to measure access blood flow in dialysis patients which are also used in other areas of medicine such as those based on ultrasound Doppler effect. Their use is not specific for applications in hemodialysis and therefore they are not discussed in this chapter. However, the very classical approach based on indicator dilution has a special appeal because it takes advantage of hemodialysis technology with regard to introducing and measuring different indicators. The original technique of creating a condition which permits to measure access flow, injecting indicator into the blood returning to the access, and measuring the dilution of this indicator in the blood drawn from the access using ultrasonic detection was developed by N. Krivitski more than 15 years ago (Krivitski 1995). This principle was subsequently adapted for other indicators such as temperature or conductivity where markers can be automatically injected through the dialysate and either measured in the blood lines or in the dialysate lines using dedicated hemodialysis technology. This chapter essentially deals with indicator dilution and with approaches derived from that technique for improved usability.

6.2 PERIPHERAL ACCESS

To provide sufficient blood flow for extracorporeal use the peripheral arterio-venous access needs to deliver access flows above 600 mL/min. This is more than the usual extracorporeal blood flow, but this magnitude is required to maintain flow also under unfavorable conditions such as low arterial pressures. Most arterio-venous accesses deliver blood flows in the range of 1500 mL/min.

The creation of a peripheral arterio-venous access has major hemodynamic consequences. For comparison, in the common central-venous and in the more rarely used arterio-arterial access (Bünger et al. 2005, Chiang et al. 2007, Krisper et al. 2011) blood is removed from the same part of the circulation to which it is returned and therefore these types of access have little hemodynamic effects. Once the extracorporeal system is filled, the removal does not affect the volume and the pressure in the central venous compartment because the removal is balanced by the return. The balance is only affected by the amount of ultrafiltration which usually is a small fraction of extracorporeal blood flow. There is no hemodynamic effect when the central venous access is not in use, however, the catheter lines which usually remain in place have to be kept patent by using special catheter locks to prevent coagulation of stagnant blood within the catheters.

The creation of an arterio-venous access establishes a direct connection between the high pressure arterial system and the low pressure venous system (see Fig. 6.1). The flow through the arterio-venous access is essentially a flow bypassing systemic tissue compartments and flow control (Bos et al. 1999, Schneditz et al. 1992, Válek et al. 2010). Cardiac output Q_{co} can be seen as the sum of two parallel flows, systemic blood flow Q_s and access blood flow Q_a:

$$Q_{co} = Q_a + Q_s \tag{6.1}$$

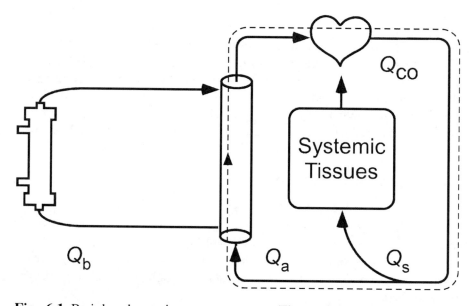

Fig. 6.1 Peripheral arterio-venous access. The peripheral arterio-venous access is a parallel circuit between arterial and venous compartments of the circulation bypassing systemic tissues and bypassing autonomic flow control (broken line). The diagram also shows the position of the extracorporeal circulation. Abbreviations: Q_{co} cardiac output, Q_s systemic blood flow, Q_a access blood flow, Q_b extracorporeal blood flow.

The peripheral arterio-venous access constitutes a parallel circuit to the systemic circulation. The parallel configuration therefore reduces the total peripheral resistance, and to maintain the same arterial blood pressure, cardiac output is increased by autonomic control. If cardiac output cannot be increased by increasing stroke volume, it rises by increasing heart rate.

The change in heart rate induced by a temporary occlusion of peripheral access flow therefore is an indirect sign for a high access flow.

Q_a is different from Q_s especially with regard to flow control. The flow through the arterio-venous access is essentially determined by the artificial and passive resistance of the connection between arterial and venous compartments and by the arterio-venous pressure gradient. Short term changes in access flow such as those seen during hemodialysis are therefore more likely related to changes in driving pressures than to changes in vascular resistance (Schneditz et al. 1998b). Therefore, for comparison of flows under different hemodynamic situations it is essential to record mean arterial pressures. The calculation of access resistance AR is approximated by the ratio of mean arterial pressure p_{mean} to access flow Q_a and allows for comparing flows under different driving pressures:

$$AR = \frac{\Delta p}{Q_a} \approx \frac{p_{mean}}{Q_a} \qquad (6.2)$$

Also, access flow is maintained throughout the lifetime of the access, whether it is used for extracorporeal therapy or not. The flow past systemic tissue compartments is a significant amount of cardiac output. The magnitude of access flow is in the range of 1.5 L/min and comparable to the magnitude of renal blood flow, but flows as high as 3 L/min and above are not unusual. This is a major fraction of cardiac output. In case of end stage kidney disease the Q_a is tacitly assumed to compensate for absent renal blood flow so that access flows in the range of 1 to 2 L are considered as acceptable. However, unlike renal blood flow, there is no auto-regulation of access blood flow which is passively following the changes in mean arterial pressure. For example, when mean arterial pressure changes with exercise, and more blood flow is required for perfusion of the working muscle, access flow is going to passively increase, stealing blood flow from the systemic circulation or from the distal parts of the circulation (Novljan et al. 2011). More important than the absolute volume flow rate is the fraction of cardiac output flowing through the peripheral arterio-venous access. This magnitude has been termed cardiopulmonary recirculation:

$$R_{cpr} = \frac{Q_a}{Q_{co}} \qquad (6.3)$$

Cardiopulmonary recirculation R_{cpr} is in the range of 20% to 30% and may reach values up to 50% (Schneditz et al. 1999). It is assumed that a value exceeding 30% is a risk factor for cardiac failure (Basile et al. 2008). Cardiovascular mortality is especially high in dialysis patients.

6.3 FLOW MEASUREMENT

Under most circumstances physiological volumes and/or volume flow rates are not accessible to direct measurement. Flows and volumes are extensive quantities and such quantities are difficult to measure in general. However, the measurement of one extensive variable, for example volume, can be replaced by another extensive variable, mass. And, to avoid measuring all the mass, the mass of a surrogate is measured; this surrogate is called an indicator. Based on principles of mass conservation the distribution volume and/or volume flow rate is determined from the amount of indicator added and from the concentration of the indicator measured in the system. Indicator dilution to measure blood flow goes back to the technique introduced by A. Fick (Fick 1870) where O_2 is used as an indicator to determine cardiac output Q_{CO} from arterio-venous oxygen differences and respiratory oxygen uptake applying principles of mass conservation:

$$Q_{co} = \frac{\dot{V}_{O_2}}{a_{O_2} - v_{O_2}} \tag{6.4}$$

The important point here is that O_2 uptake can be measured non-invasively and that arterio-venous O_2 differences are accessible to direct measurement. Notice that O_2 is an intrinsic indicator. It is assumed that all O_2 entering the blood in the lungs appears in the arterial side of the circulation without losses, that O_2 is well mixed in arterial blood so that a sample represents an equilibrated concentration and that such a representative sample can be taken from almost any peripheral artery. Also note that it is not required to sample the whole cardiac output. It is further assumed that the system is in a steady state: O_2 entering the lungs is essentially used in peripheral tissues and cleared from the blood stream so that mixed-venous concentration stays constant. Entry and removal of O_2 is in a steady state and there is no net recirculation of O_2 entering the lungs. This summarizes some requirements for an indicator: the indicator should be non-toxic, without effects on the measured entity, stable, easily measurable, and its distribution and elimination characteristics should be known.

Another classic approaches to estimate blood flow is related to clearance such as the estimation of liver blood flow from the measurement of indocyanine green (ICG, also known as cardiogreen) concentrations

(Cherrick et al. 1960, Fox et al. 1956). ICG is an exogenous dye which binds to plasma albumin upon infusion and which is readily taken up by hepatocytes and completely cleared from blood passing the healthy liver. The ICG has an absorption maximum and high extinction in the range of 805 nm and its concentration is easily measured in plasma for example during hemodialysis (Schneditz et al. 2005), but also transcutaneously. Thus, the ICG clearance can be used to determine hepatic blood flow (Hinghofer-Szalkay et al. 2008) and hepatic function non-invasively:

$$V \frac{dc}{dt} = -Kc + J_i \qquad (6.5)$$

In the steady state approach the infusion of ICG green is adjusted to obtain a constant concentration in arterial blood. Then, when the concentration of ICG is constant ($dc/dt=0$, Eq. 6.5) the ICG clearance is obtained from the infusion rate J_i and the steady state concentration c_{ss} as $K=J_i/c_{ss}$. A similar approach is used for assessing renal function and calculating glomerular filtration rate (GFR) from steady state creatinine concentration c_{ss} and endogenous creatinine generation rate G_{cr} as GFR$=G_{cr}/c_{ss}$.

An alternative to the steady state approach is to inject a known amount of indicator into the blood stream as a bolus so that the indicator disperses within the blood flow of the organ or organ system to be studied, and to measure the concentration of the indicator diluted by the blood flow passing the system. In this case it is not sufficient to determine a single concentration – the system is not in a steady state situation - but one has to sample the whole time course of concentrations, the so-called dilution curve ideally until all indicator is retrieved (see Fig. 6.2). The volume flow through the system is then obtained by the mass m of indicator injected and the area under the indicator concentration curve (AUC) sampled at the system outflow. The average concentration of indicator sampled at the outlet is given as:

$$\bar{c} = \frac{AUC}{t} \qquad (6.6)$$

and since the distribution volume V is given as:

$$V = \frac{m}{\bar{c}} \qquad (6.7)$$

the flow Q through the system is obtained by combining Eq. (6.6) and Eq. (6.7) as:

$$Q = \frac{V}{t} = \frac{m}{AUC} \tag{6.8}$$

This is the classic Stewart approach to measure flow by indicator dilution (Stewart 1897). The time course of the complete indicator concentration follows a statistical distribution function and the exact shape of this function is of theoretical interest regarding the process of indicator dispersion between sites of indicator injection and indicator measurement (Bassingthwaighte et al. 1966, King et al. 1996). Independent of its shape the AUC of the first transit is required to compute the flow through the system. In the real situation, however, the full curve corresponding to the first indicator transit often cannot be sampled without further perturbations because of so-called recirculation of indicator. Indicator leaving the organ eventually returns to the organ by way of the blood circulation and causes a second transit within some delay superimposed to late portions of the first transit. The second transit also recirculates and causes a third transit and so on. Eventually, the indicator has spread out over the whole circulation and other processes take over in its elimination. The theory provides a solution for the first transit of indicator only and all calculations are based on the first dilution curve. The separation of the first from subsequent transits is possible by extrapolation as shown by Hamilton et al. (Hamilton et al. 1928). For this reason it is important to avoid the superposition of first transits with second or higher order transits. A maximum separation is achieved by first injecting the indicator within the shortest possible time and then, by eliminating the superposition of higher transits from the late phase of the indicator dilution curve, and, last but not least, by choosing the proper indicator. The elimination of superposition can be done by extrapolating the decay of the late phase from the decay measured during early phases of the dilution curve. This also requires sensors with short response times, favorably less than 1 s. Typically, with a blood volume V_b of 5 L and with a cardiac output of 5 L/min the mean transit of indicator through the whole circulation ($\tau = V_b/Q_{co}$) is in the range of 60 s. More information on the theory of indicator dilution is found in specialized monographs (Hegglin et al. 1962, Lassen et al. 1983).

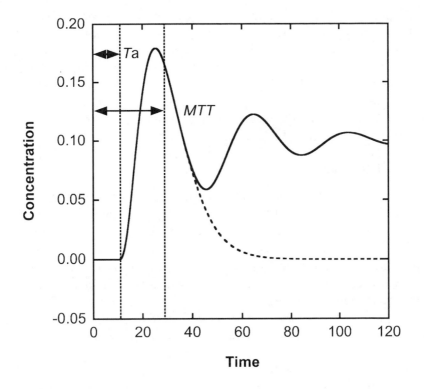

Fig. 6.2 Indicator dilution. A bolus of indicator injected at time $t=0$ appears at the measuring site at time $t=T_a$ (appearance time) and passes the measuring site with a mean transit time (MTT). The broken line shows the first transit without recirculation. The full line shows the dilution of multiple transits because of recirculation.

The classical application of indicator dilution is used to measure cardiac output where indicator such as cold saline is injected into the right atrium and the time course of the temperature change is measured distally to the injection site, in close vicinity to the injection site using the same catheter or a second catheter with a thermistor placed in the left heart or the aortic arch. Close vicinity of indicator delivery and indicator measurement is required for indicators rapidly dissipating not only within blood but also within the surrounding tissue. Because of dissipation in surrounding tissue the superposition of recirculating indicator as well as the accumulation of indicator is minimized so that measurements can be repeated without delay. However, because of dissipation in surrounding tissue it is necessary that injection and measuring sites are located close to the mixing site and the indicator is required to completely mix with blood flow between injection and measuring sites. With regard to measuring access flow the thermodilution approach had been used in the AngioFlow (AngioDynamics Inc., Latham, New York) which required the insertion of a catheter into the vascular access (Vesely et al. 2002). This device, however, is no longer available on the market.

For indicators confined to the intravascular space and only slowly removed from the blood or lost to the surrounding tissue injection and measuring sites do not have to be located in close vicinity to the mixing site. Thus, for the measurement of cardiac output using ICG which is bound to albumin and slowly removed from the blood by the liver, the indicator can be injected into the venous system far away from the central mixing site, the heart, and the diluted indicator can be measured at any suitable sampling point of the arterial system or microcirculation, for example in the finger, ear lobe, or nostrils. Notice that it is not required to sample the whole cardiac output. The measurement of a representative sample is sufficient. Apart from the delay caused by transport from the heart to the sampling point an arterial sample measured anywhere in the circulation will be representative of the mixed concentration leaving the heart (Henriques 1913). The shape of the curve is changing, but the area under the curve remains unchanged.

6.4 EXTRACORPOREAL APPLICATION

The Stewart-Hamilton principle of indicator dilution can be extended to extracorporeal applications such as hemodialysis where the blood lines may be used as catheters, and where sensors can be attached to these blood lines (see Fig. 6.3). Indicator can be injected into blood returning to the patient through the venous limb of the extracorporeal circulation and the dilution curve can be measured in arterial blood passing the arterial limb of the extracorporeal circulation.

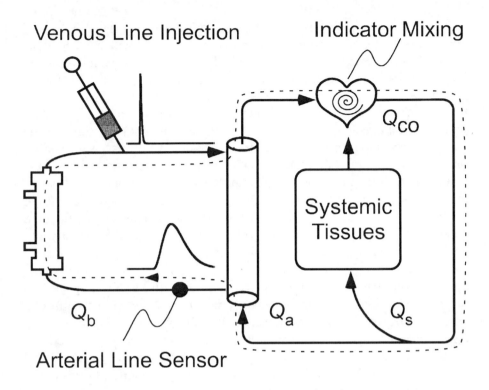

Fig. 6.3 Indicator dilution for cardiac output measurement. Indicator injected into the venous line and returned to the access with blood flow Q_b is mixing with systemic flow Q_s in the heart. The diluted indicator is sampled from the upstream part of the access and the dilution curve is measured by the arterial sensor. Notice the correct placement of blood lines and the absence of access recirculation.

This type of injection leads to a high and narrow pulse at the injection site. As this high indicator pulse is carried downstream with the blood it first mixes with extracorporeal blood flow, then with access flow, finally with the venous return from all tissues which is equal to the cardiac output. After having passed the heart a fraction of the diluted indicator eventually returns to the access. On its way through the circulation the bolus is progressively delayed and becomes wider and smaller the further downstream the concentration is measured. After a few circulations the dispersion of the indicator is complete as it becomes evenly distributed across the whole blood volume.

The requirements for indicator dilution are met when hemodialysis is done with the typical peripheral arterio-venous access which receives its inflow from a peripheral artery and which feeds into the venous system. The conditions to determine cardiac output are not met with the common central-venous or with the rare arterio-arterial access. It is also important that all of the indicator injected into the venous line flows to the heart without access recirculation, i.e. without taking the shortcut through the vascular access. The first application in hemodialysis was performed by one of us with 50 mL of isotonic saline injected into the venous limb of the extracorporeal circulation at body temperature and ultrasonic detection of diluted blood in the arterial line (Schneditz et al. 1991). Sound velocity in blood importantly depends on the concentration of plasma proteins and hemoglobin and can be used to determine the hematocrit and the water content in blood with high resolution (Schneditz et al. 1989a, b; Schneditz et al. 1990). This approach has been adapted for other sensors and is now available with the HD03 (Transonic Systems Inc. Ithaca, New York). Notice that recirculation through the access must be avoided in this setting. In case of recirculation through the access the dilution curve cannot be analyzed by usual algorithms. However, recirculation is easily detected because of the short delay between injection and indicator appearance, and because of the shape of the dilution curve. But more importantly, recirculation can be used to determine access flow.

6.4.1 Recirculation

"It's like déjà vu all over again." Yogi Berra (Berra 2011)

Under certain conditions processed blood returned to the access finds its way to the arterial line without systemic equilibration by recirculation. "Recirculation" refers to the reflux of dialyzed blood from the venous return back into the arterial line (Sherman and Kapoian 1997).

Recirculation may have different reasons, mostly because of violation of the basic requirements such as wrong needle placement. Thus, to identify access recirculation and to exclude false positive results one needs to be aware of the situations which may affect and contaminate the recirculation measurement (Schneditz 1998).

Recirculation is a local effect in the veno-venous or central-venous access (Twardowski et al. 1993). In this type of access recirculation occurs when one or more conditions to prevent admixture of cleared blood such as inadequate access flow, reversed and close placement of blood lines are violated.

6.4.2 Access Recirculation

Access recirculation into the arterial line is defined as the fraction of cleared extracorporeal blood flow that returns to the inlet of the extracorporeal blood line taking the short connection between the access needles. In this type of recirculation there is retrograde flow Q_r within the vessel in which the access needles are placed. Extracorporeal blood flow Q_b can be maintained in spite of insufficient access flow Q_a so that:

$$Q_b = Q_r + Q_a \qquad (6.9)$$

The magnitude of local or access recirculation R is given as the ratio of recirculating flow to extracorporeal blood flow as:

$$R = \frac{Q_r}{Q_b}, (Q_a \leq Q_b) \qquad (6.10)$$

Access recirculation ranges between 0 and 1 for access flows smaller or equal to Q_b. This effect is well known in hemodialysis as it reduces the efficiency of the treatment, because a fraction of cleared blood returns to the access, bypasses equilibration in the body and returns to the extracorporeal system. There are different reasons for access recirculation to occur and for the operator it is not easy to recognize local recirculation because extracorporeal blood flows are often easily achieved with acceptable arterial and venous line pressures. Therefore, different techniques have been used to measure recirculation (Schneditz and Krivitski 2004).

Local recirculation is absent with a functioning access. It occurs with inadequate access blood flow, i.e., if Q_b is larger than Q_a, and with close or reversed needle position. If wrong placement of access needles and reversed placement of blood lines can be excluded, access recirculation is an indicator of an acute access problem. On the other hand, absence of access recirculation does not necessarily exclude access problems since the presence of a significant stenosis between arterial and venous puncture sites is not detected by conventional recirculation measurements (Besarab et al. 1997). The explanation for the failure of access recirculation to detect a mid-access stenosis is as follows: With intra-access strictures which produce a significant resistance to access blood flow between arterial and venous needle puncture sites, the blood flow evades intra-access resistance during hemodialysis and takes a functional bypass through the extracorporeal circulation (van Gemert et al. 1984). Even though the access is under risk for future thrombosis because of the intra-access stricture, there is sufficient blood supply to the inlet of the arterial blood line and there is no recirculation.

6.5 ACCESS FLOW

Inspection of Eq. (6.9) and Eq. (6.10) shows that access flow can be calculated from the magnitude of local access recirculation and the extracorporeal blood flow as:

$$Q_a = Q_b(1-R), \quad (0 < R \le 1) \tag{6.11}$$

In case of access recirculation access flow is always smaller than extracorporeal blood flow. With 100% recirculation access flow is zero, but without recirculation, access flow can be equal or larger than Q_b. Access flow is not defined under the condition that $R=0$ as R will be absent with any access flow equal to or larger than blood flow. Thus, to determine access flow by this approach some degree of recirculation is required. The flow delivered by extracorporeal blood pumps is limited to 600 mL/min in most machines and rarely delivered in routine hemodialysis. Extracorporeal blood flows are in the range of 300 to 400 mL/min, so that this approach allows for determination of access flows which are below the extracorporeal blood flow. Access flow, however, is created in the range of 1000 to 1500 mL/min, and access flows in the range of 300 to 400 mL/min are already inadequate. Therefore, this technique is not really useful to monitor access blood flow.

How is recirculation related to indicator dilution and to the measurement of access flow?

The return of blood to the access using the venous line serves as a system to deliver a known amount of indicator. In case of access recirculation a fraction R of that indicator recirculates and is carried to the inflow of the arterial needle where it is diluted by access flow. The dilution is then measured in the arterial blood line. Indicator can be delivered as a bolus or as a continuous injection, and intrinsic as well as extrinsic indicators can be used.

6.5.1 Forced Recirculation

Access recirculation not only develops with insufficient access flow, but also with inadequate needle placement. If, for example the removal of blood from the access and the return of blood to the access is reversed, access recirculation develops in spite of sufficient access flow. Inadvertent reversal of blood lines is more frequent than anticipated (Shapiro and Gurevich 1997) especially in loop grafts where the direction of blood flow is not always obvious. Extracorporeal (Q_b) and access (Q_a) blood flows mix in the midsection between venous and arterial needles and the mixed blood is used to feed the extracorporeal circulation (Krivitski 1995). Forced recirculation is given as:

$$R = \frac{Q_b}{Q_a + Q_b} \qquad (6.12)$$

R ranges between 0 and 1 for all possible access flows. Notice the difference to Eq. (6.10). There is no benefit in forced recirculation other than inducing a condition where access flow can be measured by indicator dilution. This important condition was recognized by N. Krivitski who developed the current reference technique for the measurement of access flow. Rearranging Eq. (6.12) provides the relationship between access flow and the magnitude of forced recirculation as follows:

$$Q_a = Q_b \left(\frac{1}{R} - 1 \right) \qquad (6.13)$$

The smaller the recirculation under reversed line positions, the higher the access flow. Also notice the non-linearity between Q_a and R because of the $1/x$ relationship.

6.5.2 Limitations

The baseline access flow can be defined as the access flow without extracorporeal circulation. It depends on the driving pressure and the serial arrangement of arterial inflow resistance, intra-access resistance R_n constituting the section where the needles are placed, and venous outflow resistance. As soon as extracorporeal blood flow is established, blood inflow into the access is expected to increase because part of that flow with the magnitude of Q_b takes a functional bypass through the extracorporeal circuit. The extracorporeal effect on access blood flow is negligible when the flow resistance between needles is small. Usually, this is the case. However, when intra-access resistance R_n between the needles is high, establishing extracorporeal blood flow will increase access flow by a magnitude not exceeding Q_b.

Similar considerations apply to the measurement of access flow reversing the blood lines (see Fig. 6.4). Assume that in the undisturbed access with normal connection of blood lines the flow through the access is given as $Q_{a,n}$ for a given pressure gradient. For the same pressure gradient and for a constant resistance between arterial and venous needles the access flows $Q_{a,n}$ and $Q_{x,n}$ are related to each other by the magnitude of Q_b:

$$Q_{a,n} = Q_{a,x} + Q_b \qquad (6.14)$$

It therefore follows that $Q_{a,x}$, the flow measured by reversed line technique, is always smaller than $Q_{a,n}$ (Krivitski and Depner 1998). The theoretical difference ΔQ_a is given as:

$$\Delta Q_a = Q_b \frac{R_n}{R_t} < Q_b \qquad (6.15)$$

This difference will never exceed Q_b. In most cases the actual difference will depend on the ratio of the resistance between needles R_n to the total resistance R_t of the whole access loop. Usually $R_n < R_t$ so that the error ΔQ_a is only a few percent of Q_a. If $R_n = R_t$, the error is maximal but never larger than Q_b. Also notice that reversal of blood flow is not possible when access needles are placed in collateral veins.

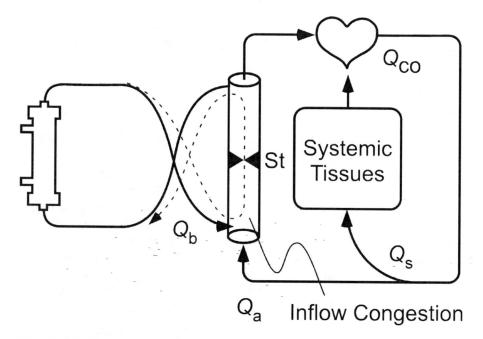

Fig. 6.4 Mid-access stenosis. In presence of significant mid-access resistance caused by stenosis (St) reversal of extracorporeal blood flow Q_b leads to a congestive backup of access flow upstream of that stenosis. Abbreviations: extracorporeal blood flow (Q_b), access blood flow (Q_a), systemic flow (Q_s), outflow stenosis (St), cardiac output (Q_{co}).

6.6 BOLUS APPROACH

Access flow can be computed from the dilution of a bolus of indicator introduced into the venous blood stream under the condition of forced recirculation (see Fig. 6.5). Under this condition blood is returned to the upstream part of the arterio-venous access while blood is withdrawn from its downstream part. The amount of indicator injected into the access (m_i) and recovered from the access (m_r) can be measured by sensors placed on venous and arterial blood lines, respectively.

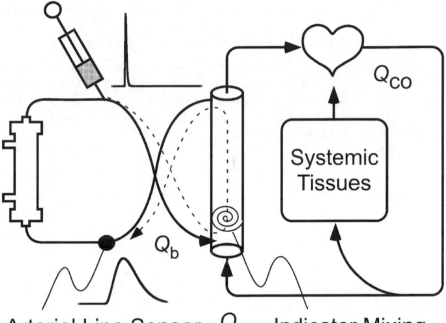

Venous Line Injection

Systemic Tissues

Q_{CO}

Q_b

Arterial Line Sensor $\quad Q_a \quad$ Indicator Mixing

Fig. 6.5 Indicator dilution for access flow measurement. Indicator injected into the venous line and returned to the access with blood flow Q_b is mixing with access flow Q_a in the upstream part of the arterio-venous access. The diluted indicator is sampled from the downstream part of the access and the dilution curve is measured by the arterial sensor. Notice the similarity to the set-up in Fig. 6.3 with the important difference that the blood line connections to the access are reversed.

Indicator added to the venous blood stream is diluted by extracorporeal blood flow, enters the upstream part of the access, and reappears in the arterial blood line withdrawn from the downstream part of the access with a delay of a few seconds because of forced access recirculation. The transit of indicator recirculating through the access takes a few seconds. The exact transit times depend on blood flow, shunt volume between the needles, and the location of injection and sampling sites in the extracorporeal circulation. The transit of indicator recirculating through the veins, the cardiopulmonary loop and the arterial branch feeding the peripheral access takes much longer. Apart from blood flow and the location of injection and sampling sites, the exact times depend on access flow, cardiac output and central blood volume. Because of this time difference the two transients caused by forced access (short loop) and cardiopulmonary (long loop) recirculation are usually well separated when injection and sampling sites are close to the access and indicator is applied by slug injection.

The separation of the two transients is crucial for the proper estimation of access flow using this technology. Minimizing the duration of the injection, injecting and measuring the indicator as close to the access as possible helps to separate the first transient through the access from the subsequent cardiopulmonary transient.

The magnitude of forced recirculation is then determined by the amount of indicator retrieved in the arterial line (m_r) during its first transit relative to the amount of indicator delivered to the access using the venous line (m_i) as:

$$R = \frac{m_r}{m_i} = \frac{AUC_a Q_{b,a}}{AUC_v Q_{b,v}} \tag{6.16}$$

where AUC is the area under the indicator concentration vs. time curve. Typically, venous line blood flow ($Q_{b,v}$) is smaller than arterial line blood flow ($Q_{b,a}$) because of ultrafiltration which has to be considered in the calculations.

The AUC measurement of the fast transients which only last a few seconds requires frequent sampling. For reasonable accuracy this can only be done by automatic sensors placed on or inserted in the extracorporeal blood lines.

6.6.1 Saline Dilution

The reference technique for measuring access flow is based on saline dilution (Krivitski 1995). The decrease in sound velocity caused by the dilution of blood with isotonic saline is utilized by the Hemodialysis Monitor (HDM03, Transonic Systems, Inc., Ithaca, New York) to calculate access flow. The magnitude of recirculation is displayed together with extracorporeal blood flow which is also measured by ultrasonic means and which is an important variable in the development of access recirculation. The technique is often improperly referred to as "ultrasound dilution". Ultrasound is not diluted but used to detect dilution.

The manufacturer currently recommends to release saline from the saline bag (connected to the arterial line upstream of the dialyzer) for a duration of four to five seconds or to inject 10 mL of saline before or into the venous bubble trap of the venous blood line. This type of administration simplifies handling, provides a smoother bolus, and causes less flow perturbation in the venous line, albeit requiring more sophisticated algorithms to separate true access recirculation from cardiopulmonary recirculation because of the dispersion of the bolus passing a significant section of the extracorporeal blood line.

In a study using 5 mL of saline as indicator volume the coefficient of variation of subsequent recirculation measurements was 9.3% (Lindsay et al. 1998). The technique stands out for its ability to separate the components of recirculation such as access and cardiopulmonary recirculation and thus to measure true access flow.

In principle, all techniques capable of measuring recirculation and separating first from subsequent transients can be used to calculate access flow from the degree of forced recirculation induced by switching of blood lines (Krivitski and Schneditz 2004).

In spite of its high accuracy and repeatability, the reference technique requires manual operation and it is time consuming so that alternatives have been investigated.

6.7 CONTINUOUS INFUSION APPROACH

These techniques are based on constant infusion or removal of indicator to reach a more or less stable concentration in the mixed blood. The indicator can be temperature, hypertonic dialysate as used for on-line clearance measurements, or a change in blood water concentration caused by ultrafiltration. The techniques are of special interest as the indicators are of inherent importance to the hemodialysis process itself. One of the difficulties with constant infusion techniques is the presence of cardiopulmonary re-circulation (Schneditz and Krivitski 2004).

6.7.1 Cardiopulmonary Recirculation

When the extracorporeal circulation is connected to a peripheral arterio-venous access, a fraction of Q_b returned to the patient reaches the inflow to the extracorporeal circulation and bypasses systemic equilibration. The magnitude of this functional bypass is given by the ratio of blood flow Q_b and systemic flow Q_s as:

$$R_{cpr,ex} = \frac{Q_b}{Q_s + Q_b} \tag{6.17}$$

The systemic flow Q_s is given as the Q_{co}-Q_a according to Eq. (6.1). The magnitude of $R_{cpr,ex}$ can be described as the extracorporeal effect of cardiopulmonary recirculation. A comparison with Eq. (6.3) shows some difference. As extracorporeal blood flow Q_b is typically smaller than access flow Q_a, $R_{cpr,ex}$ is usually smaller than R_{cpr}. Only if $Q_b=Q_a$, i.e., when all access flow enters the extracorporeal circulation, then the two measures are identical and $R_{cpr}=R_{cpr,ex}$.

Regardless whether the lines of the extracorporeal circulation are connected to the patient in the correct or in reversed fashion, cardiopulmonary recirculation is present with any extracorporeal configuration when using a peripheral arterio-venous access and it will have effects on recirculation, clearance, and hemoconcentration whether measured with correct or reversed placement of extracorporeal blood lines (see Fig. 6.3 and Fig. 6.5).

If the cardiopulmonary transient of indicator cannot be separated from recirculation (R_x) measured with reversed placement of blood lines, access flow calculated from the original formula will be erroneously low because R_x is inflated by the combined effects of forced access recirculation R and cardiopulmonary recirculation R_{cpr} (Schneditz et al. 1998a):

$$Q_a = Q_b \left(\frac{1}{R} - 1 \right) \left(\frac{1}{1 - R_{cpr}} \right) \tag{6.18}$$

Comparison with Eq. (6.13) shows that the original formula has to be corrected for a factor $1/(1-R_{cpr})$. Since R_{cpr} can reach values of 0.5 [Eq. (6.3)], Q_a will be underestimated by a factor of as much as 2 (Wang et al. 2000).

6.7.2 Double Recirculation Techniques

When two constant infusion measurements are done both with correct and with reversed placement of blood lines, and under the assumption that the ratio of Q_a/Q_{co} [Eq. (6.3)] does not change when switching the blood lines, then the effect of cardiopulmonary recirculation can be eliminated. The approach to take two measurements with correct and with reversed placement of blood lines has been termed "double recirculation technique" and is the basis to measure access flow either by thermodilution, on-line clearance, or ultrafiltration technique (Gotch et al. 1999, Mercadal et al. 1999, Schneditz et al. 1998a, Yarar et al. 1999) available in some dialysis machines.

Access flow can be calculated from recirculation obtained with correct R_n and with reversed R_x placement of blood lines. From these combined measurements it is possible to determine the magnitude of cardiopulmonary recirculation (Schneditz et al. 1998a). When the test is done for the same extracorporeal blood flow and when effects of ultrafiltration on blood flow are ignored, cardiopulmonary recirculation is obtained as follows:

$$R_{cpr} = \frac{R_n\left(1 - R_x\right)}{R_x\left(1 - R_n\right)} \tag{6.19}$$

Combination of Eq. (6.18) and Eq. (6.19) then leads to the following relationship:

$$Q_a = Q_b \frac{\left(1 - R_n\right)\left(1 - R_x\right)}{R_x - R_n} \tag{6.20}$$

This relates access flow to recirculation measurements R_n and R_x obtained by continuous infusion techniques.

6.7.2.1 Thermodilution

The fast response of temperature sensors for the bolus approach used with classic thermodilution is no longer required when temperature is used in a constant infusion approach such as with hemodialysis where temperature and temperature control is an important issue of dialysis delivery. In case of access recirculation the temperatures of venous line blood and of access inlet blood mix to give the temperature measured in the arterial blood line. The temperature of venous blood returning to the access can easily be changed by changing the dialysate temperature without changing Q_b and without affecting the flow and recirculation conditions in the vascular access. The recirculation is then determined as:

$$R = \frac{\Delta T_a}{\Delta T_v},$$ (6.21)

ΔT_a and ΔT_v relate to the changes in arterial and venous line temperatures caused by the change in dialysate temperature.

The technique to measure arterial and venous line temperatures with the required accuracy avoiding direct blood contact is utilized in the Blood Temperature Monitor (BTM, Fresenius Medical Care, Bad Homburg, Germany). The BTM is designed to measure and to control thermal balance in hemodialysis patients during their treatment (Azar 2008, Azar 2009, Rosales et al. 2000). The BTM also performs automatic recirculation measurements by measuring the change in arterial and venous line temperatures caused by a change in dialysate temperature (Kaufman et al. 1991). The technique is relatively slow since the infusion of cooled (or warmed) blood to produce a stable step change in arterial and venous line temperatures requires two to three minutes, long enough to overlap with effects caused by cardiopulmonary recirculation. The test result is available within minutes.

The standard deviation for BTM recirculation measurements is in the range of ±1.2% (full-scale) and the coefficient of variation decreases with increasing recirculation (≈5% at 30% recirculation).

Note that when measured in peripheral accesses, BTM recirculation includes a component caused by cardiopulmonary recirculation. The exact value of this component depends on the magnitude of Q_b and Q_s [Eq. 6.17)] but a threshold of 15% may help to detect 93% of accesses with (sensitivity) and reject 99% of accesses without access recirculation (specificity) (Wang et al. 2000). The same threshold applied to detect fistulae for revision yields a sensitivity of 82% and a specificity of 99%, respectively (Wang et al. 2002).

Access flow measurements by BTM thermodilution technique have a 95% confidence limit of ±70 mL/min at access flows of 500 mL/min, and the confidence limits widen as access flow increases (Ragg et al. 2003). A comparison to the bolus technique using ultrasonic detection of saline showed that the mean difference of -3.5±16.4% between the constant infusion and the bolus approaches was not significantly different from zero (Schneditz et al. 1999).

6.7.2.2 On-Line Clearance

On-line clearance K also known as ionic dialysance measures the urea clearance of the dialyzer corrected for any effects of access and cardiopulmonary recirculation (Di Filippo et al. 2001, Polaschegg, Steil et al. 1993). The measurement is performed by producing a step change in dialysate inflow conductivity, i.e. sodium concentration, and measuring the resulting step in dialysate outflow conductivity. The difference in dialysate inlet to outlet conductivities is compared and determines the clearance of the dialyzer. The duration of the step changes to reach equilibration is in the range of a minute so that effects of access and cardiopulmonary recirculation which develop within seconds are included in the measurement of on-line clearance. This technology is built into most modern dialysis machine.

Comparable to the thermodilution technique two subsequent on-line clearance measurements, one performed with correct K_n and one performed with reversed K_x placement of blood lines, can be used to calculate access blood flow under the assumption that cardiopulmonary recirculation does not change when reversing the connection of the extracorporeal blood lines (Gotch et al. 1999):

$$Q_a = \frac{1}{f_{bw}} \frac{K_n K_x}{K_n - K_x}$$
(6.22)

The flow obtained from on-line clearance measurements in Eq. (6.22) has to be corrected for blood water concentration f_{bw} which is in the range of 0.93 and depends on hematocrit and plasma protein concentration. Notice that these equations do not require explicit information on extracorporeal blood flow. Nor is this information explicitly required for the measurement of K_n or K_x, even though the values of K_n and K_x importantly depend on Q_b.

The measurement of on-line clearance is utilized in two commercial devices, the Diascan (Hospal Dasco SpA, Medolla, Italy) and the On-Line Clearance Monitor (OLC and/or OCM, Fresenius Medical Care, Germany). Both devices have been used to measure access flow by reversing the blood lines and the results have been compared to access flows measured by bolus technique using ultrasonic detection of a saline bolus. A validation of access flow calculations obtained by the Diascan showed a mean bias in the range of 100 mL/min and a 95% confidence interval of approximately 750 mL/min (Mercadal et al. 1999). The validation of access flow calculations obtained by the OLC or OCM monitor showed a rather large bias and poor reproducibility when compared to the reference technique (Eloot et al. 2010, Gotch et al. 1999, Lacson et al. 2008, Whittier et al. 2009). This discrepancy could be due to technical differences of the on-line clearance measurement in both devices, the OLC-Monitor using two separate sensors for measuring dialysate inflow and outflow conductivities, and the Diascan using only one sensor. Also, the shape of the step-changes (number, direction, magnitude, and duration of steps) which appears to be different in these devices could play a role in the observed differences.

6.7.2.3 Ultrafiltration Step

Ultrafiltration by the extracorporeal device is the third simple possibility to affect the composition of blood. Ultrafiltration removes plasma water from the blood passing the dialyzer thereby increasing the hematocrit, the hemoglobin concentration, and the plasma protein concentration in venous blood returning to the patient. When ultrafiltration rate is changed from 0 L/h to a high rate of for example 2 L/h, recirculation (access recirculation, cardiopulmonary recirculation, forced recirculation) of concentrated blood into the arterial blood line will produce a step change in arterial blood concentration which can be measured by on-line hematocrit, hemoglobin, and total protein monitors.

The magnitude of the step change in arterial line hematocrit ΔH has been shown to carry information on ultrafiltration rate Q_u, initial hematocrit H_0 and the combined effects of access and cardiopulmonary recirculation. To eliminate the effects of cardiopulmonary recirculation, and again under the assumption that CPR does not change between measurements, the change in hematocrit in the arterial line as a consequence of an abrupt change in ultrafiltration has to be measured with correct ΔH_n and with reversed ΔH_x placement of blood lines. This information can then be used to calculate the access flow (Yarar et al. 1999):

$$Q_a = Q_u \frac{H_0}{\Delta H_x - \Delta H_n} \qquad (6.23)$$

The configuration is comparable to that of determining Q_a using saline dilution and inducing forced recirculation by the reversed position of blood lines. When using ultrafiltration rate, however, the characteristics of blood are altered by removing plasma water rather than adding saline. Note that the calculation of Q_a requires an accurate estimate of Q_u but it is independent of the dialyzer blood flow.

This approach using the Crit-Line Instrument (Hemametrics, Kaysville, UT) for on-line measurement of arterial hematocrit values has been compared to the saline dilution technique. The correlation between techniques was high ($r=0.92$) and the slope in the identity plot was not different from one. Bland-Altman analysis showed that the bias of the ultrafiltration method was to systematically overestimate Q_a by 16±25%. The reproducibility of successive measurements was 13.4%.

6.8 LINE SWITCHES

In the original approach recirculation is induced by switching the blood lines connected to arterial and venous access needles. When this is done manually blood flow has to be stopped, lines have to be clamped, connections between extracorporeal blood lines and access needles have to be opened, access needles and extracorporeal blood lines have to be reconnected in a crossed flow configuration, clamps have to be opened, and blood flow has to be restarted. After having completed the manual dilution measurement, the lines have to be reconnected in their normal configuration. This manipulation is time consuming and bears the risks for contamination and malfunction. This has been recognized as a limitation and special extracorporeal blood lines have been designed to allow for a faster switch without manual disconnection. For example, a switch based on two plates holding the arterial and venous blood line segments and where the plates can be rotated against each other by 180° allows for an almost instantaneous reversal of blood flow in proximal parts of the extracorporeal circulation (Twister, Fresenius Medical Care) (see Fig. 6.6). Other systems use a double connection between arterial and venous line segments to be manually opened or clamped for normal or reversed blood flow through arterial and venous access needles (Reverso, Medisystems Cooperation, Seattle, WA). Still, some manipulation is required to reverse the blood flow. There are, however, alternatives for automatic implementation. For example, the clamping of connections could be done automatically. The condition of forced access recirculation could also be obtained by reversing the blood flow throughout the whole extracorporeal circulation such as by reversing the rotation of the blood pump. Reversing the whole extracorporeal blood flow would allow to eliminate the switch and to fully automate the access flow measurement, but a series of safety issues has to be properly addressed before such a technique can be used.

6.9 ARTERIO-VENOUS GRADIENTS

The approaches discussed so far require the injection of indicator, either directly into the venous blood line or indirectly using a change in dialysate properties such as temperature or conductivity. The injection, however, can be eliminated when the process of dialysis itself is seen as a continuous injection or removal of indicator such as thermal energy by extracorporeal cooling, removal of urea by extracorporeal clearance, or removal of plasma water by ultrafiltration. The continuous removal of these entities during extracorporeal treatments leads to distinctive arterio-venous gradients. If in presence of such gradients recirculation is induced by reversing blood lines, the concentrations and temperatures in arterial line blood are expected to change depending on the degree of recirculation (Schneditz et al. 2007a, b; Wijnen et al. 2007). As recirculation depends on access flow the change in temperatures and/or concentrations measured in the extracorporeal circulation can be used to calculate access flow without indicator injection, just from a simple line switch. Furthermore, when the switch is done almost instantaneously without manual disconnection and reversal of blood lines, the measurement is done within much shorter time.

The situation is best explained with temperature, even though temperature may not be the best indicator because thermal energy is exchanged with the environment in extracorporeal blood lines (see Fig. 6.6 and Fig. 6.7).

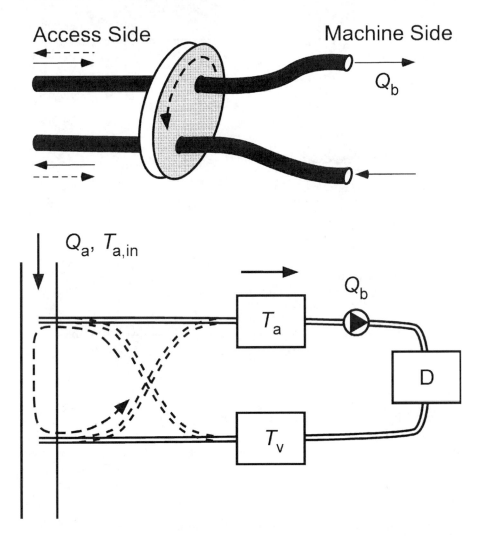

Fig. 6.6 Line switch. Top panel: Example of a line switch inserted between the access and the blood pump consisting of two plates holding the arterial and venous line segments. The plates can be rotated against each other. When the plates are rotated by 180° the flow on the access side of the switch is reversed (broken arrows). Bottom panel: If $T_a \neq T_v$ because of extracorporeal gradients, the switch leads to a change measured in T_a without injection of indicator, also see Fig. 6.7.

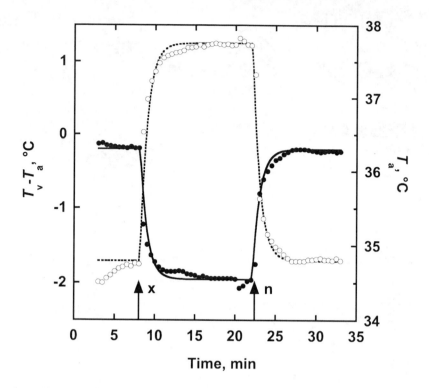

Fig. 6.7 Line switch and temperature change. Modeled (lines) and measured (symbols) temperatures in the arterial line (T_a, full circles) following
the instantaneous switch of the extracorporeal blood line (indicated as x
and n) in presence of an arterio-venous temperature gradient (open circles)
of approximately 1.8 °C. Also see Fig. 6.6.

In absence of access recirculation and with correct placement of blood
lines indicated by the subscript n:

$$T_{a,n} = T_{a,in} \qquad (6.24)$$

$T_{a,in}$ is the temperature of blood entering the access and $T_{a,n}$ is arterial
line temperature measured with normal placement of blood lines.

When blood lines are reversed (indicated by the subscript x), the temperature $T_{a,x}$ measured by the arterial line sensor is given as:

$$T_{a,x} = T_v R_x + T_{a,in}\left(1 - R_x\right) \qquad (6.25)$$

Combining Eq. (6.24) and Eq. (6.25) leads to:

$$R_x = \frac{T_{a,x} - T_{a,n}}{T_v - T_{a,n}} \tag{6.26}$$

Combining Eq. (6.13) and Eq. (6.26) and solving for Q_a yields:

$$Q_a = Q_b \frac{T_{a,x} - T_v}{T_{a,n} - T_{a,x}} \tag{6.27}$$

The measurement of access flow therefore requires the measurement of arterial and venous line temperatures with correct and reversed placement of blood lines and employs the arterio-venous temperature gradients (see Fig. 6.7). Since arterial and venous temperatures are continuously measured in the current BTM configuration, the measurement of access flow only requires to switch the connector and to measure the step-change in arterial line temperature. The technique importantly depends on the magnitude of the arterio-venous temperature gradient. The approach does not work for the condition that $T_{a,n}=T_v$. This is an unlikely condition as T_v should be smaller than $T_{a,n}$ in regular hemodialysis in order to prevent dialysis associated heat accumulation and to cool the patient during the treatment. If, however, the arterio-venous temperature gradient is considered too small then it will be useful to reduce the dialysis temperature for some time before starting the test.

When hematocrit is used as a marker, and arterio-venous hematocrit gradients develop because of ultrafiltration, it should be possible to determine access flow from ultrafiltration rate and hematocrit readings taken from a single sensor placed in the arterial line with lines in normal and in switched positions according to:

$$Q_a = Q_u \frac{H_{a,x}}{H_{a,x} - H_{a,n}} \tag{6.28}$$

There is no need to measure blood flow. Similar considerations apply to other indicators affected by ultrafiltration such as hemoglobin or blood water concentration. Notice the similarity with Eq. (6.23) and a previous relationship derived for an ultrafiltration test to measure access flow (Yarar et al. 1999).

The approach has been extended to measuring concentrations in the dialysate instead of blood (Lindsay et al. 2010, Lindsay et al. 2006). After establishing a gradient in dialysate conductivity and few minutes of equilibration throughout the extracorporeal system the conductivities λ are measured in dialysate in- and outflows with correct and reversed placement of bloodlines. The magnitude of access flow is then determined from on-line clearance K_n, blood water concentration f_{bw} and the change in conductivities caused by switching the blood lines according to the following expression:

$$Q_a = \frac{K_n}{f_{bw}} \frac{\lambda_{out,x} - \lambda_{in,n}}{\lambda_{out,n} - \lambda_{out,x}}$$
(6.29)

The major disadvantage of current techniques is that they either require manual injection of indicator or that they are slow and time consuming. The BTM and OLC techniques require two measurements with correct and reversed placement of blood lines, the algorithms require stability, and the injection of indicator takes a few minutes so that the whole procedure may take 30 minutes or longer. This is too long for everyday measurements, especially since solute clearance and treatment efficiency are reduced in the setting where blood flow is reversed. Moreover, since two measurements are required using correct and reversed placement of blood lines, the accuracy of the access flow measurement is also reduced. These shortcomings have prevented widespread application of frequent access flow measurements required to detect accesses at risk. However, at this stage of technological development, the measurement of access flow with every treatment seems almost possible.

6.10 CONCLUSION

The efficient exchange of solute between the patient and the extracorporeal system essentially depends on convective transport, and the arteriovenous access to the cardiovascular system is a vital albeit vulnerable link in this transport chain. The function of the arterio-venous access is essentially determined by its blood flow. Extracorporeal techniques are well suited to measure access flow using well-established principles of indicator dilution, as the concentration and clearance of solutes as well as the temperature and the hematocrit of blood are continuously measured with modern hemodialysis machines. These variables can be used as classic indicators. They are affected by the magnitude of access flow and by the connection of extracorporeal blood lines to the vascular system leading to different magnitudes and types of recirculation from which access flow can be calculated. Recent developments based on the measurement of such treatment variables during hemodialysis have greatly simplified the estimation of access flow so that automatic procedures done with every treatment are within technological reach today.

REFERENCES

Azar, A.T.: Biofeedback systems and adaptive control hemodialysis treatment. Saudi J. Kidney Dis. Transpl. 19(6), 895–903 (2008)

Azar, A.T.: Effect of dialysate temperature on hemodynamic stability among hemodialysis patients. Saudi J. Kidney Dis. Transpl. 20(4), 596–603 (2009)

Basile, C., Lomonte, C., Vernaglione, L., et al.: The relationship between the flow of arteriovenous fistula and cardiac output in haemodialysis patients. Nephrol. Dial. Transplant. 23(1), 282–287 (2008)

Bassingthwaighte, J.B., Ackerman, F.H., Wood, E.H.: Applications of the lagged normal density curve as a model for arterial dilution curves. Circ. Res. 18(4), 398–415 (1966)

Berra, Y.: Yogi Berra Sayings (2011),
http://www.retrogalaxy.com/sports/yogi-berra.asp

Besarab, A., Lubkowski, T., Frinak, S., et al.: Detection of access strictures and outlet stenoses in vascular accesses Which test is best? ASAIO J. 43(5), M548-M552 (1997)

Bos, W.J., Zietse, R., Wesseling, K.H., Westerhof, N.: Effects of arteriovenous fistulas on cardiac oxygen supply and demand. Kidney Int. 55(5), 2049–2053 (1999)

Bünger, C.M., Kröger, J., Kock, L., et al.: Axillary-axillary interarterial chest loop conduit as an alternative for chronic hemodialysis access. J. Vasc. Surg. 42(2), 290–295 (2005)

Cherrick, G.R., Stein, S.W., Leevy, C.M., Davidson, C.S.: Indocyanine green: observations on its physical properties, plasma decay, and hepatic extraction. J. Clin. Invest. 39, 592–600 (1960)

Chiang, J.C., Teh, L.S., Wu, H.S.: Preliminary experience with patch-enlarged brachial artery for hemodialysis access. ASAIO J. 53(5), 576–581 (2007)

Di Filippo, S., Manzoni, C., Andrulli, S., et al.: How to determine ionic dialysance for the online assessment of delivered dialysis dose. Kidney Int. 59(2), 774–782 (2001)

Eloot, S., Dhondt, A., Hoeben, H., Vanholder, R.: Comparison of different methods to assess fistula flow. Blood Purificat. 30(2), 89–95 (2010)

Fick, A.: Über die Messung des Blutquantums in den Herzventrikeln. Verh. Phys. Med. Ges. Würzburg 2, 16 (1870)

Fox, I.J., Brooker, L.G.S., Heseltine, D.W., Wood, E.H.: A new dye for continuous recording of dilution curves in whole blood independent of variations in blood oxygen saturation. Circulation 14, 937 (1956)

Gotch, F.A., Buyaki, R., Panlilio, F.M., Folden, T.: Measurement of blood access flow rate during hemodialysis from conductivity dialysance. ASAIO J. 45(3), 139–146 (1999)

Hamilton, W.F., Moore, J.W., Kinsman, J.M., Spurling, R.G.: Simultaneous determination of the pulmonary circulation times in man and of a figure related to the cardiac output. Am. J. Physiol. 84, 338–344 (1928)

Hegglin, R., Rutishauser, W., Kaufmann, G., et al.: Kreislaufdiagnostik mit der Farbstoffverdünnungsmethode. Georg Thieme Verlag, Stuttgart (1962)

Henriques, V.: Über die Verteilung des Blutes vom linken Herzen zwischen dem Herzen und dem übrigen Organismus. Biochemische Zeitschrift 56, 230–248 (1913)

Hinghofer-Szalkay, H.G., Goswami, N., Rössler, A., et al.: Reactive hyperemia in the human liver. Am. J. Physiol. Gastrointest. Liver Physiol. 295(2), G332–G337 (2008)

Kaufman, A.M., Krämer, M., Godmere, R.O., et al.: Hemodialysis access recirculation (R) measurement by blood temperature monitoring (BTM). A new technique. J. Am. Soc. Nephrol. 2, 324 (1991)

Kim, H.S., Park, J.W., Chang, J.H., et al.: Early vascular access blood flow as a predictor of long-term vascular access patency in incident hemodialysis patients. J. Korean Med. Sci. 25(5), 728–733 (2010)

King, R.B., Raymond, G.M., Bassingthwaighte, J.B.: Modeling blood flow heterogeneity. Ann. Biomed. Eng. 24(3), 352–372 (1996)

Krisper, P., Martinelli, E., Zierler, E., et al.: More may be less: increasing extracorporeal blood flow in an axillary arterio-arterial access decreases effective clearance. Nephrol. Dial. Transplant. 26(7), 2401–2403 (2011)

Krivitski, N.M.: Novel method to measure access flow during hemodialysis by ultrasound velocity dilution technique. ASAIO J. 41(3), M741–M745 (1995)

Krivitski, N.M., Depner, T.A.: Development of a method for measuring hemodialysis access flow: from idea to robust technology. Semin. Dial. 11(2), 124–130 (1998)

Krivitski, N.M., Schneditz, D.: Arteriovenous vascular access flow measurement: Accuracy and clinical implications. Contrib. Nephrol. 142, 269–284 (2004)

Lassen, N.A., Henriksen, O., Sejrsen, P.: Indicator methods for measurement of organ and tissue blood flow. In: Shepherd, J.T., Abboud, F.M. (eds.) Handbook of Physiology Section 2: The Cardiovascular System, vol. 3, pp. 21–63. American Physiological Society, Bethesda (1983)

Lacson Jr., E., Lazarus, J.M., Panlilio, R., Gotch, F.: Comparison of hemodialysis blood access flow rates using online measurement of conductivity dialysance and ultrasound dilution. Am. J. Kidney Dis. 51(1), 99–106 (2008)

Lindsay, R.M., Huang, S.H., Sternby, J., Hertz, T.: The Measurement of hemodialysis access blood flow by a conductivity step method. Clin. J. Am. Soc. Nephrol. 5(9), 1602–1606 (2010)

Lindsay, R.M., Bradfield, E., Rothera, C., et al.: A comparison of methods for the measurement of hemodialysis access recirculation and access blood flow rate. ASAIO J. 44(1), 62–67 (1998)

Lindsay, R.M., Sternby, J., Olde, B., et al.: Hemodialysis blood access flow rates can be estimated accurately from on-line dialysate urea measurements and the knowledge of effective dialyzer urea clearance. Clin. J. Am. Soc. Nephrol. 1(5), 960–964 (2006)

Lomonte, C., Basile, C.: The role of nephrologist in the management of vascular access. Nephrol. Dial. Transplant. 26(5), 1461–1463 (2011)

Marticorena, R.M., Hunter, J., Macleod, S., et al.: Use of the BioHole[TM] device for the creation of tunnel tracks for buttonhole cannulation of fistula for hemodialysis. Hemodial. Int. 15(2), 243–249 (2011)

McCarley, P., Wingard, R.L., Shyr, Y., et al.: Vascular access blood flow monitoring reduces access morbidity and costs. Kidney Int. 60(3), 1164–1172 (2001)

Mercadal, L., Hamani, A., Béné, B., Petitclerc, T.: Determination of access blood flow from ionic dialysance: theory and validation. Kidney Int. 56(4), 1560–1565 (1999)

Novljan, G., Rus, R.R., Koren-Jeverica, A., et al.: Detection of dialysis access induced limb ischemia by infrared thermography in children. Ther. Apher. Dial. 15(3), 298–305 (2011)

Polaschegg, H.D.: Automatic, noninvasive intradialytic clearance measurement. Int. J. Artif. Organs 16(4), 185–191 (1993)

Ragg, J.L., Treacy, J.P., Snelling, P., et al.: Confidence limits of arteriovenous fistula flow rate measured by the 'on-line' thermodilution technique. Nephrol. Dial. Transplant. 18(5), 955–960 (2003)

Rosales, L.M., Schneditz, D., Morris, A.T., et al.: Isothermic hemodialysis and ultrafiltration. Am. J. Kidney Dis. 36(2), 353–361 (2000)

Schneditz, D.: Recirculation, a seemingly simple concept. Nephrol. Dial. Transplant. 13(9), 2191–2193 (1998)

Schneditz, D., Fan, Z., Kaufman, A.M., Levin, N.W.: Measurement of access flow during hemodialysis using the constant infusion approach. ASAIO J. 44(1), 74–81 (1998a)

Schneditz, D., Fan, Z., Kaufman, A.M., Levin, N.W.: Stability of access resistance during hemodialysis. Nephrol. Dial. Transplant. 13(3), 739–744 (1998b)

Schneditz, D., Krivitski, N.M.: Vascular access recirculation measurement and clinical implications. Contrib. Nephrol. 142, 254–268 (2004)

Schneditz, D., Heimel, H., Stabinger, H.: Sound speed, density and total protein concentration of blood. J. Clin. Chem. Clin. Biochem. 27(10), 803–806 (1989a)

Schneditz, D., Kenner, T., Heimel, H., Stabinger, H.: A sound speed sensor for the measurement of total protein concentration in disposable, blood perfused tubes. J. Acoust. Soc. Am. 86(6), 2073–2080 (1989b)

Schneditz, D., Wang, E., Levin, N.W.: Validation of hemodialysis recirculation and access blood flow measured by thermodilution. Nephrol. Dial. Transplant. 14(2), 376–383 (1999)

Schneditz, D., Bachler, I., van der Sande, F.M.: Timing and reproducibility of access flow measurements using extracorporeal temperature gradients. ASAIO J. 53(4), 469–473 (2007a)

Schneditz, D., van der Sande, F.M., Bachler, I., et al.: Access flow measurement by indicator dilution without indicator injection: Effect of switch location. Int. J. Artif. Organs 30(11), 980–986 (2007b)

Schneditz, D., Pogglitsch, H., Horina, J., Binswanger, U.: A blood protein monitor for the continuous measurement of blood volume changes during hemodialysis. Kidney Int. 38(2), 342–346 (1990)

Schneditz, D., Probst, W., Kubista, H., Binswanger, U.: Kontinuierliche Blutvolumenmessung im extrakorporellen Kreislauf mit Ultraschall. Nieren- und Hochdruckkrankheiten 20, 649–652 (1991)

Schneditz, D., Mekaroonkamol, P., Haditsch, B., Stauber, R.: Measurement of indocyanine green dye concentration in the extracorporeal circulation. ASAIO J. 51(4), 376–378 (2005)

Schneditz, D., Kaufman, A.M., Polaschegg, H.D., et al.: Cardiopulmonary recirculation during hemodialysis. Kidney Int. 42(6), 1450–1456 (1992)

Shapiro, W., Gurevich, L.: Inadvertent reversal of hemodialysis lines - a possible cause of decreased hemodialysis (HD) efficiency. J. Am. Soc. Nephrol., 8, 173A (1997)

Sherman, R.A., Kapoian, T.: Recirculation, urea disequilibrium, and dialysis efficiency: peripheral arteriovenous versus central venovenous vascular access. Am. J. Kidney Dis. 29(4), 479–489 (1997)

Steil, H., Kaufman, A.M., Morris, A.T., et al.: In vivo verification of an automatic noninvasive system for real time Kt evaluation. ASAIO J. 39(3), M348–M352 (1993)

Stewart, G.N.: The output of the heart. J. Physiol. 22, 159–183 (1897)

Twardowski, Z.J., Van Stone, J.C., Jones, M.E., et al.: Blood recirculation in intravenous catheters for hemodialysis. J. Am. Soc. Nephrol. 3(12), 1978–1981 (1993)

Válek, M., Lopot, F., Polakovic, V.: Arteriovenous fistula, blood flow, cardiac output, and left ventricle load in hemodialysis patients. ASAIO J. 56(3), 200–203 (2010)

van Gemert, M.J., Bruyninckx, C.M., Baggen, M.J.: Shunt haemodynamics and extracorporeal dialysis: an electrical resistance network analysis. Phys. Med. Biol. 29(3), 219–235 (1984)

Vesely, T.M., Gherardini, D., Gleed, R.D., et al.: Use of a catheter-based system to measure blood flow in hemodialysis grafts during angioplasty procedures. J. Vasc. Interv. Radiol. 13(4), 371–378 (2002)

Wang, E., Schneditz, D., Kaufman, A.M., Levin, N.W.: Sensitivity and specificity of the thermodilution technique in detection of access recirculation. Nephron. 85(2), 134–141 (2000)

Wang, E., Schneditz, D., Ronco, C., Levin, N.W.: Surveillance of fistula function by frequent recirculation measurements during high efficiency dialysis. ASAIO J. 48(4), 394–397 (2002)

Whittier, W.L., Mansy, H.A., Rutz, D.R., et al.: Comparison of hemodialysis access flow measurements using flow dilution and in-line dialysance. ASAIO J. 55(4), 369–372 (2009)

Wijnen, E., van der Sande, F.M., Kooman, J.P., et al.: Measurement of hemodialysis vascular access flow using extracorporeal temperature gradients. Kidney Int. 72(6), 736–741 (2007)

Yarar, D., Cheung, A.K., Sakiewicz, P., et al.: Ultrafiltration method for measuring vascular access flow rates during hemodialysis. Kidney Int. 56(3), 1129–1135 (1999)

ESSAY QUESTIONS

1. In a typical situation, cardiac output is 5 L/min, access flow is 1.5 L/min, and extracorporeal blood flow is 0.3 L/min. How much is the systemic flow Q_s, how large is the cardiopulmonary recirculation (R_{cpr}), and how much is the cardiopulmonary recirculation of extracorporeal blood flow $R_{cpr,ex}$?

2. In the same patient the mean arterial pressure is 100 mmHg and the central venous pressure is 5 mmHg. How large is the total peripheral resistance TPR, the systemic vascular resistance SVR, and the access resistance AR? How are they related? For practical reasons, use peripheral resistance units for resistance (PRU=mmHg.s/mL).

3. In a patient with a peripheral arterio-venous access the mean arterial pressure (p_{mean}) is 120 mmHg, the cardiac output is 6 L/min and the access flow is 1 L/min. During hemodialysis cardiac output falls to 5 L/min, while p_{mean} paradoxically increases to 150 mmHg. What access flow is expected?

4. The average O_2 uptake in a 70 kg person at rest is 0.250 L/min. The arterial and mixed-venous O_2 concentrations are 0.20 and 0.15 L/L, respectively. How big is the cardiac output?

5. With a steady state ICG concentration of 1 mg/L and an infusion rate of 1.2 mg/min, how large is the expected hepatic blood flow?

6. In a study access flow was measured as 1.5 L/min at a mean arterial pressure of 150 mmHg. One week later, access flow was only 1 L/min and mean arterial pressure was 100 mmHg. Is this patient at risk to develop access thrombosis?

7. In a peripheral arterio-venous access, local recirculation was measured as 30%. The extracorporeal flow was 300 mL/min. How large is the access flow?

8. A typical recirculation is measured with an absolute accuracy of 1%. In a peripheral arterio-venous access, the forced recirculation was 30%. The extracorporeal flow was 300 mL/min. How large is the access flow? Compare the data and the result with that of $Q7$.

9. For the measurement of recirculation by thermodilution, which resolution in temperature measurements is required if the venous temperature can be changed by 2 to 3 centigrades?

10. In a study using slow thermodilution recirculation was measured as $R_1=15\%$ at a blood flow of 300 mL/min. A problem of inadvertent line reversal was suspected, the lines where reversed and the recirculation measurement was repeated. The second measurement gave a value of $R_2=35\%$. Which line position is correct? How large is the cardiopulmonary recirculation, how large is the access blood flow Q_a, the cardiac output Q_{co}, and the systemic pefusion Q_s?

MULTIPLE CHOICE QUESTIONS

Choose the best answer

1. To provide sufficient blood flow for extracorporeal use the peripheral arterio-venous access needs to deliver access flows above....

   A. 300 ml/min
   B. 400 ml/min
   C. 500 ml/min
   D. 600 ml/min

2. Most arterio-venous accesses deliver blood flows in the range of....

   A. 900 ml/min
   B. 850 ml/min
   C. 1500 ml/min
   D. 1000 ml/min

3. The calculation of access resistance AR is approximated by the ratio of....

   A. mean arterial pressure p_{mean} to access flow Q_a
   B. mean venous pressure p_{mean} to access flow Q_a
   C. mean arterial pressure p_{mean} to mean venous pressure

4. Access recirculation ranges between....

   A. 10 and 100%
   B. 0 and 100%
   C. 50 and 100%
   D. 10 and 50%

5. Recirculation occurs if....

   A. Q_b is lower than Q_a
   B. Q_b is equal to Q_a
   C. Q_b is larger than Q_a

6. The smaller the recirculation under reversed line positions, the .... the access flow.

   A. smaller
   B. higher

7. The extracorporeal effect on access blood flow is .... when the flow resistance between needles is small.

   A. negligible
   B. significant

8. The reference technique for measuring access flow is based on....

   A. access recirculation approach
   B. continuous infusion approach
   C. saline dilution approach

9. In a well-functioning peripheral arterio-venous access cardiopulmonary recirculation is....

   A. always absent
   B. always present

10. The peripheral arterio-venous access represents a segment connected to the cardiovascular system as a....

    A. parallel loop
    B. serial loop

11. In a well-functioning peripheral arterio-venous access local access recirculation is....

    A. always absent
    B. always present

12. At the same arterial pressure the total peripheral resistance is most likely increased with the creation of the following vascular access:

    A. arterio-arterial
    B. arterio-venous
    C. central venous
    D. femoral venous
    E. none of the above

13. When everything else remains unchanged, blood flow through the peripheral arterio-venous access increases with….

    A. increasing access resistance
    B. increasing mean arterial pressure
    C. increasing central venous pressure
    D. increasing blood viscosity
    E. none of the above

14. The measurement of peripheral arterio-venous access flow by indicator dilution….

    1) requires the switching of blood lines connected to the access

    2) requires the injection of indicator into the extracorporeal blood line

    3) can be determined using extracorporeal gradients

    4) is easily done off dialysis

    A. Only 1) and 3) are correct
    B. Only 2) and 4) are correct
    C. Only 1), 2), and 3) are correct
    D. Only 4) is correct
    E. All answers are correct

15. The manual measurement of peripheral arterio-venous access flow by indicator dilution….

    1) interferes with treatment efficiency

    2) requires blood sampling

    3) bears the risk of contamination

    4) only takes a few seconds

    A. Only 1) and 3) are correct
    B. Only 2) and 4) are correct
    C. Only 1), 2), and 3) are correct
    D. Only 4) is correct
    E. All answers are correct

16. The following indicators are used to measure access flow by indicator dilution:

   1) air

   2) water

   3) pressure

   4) saline

   A. Only 1) and 3) are correct
   B. Only 2) and 4) are correct
   C. Only 1), 2), and 3) are correct
   D. Only 4) is correct
   E. All answers are correct

17. Recirculation can be measured using extracorporeal line sensors for....

   1) hemoglobin

   2) hematocrit

   3) total protein concentration

   4) sound velocity

   A. Only 1) and 3) are correct
   B. Only 2) and 4) are correct
   C. Only 1), 2), and 3) are correct
   D. Only 4) is correct
   E. All answers are correct

18. For the measurement of access recirculation, the mixing site for indicator in the vascular access is located....

   1) upstream of the arterial needle

   2) downstream of the arterial needle

   3) downstream of the venous needle

   4) upstream of the venous line needle

   A. Only 1) and 3) are correct
   B. Only 2) and 4) are correct
   C. Only 1), 2), and 3) are correct
   D. Only 4) is correct
   E. All answers are correct

19. For the measurement of access flow, the mixing site for indicator in the vascular access is located…

    1) upstream of the arterial needle drawing blood from the access

    2) downstream of the arterial needle drawing blood from the access

    3) downstream of the venous needle returning blood to the access

    4) upstream of the venous line needle returning blood to the access

    A. Only 1) and 3) are correct
    B. Only 2) and 4) are correct
    C. Only 1), 2), and 3) are correct
    D. Only 4) is correct
    E. All answers are correct

20. The measurement of access flow by indicator dilution according to the bolus principle….

    1) requires the injection within a short period of time

    2) requires sensors with short response times

    3) requires separation of first and second transients

    4) requires extended observation times

    A. Only 1) and 3) are correct
    B. Only 2) and 4) are correct
    C. Only 1), 2), and 3) are correct
    D. Only 4) is correct
    E. All answers are correct

Chapter (7)

Hemodialysis Water Treatment System

Ahmad Taher Azar, Suhail Ahmad

CHAPTER OUTLINES

- Water contaminants
- Methods of hemodialysis water purification
- Disinfection of water treatment systems
- Monitoring and testing of dialysis water treatment system
- Conclusion

CHAPTER OBJECTIVES

- Discuss the purpose of water treatment for dialysis.
- Describe the major components of dialysis water treatment system.
- Identify clinical manifestations in hemodialysis patients exposed to inadequately purified water.
- Describe the methods for testing the water treatment system.

KEY TERMS

- Water softener
- Activated carbon filters
- Reverse osmosis
- Deionization
- Ultraviolet irradiator
- Disinfection
- Distribution system

ABSTRACT

Drinking water contains chemical, microbiological, and other contaminants. A healthy adult drinks about 10–12 liters of water per week, this water goes across a selective barrier of the gastrointestinal tract, and excess chemicals are removed by the healthy kidney. In contrast, with a typical three times a week hemodialysis protocol, a dialysis patient is exposed to more than 300 liters of water weekly, the water passes through the nonselective dialyzer membrane, and there is no kidney to maintain the normal balance of chemicals. Moreover, the highly permeable high-flux membrane used today increases the risk of increased load of contaminants passing through the membrane and into the blood. Some common contaminants have been shown to be injurious to patients. Thus, the water for dialysis must be purified of these contaminants prior to its use by the proportioning system of the dialysis machine to make the final dialysate. This chapter covers the purpose of water purification before it is used for dialysis. It describes the components of a water treatment system, how the system is monitored, and the common contaminants found in water.

A.T. Azar (Ed.): Modelling and Control of Dialysis Systems, SCI 404, pp. 347–378.
springerlink.com   © Springer-Verlag Berlin Heidelberg 2013

7.1 WATER CONTAMINANTS

The quality of the water used to make up dialysate solution is of crucial importance in minimizing the health hazards associated with hemodialysis (Hoenich et al. 2006, 2008, 2009). The average person drinks approximately two liters of water a day, whereas a dialysis patient is exposed to anywhere from 90 to 192 liters of water per treatment (Amato 2001). In healthy individuals, the contaminants in water are mainly excreted through the kidneys and gastrointestinal (GI) system. Hemodialysis (HD) patients on the other hand, do not have functioning kidneys to excrete the waste products from this massive water (as dialysate) exposure. The blood is separated from the water by a semipermeable membrane, the dialyzer that is selective as far as size of molecule but not contaminant specific. All small molecular weight substances present in the water have direct access to the patient's bloodstream as if they had been administered by intravenous injection. Moreover, the highly permeable high-flux membrane used today increases the risk of contaminants passing through the membrane and into the blood. Water contaminants can be divided into three major categories (Ahmad 2005):

1) **Particulate matter:** These cause turbidity and include clay, iron, sand, chalk, silica, etc.
2) **Chemicals:** These include dissolved inorganic ions and salts such as Na, Cl, Al, Ca, Mg, and Fl. Organic matter includes industrial and agricultural toxins such as fertilizers, pesticides, and oils.
3) **Microorganisms and endotoxins:** These include predominantly bacteria and occasionally fungi, viruses, protozoa, spores, and endotoxins produced by the organisms.

Table 7.1 gives the commonly present contaminants and medical syndrome caused by these in dialysis patients (AAMI 2001). Over the years, there have been many sad cases of patient harm and death due to the use of contaminated water for dialysis treatments (Levin 2001). The Association for the Advancement of Medical Instrumentation (AAMI) has recommended minimum standards for the water used in dialysis (see Table 7.2) (AAMI 2001). Thus, the water for dialysis must be purified of these contaminants prior to its use by the proportioning system of the dialysis machine.

Table 7.1 Signs and Symptoms and Possible Water Contaminant-Related Causes (AAMI 2001)

Contaminants	Symptom
Aluminum	Encephalopathy, Bone disease, Anemia
Calcium/Mg	Nausea, Vomiting, Weakness, Headache, HTN, Malaise, Cardiac Prob.
Copper	Hemolysis, Fever, Headache, Hepatitis
Chloramines	Hemolysis, Anemia, Methemoglobinemia
Fluoride	Bone Disease, Osteomalacia, Arrhythmia
Nitrate	Cyanosis, MetHb, Hypotension, Nausea
Sodium	HTN, Pulmonary edema, Headache, Thirst, Confusion, Seizure, Coma
Sulfate	Nausea, Vomiting, Acidosis
Zinc	Anemia, Nausea, Vomiting, Fever
Microbial Cont.	Chills, Fever, Septicemia, Liver Injury
Pyrogen	Pyrogenic Shock

Table 7.2 AAMI standard of water quality for dialysis (AAMI 2001)

Substance	Maximum allowable concentration (mg/l)
Aluminum	0.01
Chloramines	0.1
Copper	0.1
Fluoride	0.2
Nitrate	2.0
Sulfate	100.0
Zinc	0.1
Arsenic	0.005
Barium	0.1
Cadmium	0.001
Chromium	0.014
Lead	0.005
Mercury	0.0002
Selenium	0.09
Silver	0.005
Calcium	2.0 (0.1 mEq/L)

Table 7.2 Continued (AAMI 2001)

Substance	Maximum allowable concentration (mg/l)
Magnesium	4.0. (0.3 mEq/L)
Potassium	8.0. (0.2 mEq/L)
Sodium	70.0. (3.0 mEq/L)
Antimony	0.006
Free Chlorine	0.50
Thallium	0.002

7.2 METHODS OF HEMODIALYSIS WATER PURIFICATION

City water is supplied to the dialysis unit through water distribution system after chlorination. Often municipal authorities add other chemicals to the supply water, these include alum as a flocculant, fluoride for healthy teeth. A series of treatment components are needed to use for dialysis as shown in Fig. 7.1. Each one removes certain contaminants to make the water safe for use in dialysis. Two major types of water purification systems are in common use: (1) reverse osmosis (RO) and (2) deionizer (DI). However, to protect and prolong the lives of RO membrane or the DI resins, water goes through several steps of pretreatment. The treated water then either passes directly through a re-circulation loop in the dialysis unit (the Direct Feed System) or is collected in a storage tanks from there it is recirculated through the closed re-circulation loop. The water circulates continuously, passing through two Ultraviolet (UV) light treatment units and microfilters before reaching the dialysis stations.

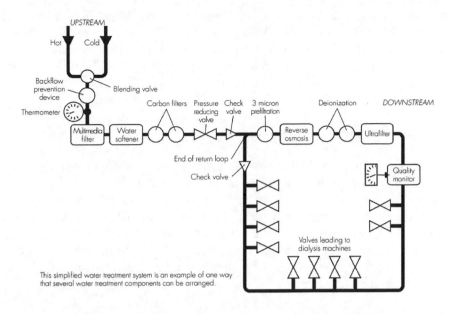

Fig. 7.1 Sample schematic of water treatment system. [Published with permission of Amgen Inc. http://www.amgen.com]

7.2.1 Pretreatment Components

7.2.1.1 Back Flow Prevention

Many local authorities require that a one way valve be placed between building water supply and water treatment equipment. This is to prevent any back flow of water from the water purification unit to building water supply, thus preventing backflow of chemicals used in the water purification into the building water. This device also protects the water purifiaction system, for example if main water pipe broke without this device water would be pulled out of the water purification unit thus preventing any damage to the components. Pressure drop across the valve must be monitored in order to diagnose plugging up of the screen used in the device.

7.2.1.2 pH Adjustment System

The ideal pH of the feed water should be 5.0–8.5 to prevent corrosion of water pipes and fixtures, particularly to prevent dissolution of lead into a potable water supply (Amato 2001). If the pH is higher than 8.5, a chemical injection system may be used to inject a small amount of hydrochloric or sulfuric acid into the feed water (Luehmann et al. 1989). This will lower the water's pH level. Such systems may also be used to reduce chloramines in feed water by injecting sodium metabisulfite (Amato 2005). Chemical injection systems have a reservoir to hold the chemicals, a metering pump, and a mixing chamber in the feed water line. These systems must have a way to control the amount of chemicals added to the water.

7.2.1.3 Temperature Blending Valve

For the water purification unit to work efficiently the feed water supplying the purification unit should be raised to certain temperature. For example reverse osmosis system may be most efficient if the feed water is at 77° F. Working in conjunction with a water heater the device mixes the hot and cold water to get feed water at the desired temperature. This unit should be monitored for proper functioning in order to prevent damage to water purification components by very hot water delivered by a malfunctioning device.

7.2.1.4 Sediment Filter

Sediment filter removes sediments such as silt, rust, and clay as water percolates through the filter. Sediment filters may be used at several points in the water treatment system: for pre-filtration of the water supply, downstream of carbon filters and at the inlet of the hemodialysis delivery system. The multimedia filter is the most common sediment filter as shown in Fig. 7.2 (Amato 2001). Large particulates of 10 microns or greater that cause the feed water to be turbid are removed by a multimedia filter, sometimes referred to as a depth bed filter (Amato 2001). Large particulates can clog the carbon and softener tanks, destroy the RO pump, and foul the RO membrane. Multimedia filters have different-sized layers of gravel. Each layer is finer than the one before, to trap smaller and smaller particles. The arrangement of the media (coarse and less dense on top of finer higher density placed deeper in the bed) enables the filter to run for longer periods of time before backwashing is necessary. The top layer is typically coarse anthracite followed by fine sand. The size of the multimedia filter shall be determined by a competent dialysis water pretreatment plant contractor or provider. The sediment filters are usually back washed to remove particulate matters usually once a day when dialysis unit is not operating. Often a timer is required so that the back flush only occurs when the dialysis unit is closed. The plugging up of the filter will increase pre-filter pressure and decrease the post filter pressure, a significant increase in the delta pressure will reflect a filter that is getting plugged and will decrease yield of water. Sediment filters should be checked each day by measuring pressure before and after the filter at normal operating flow rates (Curtis et al. 2005).

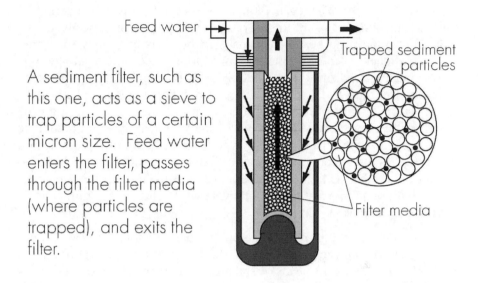

A sediment filter, such as this one, acts as a sieve to trap particles of a certain micron size. Feed water enters the filter, passes through the filter media (where particles are trapped), and exits the filter.

Fig. 7.2 Sediment Filter. [Published with permission of Amgen Inc. http://www.amgen.com]

7.2.1.5 Water Softener

Softeners work on an ion exchange basis (AWWA 1998, 1999). Its function is to remove scale-forming divalent calcium and magnesium ions from hard water. In many cases soluble iron (ferrous) can also be removed with softeners (Cappelli and Inguaggiato 2004). A standard water softener has four major components: a resin tank, resin, a brine tank to hold sodium chloride, and a valve or controller as shown in Fig. 7.3. The softener resin tank contains the treated ion exchange resin – small beads of polystyrene. The resin bead are saturated with Na on exchange sites (Keshavia 1994), these beads have great affinity for divalent cations such as calcium and magnesium. The resin has a greater affinity for multivalent ions such as calcium and magnesium than it does for sodium. Thus, when hard water is passed through the resin tank in service, calcium and magnesium ions adhere to the resin, releasing the sodium ions and water coming out of the tank has low levels of calcium and magnesium. When most of the sodium ions have been replaced by hardness ions, the resin is exhausted and must be regenerated. Regeneration is achieved by passing a concentrated NaCl solution through the resin tanks, replacing the hardness ions with sodium ions. The resin's affinity for the hardness ions is overcomed by the concentrated NaCl solution. The regeneration process can be repeated indefinitely without damaging the resin. Regeneration cycle is critical, it needs to take place before the resin beads are exhausted but it is extremely important that the softener water must not be allowed to proceed further into the water treatment system since it will be loaded with calcium and magnesium. A mechanism must installed to ensure that regenerating tank is locked out of the water treatment system, to prevent product water passing into the water treatment system. Most popular water softeners have an automatic regenerating system. The most basic type has an electric timer that flushes and recharges the system on a regular schedule. The timer should be set to activate when the facility is not operating, and monitored daily to make sure it will not go into a regeneration cycle while unit is dialyzing patients and using treated water.

A second type of control uses a computer that monitors how much water is processed. When certain volume of water has passed through the resin tank to have depleted the beads of sodium, the computer triggers regeneration. These softeners often have reserve resin capacity, so that some soft water will be available during recharging.

A third type of control uses a mechanical water meter to measure water usage and initiate recharging. The advantage of this system is that no electrical components are required and the mineral tank is only recharged when necessary. Often two softener tanks are used and when one is being recharged it is locked out and the other tank is used for water treatment. When it is equipped with two mineral tanks, softened water is always available. The timer must be checked at the beginning of the day to ensure that it is operating as programmed. The softener needs constant monitoring of the quality of softness/hardness and if the hardness increases above 1 grains per gallon (17.2 parts per million), the resins must not be used and be regenerating by flushing with brine (Ahmad 2005). The water softener also is a major site for microorganism growth and potential for downstream seeding. To prevent this, periodic back-flushing and use of sodium hypochlorite solution is employed (Ahmad 2005). Increased concentrations of calcium and magnesium scale the reverse osmosis membrane thus reducing its efficiency, similarly high load of these divalents overwhelm deionizer beds thus releasing toxic levels of other ions such as fluoride into the product water thus exposing patients to harm.

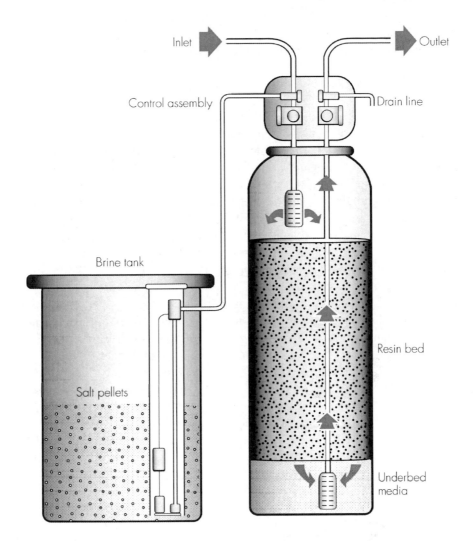

Fig. 7.3 Water Softener. [Published with permission of Amgen Inc. http://www.amgen.com]

7.2.1.6 Brine Tank

The brine tank is a plastic tank that contains a brine, water saturated with salt. The brine solution is typically made with salt or sodium chloride. The salt level in the brine tank should be inspected daily and maintained as needed (Amato 2001). Monitor the brine tank for a "Salt Bridge"- where salt pellets are visible above the water level, ensuring saturated solution for regeneration. The brine tank should be made of opaque housing to prevent algae growth and the salt level must be inspected at least once a day.

7.2.1.7 Activated Carbon

Activated carbon (AC) column as shown in Fig. 7.4 is mainly used to remove chlorine, chloramines, pesticides, industrial solvents, and some trace organic substances. Activated carbon is available in two different forms: powdered (PAC) and granular (GAC) (AWWA 1998, 1999). Powdered activated carbon (PAC) has a relatively smaller particle size when compared to granular activated carbons and consequently, presents a large surface to volume ratio, however it is not commonly used because of channeling and pressure related issues. Granular activated carbon (GAC) adsorbs many dissolved organics and eliminates chlorine, chloramines or other halogens in water (Cappelli and Inguaggiato 2004). This is important because chloramines can damage the RO membranes and are not effectively removed by thigh levels of chloramines can cause severe hemolytic anemia in dialysis patients and need to be removed effectively by activated carbon. A minimum of 10 minutes of Empty Bed Contact Time (EBCT) to ensure effective removal of chloramines to a desirable level below 0.1 ppm. Volume of AC needed to get 10 minutes of EBCT is dependent on the flow rate of the water and can be calculated by the following formula:

$$EBCT = \frac{V}{Q} \qquad (7.1)$$

Where V is the volume of carbon in cubic feet and Q is the maximum water flow rate in ft^3/min.

Since the number of gallons per cubic feet = 7.48, then:

$$EBCT \ (gallon/min) = 10 = \frac{V \times 7.48}{Q} \Rightarrow V = \frac{10 \times Q}{7.48} \qquad (7.2)$$

Most set up contains two AC tanks connected in series and water exiting the first tank is tested for chloramine, it is below 0.1 mg/dL, nothing else needs to be done. If chloramine exceeds this level then carbon tank needs to be changed and water from the second tank is monitored closely, used if it below the 0.1 mg/dL level. If level is higher, the water system cannot be used until the new carbon is placed in.

GAC does not remove sediment / particulate material very well, so they are often preceded by a sediment filter. Sediment pre-filters also prolong the activate carbon cartridge life by eliminating gross contaminants that would otherwise clog the activated carbon thereby reducing the surface area available for absorption. Carbon block filters are generally better than GAC filters at removing sediment. Exhaustion of the charcoal column has led to several significant incidences of chloramine toxicity. It is, therefore, required that treated water is checked for chloramines at least three times a day to ensure proper functioning of the carbon filter. AC columns are one of the only low-cost methods available to remove low-molecular weight (<100 MW) organics and chlorine.

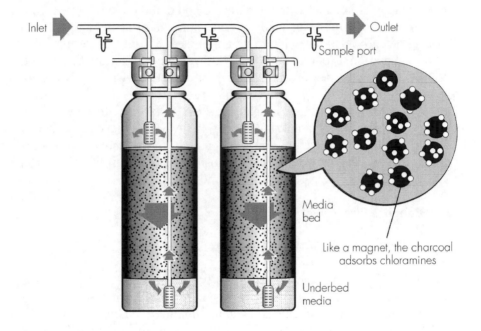

Fig. 7.4 Activated Carbon column. [Published with permission of Amgen Inc. http://www.amgen.com]

AC filters may become a breeding site for bacteria and pyrogenic materials. The carbon must be sanitized or changed periodically to avoid bacterial growth, and when all adsorption sites are used up it must be reactivated by a controlled heat process. This is not easily reactivated in the field. The suspended solids accumulated in the bed from most water sources require frequent backwashing of the filter unless installed after reverse osmosis or ultrafiltration. The two most important factors affecting the efficiency of activated carbon filtration are the amount of carbon in the unit and the amount of time the contaminant spends in contact with it. The lower the flow rate of the water, the more time that contaminants will be in contact with the carbon, and the more absorption that will take place.

Particle size also affects removal rates. Activated carbon filters are usually rated by the size of the particles they are able to remove, measured in microns, and generally range from 50 microns (least effective) down to 0.5 microns (most effective). A typical counter-top or under-the-counter filter system has from 12 to 24 ounces of activated carbon. Carbon tanks should be back-washed at frequent intervals, (at least weekly) to reduce the impact of channel formation, to remove debris and expose un-reacted charcoal surface. Biological fouling is inherent problem with GAC because it is an organic medium, and with the chlorine and chloramine removed from the water, bacteria grow. Channelling, accumulation of debris and bacteria all cause the carbon surface area to be underused. Therefore, carbon tanks are backwashed on a routine basis to "fluff" the bed, clean the debris out, and expose unused sides of the carbon particles. Back-washing does not 'regenerate' the carbon when it is exhausted, it simply exposes unused sides of the carbon. Exhausted tanks are best replaced with new carbon granules. If the carbon tank cannot be back-washed, the carbon media should be changed on a more frequent basis. Carbon also releases very small particles of carbon called 'fine', a post carbon filter usually 5 micron in size placed to remove particles, debris and 'fine'.

7.2.2 Primary Treatment Components

7.2.2.1 Reverse Osmosis System

The RO system is the most fragile, costly but most effective part of the water treatment system. Reverse osmosis is a water purification process from both organic and inorganic solutes, including organisms and endotoxins in which water is forced by pressure through a semi-permeable membrane (Ahmad 2005). In normal osmosis, water flows from a less concentrated solution through a semi-permeable membrane to a more concentrated solution (see Fig. 7.5). In the RO system since only pure water molecules are forced across the membrane the feed water side contains more solute having higher osmolarity which should move water to this side. Enough pressure forces the water against osmolarity hence the name. Thus, reverse osmosis uses pressure to reverse normal osmotic flow. Water flows from a more concentrated solution through a semi-permeable membrane to a less concentrated solution (see Fig. 7.5).

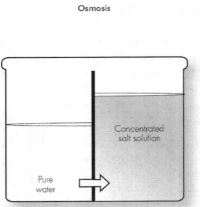
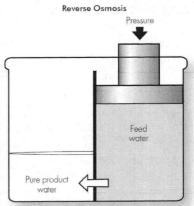

Osmosis

Reverse Osmosis

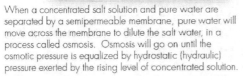

When a concentrated salt solution and pure water are separated by a semipermeable membrane, pure water will move across the membrane to dilute the salt water, in a process called osmosis. Osmosis will go on until the osmotic pressure is equalized by hydrostatic (hydraulic) pressure exerted by the rising level of concentrated solution.

If enough pressure is exerted on the concentrated solution to overcome osmosis, reverse osmosis occurs. Pure water is forced out of the concentrated solution.

Fig. 7.5 Concept of osmosis and reverse osmosis. [Published with permission of Amgen Inc. http://www.amgen.com]

In normal filtration system such as in sand filters, multi-media filters, bag filters or cartridge filters, feedwater flows in perpendicular with the filter media. While filtered water comes out of the system, large suspended solids being removed from water remain in the surface of the filter media. As this process continues, problem occurs as the desired amount of water becomes less and less and the pressure drop becomes larger while fouling increases. The only means to relieve the trouble is to clean or backwash or otherwise replace the components. This method consumes a lot of time and costs amount of money. Reverse osmosis system presents several advantages over a normal filtration system. It utilizes a *crossflow* filtration to supply a continuous flow operation without interference of frequent system cleaning or backwash or even frequent replacement of component. As the feedwater passes through the membrane, water flows into two outlets separating the purified water from the concentrated water. The purified water is called permeate (product water) while the concentrated water is considered as the concentrate (reject water). The dissolved ions and suspended solids are carried into the concentrated stream, thus reducing the rate of fouling in the system. This means that system benefits a continuous operation and lessens the schedule for cleaning or backwashing and therefore prolonging the life of the system.

7.2.2.1.1 Basic components of Reverse Osmosis Systems

A) Prefilters: There may be more than one pre-filter used in a Reverse Osmosis system. Typically, pre-filters range in pore size from 1 to 5 microns. These are used to remove sand silt, dirt, fine and other sediment. Additionally, carbon filters may be used to remove chlorine, which can have a negative effect on TFC (Thin Film Composite) & TFM (Thin Film Material) membranes. Carbon pre filters are not used if the RO system contains a CTA (Cellulose Tri-Acetate) membrane. Gauges should be placed before and after the prefilter and pre- and post filter pressures and delta pressure monitored to assess the clogging. Prefilters are low-cost and should be changed on a regular basis.

B) RO pump and motor: The RO pump increases water pressure across the RO membrane to increase both product water flow (RO yield) and rejection characteristics of the RO membrane (Amato 2001).

C) Reverse Osmosis Membrane: The Reverse Osmosis Membrane is the heart of the system. The membrane separates the pure water or permeates from the feed and "rejected" water, the pure water is allowed to circulate through the dialysis unit to be used for the dialysate proportioning; the rejected water is drained out (see Fig. 7.6). Sometimes a part of rejected water is mixed with the feed water entering the RO. RO membranes are manufactured into various configurations – tubular, hollow-fiber, flat-sheet or spiral-wound (Baker 1990; Strathmann 1990; Bhattacharyya et al. 1992). Due to relative efficiency and economy, spiral-wound membranes (called sepralators) are by far the most popular for crossflow water purification.

- **Spiral-wound Membrane**: The most commonly used membrane is a spiral wound of which there are two options: the CTA, which is chlorine tolerant, and the TFC/TFM (Thin Film Composite/Material), which is not chlorine tolerant (see Fig. 7.6). Thin film composite (TFC) RO membranes made of polyamide (PA) are the most common type used in HD. These RO membranes are made with a thin, dense, semipermeable membrane over a thick porous substructure for strength and spiral wound around a permeate collecting tube. The spiral design allows for a large surface area in a small space (Baker 1990; Strathmann 1990; Bhattacharyya et al. 1992). Spiral-wound module uses a sandwich of flat sheet membranes and supports, wrapped spirally around a collection tube (see Fig. 7.7). The feed flows in against one end of the rolled spiral and along one side of the membrane sandwich. The support layers are designed to minimize pressure drop and allow a high packing density. Spacers between membrane layers promote turbulent flow to ensure low fouling and longer life. Additionally, the spiral-wound modules can be designed by equipment suppliers to promote turbulence and therefore increase the mass transfer across the membrane or to provide an uninterrupted flow path to decrease membrane fouling. Spiral wound modules offer greater packing densities, but maintenance is difficult.

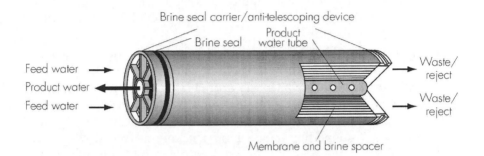

Fig. 7.6 RO membrane configuration. [Published with permission of Amgen Inc. http://www.amgen.com]

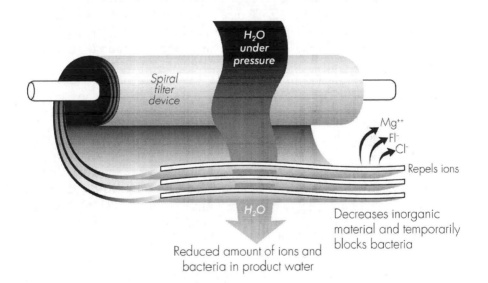

Fig. 7.7 Spiral-wound RO module. [Published with permission of Amgen Inc. http://www.amgen.com]

- **Hollow Fine-Fiber Membranes** consist of hollow fibers each roughly the size of a human hair. Thousands of fibers are closely bundled in each housing (Baker 1990; Strathmann 1990; Bhattacharyya et al., 1992). The pressurized feed flows slowly over the outside of the fibers and pure water permeates to the center. Then the water is collected out of potted tube sheet. In the early 1970's hollow fine-fiber water purification systems gained popularity because of their high productivity resulting from very high membrane surface areas. The major disadvantage of this element is the amount of pre-filtration required to keep the tightly-packed membrane surface free of severe fouling due to the laminar flow in the element.

- **Hollow Fat-Fiber Membranes** are only used in ultrafiltration and microfiltration due to burst-strength limitations (Baker 1990; Strathmann 1990; Bhattacharyya et al. 1992). The pressurized feed flow is on the inside of the fiber and water permeates to the outside of the fiber. The fibers are potted at each end in housing. Their self-supporting nature limits maximum feed flows. 70 psi (4.8 bar) is the pressure limit through elements constructed with these small fibers.

The efficacy of the membrane is continuously monitored by measuring the resistance to electrical current through the product (permeate) and feed water. A membrane that rejects > 85% of conductant water is considered to be functioning well, if this rejection rate goes below 85%, the membrane needs to be changed (Curtis et al. 2005). The % rejection ratio is calculated by the following formula:

$$\text{Rejection Ratio (RR)} = 1 - \frac{\text{Permeate water conductivity}}{\text{feed-water conductivity}} \times 100 \qquad (7.3)$$

This rejection ratio need to be individualized based on the feed water conductivity. Thus feed water with very low conductivity will have a lower rejection ratio at which the membrane should be changed than water feeding RO having higher conductivity. It is, therefore, to monitor the trends in RR to decide the need for changing the membrane.

Similarly the percent recovery is also a good measure to assess the performance of the RO membrane:

$$\text{Percent Recovery} = \frac{\text{Permeate flow rate}}{\text{Permeate + Rejection flow rate}} \times 100 \qquad (7.4)$$

RO membranes should be cleaned and disinfected at least quarterly to insure proper functioning, extend the life of the membrane and reduce the bacterial growth in the system that can harm patients (Amato 2001).

7.2.2.2 Deionization (DI)

Deionization can be used as an alternative process to reverse osmosis, or sometimes it is used to further purify water after the reverse osmosis process (Keshavia 1994). Ion exchange deionizers use synthetic resins similar to those in water softeners. Typically used on water that has been prefiltered, DI uses a two-stage process (two beds or mixed bed DI) to remove virtually all ionic material in water. Two types of synthetic resins are used as shown in Fig. 7.8: one to exchange positively-charged ions (cations) for H^+ and another to exchange negatively-charged ions (anions) for OH^- (Amato 2001). Cation exchange resins (hydrogen cycle) release hydrogen (H^+) in exchange for cations such as calcium, magnesium and sodium. Anion exchange resins (hydroxide cycle) exchange hydroxide (OH^-) ions for anions such as chloride, sulfate, Nitrate and bicarbonate. The displaced H^+ and OH^- combine to form pure H_2O. Resins have limited capacities and must be regenerated upon exhaustion. This occurs when equilibrium between the adsorbed ions is reached. Cation resins are regenerated by treatment with acid which replenishes the adsorption sites with H^+ ions. Anion resins are regenerated with a base which replenishes the resin with (OH^-) ions. Regeneration can take place off-site with exhausted resin exchanged with deionizers brought in by a service company. Regeneration can also be accomplished on-site by installing regenerable-design deionizer equipment and by proper use of the necessary chemicals. The two basic configurations of deionizers are *two-bed* and *mixed-bed* (Amato 2001). Two-bed deionizers have separate tanks of cation and anion resins. In mixed-bed deionizers, the two resins are blended together in a single tank or vessel. Generally mixed-bed systems will produce higher-quality water, but with a lower total capacity than two-bed systems (Amato 2005). Deionization can produce extremely high-quality water in terms of dissolved ions or minerals, up to the maximum purity of 18.3 mega ohms/cm resistance. However, it generally cannot remove organics, and can become a breeding ground for bacteria actually diminishing water quality if organic and microbial contaminations are critical. Failure to regenerate the resin at the proper time may result in salts remaining in the water or even worse, being released from the resin resulting in water containing life-threatening toxic levels of certain ions such as fluoride. Even partially-exhausted resin beds can increase levels of some contaminants due to varying selectivity for ions, and may add particulates and resin fines to the deionized water.

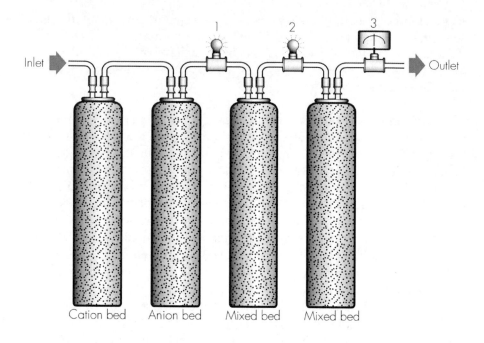

Fig. 7.8 Deionization Tanks. [Published with permission of Amgen Inc. http://www.amgen.com]

7.2.2.3 Ultraviolet Irradiator (UV)

Ultraviolet radiation is actually high energy light. The wavelengths in the ultraviolet spectrum are too short for the human eye to resolve and ultraviolet light is therefore invisible. With regard to biological effect, UV radiation is divided into three spectral ranges. The ultraviolet spectrum ranges from 40 to 400 Nanometers (nm), with the most effective spectral region for germicidal purposes being between 250 and 265 nm (AAMI 2001). At the proper level of intensity, ultraviolet light is fatal to all microorganisms known to inhabit water. Mercury arc lamps generate the ultraviolet radiation for water disinfection, with low pressure lamps being the most common and effective type. Since normal glass blocks ultraviolet, the lamp and its protective sleeve are generally made of fused silica or quartz, which readily transmit the germicidal ultraviolet rays. Low pressure mercury arc lamps are efficient producers of ultraviolet rays in the range lethal to microbes. About 50% of the input energy is converted to ultraviolet rays having a wavelength of 254 nm. This wavelength is very effective in the destruction of all known micro-organisms. Studies show that DNA molecules in the nucleus of the organism absorb ultraviolet light. The organism is inactivated when sufficient dosage has been absorbed to modify the molecular structure in the DNA. This results when exposure to ultraviolet light causes two thymine molecules to form an inappropriate bond, or dimer. The effect of numerous thymine dimers forming along the DNA chain inhibits replication of the organism. It may not be killed instantly, but the scrambling of the genetic material in the nucleus prevents reproduction, rendering it non-viable and harmless to humans (Amato 2001). The amount of energy required to produce this effect in a given organism is referred to as the lethal dosage. If the dosage is not optimized, then complete inhibition of replication will not occur. On the other hand, an insufficient UV dosage may cause limited damage to the DNA, which then can, under favorable conditions, repair using repair enzymes. That's why it is extremely critical to impart the optimum UV dosage to prevent repair. The ultraviolet system should be designed such that it can handle the known flow rate of the water system and it should be sized to match the maximum expected peak flow. These measures would eliminate the possibility of inadequate treatment by preventing a flow rate through the treatment chamber that exceeds the disinfection capability of the unit.

The typical UV treatment device consists, of a cylindrical chamber housing the UV bulb along its central axis. A quartz glass sleeve encases the bulb; water flow is parallel to the bulb, which requires electrical power. A flow control device prevents the water from passing too quickly past the bulb, assuring appropriate radiation contact time with the flowing water. It has been reported that turbulent (agitated) water flow provides more complete exposure of the organism to UV radiation. The UV system housing should be made of stainless steel to protect any electronic parts from corrosion. To assure they will be contaminant-free, all welds in the system should be plasma-fused and purged with argon gas. The major differences in UV treatment units are in capacity and optional features. In some situations, monitoring devices should be an integral part of the ultraviolet system employed, since the effectiveness of an ultraviolet sterilizer is governed by the amount of radiation that actually penetrates the water. Most suppliers provide some form of a sensing circuit, but a Fail-Safe system is preferable and often required by regulation in critical applications. A Fail-Safe system should include monitoring of ultraviolet levels in the treatment chamber, linked to audible or visual alarms and a water shut-off system. Lamp function/failure monitors should be part of the system, and should also be capable of activating alarms and shut-off switches. These systems ensure that only properly disinfected water leaves the treatment chamber. The wiring and electronic circuitry for monitoring systems should be protected from moisture and harsh environments. In many applications, a remote electrical enclosure is desirable or mandatory. Although ultraviolet disinfection units require a minimum of care, design consideration should be given to ease of service. The lamps should be readily accessible, and the quartz sleeves should not require any special skills or tools for cleaning or replacement.

7.2.2.4 Submicron and Ultrafilters

Submicron filters are membrane filters that reduce the level of bacteria in product water. An ultrafilter, installed at the point where the water is used, is a further means of ensuring that water of high microbiologic quality is provided to the dialysis equipment (see Fig. 7.9). However, these ultrafilters will reduce the flow rate and, therefore, decrease the flow velocity; thus, they have to be carefully thought out and designed into the system. Other points of use that require ultrafiltration are the reuse equipment and the bicarbonate filling station. Ultrafilters need to be disinfected and/or replaced on a routine basis or they will grow bacteria and shed endotoxin. Bacterial levels should be tested monthly at the points where all dialysis systems connect to the loop. This includes reuse systems, dialysis machines, bicarbonate filling stations, etc. Bacteria levels shall not exceed 200 colony forming units/ml (CFU/ml) with an action level of 50 CFU/ ml (Amato 2001). If 50 CFU/ml is reported, then an action should be taken such as disinfecting the RO and/or loop and resampling. For endotoxins, the AAMI recommendation is less than 2.0 endotoxin units (EU)/ml with an action level of 1.0 EU/ml (AAMI 2001).

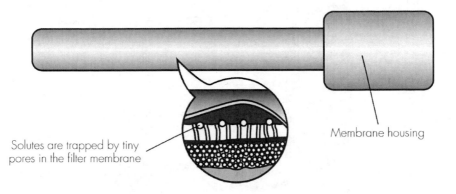

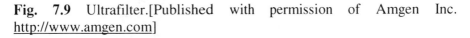

Fig. 7.9 Ultrafilter.[Published with permission of Amgen Inc. http://www.amgen.com]

7.2.3 Distribution System

Distribution systems can be divided into two categories, direct feed and indirect feed (Amato 2001). The direct feed system delivers product water directly from the RO system to the product water loop for distribution. Unused product water is sent back to the RO system. The indirect feed system uses a storage tank to hold product water and send it to the product water loop for use (see Fig. 7.10). Unused product water is returned to the storage tank. If a storage tank is used, it should be no bigger than necessary, have a tight-fitting lid and a conical bottom, drain from the lowest point, and be designed for easy disinfection of all its internal surfaces (Ward 2007). A continuous loop is the recommended design by AAMI for a water distribution piping system (AAMI 2001; Amato 2001). The piping material is commonly nonplasticized polyvinyl chloride (PVC), joined by solvent welding. Other materials, such as cross-linked polyethylene or polyvinylidene fluoride (PVDF), may be needed if the distribution system incorporates hot water or ozone disinfection (Ward 2007). A new material being used to make distribution loop is Gortex that has the potential advantage of lower risk of biofilm formation due to its non-sticky nature. The loop is usually a single long tube with less number of joints. The loop should not have dead ends or multiple branches, as these raise the risk of contamination (Amato 2001).

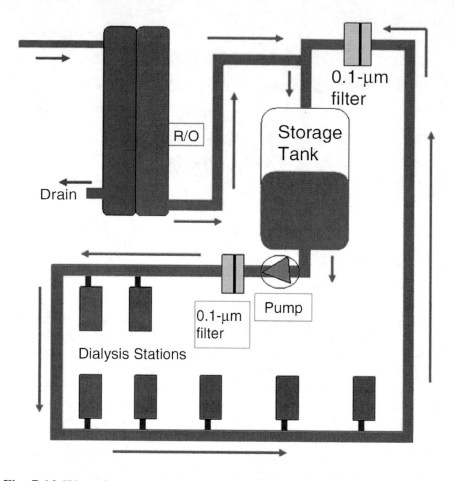

Fig. 7.10 Water loop connected to a storage tank. Adapted from Ahmad S (2005) Essentials of water treatment in hemodialysis. Hemodial Int; 9(2):127-34, with permission]

7.3 DISINFECTION OF WATER TREATMENT SYSTEMS

When starting a new water treatment system it is recommended to disinfect on a weekly basis to sanitize the resins, RO, filters, and the pipe system, until a stable disinfection is achieved as checked by culture and endotoxin measurements. Afterward, the periodicity of disinfection cycles should be adapted to the configuration of the system and on the results of the microbiological monitoring. The most common type of water treatment system disinfection is chemical (e.g., bleach). Ozone and heat can also be used. The optimal periodicity of disinfection measures should be established according to the degree and the kinetics of recontamination after a disinfection procedure (EBPG 2002). Starting early and effective disinfection procedures is the only means to prevent microbial biofilm formation in the pipe system (Man et al. 1998; Cappelli et al. 2000; Smeets et al. 2003). Periodicity, type of disinfection, concentration, and time of exposure to the agent are dependent upon the nature of the material composing the dialysis fluid circuit and must be done in accordance with manufacturer recommendations to prevent damaging effects (Gorke and Kittel 2002). A complete disinfection of the water treatment system including RO and/or deionizer and distribution loop at least once per month appears highly desirable. Periodic changes of water treatment components such as resins (softeners, deionizer), activated carbon, and filters should be performed according to microbiological results and to their life expectancy (Mayr et al.1985). This is an efficient way to prevent downstream seeding from highly contaminated resins.

7.4 MONITORING AND TESTING OF DIALYSIS WATER TREATMENT SYSTEM

Water treatment monitoring is an area of concern and a chance for quality improvement across the nation. The only way to know if the center's system is working properly is to set up and follow an effective monitoring program (Pontoriero et al. 2003; Hoenich and Levin 2003; James 2006). Each component must be checked to be sure it is working properly.

7.4.1 Water Hardness

The first test that is done for any dialysis water pre-treatment system is feed water hardness. Hardness is the presence of calcium (Ca^{2+}) and magnesium (Mg^{2+}) ions in a water supply. It is usually expressed as Grains Per Gallon (GPG) or Parts per Million (PPM) (Amato 2001; Curtis et al. 2005). Water hardness of both feed and product water should be less than 35 mg/L [2 GPG] (Amato 2001). AAMI guideline recommends acceptable hardness for product water as 1 GPG (17.2 g/L) or lower, if hardness increases above 1 PPM the softener must be regenerated. Hardness shall be tested early to assist in the design of the water pre-treatment system, including whether a softener is required, and the volume of the vessel if it is required. Once the softener has been installed and in operation the product water hardness shall be tested and recorded to verify the operation of the softener. Water hardness does not greatly vary thereafter, as it depends on catchment area soil constituents and town water factors.

Product water hardness must be monitored daily. Water hardness of feed water may be tested and recorded monthly so trends can be monitored and corrective action taken as necessary (Amato 2001; Pontoriero et al. 2005).

7.4.2 Chlorine and Chloramine

Chlorine and Chloramine are removed from water by passing the water through a bed of (activated charcoal) carbon. The water needs to be in contact with the carbon for this to occur. The contact time is a critical factor in determining the efficiency of the carbon to absorb the Chlorine and Chloramine. The longer the contact time the less Chlorine and Chloramine there will be in the water post carbon. Tests for Chlorine and/or chloramine shall be done and recorded at least once per dialysis shift. The chlorine and/or chloramine tests shall, as a minimum, be done using the manual process photometer method but in addition an In-line Total Chlorine Meter is highly recommended. In-line Chlorine Meters continuously measure the total chlorine concentration in the sample water (between the two carbon tanks). When total chlorine tests are used as a single analysis the maximum level for both chlorine and chloramine should not exceed 0.1 mg/L. Since there is no distinction between chlorine and chloramine, this safely assumes that all chlorine present is chloramine (AAMI 2004). The AAMI maximum level for chlorine is 0.5 mg/L and for chloramine is 0.1 mg/L. If using an In-line Chlorine Meter, the acceptable maximum level for total chlorine is 0.1 mg/L. When trending of test results indicate an increase in the level of chlorine then the carbon shall be replaced earlier than twelve monthly. The water must be flowing through the carbon tank for a minimum of 15 minutes before the chlorine/chloramines test is done to prevent false negative results.

7.4.3 Microbiological Monitoring

Microbiological monitoring includes cultures of water and dialysis fluid samples to determine the number of colony-forming units per millilitre (CFU/ml). Periodicity of sampling must be determined according to the design of the water treatment chain and the configuration of the dialysis-proportioning machine. However, it is strongly recommended that a microbiological check up should be performed monthly both on water and on dialysis fluid to provide a representative picture of the dialysis fluid purity (Vorbeck-Meister et al. 1999; Ledebo and Nystrand 1999; Arvanitidou et al. 2000). The most sensitive methods to detect water-borne bacteria and endotoxin should be used to detect and quantify the degree of dialysis fluid contamination (Bland 1995; Nystrand 1999). Bacterial levels shall be tested monthly at a minimum from two points, at the first outlet in the distribution loop (usually the first dialysis station) and the last outlet in the distribution loop (last station), if these contain action level values then other sites must be sampled to isolate the contamination site. In addition the dialysis machines, bicarbonate filling stations, reuse room, preventive maintenance stations etc. should also be monitored with culture and endotoxin tests. Bacteria in dialysis water must not exceed the AAMI standard of 200 colony forming units (CFU) (measure of the number of living bacteria) and the endotoxin level should not exceed 2 EU. The AAMI action level for bacteria in water for dialysate is 50 CFU/Ml (AAMI 2001). For ultrapure (sterile, non-pyrogenic) dialysate, the level should be less than 0.1 CFU/mL. An "action level" is the point when measures must be taken to meet AAMI standards (AAMI 2004). The new ISO/AAMI guidlenes have decreased these values to acceptable colony count of 100 CFU and action level to 25 CFU. The acceptable endotoxin level has been decreased to 1 EU and action level to 0.5 EU. The center must show that some action (e.g., disinfection, retesting) has been taken to lower the bacteria count if the action level is reached. Endotoxins should be measured 6-monthly. The endotoxin level should be less than 2 EU/mL (endotoxin units/ml) with an action level of 1 EU/mL. To be considered ultrapure dialysate, the endotoxin level should be less than 0.03 EU/mL (AAMI 2004).

7.4.4 Chemical Contaminant

Monitoring chemical contaminants in dialysis fluids is mandatory to minimize the risk of dialysate-related toxicity either in acute or chronic conditions. For the purpose of testing of chemical contaminants and heavy metal levels, it may be sufficient to collect sample(s) at a point chosen so that the effects of the water pre-treatment system and the piping are completely included. Chemical Contaminant and Heavy metal testing shall be done as part of the commissioning procedure for any new water pre-treatment system. Once the water pre-treatment system is in operation, testing shall be done six monthly or at the time of carbon /RO change, whichever is earlier (Curtis et al. 2005; Pontoriero et al. 2005). The water treatment system must operate within the AAMI standards at all times. AAMI has set the highest allowable levels of contaminants that can be in the product water (see Table 7.2).

7.5 CONCLUSION

Appropriate water quality is one of the most important aspects of ensuring safe and effective delivery of hemodialysis. Hemodialysis may expose the patient to more than 300 L of water per week across the semipermeable membrane of the dialyzer. Healthy individuals seldom have a weekly oral intake of water above 12 L. The near 30 times increase in water exposure to dialysis patients requires control and monitoring of water quality to avoid excesses of known or suspected harmful elements being carried in the water and transmitted to the patient. Moreover, all patients undergoing dialysis in a unit are using water from one source, consequently are at risk with water related catastrophe. Several such catastrophes have caused many deaths in past and must be prevented at all cost. In fact water is the single most exposure to injury including fatality in hemodialysis treatement. The water to be used for the preparation of hemodialysis fluids needs treatment to achieve the appropriate quality. The water treatment is provided by a water pre-treatment system which may include various components such as sediment filters, water softeners, carbon tanks, microfilters, ultraviolet disinfection units, reverse osmosis units, ultrafilters and storage tanks. The components of the system will be determined by the quality of feed water and the ability of the overall system to produce and maintain appropriate water quality. Failure to ensure adequate water quality may have dire consequences to patient safety and welfare. Patients undergoing hemodialysis may show signs and symptoms caused by water contamination, which can lead to patient injury or death.

REFERENCES

Ahmad, S.: Essentials of water treatment in hemodialysis. Hemodial. Int. 9(2), 127–134 (2005)

Amato, R.L.: Water treatment for hemodialysis, including the latest AAMI standards. Nephrol. Nurs. J. 28(6), 619–629 (2001)

Amato, R.L.: Water treatment for hemodialysis: updated to include the latest AAMI Standards for Dialysate (RD52:2004). Nephrol. Nurs. J. 32(2), 151–169 (2005)

Arvanitidou, M., Spaia, S., Velegraki, A., et al.: High level of recovery of fungi from water and dialysis fluid in haemodialysis units. J. Hosp. Infect. 45(B), 225–230 (2000)

Association for the Advancement of Medical Instrumentation (AAMI), Dialysate for Hemodialysis (ANSI/AAMI RD52:2004). Arlington, VA, American National Standard (2004)

Association for the Advancement of Medical Instrumentation, AAMI (2001) Hemodialysis systems (ANSI/AAMI RD62: 2001), vol. 3. Arlington, VA

AWWA. In: Water Treatment Plant Design, 3rd edn. McGraw-Hill (1998)

AWWA. In: Letterman, R.D. (ed.) Water Quality and Treatment, 5th edn. McGraw-Hill, Inc., New York (1999)

Baker, R.: Membrane and Module Preparation. In: Membrane Separation Systems, vol. 2, US DOE Report, DOE/ER/30133-H1 (1990)

Bhattacharyya, D., Williams, M., Ray, R., McCray, S.: Reverse Osmosis. In: Ho, W., Sirkar, K. (eds.) Membrane Handbook, pp. 263–390. Van Nostrand Reinhold, New York (1992)

Bland, L.A.: Microbiological and endotoxin assays of haemodialysis fluids. Adv. Ren. Replace Ther. 2(C), 70–79 (1995)

Cappelli, G., Ballestri, M., Perrone, S., et al.: Biofilms invade nephrology: effects in hemodialysis. Blood Purif. 18(3), 224–230 (2000)

Cappelli, G., Inguaggiato, P.: Water treatment for contemporary haemodialysis. In: Horl, W.H. (ed.) Replacement of Renal Function by Dialysis, 5th edn. Springer, Heidelberg (2004)

Curtis, J., Byers, L., Roshto, B., Roshto, B.: Monitoring Your Dialysis Water Treatment System. Northwest Renal Network, Seattle (2005)

European Best Practice Guidelines (EBPG). Section IV Dialysis Fluid Purity Nephrol. Dial. Transplant. 17(suppl. 7), 45–62 (2002); official publication of the European Dialysis and Transplant Association European Renal Association

Gorke, A., Kittel, J.: Routine disinfection of the total dialysis fluid system. EDTNA ERCA J. 28(3), 130–133 (2002)

Hoenich, N.A., Levin, R.: The implications of water quality in hemodialysis. Semin. Dial. 16(6), 492–497 (2003)

Hoenich, N.A., Ronco, C., Levin, R.: The importance of water quality and haemodialysis fluid composition. Blood Purif. 24(1), 11–18 (2006)

Hoenich, N., Thijssen, S., Kitzler, T., Levin, R., Ronco, C.: Impact of water quality and dialysis fluid composition on dialysis practice. Blood Purif. 26(1), 6–11 (2008)

Hoenich, N.A., Levin, R., Ronco, C.: How do changes in water quality and dialysate composition affect clinical outcomes? Blood Purif. 27(1), 11–15 (2009) (Epub. January 23, 2009)

James, R.: Monitoring of dialysis water systems–is there a need for increased sampling? EDTNA ERCA J. 32(2), 74–77 (2006)

Keshavia, P.: Water treatment for hemodialysis. In: Henderson, L.W., Thuma, R.S. (eds.) Quality Assurance in Dialysis, pp. 85–87. Kluwer Academic Publishers, The Netherlands (1994)

Ledebo, I., Nystrand, R.: Defining the microbiological quality of dialysis fluid. Artif. Organs 23(1), 37–43 (1999)

Levin, R.: The role of water in dialysis: why does it need to be more than "clean"? Nephrol. News Issues 15(2), 21–22 (2001)

Luehmann, D., Keshaviah, P., Ward, R., et al.: A manual on water treatment for hemodialysis. FDA, Rockville (1989)

Man, N.K., Degremont, A., Darbord, J.C., et al.: Evidence of bacterial biofilm in tubing from hydraulic pathway of hemodialysis system. Artif. Organs 22(7), 596–600 (1998)

Mayr, H.U., Stec, F., Mion, C.: Standard methods for the microbiological assessment of electrolyte solution prepared on line for haemofiltration. Proc. Eur. Dial Transplant. Assoc. Eur. Ren. Assoc. 21(B), 454–460 (1985)

Nystrand, R.: Standards and standardization of detection methods for bacteria and endotoxin in water and dialysis fluid. Nieren und Hochdruckkrankheiten 28, 43–48 (1999)

Pontoriero, G., Pozzoni, P., Andrulli, S., Locatelli, F.: The quality of dialysis water. Nephrol. Dial. Transplant. 18(Suppl. 7), vii21–vii25 (2003); discussion vii56

Pontoriero, G., Pozzoni, P., Tentori, F., et al.: Maintenance and monitoring of water treatment system. G. Ital. Nefrol. 22(6), 562–568 (2005)

Smeets, E., Kooman, J., van der Sande, F., et al.: Prevention of biofilm formation in dialysis water treatment systems. Kidney Int. 63(4), 1574–1576 (2003)

Strathmann, H.: Synthetic Membranes and Their Preparation. In: Porter, M. (ed.) Handbook of Industrial Membrane Technology, pp. 1–60. Noyes Publications, Park Ridge (1990)

Vorbeck-Meister, I., Sommer, R., Vorbeck, F., Horl, W.H.: Quality of water used for haemodialysis: bacteriological and chemical parameters. Nephrol. Dial. Transplant. 14(3), 666–675 (1999)

Ward, R.A.: Water Treatment Equipment for In-Center Hemodialysis: Including Verification of Water Quality and Disinfection. In: Nissenson, A.R., Fine, R.N. (eds.) Handbook of Dialysis Therapy, 4th edn. Elsevier, Saunders, Philadelphia (2007)

ESSAY QUESTIONS

1. List some of the common water contaminants
2. What are the two major types of water purification systems?
3. List the pretreatment components of dialysis water treatment system

4. What are the major components of a standard water softener?
5. List the primary water treatment components
6. Compare between the various types of automatic regenerating system of water softeners
7. What are the basic components of reverse osmosis systems?
8. What is the main advantage of reverse osmosis system over a normal filtration system?
9. Describe the two types of synthetic resins used in deionizers.
10. List the main two categories of distribution systems
11. What are the main testing of dialysis water treatment system

MULTIPLE CHOICE QUESTIONS

Choose the best answer

1. The dialysis patient is exposed to … liters of water per treatment
    A. 300-400 liters
    B. 25-150 liters
    C. 90 to 192 liters
    D. 200-350 liters

2. Signs and Symptoms when patients exposed to hard water (calcium and magnesium) are …
    A. Arrhythmia
    B. Hemolysis
    C. Nausea and vomiting
    D. Encephalopathy

3. The ideal pH of the feed water should be …
    A. 5.0–8.5
    B. 125 ml/min/1.73 m^2
    C. 110 ml/min/1.73 m^2
    D. 130 ml/min/1.73 m^2

4. The multimedia filter is…
    A. The most common sediment filter
    B. The most common Carbon filter
    C. The most common Sand Filters
    D. The most common Neutralizing Filters

5. It is recommended that treated water is checked for chloramines at least
... a day to ensure proper functioning of the carbon filter.
   A. twice
   B. three times
   C. four times
   D. one time

6. Carbon tanks should be back-washed at least ... to reduce the impact of
channel formation.
   A. Daily
   B. Monthly
   C. Weekly
   D. Annulay

7. Typically, RO pre-filters range in pore size from...
   A. 2-10 microns
   B. 10-20 microns
   C. 5-15 microns
   D. 1 to 5 microns

8. RO systems typically operate between...
   A. 200-250 PSI
   B. 300-400 PSI
   C. 450-500 PSI
   D. 150-200 PSI

9. The most commonly RO membrane used is ...
   A. Tubular membrane
   B. spiral-wound membrane
   C. hollow-fiber membrane
   D. flat-sheet membrane

10. A membrane that rejects greater than ... of conductant water is consi-
dered to be functioning well.
   A. 70 %
   B. 90 %
   C. 85 %
   D. 80 %

11. The basic configurations of deionizers are …
    A. Two-bed
    B. Mixed-bed
    C. Three bed
    D. A and B

12. The ultraviolet spectrum ranges from … nm
    A. 40 to 400
    B. 50 to 300
    C. 60 to 200
    D. 100 to 400

13. RO membranes should be cleaned and disinfected at least … to insure proper functioning.
    A. weekly
    B. quarterly
    C. monthly
    D. annually

14. The most effective spectral region for germicidal purposes being between … nm.
    A. 350 and 365
    B. 100 and 150
    C. 250 and 265
    D. 500 and 550

15. Bacteria levels shall not exceed … colony forming units/ml (CFU/ml) with an action level of 50 CFU/ml.
    A. 100
    B. 300
    C. 50
    D. 200

16. Deionization tanks should be followed by…
    A. Ultraviolet Irradiator (UV)
    B. Submicron Filter
    C. Multimedia Filter
    D. Ultrafilter

17. Water hardness of both feed and product water should be less than ... mg/L
    A. 50
    B. 35
    C. 25
    D. 45

18. Chlorine and Chloramine are removed from water by passing the water through ...
    A. Multimedia Filter
    B. Ultrafilter
    C. Activated Carbon Filter
    D. Submicron Filter

19. The AAMI maximum level for chlorine and chloramines ... is mg/L respectively
    A. 0.5 and 0.1
    B. 0.1 and 0.5
    C. 0.2 and 0.5
    D. 0.5 and 0.2

20. To be considered ultrapure dialysate, the endotoxin level should be less than ... EU/mL.
    A. 0.07
    B. 0.03
    C. 0.05
    D. 0.01

Chapter (8)

Dialyzer Performance Parameters

Ahmad Taher Azar

<table>
<tr><td>

CHAPTER OUTLINES

- Performance characteristics of dialyzers.
- Factors affecting solute clearance on hemodialysis.
- High efficiency dialysis.
- Conclusion

CHAPTER OBJECTIVES

- Identify the performance parameters of dialyzers.
- Discuss how to calculate the in vivo dialyzer urea clearance.

</td><td>

- Identify the ultrafiltration characteristics of dialyzers.
- Describe the major factors affecting solute removal during dialysis.

KEY TERMS

- Clearance
- Ultrafiltration coefficient (K_{uf})
- Transmembrane Pressure (TMP)
- Dialyzer Flux
- Backtransport
- Priming Volume
- Mass transfer coefficient of (K_oA).
- Sieving Coefficient (S)

</td></tr>
</table>

ABSTRACT

In a given treatment modality, the performance characteristics of the dialyzer determine the quantity and nature of uremic toxins removed from the patient's blood, provided that an adequate treatment time and flow conditions are prescribed. Dialyzer selection may be the most difficult task facing a dialysis facility. Practitioners must understand the functions of a dialyzer, membrane biocompatibility, implications of poor technique, financial and quality implications of dialyzer reprocessing, and matching the patient to the dialyzer's capabilities. Dialyzer membranes are a vital contributor to the success or failure of hemodialysis therapies and hemodialysis adequacy. Matching a dialyzer to patient requirements is crucial to meet the prescribed clearance goals.

A.T. Azar (Ed.): Modelling and Control of Dialysis Systems, SCI 404, pp. 379–425.
springerlink.com   © Springer-Verlag Berlin Heidelberg 2013

8.1 PERFORMANCE CHARACTERISTICS OF DIALYZERS

Although dialyzer performance is traditionally focused on urea clearance (whereby urea is simply used as a generic low molecular weight solute for the quantification of dialysis dose), the removal of larger molecules from the blood has gained more and more attention over the past years. Generally, molecules of molecular weight below 300-500 Da are termed "small solutes", while there is more ambiguity concerning the classification of larger molecules into "middle molecules" and "large solutes". Table 8.1 shows the classification of small, middle, and large molecules as defined by the European Uremic Toxin Work Group (EUTox) categorisation of small, middle and large molecules used throughout this book; the range of molecular weights taken to define "middle molecules" is such that the much-discussed solute β2-microglobulin (MW 11,818) falls into the "middle molecule" class.

Table 8.1 Categorization of small, middle and large molecules.

Classification of solutes	Molecular weight range (Daltons)
Small molecules e.g. urea (60), creatinine (113), phosphate (134)	< 500
Middle Molecules e.g. vitamin B_{12} (1355), vancomycin (1448), inulin (5200), endotoxin fragments (1000-15000), Parathromone (9425), β2-microglobulin (11818)	500-15000
Large molecules e.g. myoglobin (17000), Retinol-Binding Protein (RBP) (21000), EPO (34000), albumin (66000), Transferrin (90000)	>15000

The removal of middle molecules gained more and more attention over the past years due to its important role in uremic toxicity (Woods and Nandakumar 2000). Traditionally, however, dialysis efficiency in the clinical practice is only focused on the removal of urea. Because the diffusion rate of solutes was found inversely proportional to the square root of the solute molecular weight, only low molecular weight (LMW) molecules are removed by diffusion. Middle molecular weight solutes (MMW) are mainly removed by convection, and the contribution of convection to total solute removal increases with increasing molecular size (Ofsthun and Zydney 1994).

When ultrafiltration becomes non-negligible, diffusion and convection interfere continuously with each other. Convection causes an accumulation of large solutes (i.e. larger than the membrane cut-off) at the membrane surface, influencing the diffusion length and the concentration gradient over the membrane. On the other hand, diffusion changes the local solute concentrations, which has an impact on their netto convective transport. As a consequence, it is impossible to specify the exact contribution of convection to the overall dialyzer clearance. It is however certain that the ultrafiltration flow has a larger impact on large solutes, which are not easily diffusing through the membrane (Ofsthun and Zydney 1994). Finally, the larger middle molecules (e.g. β_2 microglobulin – MW11818) can also be removed by adsorption at the membrane. This phenomenon is however dependent on the membrane type, and is especially observed with polymethylmethacrylate (PMMA) and some polyacrylonitrile (PAN) membranes. With the latter membrane, it is usually noticed that adsorption is overruling in the early stages of the dialysis treatment, while convection becomes dominant in the later stage (Clark et al. 1999). Furthermore, solute removal by adsorption and convection are both enhanced by the use of high ultrafiltration flows (Ronco et al. 1997). The dialyzer performance data of paramount interest to the physician in everyday clinical practice are then (a) its ability to remove urea and other low molecular weight molecules normally eliminated in the urine (small solute clearance), (b) its coefficient of ultrafiltration (flux), (c) its proficiency in expelling middle molecules, and (d) its ability to retain albumin and larger substances.

8.1.1 Clearance

Clearance is likely the most useful and important characteristic of a dialyzer, because it is a critical factor in determining the dialysis prescription. It is reported in terms of clearance of solutes such as urea, creatinine, phosphate (PO_4), uric acid, beta-2-microglobulin, and vitamin B_{12}. Clearance depends on the thickness and surface area of the membrane and on the density, characteristics, and size of the pores.

- **Urea clearance** is the most commonly used measure, since it is used in the calculation of the dose of dialysis. The clearance data provided by the manufacturer usually comes from in *vitro* experiments using water and is always higher than the blood clearance obtained in *vivo*. Therefore, the manufacturer's in vitro data must not be used to determine the dialysis prescription using urea kinetics.

- **Creatinine clearance** is 70–95% of urea clearance. It provides no clinically useful additional information, as the clearances for the two molecules are almost always proportional, regardless of membrane or dialyzer type.

- **Phosphate and uric acid clearances** are not always reported but can be useful in treating markedly elevated phosphate or uric acid levels. In vitro phosphate clearance values for dialyzers of comparable ultrafiltration coefficient and surface area range from 101 to 160 mL/min for low-flux dialyzers and 140 to 180 mL/min for high-flux dialyzers of surfaces areas between 1.3 to 1.35 m^2, for example. Membranes with a negative surface charge, such as PMMA, tend to be at the lower end of the range of phosphate clearances. It has been postulated that this is the result of clearance-inhibiting charge interactions between the negatively charged phosphate ion and the negatively charged PMMA and polyacrylonitrile membranes (Okada et al. 1989). Phosphate clearance has been shown to be more sensitive to the ultrafiltration rate and the dialyzer surface area than creatinine or urea clearances (Zucchelli and Santoro 1987) The kinetics of phosphate removal during clinical dialysis are more complicated than in these in vitro measurements: phosphate transport out of cells places a limit on the amount of phosphate accessible for removal by the dialyser during treatment. However, phosphate is an intracellular ion and, using a dialyzer with a high phosphate clearance, the plasma value can fall quickly without a major impact on total body removal of this ion.

- **Vitamin B_{12}:** Although the diffusive clearance of vitamin B_{12} is frequently used as a marker for larger middle molecules removal, its relevance for the clinical assessment of dialyzer performance is further reduced by the fact that it cannot be measured with whole blood or in vivo due to its extensive binding to plasma proteins (Clark et al. 1999).

- **β_2-microglobulin:** Recently, β_2-microglobulin clearance has also been used rather than vitamin B_{12} as a method of assessing membrane characteristics, particularly the flux of the membrane. However, in vitro values of β_2-microglobulin clearance are very rarely supplied in dialyzer data sheets - membrane ultrafiltration coefficients and vitamin B_{12} clearances, although insubstantial measures for middle molecule removal, are the parameters commonly employed in practice.

Recently, a more reliable alternative to these - the membrane sieving coefficient for β_2-microglobulin - has gained acceptance by both dialyzer producers and the medical community. This will be described in the next section.

8.1.1.1 In Vivo Dialyzer Clearance Calculation

In vitro dialyzer clearances measured using aqueous solutions are generally higher than those measured using blood under otherwise identical conditions. This is because only a fraction of the blood is available for solute removal during its passage through the dialyzer, as cells and plasma proteins occupy space, and because, depending on the cell permeability for individual solutes, the distribution space of some solutes is compartmentalized. For most dialyzers, in vivo clearance is 5-25% less than in vitro clearance. By consideration of the mass balance across the dialyzer, the clearance may be expected in terms of concentration gradients and flow rates such that:

Solute transferred from blood side to dialysate side =

Solute mass entering dialyzer - Solute mass leaving dialyzer   (8.1)

In the presence of ultrafiltration (Q_F):

$$\underbrace{Q_F}_{\text{Ultrafiltration rate}} = \underbrace{Q_{Bi}}_{\text{Blood inlet flow}} - \underbrace{Q_{Bo}}_{\text{Blood outlet flow}} \quad \text{mL/min} \quad (8.2)$$

Since the clearance of a dialyzer is defined as its volumetric rate of removal of a particular blood solute, i.e. the amount of solute removed from the blood per unit time, divided by the incoming blood concentration, therefore the *in vivo dialyzer clearance in the blood side* can be calculated as (Sargent and Gotch 1996):

$$K_B = Q_B \underbrace{\left(\frac{C_{Bi} - C_{Bo}}{C_{Bi}} \right)}_{\text{Diffusive term}} + \underbrace{Q_F \left(\frac{C_{Bo}}{C_{Bi}} \right)}_{\text{Convective term}} \quad \text{mL/min} \quad (8.3)$$

The nomenclature is: K_B for blood clearance; Q_B for blood flow rate; C_{Bi} for urea concentration at the dialyzer inlet; C_{Bo} for urea concentration at the dialyzer outlet; Q_F for ultrafiltration rate. The first parts of both equations reflect solute clearance by diffusion, while the last parts represent the convective components of solute transport.

Since the solutes removed are in the dialysate (by neglecting adsorption on the membrane), the equivalent *in vivo dialyzer clearance in the dialysate side* can be calculated as (Sargent and Gotch 1996):

$$K_D = Q_{Di}\left(\frac{C_{Di} - C_{Do}}{C_{Bi}}\right) + \underbrace{Q_F\left(\frac{C_{Do}}{C_{Bi}}\right)}_{} \tag{8.4}$$
$$\underbrace{\hphantom{K_D = Q_{Di}\left(\frac{C_{Di} - C_{Do}}{C_{Bi}}\right)}}_{\text{Diffusive term}} \underbrace{\hphantom{Q_F\left(\frac{C_{Do}}{C_{Bi}}\right)}}_{\text{Convective term}}$$

Where Q_{Di} is the dialysate flow rate, C_{Di} is the dialysate concentration at the dialyzer inlet; C_{Do} is the dialysate concentration at the dialyzer outlet.

To account for fluid removal, it is necessary to modify Eq. (8.3) such that it becomes:

$$K = \underbrace{Q_{Bin}\left(\frac{C_{Bi} - C_{Bo}}{C_{Bi}}\right)}_{\text{Diffusive term}} + \underbrace{Q_F\left(\frac{C_{Bo}}{C_{Bi}}\right)}_{\text{Convective term}} \qquad \text{mL/min} \tag{8.5}$$

It should be noted that this correction does not provide a quantification of solute transport via convection but merely corrects the diffusion equation for differences in the flow rates entering and leaving the dialyzer. In the absence of ultrafiltration, Eq. (8.3) and Eq. (8.4) are reduced to their first part as:

$$K_B = Q_{Bi}\left(\frac{C_{Bi} - C_{Bo}}{C_{Bi}}\right) \tag{8.6}$$

and

$$K_D = Q_{Di}\left(\frac{C_{Di} - C_{Do}}{C_{Bi}}\right) \tag{8.7}$$

For the quantification of clearance in the presence of convection using dialyzers with highly permeable membranes, note that ultrafiltration from blood to dialysate increases solute flow. Therefore, in this case it is possible to represent dialyzer clearance as (Jaffrin 1995; Leypoldt 2000):

$$K = K_D + T_r Q_F \tag{8.8}$$

Where K_D is a pure diffusive clearance (no ultrafiltration, equivalent to $Q_{Bi} = Q_{Bo}$), Q_F is the ultrafiltration flow rate, and T_r is the transmittance coefficient, defined as a function of flow conditions and membrane properties. Granger et al first derived simple expressions for the transmittance coefficient by considering ultrafiltration (or convective solute transport) and diffusive solute transport to occur sequentially rather than simultaneously (Granger et al. 1978). Based on certain experimental data, these investigators suggested that the following expression best represented the increase in solute clearance with increasing ultrafiltration rate (Leypoldt 2000):

$$T_r = S\left(1 - \frac{K_D}{Q_{Bi}}\right) \tag{8.9}$$

Where S is the sieving coefficient, K_D is the diffusive dialyzer clearance and Q_{Bi} is the arterial blood flow rate. This equation was recently rediscovered by Waniewski et al (1991) who expressed the sieving coefficient in terms of fundamental membrane-transport parameters; however, their expression for S is not constant. A more simple formula was proposed by Sargent and Gotch (Sargent and Gotch 1996) and Werynski (Werynski 1979) for solutes whose sieving coefficient was equal to one (Leypoldt 2000):

$$T_r = 1 - \frac{K_D}{Q_{Bi}} \tag{8.10}$$

This expression can be considered to be a special case of Eq. (8.9). An expression for the transmittance coefficient that is universal for all solutes and is a quadratic function of the ultrafiltration rate has been proposed by Jaffrin (Jaffrin 1995). Substituting from Eq. (8.10) into Eq. (8.8) leads to Eq. (8.5) as follows:

$$K = Q_{Bi}\left(\frac{C_{Bi} - C_{Bo}}{C_{Bi}}\right) + \left(1 - \frac{C_{Bi} - C_{Bo}}{C_{Bi}}\right)Q_F$$

$$\Rightarrow K = Q_{Bin}\left(\frac{C_{Bi} - C_{Bo}}{C_{Bi}}\right) + Q_F\left(\frac{C_{Bo}}{C_{Bi}}\right)$$

Example 8.1

Calculate the blood flow rate at the dialyzer outlet if the flow rate at the dialyzer inlet is 300 mL/min and the patient needs to lose 4.5 kg during a 4-h dialysis treatment session.

Solution

The ultrafiltration rate is:

Q_f = (Weight gain × 1000) / dialysis time (min)
   = (4.5 × 1000) / 240 = 18.75 mL/min

According to Eq. (8.2) in the presence of ultrafiltration (Q_F):

$$\underbrace{Q_F}_{\text{Ultrafiltration rate}} = \underbrace{Q_{Bi}}_{\text{Blood inlet flow}} - \underbrace{Q_{Bo}}_{\text{Blood outlet flow}}$$

Thus, the blood flow rate at the dialyzer outlet is:

$$Q_{Bo} = Q_{Bi} - Q_F \Rightarrow Q_{Bo} = 300 - 18.75 = 281.25 \text{ mL/min}$$

Note that at zero ultrafiltration the flow rates at the dialyzer blood inlet (Q_{Bin}) and outlet (Q_{Bout}) are equal.

Example 8.2

Calculate the clearance of urea in a patient for whom the arterial urea concentration sample C_{Bi} is 95 mg/dL, the venous urea concentration sample C_{Bo} is 25 mg/dL, the blood flow rate Q_b is 300 mL/min and the patient needs to lose 2.5 kg during a 4-h run.

Solution

The ultrafiltration rate is:

$Q_f =$ (Weight gain × 1000) / dialysis time (min)

$= (2.5 \times 1000) / 240 = 10.42 \text{ mL/min}.$

The in vivo urea clearance is:

$$K_B = Q_B \underbrace{\left(\frac{C_{Bi} - C_{Bo}}{C_{Bi}} \right)}_{\text{Diffusive term}} + \underbrace{Q_F \left(\frac{C_{Bo}}{C_{Bi}} \right)}_{\text{Convective term}}$$

$$K_B = 300 \times \left(\frac{95 - 25}{95} \right) + 10.42 \times \left(\frac{25}{95} \right) = 223.79 \text{ mL/min}$$

Therefore, during each minute of dialysis, 223.79 mL of this patient's blood has been cleared of urea.

8.1.2 UF Characteristic

8.1.2.1 Ultrafiltration Coefficient (K_{UF})

Because the spent dialysate effluent pump creates negative pressure on the dialysate compartment of the membrane unit and the blood pump creates positive pressure in the blood compartment, there is a net hydrostatic pressure gradient between the compartments as shown in Fig. 8.1 (Hamilton 1998). This pressure difference across the dialyzer membrane is called transmembrane pressure (TMP). This transmembrane pressure (TMP) can be controlled by varying the pressure in the dialysate or blood compartments (Henderson 1996). Increasing negative dialysate pressure will increase ultrafiltration. The plasma oncotic pressure opposes ultrafiltration. Thus, fluid moves only when TMP exceeds the plasma oncotic pressure.

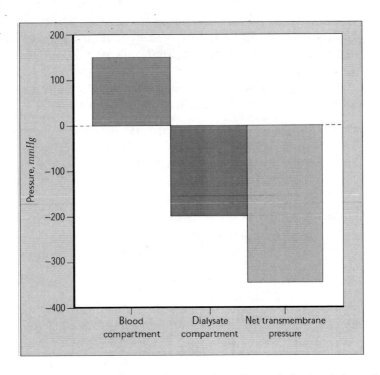

Fig. 8.1 Hydrostatic Ultrafiltration During Hemodialysis. Adapted from Hamilton RW. Principles of Dialysis: Diffusion, Convection, and Dialysis Machines. In Schrier RW, editor. Atlas of diseases of the kidney, Current Medicine, Philadelphia: Blackwell Science; 1998; with permission.

The ultrafiltration coefficient (K_{Uf}) is the number of mL of fluid transferred across the membrane per hour when 1 mmHg of TMP is applied (Cheung and Leypoldt 1997). This value varies among different membrane types, with cellulosic membranes as a group having lower K_{Uf} values than synthetic membranes (MacLeod et al. 2001). However, with the versatility of cellulose-based membranes, alterations in the manufacturing process have allowed production of cellulose hollow fibers with high K_{Uf} values suitable for all clinical uses. In practice, the membrane ultrafiltration coefficient (K_{UF}) is used to characterize the water permeability of a dialyzer as follows:

- If the K_{Uf} is 2.0, the permeability to water is low. To remove 1,000 mL per hour, 500 mmHg TMP will be needed.
- If the K_{Uf} is 4.0, the permeability to water is moderate, and the required TMP will be only 250 mmHg.
- If the K_{Uf} is 8.0, the TMP will have to be only 125 mmHg. When the K_{Uf} is large (when water permeability is high), small errors in setting the TMP will result in large errors in the amount of ultrafiltrate removed. For this reason, dialyzers with a K_{Uf} greater than 6.0 (certainly those with a K_{Uf} greater than 8.0) should be used only with dialysis machines that contain special pumps and circuits that directly control the ultrafiltration rate (Daugirdas et al. 2007).

Ultrafiltration coefficient is therefore the product of the hydraulic permeability (L_h) and the surface area (A) of the membrane embedded in the particular dialyzer casing, i.e. (Korwer et al. 2004):

$$K_{UF} = L_h \times A \qquad (8.11)$$

The membrane's hydraulic permeability depends on the membrane porosity (ρ); this is a function of pore number and size, but is particularly sensitive to the latter, being defined as (Clark et al. 1999):

$$\rho = N \cdot \pi \cdot r_p^2 \qquad (8.12)$$

Where, ρ is the membrane porosity, N is the number of pores and r is the pore radius. The overall water flux (Q_{UF}) (mL/min) in a dialyzer can be written as a function of the difference in hydraulic (ΔP) and oncotic pressure ($\Delta \pi$) between the blood and dialysate compartment (Ronco 1990):

$$Q_{UF} = \iint_A (\Delta P - \Delta \pi) \cdot K_{UF} \cdot dA \qquad (8.13)$$

Assuming the ultrafiltration coefficient of the membrane K_{UF} (mL/h/mmHg/m²) to be constant over the surface area A and ΔP to be identical at any point in a cross section of the dialyzer, Eq. (8.13) can be simplified to (Henderson 1996; Sargent and Gotch 1996):

$$Q_{UF} = K_{UF} \cdot \int_L (\Delta P - \Delta \pi)_x \cdot \frac{dx}{L} = K_{UF} \times TMP \qquad (8.14)$$

Where L is the dialyzer length, K_{UF} is the ultrafiltration coefficient of the dialyzer (mL/h/mmHg) and TMP is the transmembrane pressure (mmHg). The transmembrane pressure is determined by the mean hydrostatic pressure in the dialysate (P_d) and blood compartment (P_b) and the oncotic pressure (P_o) in the blood compartment according to:

$$TMP = P_B - (P_o - P_D) \qquad (8.15)$$

Thus, a specified transmembrane pressure gradient (whether applied directly or resulting from automatic ultrafiltration control units) will trigger a filtrate flow through the membrane, and the size of this filtrate flow is dependent on the ultrafiltration coefficient of the particular membrane. The ultrafiltration rate per unit membrane area is approximately proportional to the fourth power of the mean membrane pore radius. Thus small changes in pore size have large effects on the membrane K_{UF}. As is clear from Eq. (8.11), the K_{UF} is a direct function of the membrane surface area. Consequently, the K_{UF} of membranes of varying surface area can be easily compared by simply dividing the values by the effective surface area (i.e. the total membrane surface area minus the loss of area due to the presence of potting compound). As the surface area is an integral part of the definition of membrane ultrafiltration coefficient, knowledge of the ultrafiltration coefficient makes information on the surface area redundant for the attending physician, at least for fluid removal considerations (not true for solute removal and biocompatibility (Korwer et al. 2004).

The relationship between TMP and ultrafiltration rate is linear at relatively low TMPs for all membranes whereas a plateau in ultrafiltration rate occurs at relatively high TMP values as shown in Fig. 8.2 (Palmer 1998). Normally, the ultrafiltration rate is measured at various different TMPs, and the dialyzer K_{UF} is defined as the slope of the linear portion of the UFR versus TMP curve. Alternatively, some device manufacturers calculate the K_{UF} from the ultrafiltration rate measured at a specific TMP, i.e. according to Eq. (8.14). Values may vary from that stated by the manufacturer (in vitro values). In practice, the in vivo K_{Uf} is often somewhat lower (5%-30%) (Daugirdas et al. 2007). In vivo ultrafiltration coefficients of dialyzers can differ from the published in vitro values for a number of reasons. One is the inexactness of the in vitro values stated by the manufacturer: variations between produced batches exist and values are influenced by storage conditions (e.g. temperature and humidity). Consequently, variations of up to +20% are officially permitted. Such deviations from the stated in vitro values will be reflected in different in vivo values. Different in vivo ultrafiltration coefficients can also result from deviations of the patient's blood composition from that of the test medium (i.e. hematocrit and protein contents different from 32% and 60 g/L, respectively) and from factors that affect membrane hydraulic permeability and surface area. As the blood moves through the dialyzer, water is continually removed by filtration; the resultant increases in blood hematocrit and percentage plasma protein content along the length of the dialyzer and as dialysis progresses are such that the plasma oncotic pressure can be augmented to an extent which reduces the membrane ultrafiltration coefficient.

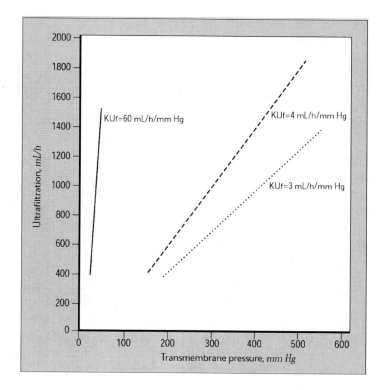

Fig. 8.2 Relationship between ultrafiltration rate and transmembrane pressure. Adapted from Palmer BF (1998) The Dialysis Prescription and Urea Modeling. In Schrier RW, editor. Atlas of diseases of the kidney, Current Medicine, Philadelphia: Blackwell Science; with permission.

Example 8.3

If the clinician wishes to remove 4 kg of fluid during a 4 hour dialysis, calculate:

a) The ultrafiltration rate.
b) TMP when using a dialyzer with a K_{Uf} of 5 mL/h/mmHg.

Solution

a) *The ultrafiltration rate is:*
$$Q_F = (4 \times 1000) / 4 = 1000 \text{ ml/h}$$
Add the volume of saline that will be given at the end of dialysis (usually 300 ml) and the amount of ingested fluid during dialysis (e.g., 100ml). This means that 4.4 L will have to be removed during 4 hours dialysis.

b) When using a dialyzer with K_{UF} value of 5.0 ml/hour, the TMP will need to be set at:
$$TMP = 1000 / 5 = 200 \text{ mmHg}$$

Example 8.4

A dialyzer with a K_{UF} of 4 mL/h/mmHg is used for a dialysis treatment. The pre-pump arterial pressure is -120 mmHg, the post-pump arterial pressure is not measured, the venous pressure is 120 mmHg, and the patient needs to lose 3.6 kg during a 3-h run. What should be the dialysate pressure to achieve the above UF goal if no UF modeling is used? Neglect the oncotic pressure.

Solution

The ultrafiltration rate is:
$$Q_F = (3.6 \times 1000) / 3 = 1200 \text{ mL/h}$$
$$\because Q_{UF} = K_{UF} \times TMP$$
$$\therefore 1200 = 4 \text{ ml/h/mmHg} \times TMP \implies TMP = 300 \text{ mmHg}$$

According to Eq. (8.15) and by neglecting the oncotic pressure:

$$\text{TMP} = P_B - P_D \Rightarrow 300 \text{ mmHg} = 120 - P_D$$
$$\therefore P_D = -180 \text{ mmHg}$$

This means that the dialysate side would have to supplement the blood side pressure by having a negative pressure.

8.1.2.2 Dialyzer Flux

Although numerous classification schemes of HD membranes have been proposed (Akizawa et al. 1995), they are traditionally classified according to water flux. The term flux defines the ability to ultrafilter plasma water. The flux of a dialyzer is defined by its K_{Uf}. Clinically, the flux of the dialysis membrane is more frequently defined by its ability to remove middle molecules (often using β_2-microglobulin as the marker) (Clark et al. 1999). Low-flux dialyzers have small pores, which severely restrict the transport of β_2-microglobulin; while high-flux dialyzers permit the transport of β_2-microglobulin to various extents. Modified cellulosic membranes and synthetic membranes can both be configured into either high-flux or low-flux dialyzers.

High-flux dialyzers have K_{Uf} ranging between 20–60 mL/mmHg/hour, while low flux dialyzers have K_{Uf} < 10 mL/mmHg/hour and medium-flux dialyzers have K_{Uf} that range between 10–19 mL/mmHg/hour (Palmer 1998; Clark et al. 1999). High efficiency dialyzers and cellulosic dialyzers have K_{Uf} of 5–15 mL/mmHg/hour and 3–5 mL/ mmHg/hour respectively. While low flux dialyzers were originally designed as diffusive exchangers, high flux dialyzers have the therapeutic advantage of an increased solute removal by ultrafiltration. Their open pore structure results in high rates of small molecule diffusion and middle molecule diffusion and convection.

8.1.3 Backtransport

Backtransport has been divided into backdiffusion and backfiltration (Klinkmann et al. 1993). The former is driven by the concentration gradient of a given substance and can occur in any dialyzer. Bicarbonate transfer from dialysate to blood is one example of therapeutic backdiffusion, whereas endotoxin transfer would represent an example of pathologic backdiffusion. The term backfiltration is a convective phenomenon describes the movement of fluid from the dialysis fluid compartment into the blood compartment of the dialyzer in that section of the dialyzer distant from the blood inlet port. The driving force is a trans-membrane pressure gradient, which is such that the dialysis fluid pressure is higher than the blood pressure - this is in the reverse direction of the TMP set (either manually or automatically by ultrafiltration control units) for the removal of fluid from the patient's blood. At the blood inlet port, the blood pressure will always exceed the dialysis fluid pressure, so filtration from blood to dialysis fluid occurs (Ronco 1990; Ofsthun and Leypoldt 1995). However, pressures drop along the length of the dialyzer (from inlet to outlet) and the blood pressure may become lower than the dialysis fluid pressure at some point in the dialyzer as shown in Fig. 8.3. The role played by the membrane ultrafiltration coefficient in this scenario is fairly straightforward: the higher the ultrafiltration coefficient (i.e. the more "open" a membrane is), the less TMP is necessary to instigate fluid movement across the membrane; and the lower the TMP, the more difficult it becomes to avoid crossing of the blood and dialysis fluid compartment hydrostatic pressure profiles. Such a crossing of the pressure profiles does not normally occur during low-flux dialysis, but is unavoidable during high-flux dialysis, and irrevocably results in backfiltration of dialysis fluid into patient blood during treatment. The volume of backfiltered fluid was originally estimated from measurements of the pressure ratios at the blood and dialysis fluid ports (Korwer et al. 2004). Backfiltration almost never occurs under conditions of low-flux dialysis, and its occurrence during high-flux treatments depends on the transmembrane pressure used. It is a crucial issue for device safety, because any contamination of dialysate or wash-out from the membrane can reach the blood side. Forward and backfiltration coefficients are different in vitro and even more different in vivo because of the protein layer in the blood compartment and the structure of the membrane (Ronco 1990).

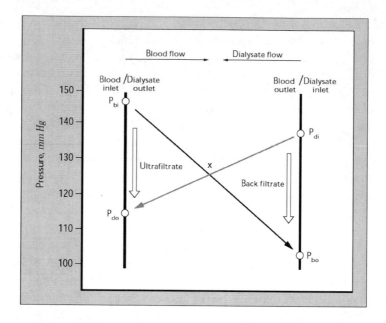

Fig. 8.3 The principle of Backfiltration. Adapted from Ambalavanan S., Rabetoy G., Cheung A (1999) High efficiency and high flux hemodialysis. In: Schrier R.W. (ed) Atlas of Diseases of the Kidney, Vol.5, pp. 3.1-3.10; Philadelphia, Current Medicine; with permission.

8.1.4 Dialyzer Efficiency (K_oA)

The efficiency of solute clearance is measured by the K_oA (mass transfer urea coefficient), and is provided for each dialyser by the manufacturer. This parameter is the optimum value of small molecular clearance (usually urea) under conditions of infinite blood and dialysate flows (i.e., the maximum clearance possible at infinite blood and dialysate flow rates) (Choong et al. 1999). K_oA is the calculated product of the mass transfer coefficient (K_o) and membrane surface area (A), with its unit in mL/min. The mass transfer coefficient of a dialyzer (K_oA) is related to the clearance by the mathematical relationship (Sargent and Gotch 1996):

$$K_d = Q_B \left[\frac{\exp\left[\dfrac{K_oA}{Q_B}\left(1 - \dfrac{Q_B}{Q_D}\right)\right] - 1}{\exp\left[\dfrac{K_oA}{Q_B}\left(1 - \dfrac{Q_B}{Q_D}\right)\right] - \dfrac{Q_B}{Q_D}} \right] \tag{8.16}$$

Where K_o is the mass transfer coefficient, A is the surface area, Q_B is the Blood flow rate, Q_D is the dialysate flow rate, ln is the natural log and K_d is the mean of blood and dialysate side urea clearance. Rearranging Eq. (8.16), K_oA can be calculated using Michaels formula (Michaels 1966):

$$K_oA = \frac{Q_BQ_D}{Q_B-Q_D} \ln\left[\frac{1-\frac{K_d}{Q_B}}{1-\frac{K_d}{Q_D}}\right] \qquad (8.17)$$

K_oA was considered to be constant, i.e. independent of blood and dialysis fluid flow. In practice, however, this has been shown not to be the case because increasing the dialysate flow rate results in an alteration of the koA characteristics due to a better flow distribution within the fiber bundle for hollow fiber dialyzers (Hoenich and Ronco 2008).

Dialyzers with K_oA values less than 500 mL/min are generally used only for low-efficiency dialysis or for small patients. Dialyzers with K_oA values of 500 mL/min to 600 mL/min represent moderate efficiency dialyzers, suitable for routine therapy. Dialyzers with K_oA values greater than 600 mL/min are considered high-efficiency dialysis. Generally, the high-flux dialyzers also have high-efficiency membranes and vice versa. However, theoretically, the two could be very different (see Fig. 8.4). The term "high efficiency" actually had its origin as a therapy, first described by Keshaviah et al (1986), rather than a specific type of dialyzer. Alternatively, K_oA can be calculated from a clearance versus K_oA nomogram computed from the in vitro clearances published by the dialyzer manufacturer as shown in Fig. 8.5 and the calculation steps are also summarized in Daugirdas et al (2007). Actually, industry reported K_oA should be reduced by 20%-30% for a true in vivo clearance, but this will vary by manufacturer.

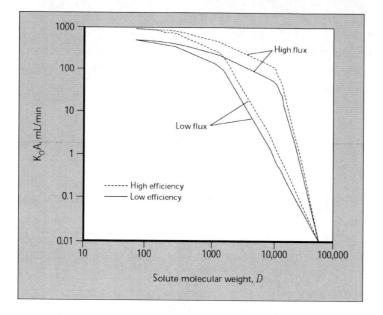

Fig. 8.4 Theoretic K_oA profile of high- and low-flux dialyzers and high and low-efficiency dialyzers. Adapted from Ambalavanan S., Rabetoy G., Cheung A (1999) High efficiency and high flux hemodialysis. In: Schrier R.W. (ed) Atlas of Diseases of the Kidney, Vol.5, pp. 3.1-3.10; Philadelphia, Current Medicine; with permission.

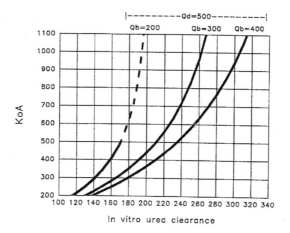

Fig. 8.5 Nomogram of relationship between mass transfer area coefficient (K_oA) and in vitro urea clearance. Adapted from Daugirdas JT, Depner TA (1994) A nomogram approach to hemodialysis urea modeling. Am J Kidney Dis.; 23(1):33-40, with permission from Elsevier.

Example 8.5

Calculate the dialyzer efficiency K_oA if the blood flow rate is 300 mL/min, the dialysate flow rate is 500 mL/min and the in vitro dialyzer clearance is 228 mL/min. What is the type of this dialyzer according to the calculated K_oA?

Solution

According to Eq. (8.17), the dialyzer K_oA is:

$$K_oA = \frac{300 \times 500}{300 - 500} \ln \left[\frac{1 - \dfrac{228}{300}}{1 - \dfrac{228}{500}} \right] = (-750 \text{ mL/min}) \ln \left[\frac{0.24}{0.544} \right]$$

$$= (-750 \text{ mL/min}) \times (-0.818) = 613.73 \approx 614 \text{ mL/min}$$

According to the calculated K_oA, the dialyzer is moderate efficiency.

K_oA also allows easy comparison of the solute removal characteristics of dialyzers of different sizes. Daugirdas and Depner developed an algorithm by using K_oA to estimate the expected in vivo clearance of a dialyzer based upon in vitro clearance and the nominal blood and dialysis fluid flows as shown in Fig. 8.6 and can be calculated mathematically (Daugirdas and Depner 1994; Daugirdas et al. 2007).

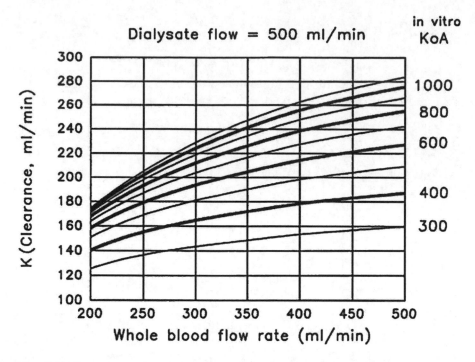

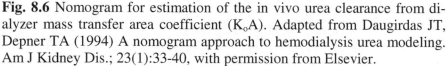

Fig. 8.6 Nomogram for estimation of the in vivo urea clearance from dialyzer mass transfer area coefficient (K_oA). Adapted from Daugirdas JT, Depner TA (1994) A nomogram approach to hemodialysis urea modeling. Am J Kidney Dis.; 23(1):33-40, with permission from Elsevier.

Example 8.6

A low flux dialyzer has in vitro clearance of 237 mL/min at dialysate flow rate $Q_D = 500$ mL/min and blood flow rate of 300 mL/min.

a) Calculate the in vivo dialyzer clearance during 4-hours dialysis for a patient has arterial urea concentration C_{Bi} of 104 mg/dL, venous urea concentration C_{Bo} of 35 mg/dL, and the weight gain is 5 kg.

b) Compare the result obtained in (a) with the in vivo dialyzer clearance using Daugirdas and Depner adjustment method.

Solution

The ultrafiltration rate is:

Q_f = (Weight gain × 1000) / dialysis time (min)
  = (5 × 1000) / 240 = 20.8 mL/min.

a) The in vivo urea clearance is:

$$K_{in-vivo} = Q_B \underbrace{\left(\frac{C_{Bi} - C_{Bo}}{C_{Bi}}\right)}_{\text{Diffusive term}} + \underbrace{Q_F \left(\frac{C_{Bo}}{C_{Bi}}\right)}_{\text{Convective term}}$$

$$K_{in-vivo} = 300 \times \left(\frac{104 - 36}{104}\right) + 20.8 \times \left(\frac{36}{104}\right) = 203.35 \text{ mL/min}$$

Thus, the in vivo urea clearance is lower than the in vitro by about 14.2 %.

b) The K_oA of the dialyzer is calculated:

$$K_oA = \frac{300 \times 500}{300 - 500} \ln \left[\frac{1 - \dfrac{237}{300}}{1 - \dfrac{237}{500}}\right] = (-750 \text{ mL/min}) \ln \left[\frac{0.21}{0.526}\right]$$

$$= (-500 \text{ mL/min}) \times (-0.918) = 688.65 \approx 689 \text{ mL/min}$$

By reducing K_oA by 10% (Daugirdas et al. 2007), the adjusted K_oA will be 620.1 mL/min.

According to Daugirdas et al (2007), the blood flow must be adjusted to compensate for pre-pump negative pressure as follows:

$$\text{Adjusted Blood flow rate} = \text{unadjusted Blood flow rate} \times$$
$$\underbrace{\left[1.0 - \frac{\text{unadjusted Blood flow rate} - 200}{2000}\right]}_{\text{Adjustment Factor}} \quad (8.18)$$

$$Q_{Badj} = 300 \times \left[1.0 - \frac{300 - 200}{2000}\right] = 285 \text{ mL/min}$$

The adjusted diffusive blood water clearance (K_{difadj}) can be calculated as follows (Daugirdas et al. 2007):

$$K_{difadj} = 0.894 \times Q_{Badj} \times \frac{Z - 1}{Z - \dfrac{Q_{Badj}}{Q_D}} \quad (8.19)$$

where
$$Z = \exp\left[\frac{K_o A}{Q_B}\left(1 - \frac{Q_B}{Q_D}\right)\right] \qquad (8.20)$$

$$\therefore K_{difadj} = 0.894 \times 285 \times 0.783 = 199.46 \text{ mL/min}$$

Then, the total in vivo urea clearance can be calculated as follows (Daugirdas et al. 2007):

$$K_{\text{Total invivo}} = \left[1 - \frac{Q_f}{0.894 \times Q_{Badj}}\right] \times K_{difadj} + Q_f \qquad (8.21)$$

$$K_{\text{Total invivo}} = \left[1 - \frac{20.8}{0.894 \times 285}\right] \times 199.46 + 20.8 = 203.94 \approx 204 \text{ mL/min}$$

In this practical example, the in vivo urea clearance is approximately similar to urea clearance calculated by Daugirdas and Depner adjustment method.

8.1.5 Dialyzer Surface Area

Surface area is a key to how well a dialyzer can remove solutes. If all other aspects are equal, dialyzers with more surface area can expose more blood to dialysate. This means more solutes can be removed from the blood. While dialyzer manufactures usually publish the effective membrane surface areas as measured in the dry state, surface areas change in vivo due to wetting of the membrane with saline, blood or dialysis fluid (e.g. swelling of hollow-fiber cellulose by 13.5% in internal diameter and 100% in wall thickness). However, such changes in surface area can be ignored with respect to their effect on the membrane ultrafiltration coefficient, as standard K_{UF} determinations are conducted on wet membranes after allowing at least 10 minutes for swelling (Korwer et al. 2004).

8.1.6 Molecular Weight Cutoff

Each membrane has a molecular weight cutoff which determines the largest molecule that can pass through the membrane. Molecular weight is measured in Daltons (Da). It is the average weight of a molecule, expressed as the sum of the atomic weights of all the atoms in the molecule.

Larger molecules have higher molecular weights; smaller molecules have lower ones (see Table 8.1). Knowing the range of molecular weights that each membrane will allow through helps doctors choose membranes that will remove certain molecules from the blood. Dialyzers can be chosen with molecular weight cutoffs ranging from 3,000 Da to more than 15,000 Da (Curtis 2001).

8.1.7 Priming Volume

The volume of blood within the dialyzer is known as priming volume (Khandpur 2003). The priming volume of most of dialyzers is usually between 60 and 120 mL. It is related to the area of the membrane and in general is less than the volume of blood contained in the blood tubing sets. Requirements of low priming volume permit the use of patients own blood to prime the circuit without serious hypovolemic effects (Khandpur 2003). In a typical adult patient, this parameter is not of great clinical importance. However, it could be important in pediatric or small adult patients.

8.1.8 Sterilization

Today, the three primary methods of sterilization are ethylene oxide gas, steam autoclaving, or gamma irradiation. Steam and irradiation pose least risk to patients, as ethylene oxide must be thoroughly rinsed out prior to use. The type of membrane being used is another factor that influences the manufacturer's choice of sterilization. Some membranes cannot be sterilized by heat-based methods (e.g., cellulose acetate and polyacrylonitrile). Although the dialyzers produced are sterile, their adequate rinsing prior to use by the patient is a mandatory requirement to ensure that sterilant byproducts and microorganisms destroyed by the sterilization process are removed.

8.2 FACTORS AFFECTING SOLUTE CLEARANCE ON HEMODIALYSIS

8.2.1 Blood Flow Rate

Blood flow is usually maintained at 200-500 mL/min. For any dialyzer, the general relationship between blood flow rate and solute removal is curvilinear. Increasing blood flow increases solute clearance, but the increase is not proportional to the increased blood flow, as the efficiency of diffusion is reduced as blood flow increases. At low blood flow rates, the solute removal or clearance cannot exceed the blood flow rate. At higher blood flow rates, increases in clearance rates progressively decrease as the characteristics of the dialysis membrane become the limiting factor (Palmer 1998). The blood flow rate influences the clearance of small molecules and therefore said to be flow-limited because their clearance is highly flow-dependent as shown in Fig. 8.7 (Palmer 1998). However, there are exceptions to this; for example, phosphate as small molecule (MW 145 daltons) whose removal is influenced both by its behavior within the body (high body mass transfer resistance) and its hydration radius. Because of this, phosphate mass transfer per dialysis session remains inadequate despite the use of high-flux membrane and high-efficiency modalities. In general, a 100% increase in blood flow may only increase urea clearance by 20-50%, with less effect on larger MW molecules (Daugirdas et al. 2007). However, use of high blood flows can increase the risk of recirculation if the vascular access is problematic, and is not recommended for some patient groups due to the danger of inducing a disequilibrium syndrome, e.g. children, elderly and diabetic patients, and patients with severe acidosis and/or high urea levels (Daniels et al. 1992). The decision on which blood flow to use will then depend on the type of dialysis being performed (e.g. high-efficiency), on the quality of the vascular access, and on the ability/inability of the patient to tolerate higher blood flows (Korwer et al. 2004).

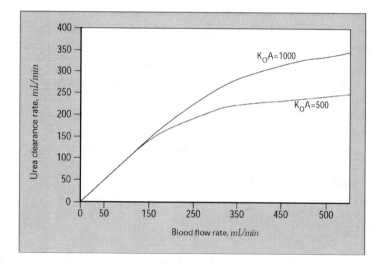

Fig. 8.7 Comparison of urea clearance rates between low- and high-efficiency hemodialyzers (urea K_oA = 500 and 1000 mL/min, respectively). The urea clearance rate increases with the blood flow rate and gradually reaches a plateau for both types of dialyzers. The plateau value of K_oA is higher for the high-efficiency dialyzer. At low blood flow rates (<200 mL/min), however, the capacity of the high-efficiency dialyzer cannot be exploited and the clearance rate is similar to that of the low-flux dialyzer. Adapted from Ambalavanan S., Rabetoy G., Cheung A (1999) High efficiency and high flux hemodialysis. In: Schrier R.W. (ed) Atlas of Diseases of the Kidney, Vol.5, pp. 3.1-3.10; Philadelphia, Current Medicine; with permission.

Example 8.7

If the in-vitro clearance of high flux dialyzer at blood flow rate (Q_B) of 300 and dialysate flow rate (Q_D) of 500 mL/min is 242 is mL/min.

a) Calculate the in-vitro dialyzer clearance at blood flow rate of 250 mL/min and at the same dialysate flow rate.

b) What is the percentage change in dialyzer clearance due to the reduction in blood flow rate?

Solution

Step 1 Calculate the in-vitro dialyzer K_oA at Q_B of 300 mL/min, Q_D of 500 mL/min and K_D of 242 mL/min according to Eq. (8.17):

$$K_oA_{in-vitro} = \frac{300 \times 500}{300 - 500} \ln \left[\frac{1 - \dfrac{242}{300}}{1 - \dfrac{242}{500}} \right] = \left(-750 \text{ ml/min} \right) \ln \left[\frac{0.193}{0.516} \right]$$

$$= \left(-750 \text{ ml/min} \right) \times \left(-0.9834 \right) = 737.55 \text{ ml/min}$$

Step 2 Adjust the K_oA according to Daugirdas and Depner adjustment method if the required Q_D > 500 mL/min as discussed previously. Since the required Q_D is 500 mL/min, so the adjusted K_oA and the $K_oA_{in-vitro}$ are equal (Daugirdas et al. 2007).

Step 3 Use the adjusted K_oA to calculate the required in vitro dialyzer clearance for any combination of blood and dialysate flow rates using Eq. (8.16) as follows (Daugirdas et al. 2007):

$$K_{in-vitro} = 250 \times \left[\frac{\exp\left[\dfrac{737.55}{250} \left(1 - \dfrac{250}{500} \right) \right] - 1}{\exp\left[\dfrac{737.55}{250} \left(1 - \dfrac{250}{500} \right) \right] - \dfrac{250}{500}} \right] = 217.71 \text{ mL/min}$$

b) Thus, reducing the blood flow rate from 300 mL/min to 250 mL/min reduces the in-vitro dialyzer clearance by about 10.04 %

8.2.2 Dialysate Flow Rate

Dialysate flow rates are usually maintained at 500 mL/min. Increasing dialysate flow rate increases clearance (Leypoldt et al. 1997; Leypoldt 1998), but the increases in clearance are more substantial at the higher blood flow rate and when a high-efficiency dialyzer is used (Daugirdas et al. 2007). Leypoldt et al (1997) showed that increasing dialysate flow rate from 500 to 800 mL/min in a variety of dialyzers increased urea K_oA by 14% in vitro. They suggested this increase could result from improved flow distribution through the dialysate compartment or decreased dialysate boundary layer resistance to mass transfer. Early investigations showed that the optimal choice of dialysis fluid flow with regard to solute clearance is approximately twice the blood flow - values higher than $2\text{-}Q_B$ were long believed to have only a slight enhancing effect on small solute clearance (Clark and Shinaberger 2000). In vitro and in vivo study has proven the positive effect of increasing dialysis fluid flow to between $2\text{-}Q_B$ and $3\text{-}Q_B$ on solute clearance (Ouseph and Ward 2001). Hauk et al (2000) found a greater than predicted increase in urea Kt/V when dialysate flow rate was increased from 500 to 800 mL/min. Depner et al (2004) found only a $5.5 \pm 1.5\%$ increase in K_oA when the dialysate flow rate was increased from 500 to 800 mL/min. A recent study showed that a dialysate flow rate of 800 mL per minute increases urea clearance by about 11.5% when a high-efficiency dialyzer is used and when the blood flow rate is 300 mL per minute (Azar 2009). For example, at a Q_B of 300 mL/min, increasing Q_D from 500 to 800 mL/min results in an increase in K_oA (originally believed to be fixed for each dialyzer) and, consequently, an increase in small solute clearance (Leypoldt and Cheung 1999) (see Fig. 8.8). It was postulated that the higher dialysis fluid flow (a) decreases the thickness of the stagnant dialysis fluid layer at the outer membrane surface, thus reducing the total membrane-associated resistance to solute movement and (b) acts to more equally distribute flow around the hollow fibres in bundles which do not already have spacer yarn or wave structure, thus yielding a larger effective membrane surface area (Ouseph and Ward 2001). The consequence is that use of dialysis fluid flows higher than the traditional 500 mL/min have been recommended to optimize dialyzer performance (Azar 2009). Many modern dialysis machines offer a choice of Q_D of 300, 500 or 800 mL/min. Increasing dialysis fluid flow to over 2 times the blood flow means more dialysis fluid concentrate is required per dialysis, and thus increases the cost of treatment. Recent developments in dialyzer design improve the distribution of dialysis fluid around the individual fibres and hinder the formation of stagnant fluid layers; use of such designs could well have the same beneficial effect on solute clearance as increasing the dialysis fluid flow above twice the blood flow (Leypoldt et al. 2003). The use of fibers with undulations has been shown to improve dialysate flow distribution compared to straight fibers performance (Ronco et al. 2002). Moreover, Yamamoto and colleagues have shown that the design of the baffles at the inlet to the dialysate compartment also influences both dialysate flow distribution and dialyzer (Yamamoto et al. 2007, 2009). Recent study showed that increasing the dialysate flow rate from 500 to 800 mL/min had only a modest impact on dialyzer performance, limited to the theoretical increase predicted by the Michaels equation for a constant K_oA (Bhimani et al. 2010). This finding suggests that increasing the dialysate flow rate beyond 500–600 mL/min may provide only a marginal benefit in terms of delivered Kt/V.

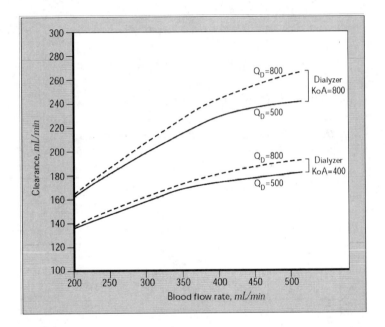

Fig. 8.8 Relationships between dialysate flow rates and urea clearance in hemodialysis. Adapted from Palmer BF (1998) The Dialysis Prescription and Urea Modeling. In Schrier RW, editor. Atlas of diseases of the kidney, Vol. 5; pp. 6.1-6.8; Current Medicine, Philadelphia: Blackwell Science; with permission.

Example 8.8

Using the same data in Example 8.7,

a) Calculate the in-vitro dialyzer clearance at the same blood flow rate of 300 mL/min and at dialysate flow rate of 800 mL/min.
b) What is the percentage change in dialyzer clearance due to the increase in dialysate flow rate?

Solution

Step 1 The in-vitro dialyzer K_oA at Q_B of 300 mL/min, Q_D of 500 mL/min and K_D of 242 mL/min is 737.56 mL/min.

Step 2 Since the required Q_D is 800 mL/min, so the adjusted K_oA is calculated using Daugirdas and Depner adjustment method as follows (Daugirdas et al. 2007):

$$K_oA_{\text{Adjusted}} = K_oA_{\text{in-vitro}} \times \text{multplication Factor}$$

Using the look up Table (see Table 8.2) based on Daugirdas et al (2007):

Table 8.2 Effect of dialysate flow rate on dialyzer clearance efficiency K_oA (Daugirdas et al. 2007)

Dialysate flow rate (mL/min)	Multiplication factor
500	1
600	1.033
700	1.066
800	1.099
900	1.132
1000	1.165

Thus, the multiplication factor is 1.099.

$$K_oA_{\text{Adjusted}} = K_oA_{\text{in-vitro}} \times 1.099 = 810.58 \text{ mL/min}$$

Step 3 The required in vitro dialyzer clearance at dialysate flow of 800 mL/min and blood flow rate of 300 mL/min is:

$$K_{in-vitro} = 300 \times \left[\frac{\exp\left[\frac{810.58}{300}\left(1 - \frac{300}{800}\right)\right] - 1}{\exp\left[\frac{810.58}{300}\left(1 - \frac{300}{800}\right)\right] - \frac{300}{800}} \right] = 262.78 \text{ mL/min}$$

b) Thus, increasing the dialysate flow rate from 500 mL/min to 800 mL/min increases the in-vitro dialyzer clearance by about 8.59 %

8.2.3 Surface Area

Surface areas of dialyzers vary between as little as 0.3 m^2 and as much as 2.6 m^2, but most are in the 0.8 -1.4 m^2 range. As small solute clearance is achieved by diffusion, it is governed by Fick's Law and is, consequently, a direct function of solute diffusivity and membrane surface area. Assuming equal blood, dialysis fluid and ultrafiltration, small solute clearance has been shown to increase linearly with surface area up to about 1.2 -1.4 m and to then flatten off. Thus only dialyzers of comparable surface areas should be used when comparing filter clearances. Alternatively, comparison of dialyzers of different surface area can be conducted using formulae involving mass transfer coefficient of a dialyzer (K_oA). Augmented diffusive clearances can also be achieved nowadays with the use of thinner membranes or with dialyzers of more efficient design, such that dialysis fluid flow around the individual fibres is optimized. Therefore, focus on surface area is considered by some to be of less significance for small solutes, which are predominately removed from patient blood by diffusion, than for larger solutes (Locatelli et al. 2000). As solute size increases, solute diffusivity decreases and convection contributes more and more to total clearance. Here ultrafiltration rate (Q_F) is all-important, and membrane surface area is an integral part thereof (Eq. (8.11) and Eq. (8.14)). Consequently, total clearance (i.e. diffusive plus convective clearance) of middle or large solutes is more sensitive to membrane surface area than small solute clearance at a given blood and dialysis fluid flow (Mandolfo et al. 2003).

8.2.4 Time of Dialysis

Length of a dialysis session is the single most important determinant of solute clearance. Shortening of the dialysis time by high flux dialysis may be ultimately limited by the ability to correct the intradialytic weight gain while maintaining cardiovascular stability. As a general rule, it has been noted that when patients intradialytic weight gain more than 5 kg and the dialysis time shortened to less than 3 hours, a significant increase in hypotension may occur.

8.2.5 Erythrocytes and Hematocrit

Blood water is the solvent for most materials, diffusively transported by the dialyzer. In general blood water can be considered to be divided into extracellular or plasma water and intercellular or red cell water. Urea is dissolved in erythrocytes and plasma water. Approximately 93% of plasma is water and about 72% of an erythrocyte is water. As the mass ratio between red blood and plasma is 0.894, the whole-blood clearance should be multiplied by 0.894 to account for blood water content of both plasma and erythrocytes together (Daugirdas et al. 2007). Because some urea associates with the non-water portion of erythrocytes, one normally considers urea to be dissolved in a volume equal to 80% of the erythrocyte volume. Solutes other than urea do not always distribute in erythrocytes, and transport out of the erythrocyte can be delayed as blood traverses the dialyzer within 10 to 30 seconds. So the presence of erythrocytes has little effect on urea clearance because urea diffuses into and out of erythrocytes quickly (Bagnasco 2006). As the red cell mass usually makes up 30% to 40% of a patient's blood volume, distribution and transport of solutes in erythrocytes can have negatively affected by hematocrit increases than the clearance of urea (Ronco et al. 2001). Lim et al (1990) showed that varying hematocrits from 16 to 44% did not adversely affect urea nitrogen clearance, but did significantly reduce creatinine and phospbate clearances. Any substance that has a slow coefficient of transfer from the red cells to the serum, and is dependent on serum water clearance, notably phospbate and creatinine, will be significantly and proportionately reduced by increased hematocrit levels. Therefore, as the hematocrit is increased from 20% to 40%, creatinine removal decreases by about 8% and a trivial reduction of the blood water urea clearance will occur (Daugirdas et al. 2007). The increase in hematocrit results in an increase in the viscosity of blood, which further increases the red cell mass and the whole blood volume. This leads to an increase in obligatory fluid loss and perhaps back diffusion of dialysate, leading thereby to decrease in clearances and the efficiency of high hematocrit hemodialysis. This in part explains the difference between in vitro and in vivo clearances, an effect that should be kept in mind when developing and applying kinetic models for solutes other than urea. Sargent and Gotch (Sargent and Gotch 1996) derived a correction factor for blood water flow rate (Q_B) which considers the impact of hematocrit on the clearance of such solutes, and of solutes for which the red blood cell membrane is impermeable and which are distributed exclusively in plasma water (e.g. inulin, β_2-microglobulin) as follows:

$$\text{Plasma water flow rate} = Q_B\left(1 - \frac{HCT}{100}\right)F_P \qquad (8.22)$$

$$\text{Red cell water flow rate} = Q_B\frac{Hct}{100}F_R \qquad (8.23)$$

Where HCT is the hematocrit, F_P is the plasma water fractions, and F_R is the red cell water fraction. The effective blood water flow rate is:

$$Q_e = Q_B\left[F_P - \frac{Hct}{100}(F_P - F_R)\right] \qquad (8.24)$$

The contribution of red blood cell to overall mass transfer can be modified by a coefficient γ which represents the fraction of red blood cell water that participated in the transfer during a transit of the dialyzer as follows:

$$Q_e = Q_B\left[F_P - \frac{Hct}{100}(F_P - \gamma F_R)\right] \qquad (8.25)$$

If the red blood cell membrane material is transparent, then γ will be 1.0. Donan ratio (R_D) must be added to Eq. (8.25) for charged particles (Sargent and Gotch 1996; Gotch et al. 2003):

$$Q_e = Q_B\left[F_P - \frac{Hct}{100}(F_P - F_R\gamma R_D)\right] \qquad (8.26)$$

Where

$$R_D = \frac{\text{anion concentration in red cells}}{\text{anion concentration in plasma water}} \qquad (8.27)$$

For bicarbonate, $\gamma = 1.0$ because the bicarbonate ion is charged particle for which the red cell membrane is very permeable and therefore the bicarbonate concentration in red cell eater will be lower than plasma water (i.e. $R_D < 1.0$). For bicarbonate concentration Eq. (8.26) becomes (Sargent and Gotch 1996; Gotch et al. 2003):

$$Q_e = Q_B\left[F_P - \frac{Hct}{100}(F_P - F_R R_D)\right] \qquad (8.28)$$

If $F_P = 0.93$, $F_R = 0.72$ and $R_D = 0.69$, then Eq. (8.28) becomes:

$$Q_e = 0.93 \times Q_B - 0.443 \times \frac{Hct}{100} \qquad (8.29)$$

The effective blood flow rate Q_e can then be used instead of Q_B in Eq. (8.17) to calculate mass transfer coefficient of a dialyzer (K_oA).

Example 8.9

If the blood flow rate Q_B is 300 mL/min at the hematocrit value of 35%, calculate:

a) Plasma water flow rate
b) Erythrocyte water flow rate
c) Whole blood water flow

Solution

According to Eq. (8.22), the plasma water flow rate is:

a) Plasma water flow rate $= 300 \times \left(1 - \dfrac{35}{100}\right) \times 0.93 = 181.35$ mL/min

Here F_P (plasma water fraction) is 0.93 because 93% of plasma is water.

According to Eq. (8.23), the erythrocyte water flow rate is:

b) Erythrocyte water flow rate $= 300 \times \dfrac{35}{100} \times 0.72 = 75.6$ mL/min

Here F_R (erythrocyte water fraction) is 0.72 because about 72% of an erythrocyte is water.

c) Thus, the whole blood water flow rate effective for urea clearance is calculated according to Eq. (8.28):

$$Q_e = 300 \times \left[0.93 - \frac{0.35}{100}(0.93 - 0.72)\right] = 256.95 \text{ mL/min}$$

Or

Q_e can be calculated by adding the plasma water flow rate to the erythrocyte water flow rate as follows:

$$181.35 \text{ mL/min} + 75.6 \text{ mL/min} = 256.95 \text{ mL/min}$$

Example 8.10

If the blood water concentration of urea is 105 mg/dL at dialyzer inlet and 30 mg/dL at dialyzer outlet, and the ultrafiltration rate during treatment is 12.5 mL/min.

a) Using the same data in Example 8.2 calculate the urea clearance of whole to take the effective blood flow rate into account.

b) Compare the results obtained in (a) without correcting the blood flow rate.

Solution

a) *The in vivo urea clearance after taking the effective whole blood water flow rate into account can be calculated as:*

$$K_B = Q_e \left(\frac{C_{Bi} - C_{Bo}}{C_{Bi}} \right) + Q_F \left(\frac{C_{Bo}}{C_{Bi}} \right)$$

$$= 256.95 \times \left(\frac{105 - 30}{105} \right) + 12.5 \times \left(\frac{30}{105} \right) = 187.11 \text{ mL/min}$$

b) The *in vivo urea clearance without* correcting the blood flow rate is:

$$K_B = Q_B \left(\frac{C_{Bi} - C_{Bo}}{C_{Bi}} \right) + Q_F \left(\frac{C_{Bo}}{C_{Bi}} \right)$$

$$= 300 \times \left(\frac{105 - 30}{105} \right) + 12.5 \times \left(\frac{30}{105} \right) = 217.86 \text{ mL/min}$$

Thus, the correction for blood water becomes important when using the dialyzer clearance to compute how much urea is being removed during a dialysis session (Daugirdas et al. 2007). In this example, not making the blood water correction will cause overestimation of the amount of urea removal by about 16%.

8.2.6 Sieving Coefficient (S)

The sieving coefficient is the permeability of dialysis membranes to a particular solute and not its diffusability. The sieving coefficient is defined as the ratio of ratio of the solute concentration in the ultrafiltrate (C_F) to that in incoming blood (C_{Bi}) (Henderson 1996):

$$S = \frac{C_F}{C_{Bi}} \tag{8.30}$$

The sieving coefficient remains near 1.0 for substances up to 1 kilodalton but is lower for larger molecular weight substances and reflect lower clearances via convection. A sieving coefficient (S) of 1 for a given substance represents unhindered transport through the membrane, while a value of zero means that the membrane is impermeable for this substance, resulting in zero diffusion as well. It is obvious that the smaller pores in the low flux membranes hamper the transport of middle molecules over the membrane. This results in a sieving coefficient of only 0.7 and 0.1 for vitamin B_{12} (MW1355) and inulin (MW 5200), respectively, in the low flux Fresenius polysulphone dialyzers (see Fig. 8.9). The high flux polysulphone membranes, however, allow free passage of molecules with a molecular weight less than or equal to inulin. Even β_2- microglobulin (MW11818), a molecule of the higher middle molecule range, is removed with a sieving coefficient approaching 0.65

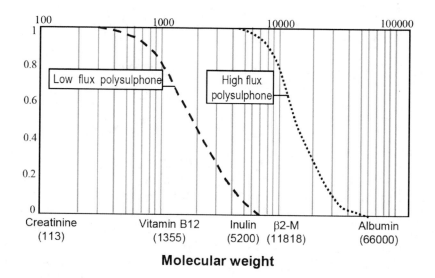

Fig. 8.9 Sieving coefficient profiles (S) of low and high flux polysulphone dialyzers as a function of molecular weight. Courtesy of Korwer U, Schorn E.B, Grassmann A., Vienken J (2004) Understanding Membranes and Dialyzers. PABST Science Publishers.

Determination of solute sieving coefficients does not require accurate measurements of blood or dialysate flow rates. However, the sieving coefficient of a membrane may not accurately reflect its ability to remove a given solute if there is increased adsorption. If a solute exhibits a high affinity for a membrane, it will be adsorbed with minimal transversing of the solute into the dialysate and the sieving coefficient will be low. As the membrane becomes saturated with the solute more will appear in the ultrafiltrate and there is an increase of the sieving coefficient. Dialyzer products must use a more accurate formula incorporating the average plasma solute concentration to calculate the sieving coefficient (S) for membranes (Klinkmann and Vienken 1995):

$$S = \frac{2C_F}{(C_{p_i} + C_{p_o})}$$ (8.31)

Where C_F is the concentration in filtrate plasma, C_{pi} is the concentration in incoming plasma and C_{po} is the concentration in outgoing plasma.

In vivo values for the sieving coefficient are different from the in vitro derived values. This is also due to the different composition of the patient's blood and the different flow conditions. Depending on the membrane type, different combinations of diffusion, convection and adsorption can occur, such that the sieving coefficient may differ significantly in between different dialyzers. Furthermore, as the relative contribution of convection and adsorption to overall solute removal can change during the dialysis session, the sieving coefficient may also decrease, increase or remain constant when blood-membrane contact time increases.

8.3 HIGH EFFICIENCY DIALYSIS

8.3.1 Characteristics of High-Efficiency and High Flux Dialysis

The use of high-efficiency and high-flux dialysis permits short high-efficiency hemodialysis to be accomplished. High-efficiency dialysis is arbitrarily defined by a high K_oA (> 600 mL/min), high clearance rate of urea (> 210 mL/min), high blood flow ($\geq$ 350 mL/min) and high dialysate flow ($\geq$ 500 mL/min) (Ambalavanan et al. 1999). High-efficiency membranes can be made from either cellulosic or synthetic materials. Depending on the membrane material and surface area, the removal of water (as measured by the ultrafiltration coefficient or K_{UF}) and molecules of middle molecular weight (as measured by β_2-microglobulin clearance) may be high or low (Collins 1996). High blood and dialysate flow rates are necessary to achieve optimal performance of high-efficiency dialyzers. Bicarbonate-containing dialysate is necessary to prevent symptoms associated with acetate intolerance (i.e., nausea, vomiting, headache, and hypotension), worsening of metabolic acidosis, and cardiac arrhythmia. Table 8.3 provides a comparison of the various characteristics of conventional, high-efficiency and high-flux dialysis.

Table 8.3 Comparison of the various characteristics of conventional, high-efficiency and high-flux dialysis (Ambalavanan et al. 1999).

Characteristics	Conventional Efficiency	High Efficiency	High Flux
K_oA	500-600 mL/min	> 600 mL/min	> 600 mL/min
Urea Clearance	< 210 mL/min	> 210 mL/min	210 mL/min
K_{UF}	< 20 mL/h/mmHg	Variable	> 20 mL/h/mmHg
β_2-microglobulin Clearance	< 10 mL/min	Variable	> 20 mL/min

High flux dialysis on the other hand is characterized by a high ultrafiltration coefficient (K_{UF} > 20 mL/h/mm Hg). Because of the high ultrafiltration coefficients of high-flux membranes, high-flux dialysis requires an automated ultrafiltration control system to avoid accidental profound intravascular volume depletion. Because high-flux membranes tend to have larger pores, clearance of middle molecular weight molecules is usually high. Urea clearance can be high or low, depending on the urea K_oA of the dialyzer (Ambalavanan et al. 1999). The high flux membranes are semisynthetic or synthetic thermoplastics that permit some passage of molecules exceeding 10,000 daltons or more. In addition, significant adsorption of protein and peptides from the blood onto the membrane may occur with these membranes. When the high-flux membrane is chemically modified such that the hydraulic permeability and the permeability to high-molecular-weight substances is reduced, a high-efficiency membrane is created. Another important aspect of high flux dialysis is that higher blood and dialysate flows are used. With conventional dialysis, increasing the rate of blood flow (for example above 300 mL/min) minimally increases the amount of dialysis. In contrast, with high flux dialyzers, when blood flow is increased up to 450 mL/min, significant improvements in dialysis efficiency can be obtained. Similarly, increasing the rate of dialysate flow allows faster removal of the toxins that are being cleared. Thus, with respect to these low-molecular-weight substances high-flux and high efficiency dialyzers have similar performance characteristics. They differ in their respective clearance rates of high-molecular substances.

8.3.2 Benefits of High-Efficiency and High Flux Dialysis

Potential benefits of high efficiency and high flux dialysis are summarized in Table 8.4. Limited controlled clinical studies demonstrated that synthetic high-flux dialyzers were associated with improvements in neutrophil functions and plasma lipolytic activities, compared with low-flux cellulosic membranes (Cheung et al. 2003). In addition, in observational studies, high-flux dialyzers were associated with lower rates of amyloidosis (Ayli et al. 2005) and death (Woods and Nandakumar 2000), compared with low-flux dialyzers. Since high flux dialysis is so much more efficient, it can allow significant reduction of dialysis times, often by 25 percent. Thus, the patient receives adequate dialysis, but minimizes the discomfort of long dialysis times. However, it is important to note that adequacy of dialysis must be maintained. Some patients may not be able to greatly shorten dialysis times when switching from conventional to high flux dialysis. Because treatment dose is affected by the combination of dialyzer clearance and time spent on the treatment modality, strict adherence to the recommended guidelines for urea clearance is essential for short hemodialysis to be safe and effective.

Table 8.4 Benefits of High-Efficiency and High Flux Dialysis

► Higher clearance of small solutes, such as urea, compared with conventional dialysis without increase in treatment time
► Reduced morbidity and hospital admissions
► Potentially higher patient survival rates
► Reduced complement activation
► Decreased inflammation
► Decreased protein catabolism
► Reduced hypersensitivity reactions to dialyzer
► Improved neutrophil and lymphocyte function
► Reduced infection
► Improved nutritional status
► Improve neuropathy

Specifically, any reduction in treatment time must be counterbalanced by a proportionate increase in the dialyzer clearance of low molecular weight substances to prevent underdelivery of dialysis. To achieve this, blood-flow rates should be maintained at 350 to 450 mL/min to optimize dialyzer performance. In addition, up to 10% more clearance can be obtained by increasing dialysate flow from 500 to 800 mL/min (Azar 2009).

Another requirement for successful short hemodialysis is sufficient removal of interdialytic weight gain (IDWG) without causing cardiovascular instability or patient discomfort. Rapid ultrafiltration rates (UFRs) can be associated with hypotension and hemodynamic instability, especially if the UFR exceeds the rate of vascular refilling. A Dialysis Outcomes and Practice Patterns (DOPP) study analysis showed that UFRs of greater than 10 mL/hr/kg were associated with a 9% increased mortality risk (Collins and Keshaviah 1995). Patients at particular risk for hemodynamic complications include those with underlying cardiac disease—namely, cardiac ischemia, arrhythmias, systolic or diastolic dysfunction—as well as those with autonomic dysfunction and persistent excessive IDWG. Therefore, educating patients about intradialytic weight gain is essential when utilizing short hemodialysis. Short hemodialysis is attractive because it offers the potential for reduced labor costs as well as patient and staff convenience. However, the same requirements for adequacy must apply to these shortened treatments as with conventional hemodialysis: to ensure effective solute removal and volume control without compromising patient well-being. At present, most studies evaluating the adverse effects of shortened dialysis time on morbidity and mortality are limited by confounding issues such as delivery of inadequate dialysis; inconsistencies among membrane characteristics with regard to efficiency, flux, and biocompatibility, as well as lack of long-term follow-up. Data in support of extended dialysis sessions are accumulating and suggest that these modalities may offer significant advantages over conventional therapies.

8.3.3 Limitations of High-Efficiency and High Flux Dialysis

Removal of a large volume of fluid over a short time period (2–2.5 h) increases the likelihood of hypotension, especially in patients with poor cardiac function or autonomic neuropathy. The loss of a fixed amount of treatment time has a proportionally greater impact during a short treatment time than during a long treatment time. Thus, the margin of safety is narrower if a short treatment time is used in conjunction with high-efficiency dialysis compared with conventional hemodialysis with a longer treatment time. Although unproved, high blood flow rates may predispose patients to vascular access damage. Rapid solute shifts potentially precipitate the dialysis disequilibrium syndrome in those patients with a very high blood urea nitrogen concentration, especially during the first treatment ((Ambalavanan et al. 1999). On the other hand, the major possible disadvantage of high flux dialysis regards pyrogen reactions (Cheung et al. 2003; Lonnemann et al. 2001). These reactions, characterized by high temperatures in patients during dialysis treatments, are caused by small pieces of dead bacteria that can be found in the dialysate. Although these reactions are not dangerous, they are uncomfortable for patients, and typically require short hospitalizations for observation. Some nephrologists feel that because high flux dialyzers have larger pores, the bacterial particles can pass more easily into the patient's bloodstream, and that patients on high flux dialysis have more frequent pyrogen reactions.

8.4 CONCLUSION

Small molecules are solely removed by diffusion while middle molecules are mainly dragged by the ultrafiltration flow (convection). Furthermore, each membrane is characterized by different contributions of diffusion and convection to the overall solute removal. As a consequence, some membranes will be found more appropriate for the removal of a specific solute than others. It is the clinician's challenge to find the optimal dialyzer for each patient individually. In general, the performance of a dialyzer depends on different aspects, which can be summarized as follows: first, the proficiency to remove urea and other small molecules that are normally eliminated by the native kidneys; second, the ultrafiltration flux for water removal, determined by the transmembrane pressure and the ultrafiltration coefficient of the membrane; third, the corresponding removal of the middle molecules expelled with the filtration fluid, and fourth, the ability to retain important proteins, such as albumin, and other large molecules. There are several reasons to use high-efficiency and high-flux dialyzers. Each of these dialyzer types has a low molecular- weight solute clearance rate far greater than that of conventional dialyzers. They are useful in large patients with high urea volumes to ensure delivery of an adequate level of therapy. In addition, the high-flux dialyzers also clear higher-molecular weight substances—including substances proven to produce toxicity [such as β_2-microglobulin (MW 11,800 daltons). The surfaces of these membranes are more biocompatible, and cause less activation of complement and less neutropenia and immune cell dysfunction during dialysis. Several studies have suggested that biocompatible membranes have a favorable impact on morbidity and mortality of hemodialysis patients. However, the primary motivation behind the use of the efficient dialyzers is often the facilitation of shorter dialysis times. Patients are not required to make any changes from their point of view in using high flux dialysis. Typically, they actually feel better, especially in terms of having less post-dialysis fatigue. High flux dialysis requires only minor technical adjustments in the dialyzing system, and will continue to be adopted by more and more dialysis centers.

REFERENCES

Akizawa, T., Kinugasa, E., Ideura, T.: Classification of dialysismembranes by performance. Contrib. Nephrol. 113, 25–31 (1995)

Ambalavanan, S., Rabetoy, G., Cheung, A.: High efficiency and high flux hemodialysis. In: Schrier, R.W. (ed.) Atlas of Diseases of the Kidney. Current Medicine, vol. 5, pp. 3.1–3.10, Philadelphia (1999)

Ayli, M., Ayli, D., Azak, A., et al.: The effect of high-flux hemodialysis on dialysis-associated amyloidosis. Ren. Fail. 27(1), 31–34 (2005)

Azar, A.T.: Increasing Dialysate Flow Rate Increases Dialyzer Urea Clearance and Dialysis Efficiency: An In Vivo Study, Saudi J Kidney Dis. Transplant. 20(6), 1023-1029 (2009)

Bagnasco, S.M.: The erythrocyte urea transporter UT-B. J. Membr. Biol. 212(2), 133–138 (2006)

Bhimani, J.P., Ouseph, R., Ward, R.A.: Effect of increasing dialysate flow rate on diffusive mass transfer of urea, phosphate and beta2-microglobulin during clinical haemodialysis. Nephrol. Dial. Transplant. 25(12), 3990–3995 (2010)

Collins, A.J., Keshaviah, P.: High-efficiency, high flux therapies in clinical dialysis. In: Nissenson, A.R. (ed.) Clinical Dialysis, 3rd edn., pp. 848–863 (1995)

Collins, A.J.: High-flux, high-efficiency procedures. In: Henrich, W. (ed.) Principles and Practice of Hemodialysis, pp. 76–88. Appleton & Large, Norwalk (1996)

Choong, L., Leypoldt, J.K., Cheung, A.: Dialyzer mass transfer-area coefficients during clinical hemodialysis are dependent on both blood flow and dialysate flow rates (abstract). J. Am. Soc. Nephrol. 10, 189A (1999)

Cheung, A.K., Levin, N.W., Greene, T., et al.: Effects of high-flux hemodialysis on clinical outcomes: results of the HEMO study. J. Am. Soc. Nephrol. 14(12), 3251–3263 (2003)

Cheung, A.K., Leypoldt, J.K.: The hemodialysis membranes: a historical perspective, current state and future prospect. Semin. Nephrol. 17(3), 196–213 (1997)

Clark, W.R., Hamburger, R.H., Lysaght, M.J.: Effect of membrane composition and structure on solute removal and biocompatibility in hemodialysis. Kidney Int. 56(6), 2005–2015 (1999)

Clark, W.R., Shinaberger, J.H.: Effect of Dialysateside Mass Transfer Resistance on Small Solute Removal in Hemodialysis. Blood Purif. 18(4), 260–263 (2000)

Curtis, J.: Splitting fibers: understanding how dialyzer differences can impact adequacy. Nephrol. News Issues 5(6), 36–39 (2001)

Daniels, I.D., Berlyne, G.M., Barth, R.H.: Blood flow rate and access recirculation in hemodialysis. Int. J. Artif. Organs 15(8), 470–474 (1992)

Daugirdas, J.T., Blake, P.G., Ing, T.S.: Handbook of Dialysis, 4th edn. Lippincott, Williams and Wilkins, Philadelphia (2007)

Daugirdas, J.T., Depner, T.A.: A nomogram approach to hemodialysis urea modeling. Am. J. Kidney Dis. 23(1), 33–40 (1994)

Depner, T.A., Greene, T., Daugirdas, J.T., et al.: Dialyzer performance in the HEMO study: in vivo KoA and true blood flow determined from a model of cross-dialyzer urea extraction. ASAIO J. 50(1), 85–93 (2004)

Gotch, F.A., Panlilio, F., Sergeyeva, O., et al.: Effective diffusion volume flow rates (Qe) for urea, creatinine, and inorganic phosphorous (Qeu, Qecr, QeiP) during hemodialysis. Semin. Dial. 16(6), 474–476 (2003)

Granger, A., Vantard, G., Vantelon, J., Perrone, B.: A mathematical approach of simultaneous dialysis and filtration (SDF). In: Proc. Eur. Soc. Artif. Organs, vol. 5, pp. 174–177 (1978)

Hauk, M., Kuhlmann, M.K., Riegel, W., et al.: In vivo effects of dialys-ate flow rate on Kt/V in maintenance hemodialysis patients. Am. J. Kidney Dis. 35(1), 105–111 (2000)

Hamilton, R.W.: Principles of Dialysis: Diffusion, Convection, and Dialysis Machines. In: Schrier, R.W. (ed.) Atlas of Diseases of the Kidney. Current Medicine, vol. 5, pp. 1.1–1.6. Blackwell Science, Philadelphia (1998)

Henderson, L.W.: Biophysics of Ultrafiltration and Hemofiltration in Replacement of renal function by dialysis. In: Jacobs, C., Kjellstrand, C.M., Koch, K.M., Winchester, J.F. (eds.), pp. 114–145. Kluwer Aca-demic Publisher (1996)

Hoenich, N.A., Ronco, C.: Selecting a Dialyzer: Technical and Clinical Considerations. In: Nissenson, A.R., Fine, R.N. (eds.) Handbook of Dialysis Therapy, 4th edn., pp. 263–278. Hanley &Belfus, Inc., Philadelphia (2008)

Jaffrin, M.Y.: Convective mass transfer in hemodialysis. Artif. Organs 19(11), 1162–1171 (1995)

Keshaviah, P., Luehmann, D., Ilstrup, K., Collins, A.: Technical requirements for rapid high efficiency therapies. Artif. Organs 10(3), 189–194 (1986)

Khandpur, R.S.: Handbook of Biomedical Instrumentation, 2nd edn. McGraw-Hill Professional (2003)

Klinkmann, H., Vienken, J.: Membranes for dialysis. Nephrol. Dial. Transplant. 10(suppl. 3), 39–45 (1995)

Klinkmann, H., Ebbinghausen, H., Uhlenbusch, I., Vienken, J.: High flux dialysis, dialysate quality and backtransport. In: Bonomini, V. (ed.) Evolution in Dialysis Adequacy. Contr. Nephrol., vol. 103, pp. 89–97 (1993)

Korwer, U., Schorn, E.B., Grassmann, A., Vienken, J.: Understanding Membranes and Dialyzers. PABST Science Publishers (2004)

Leypoldt, J.K., Cheung, A.K., Chirananthavat, T., et al.: Hollow fiber shape alters solute clearances in high flux hemodialyzers. ASAIO J. 49(1), 81–87 (2003)

Leypoldt, J.K.: Solute fluxes in different treatment modalities. Nephrol. Dial. Transplant. 15(suppl. 1), 3–9 (2000)

Leypoldt, J.K., Cheung, A.: Effect of low dialysate flow rates on hemodialyzer mass transfer area coefficients for urea and creatinine. Home HD Int. 3, 51–54 (1999)

Leypoldt, J.K., Cheung, A.K., Agodoa, L.Y., et al.: Hemodialyzer mass transfer-area coefficients for urea increase at high dialysate flow rates. Kidney Int. 51(6), 2013–2017 (1997)

Leypoldt, J.K.: Effect of Increasing Dialysate Flow Rate on KoA and Dialyzer Urea Clearance. Semin. Dial. 11(3), 195–196 (1998)

Lim, V.S., Flanigan, M.J., Fangman, J.: Effect of hematocrit on solute removal during high efficiency hemodialysis. Kidney Int. 37(6), 1557–1559 (1990)

Locatelli, F., Valderrabano, F., Hoenich, N., et al.: Progress in dialysis technology: membrane selection and patient outcome. Nephrol. Dial. Transplant. 15(8), 1133–1139 (2000)

Lonnemann, G., Sereni, L., Lemke, H.D., Tetta, C.: Pyrogen retention by highly permeable synthetic membranes during in vitro dialysis. Artif. Organs 25(12), 951–960 (2001)

MacLeod, A., Daly, C., Khan, I., et al.: Comparison of cellulose, modi-fied cellulose and synthetic membranes in the haemodialysis of patients with end-stage renal disease. Cochrane Database Syst. Rev. 3:CD003234 (2001)

Mandolfo, S., Malberti, F., Imbasciati, E., Cogliati, P., Gauly, A.: Impact of blood and dialysate flow and surface on performance of new polysulfone hemodialysis dialyzers. Int. J. Artif. Organs 26(2), 113–120 (2003)

Michaels, A.S.: Operating parameters and performance criteria for hemodialyzers and other membrane-separation devices. Trans. Am. Soc. Artif. Intern. Organs 12, 387–392 (1966)

Ofsthun, N.J., Zydney, A.L.: Importance of convection in artificial kid-ney treatment. In: Maeda, K., Shinzato, T. (eds.) Effective Hemodiafiltration: New Methods, pp. 54–70. Karger Publisher, Basel (1994)

Ofsthun, N.J., Leypoldt, J.K.: Ultrafiltration and backfiltration during hemodialysis. Artif. Organs 19(11), 1143–1161 (1995)

Okada, M., Takesawa, S., Watanabe, T., et al.: Effects of zeta potential on the permeability of dialysis membranes to inorganic phosphate. ASAIO Trans. 35(3), 320–322 (1989)

Ouseph, R., Ward, R.A.: Increasing dialysate flow rate increases dialyzer urea mass transfer-area coefficients during clinical use. Am. J. Kidney Dis. 37(2), 316–320 (2001)

Palmer, B.F.: The Dialysis Prescription and Urea Modeling. In: Schrier, R.W. (ed.) Atlas of Diseases of the Kidney, Current Medicine, vol. 5, pp. 6.1–6.8. Blackwell Science, Philadelphia (1998)

Ronco, C., Brendolan, A., Crepaldi, C., et al.: Blood and dialysate flow distributions in hollow fiber hemodialyzers analyzed by computerized helical scanning technique. J. Am. Soc. Nephrol. 13, S53–S61 (2002)

Ronco, C., Ghezzi, P.M., Metry, G., et al.: Effects of hematocrit and blood flow distribution on solute clearance in hollow fiber hemodialyzers. Nephron 89(3), 243–250 (2001)

Ronco, C., Heifetz, A., Fox, K., et al.: Beta 2-microglobulin removal by synthetic dialysis membranes. Mechanisms and kinetics of the molecule. Int. J. Artif. Organs 20, 136–143 (1997)

Ronco, C.: Backfiltration in clinical dialysis: nature of the phenomenon, mechanisms and possible solutions. Int. J. Artif. Organs 13, 11–21 (1990)

Sargent, J.A., Gotch, F.A.: Principles and biophysics of dialysis in Replacement of renal function by dialysis. In: Jacob, C., Kjellstrand, C.M., Koch, K.M., Winchester, J.F. (eds.), 4th edn., pp. 188–230. Kluwer Academic Publiher, Dordrecht (1996)

Waniewski, J., Werynski, A., Ahrenholz, P., et al.: Theoretical basis and experimental verification of the impact of ultrafiltration on dialyzer clearance. Artif. Organs 15(2), 70–77 (1991)

Werynski, A.: Evaluation of the impact of ultrafiltration on dialyzer clearance. Artif. Organs 3(2), 140–142 (1979)

Woods, H.F., Nandakumar, M.: Improved outcome for haemodialysis patients treated with high-flux membranes. Nephrol. Dial. Transplant. 15, 36–42 (2000)

Yamamoto, K., Matsukawa, H., Yakushiji, T., et al.: Technical evaluation of dialysate flow in a newly designed dialyzer. ASAIO J. 53(1), 36–40, 14 (2007)

Yamamoto, K., Matsuda, M., Hirano, A., et al.: Computational evaluation of dialysis fluid flow in dialyzers with variously designed jackets. Artif. Organs 33(6), 481–486 (2009)

Zucchelli, P., Santoro, A.: Inorganic phosphate removal during different dialytic procedures. Int. J. Artif. Organs 10(3), 173–178 (1987)

ESSAY QUESTIONS

1. Define Transmembrane pressure (TMP) and Ultrafiltration coefficient (Kuf).
2. List the main classifications of dialyzers according to water flux
3. What are the main classifications of dialyzer efficiency?
4. Differentiate between backdiffusion and backfiltration
5. Define the mass transfer urea coefficient (K_oA) and the Priming Volume of dialyzer
6. List the three primary methods of dialyzer sterilization
7. What are the main factors affecting solute clearance on hemodialysis?
8. Define the sieving coefficient of a dialyzer
9. Compare between the various characteristics of conventional, high-efficiency and high-flux dialysis
10. List the main benefits of High-Efficiency and High Flux Dialysis

MULTIPLE CHOICE QUESTIONS

Choose the best answer

1. Molecules of molecular weight 1355 Da are termed…
   A. Small molecules
   B. Middle molecules
   C. Large molecules

2. The diffusion rate of solutes is … to the square root of the solute molecular weight.
   A. Inversely proportional
   B. Directly proportional

3. For most dialyzers, in vivo clearance is … less than in vitro clearance.
   A. 20-40 %
   B. 50-60 %
   C. 30-40 %
   D. 5-25%

4. The relationship between TMP and ultrafiltration rate is … at relatively low TMPs
   A. Non-linear
   B. Linear

5. If the K_{Uf} is 2.0, the permeability to water is …
   A. High
   B. Moderate
   C. Low

6. Dialyzers with a K_{Uf} greater than 6.0 (certainly those with a K_{Uf} greater than 8.0) should be used only with dialysis machines that contain special pumps and circuits that directly control the …
   A. Transmembrane Pressure
   B. Ultrafiltration Rate
   C. Dialysate Flow rate
   D. Blood flow rate

7. High-flux dialyzers have K_{Uf} ranging between … mL/mmHg/hour.
   A. 5-10
   B. 10-20
   C. 20-40
   D. 20-60

8. The efficiency of solute clearance is measured by the…
   A. K_oA
   B. BFR
   C. DFR
   D. TMP

9. Dialyzers with K_oA values less than 500 are generally used only for …
   A. High-Efficiency
   B. Medium-Efficiency
   C. Low-Efficiency

10. At zero ultrafiltration the flow rates at the dialyzer blood inlet (Q_{Bin}) and outlet (Q_{Bout}) are …
   A. Equal
   B. Non-equal

11. If the flow rates at the dialyzer blood inlet $Q_{Bin} = 300$ mL/min; ulrafiltration rate $Q_{uf} = 20$ mL/min and the dialyzer clearance $K = 210$ mL/min, then the flow rates at the dialyzer blood outlet Q_{Bout} is…

   A. 300 mL/min
   B. 280 mL/min
   C. 320 mL/min
   D. 210 mL/min

12. Increasing dialysate flow rate increases clearance, but the increases in clearance are more substantial at…
 A. Lower blood flow rates
 B. Moderate blood flow rates
 C. Higher blood flow rates

13. Approximately … of plasma is water
 A. 95%
 B. 75%
 C. 85%
 D. 93%

14. Approximately … of an erythrocyte is water.
 A. 75%
 B. 72%
 C. 90%
 D. 93%

15. The increase in hematocrit results in an … in the viscosity of blood
 A. Increase
 B. Decrease

16. The sieving coefficient remains near … for substances up to 1 kilodalton but is lower for larger molecular weight substances.
 A. 2.0
 B. 0.5
 C. 0.7
 D. 1.0

17. A Dialysis Outcomes and Practice Patterns (DOPP) study analysis showed that UFRs of greater than 10 mL/hr/kg were associated with a … increased mortality risk.
 A. 15%
 B. 12%
 C. 9%
 D. 5%

18. Removal of a large volume of fluid over a short time period (2–2.5 h) increases the likelihood of…
 A. Hypertension
 B. Hypotension
 C. Hemolysis
 D. Anemia

19. If the blood flow rate is 300 mL/min, the dialysate flow rate is 500 ml/min and the in vitro dialyzer clearance is 210 mL/min., then the dialyzer efficiency K_oA is…

    A. 494 ml/min

    B. 500 ml/min

    C. 450 ml/min

    D. 485 ml/min

20. If the blood flow rate Q_B is 250 mL/min at the hematocrit value of 30%, the whole blood water flow is…

    A. 210 ml/min

    B. 220 ml/min

    C. 217 ml/min

    D. 225 ml/min

Chapter (9)
Dialyzer Structure and Membrane Biocompatibility

Orfeas Liangos, MD, FACP, FASN; Bertrand L. Jaber, MD, MS, FASN

CHAPTER OUTLINES

- Introduction
- Overview of Dialyzer Structure
- Materials Used for Artificial Kidney Membranes
- Key Features of Biocompatibility
- Clinical Implications of Dialysis Membrane Biocompatibility
- Conclusion

CHAPTER OBJECTIVES

- Provide an overview of basic artificial kidney configurations
- Describe dialyzer membrane materials
- Discuss biocompatibility of specific materials and their potential clinical importance

KEY TERMS

- Hollow fiber dialyzers
- Substituted/unsubstituted cellulose dialyzer membranes
- Synthetic dialyzer membranes
- Biocompatibility
- Complement activation
- Coagulation
- Inflammation

ABSTRACT

The objectives of this chapter are to provide an overview of the dialyzer structure with emphasis on advances in dialyzer performance and novel design features. This is followed by an in-depth review of the various biomaterials used for dialyzer membranes, namely unsubstituted cellulose, substituted or modified cellulose and synthetic polymers, with a discussion of their physical, chemical and biological properties. Key features of biocompatibility of dialyzer membranes including activation of the complement system and coagulation cascade, and activation of platelets and leukocytes are then discussed. Emphasis is given to the clinical relevance of dialysis membrane biocompatibility and specific syndromes are highlighted including hemodialysis-induced hypoxemia, dialyzer reactions, β_2-microglobulin deposition, protein catabolism, susceptibility to infection due to immune dysfunction, and survival of patients with kidney failure.

A.T. Azar (Ed.): Modelling and Control of Dialysis Systems, SCI 404, pp.427–480.
springerlink.com © Springer-Verlag Berlin Heidelberg 2013

9.1 INTRODUCTION

Performing a hemodialysis treatment requires the use of an extracorporeal blood circuit. The latter consists of a dialyzer cartridge, bloodlines and a vascular access. While traveling through the circuit, blood comes into contact with a host of substances that originate from the dialysis membrane, including sterilant residue from the manufacturing process, substances that leach from the dialyzer, germicide and cleansing agent residue in case that reprocessing techniques were used, as well as potential contaminants present in the dialysate. Exposure of blood to each of the above components can result in pathophysiological perturbations in the patient. Following a brief overview of dialyzer structure, this chapter focuses on dialyzer membranes and biocompatibility properties. Although to date, no precise, uniformly agreed-upon definition of the term "biocompatibility" exists, there is general consensus that a biocompatible dialysis membrane can be defined as one that elicits little or no pathophysiological reaction as the result of blood contact with the biomaterial. Reactions resulting from fluid or electrolyte shifts during dialysis are not within the scope of this discussion. Therefore, this chapter restricts its focus on alterations of cellular and non-cellular blood components induced by the blood-membrane interaction during hemodialysis. A graphical sketch summarizing the blood-membrane interaction is shown in Fig. 9.1 and will be discussed in further detail in this chapter.

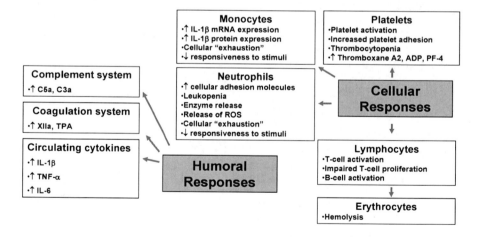

Fig. 9.1 Biological responses elicited by blood-dialysis membrane interactions. Overview of pathophysiological responses of blood components as a result of contact with the dialyzer membrane. Humoral responses referring to complement, coagulation and circulating cytokines are outlined on the left, whereas cellular responses referring to the various cell lines in peripheral blood are shown on the right side of the figure.

9.2 OVERVIEW OF DIALYZER STRUCTURE

In the past several years the hollow-fiber or capillary dialyzer design has all but replaced other dialyzer configurations, such as the parallel plate dialyzer, and is now considered to be the preferred artificial kidney configuration. Its basic design consists of a tightly packed bundle of hollow fibers, that carry blood in their lumens, and that are formed of membranes rendered semi-permeable through a design containing a large number of microscopic pores of a defined size. Each end of the fiber bundle is embedded into small chambers at the outer ends of the dialyzer, from which ports originate in an axial orientation and allow for connection with the bloodlines of the extracorporeal circuitry. The fiber bundle itself is contained in a cylindrical shell at the two ends of which ports originate, oriented at a 90-degree angle from the fiber bundle, and through which the dialysate is typically guided in counter-current fashion to the direction of the blood flow.

Although not much change has occurred to this basic design in recent years, minor modifications in the shape of the hollow fibers, dialysate compartment or blood collection chamber at the ends of the dialyzer can cause significant improvements in blood and dialysate distribution and/or internal filtration and thus improve dialyzer performance. Non-homogenous distribution of blood and dialysate flow within the cross-section of the fiber bundle can be alleviated by using various fiber design features. Examples of these are the Moiré or undulating fiber structure, externally irregular fiber surfaces, nonparallel orientation of the fibers or use of spacer yarns between the fibers. Such designs prevent contact or excess packing between adjacent fibers and thus allow for better matching of blood and dialysate flow across all sections of the fiber bundle (Ronco et al. 2002b; Ronco et al. 2006).

Other important design features influencing dialyzer performance are dialyzer jacket taper, i.e. smaller internal diameter of the dialyzer jacket in the center than at the ends, and a circumferential baffle surrounding the dialysate inlet, allowing for more uniform dialysate fluid flow in-between the hollow-fiber bundle. In this case, a specifically short jacket taper length of approximately 50 mm might provide best dialysate and blood contact and least degree of channeling (Fukuda et al. 2006). Such design features of the dialyzer jacket structure may optimize dialysis fluid flow and increase dialyzer performance (Fukuda et al. 2006; Yamamoto et al. 2009).

A short jacket taper design may also optimize internal filtration effects within the dialyzer and thereby the convective removal of solutes (Fujimura et al. 2004). Similar enhancement of internal filtration rates can be achieved through placement of an O-ring around the fiber bundle in the middle section of the dialyzer jacket (Ronco et al. 1998). Internal filtration is thought to result from filtration and backfiltration phenomena between the blood and dialysate side during flow along the fiber bundle, and can enhance the removal of middle-to-high molecular weight solutes (Ronco et al. 1998). This enhancement can also be achieved through a more dense fiber packing and narrower lumens of the individual fibers, which increase the resistance against blood and dialysate flow through the dialyzer (Ronco et al. 2002a). Finally, the membrane ultra-structure and its ability to trap molecules may be an important determinant of middle and large molecular weight solute removal, going beyond chemical composition or pore size of the membrane (Ouseph et al. 2008). Thus, there might be differences in the performance of otherwise seemingly comparable dialyzers, when based on pore size, surface area and biomaterial used. In summary, despite the lack of major changes in the basic configuration of dialyzers in recent years, improvements in certain details of dialyzer design have had a tangible positive impact on their performance as assessed by their clearance of uremic solutes across various molecular weights.

9.3 MATERIALS USED FOR ARTIFICIAL KIDNEY MEMBRANES

Dialyzer membrane materials can be classified into three groups: Unsubstituted cellulose, substituted (modified) cellulose, and synthetic (Lyman 1983; Macleod et al. 2005) (see Table 9.1).

Table 9.1 Common commercially available dialyzers in the U.S.

Biomaterial	Chemical structure	Common name
Cellulose		Cuprophan
DEAE-substitued cellulose		Hemophan
Cellulose diacetate and triacetate		CA, CTA
Multi-layer vitamin E-coated cellulose		Excebrane
Polysulfone		F-series Optiflux-series
Polyamide		Polyflux-series
Polyacrylonitrile and methallyl sulfonate		AN-69
Polyacrylonitrile and methacrylate		PAN
Polymethylmethacrylate		PMMA

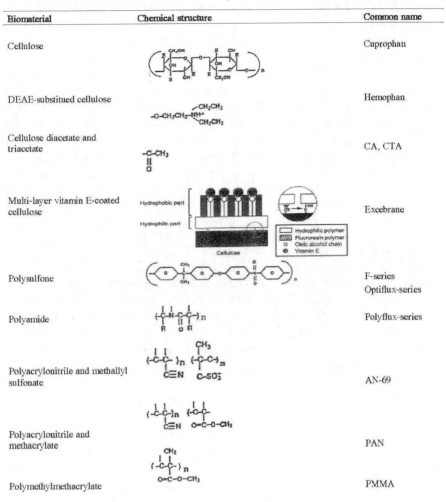

Reproduced from Jaber BL, Pereira BJG (2005) Biocompatibility of Hemodialysis Membranes. In: Pereira BJG, Sayegh MH, Blake P (eds) Chronic Kidney Disease, Dialysis, & Transplantation. Companion to Brenner & Rector's the Kidney, 2nd edn. Elsevier Saunders, Philadelphia, (Jaber B and Pereira B 2005) with permission.

9.3.1 Unsubstituted Cellulose

Cellulose membranes are composed of regenerated cellulose chemically consisting of linear chains of glucose rings with free surface hydroxyl groups. The first hemodialysis membranes used clinically were tubes of cellophane, originally manufactured to serve as sausage casings. Unfortunately, these cellophane tubings were prone to rupture and leakage, requiring continuous supervision and immediate repair if needed. Virtually all hemodialysis membranes used until the late 1960s were made from cellophane or similar materials. Following this era, Cuprophan (CU) membranes were developed by a modification of the process used for preparing cellophane, the cuprammonium process. Since then, cuprammonium membranes have been widely used for hemodialysis due to their mechanical strength, minimal thickness and good diffusive transport properties for small solutes. It is of importance to note that the name Cuprophan itself is trade-marked to a specific manufacturer and that several other cuprammonium membranes have been manufactured by various other companies and are not all identical. Cuprammonium or other regenerated cellulose membranes are still widely used in many countries throughout the world due to their low cost (Lysaght 1995). In the U.S. however, these membranes have been largely replaced in favor of substituted cellulose and synthetic membranes (USRDS 2004).

Due to the large number of free hydroxyl groups on the cellulose monomer, regenerated cellulose membranes are highly hydrophilic. In addition, porosity is relatively uniform throughout the thickness of the membrane. While early cuprammonium membranes had low permeability to solutes larger than urea, cuprammonium membranes with higher permeability to larger solutes have later become available.

9.3.2 Substituted (Modified) Cellulose

Substituted or modified cellulose membranes result from the substitution of the free hydroxyl groups on the surface of cellulose membranes. When using acetyl residues to substitute the free surface hydroxyl groups on a cellulose membrane, cellulose acetate (CA), also known as diacetate (80% substitution), or cellulose triacetate (CTA) (90% substitution) membranes are formed, according to the increasing fraction of substituted hydroxyl moieties, respectively. CA and CTA membranes are more hydrophobic than regenerated cellulose membranes because of acetylation of the hydroxyl moieties on the cellulose monomer. Use of the tertiary amino residue diethylaminoethyl (DEAE) to substitute 1% of the hydroxyl moieties in cellulose is the basis for the Hemophan membrane (Falkenhagen et al. 1987; Henne et al. 1979; Spencer et al. 1985). All of the above modified cellulose membranes are morphologically homogeneous under scanning electron microscopy. In general, substituted or modified cellulose membranes have a substantially lower complement activating potential if compared with unsubstituted cellulose. It remains unsettled, however, if the reduction in free hydroxyl groups is causal to the observed lower degree of complement activation by substituted cellulose membranes (see below). Further modification of the cellulose molecule by covalent binding of synthetic block polymers to the hydroxyl groups on cellulose has created a new type of membrane, the Excebrane, in which oleyl alcohol and vitamin E moieties incorporated into the synthetic surface are claimed to reduce thrombosis and provide anti-oxidant effects (Galli et al. 1999, 1998). Use of Excebrane membranes has been associated with lower levels of proinflammatory cytokine interleukin-6 (IL-6), and decreased activation of mononuclear cells (Girndt et al. 2000; Pertosa et al. 2002). In a meta-analysis, conversion to Excebrane dialyzers was associated with improvement in circulating biomarkers of lipid peroxidation (Sosa et al. 2006). However, the clinical significance of these findings remains unclear.

9.3.3 Synthetic (Non-cellulose) Polymers

Various synthetic membranes were developed during the 1970s primarily for use in hemofiltration, although many are now used for hemodialysis. The AN69^{TM} membrane consists of a copolymer of acrylonitrile and methallyl sulfonate, which contains negatively charged ionizable groups, and has a morphologically homogeneous architecture (Konstantin 1993). Such properties, although originally considered desirable because they parallel those of the negatively charged glomerular basement membrane (Anderson et al. 1991), may actually result in certain bioincompatible characteristics of this particular biomaterial. The synthetic polymers polysulfone (PS) and polyamide (PA) are also used to manufacture hemodialysis membranes and feature a highly asymmetric and hydrophobic microarchitecture. Initially, these materials required an additional supporting layer to reinforce the thin and highly porous surface layer, resulting in relatively low diffusion rates for small solutes. This disadvantage was alleviated by adding polyvinylpyrolidone into the manufacturing process (Göhl et al. 1992; Streicher and Schneider 1985). The microarchiteture of these membranes was asymmetric (Konstantin 1993; Radovich 1995), resembling a sponge- or foam-like structure. PS membranes with various porosities are now commercially available. Other synthetic membranes currently used clinically are polyacrylonitrile (PAN), polymethylmethacrylate (PMMA), polyethersulfone (PES), and polycarbonate (Bonomini and Berland 1995; Hoenich 2007). Except for polycarbonate, the synthetic membranes listed above are hydrophobic and cause adsorption of cells and proteins onto their surfaces. A hydrophilic membrane such as polycarbonate, however, does not cause adsorption (Kjellstrand et al. 1991), but rather activation of cells and proteins. Hydrophobic or hydrophilic membrane properties can be altered and alleviated through changes in the manufacturing process, thereby increasing their biocompatibility (Vienken et al. 1995).

A common feature of synthetic membranes is their relatively large pore size resulting in high ultrafiltration coefficients (K_{UF} > 14 ml/hour/mm Hg) and high clearances for middle molecules (β2 microglobulin clearance > 20 ml/min), also referred to as "high flux". However, high flux and synthetic membranes are not synonymous. For example, cellulose membranes, often termed "conventional" or low-flux because of their relatively smaller pore size and lower β2 microglobulin clearance characteristics, can also be configured to have larger pore sizes. Similarly, low-flux membranes can also be manufactured from synthetic membranes. If small molecular weight clearance such as urea clearance is enhanced by larger surface area in a dialyzer, it is then often referred to as "high efficiency". The efficiency of a dialyzer in removing urea can be described by a constant referred to as mass transfer urea coefficient or KoA. This constant determines the inter-relationship between urea clearance and the blood and dialysate flow rate. High-efficiency dialyzers typically have KoA values that are greater than 600-700 mL/min. Adequate dialyzer prescription by the clinician requires a detailed knowledge of membrane properties, which is complex due to the differences in clearance, flux and biocompatibility characteristics.

9.4 KEY FEATURES OF BIOCOMPATIBILITY

9.4.1 Complement Activation

Complement activation is considered to be an important feature of bio-compatibility. Therefore, membranes are often classified as biocompatible or bioincompatible based on their degree of complement activation. Complement activation can occur via two distinct pathways, the classical or the alternative pathway (Muller-Eberhard 1988). Both pathways will, via activation of C3 and under conducive conditions, lead to activation of the terminal complement components C5, C6, C7, C8 and C9. Complement activation by cellulose membranes occurs primarily through the alternative pathway (Chenoweth et al. 1983a; Cheung et al. 1989; Craddock et al. 1977). Mechanisms leading to complement activation on other membranes are less well understood.

9.4.1.1 Role of Complement Activation Products

Activation of C3 causes generation of the anaphylatoxin C3a (M_r ~9 kDa) (Muller-Eberhard 1988) along with larger fragments such as C3b (M_r

~186 kDa) and its degradation product iC3b. The latter, larger fragments may also modulate cellular functions (Fearon and Wong 1983), for example, iC3b mediates cell adherence (Cheung et al. 1991) and induce the release of proteolytic enzymes (Cheung et al. 1993) by neutrophils. Therefore the degree of complement activation during hemodialysis cannot be assessed only by measuring plasma C3a and C5a, for example, since these smaller markers (C3a and C5a) may be lost into the dialysate, taken up by circulating neutrophils, or be adsorbed onto the dialysis membrane, whereas the larger iC3b fragment may remain in the plasma and exert its biological effects. Anaphylatoxins C3a and C5a are important proinflammatory mediators and as such cause a host of localized and systemic pathobiological responses. Just a few of these are vasospasm, increased vascular permeability (Lepow et al. 1970), mast cell histamine release (Johnson et al. 1975), smooth muscle contraction (Cochrane and Muller-Eberhard 1968), neutrophil degranulation (Showell et al. 1982), and cytokine biosynthesis and release by monocytes. In animal studies, C3a also causes noxious effects on the heart such as tachycardia, left ventricular failure, and coronary vasoconstriction (del Balzo et al. 1985). Complement factor C5a has been shown to induce neutrophil chemotaxis, aggregation (Craddock et al. 1977; Hammerschmidt et al. 1981; Yancey et al. 1985), attachment to endothelial cells, leukotriene release (Camussi et al. 1984; Stimler et al. 1982), oxygen radical formation (Sacks et al. 1978), release of intra-granular enzymes (Goldstein et al., 1973; Hammerschmidt et al. 1981; Wright and Gallin 1979), and altered expression of inflammatory cell surface receptors (Arnaout et al. 1985). C5a has also been shown to release β_2-microglobulin from peripheral blood mononuclear cells (PBMC) (Zaoui et al. 1990). Serum based carboxypeptidase N is involved in the degradation of anaphylatoxins C3a and C5a (Bokisch and Muller-Eberhard 1970) into desarginine derivatives. These degradation products, although considerably less spasmogenic (Bokisch and Muller-Eberhard 1970; Gerard and Hugli, 1981; Hugli 1981), still retain certain leukocyte-directed activities.

9.4.1.2 Hemodialysis Membrane-Associated Complement Activation

Cuprophan and unsubstituted cellulose membranes are considered to be most potent in complement activation (Chenoweth et al. 1983a, b; Falkenhagen et al. 1993). Plasma C3a$_{desArg}$ concentration as a measure of complement activation usually peaks shortly after initiation of the dialysis treatment and declines almost to pretreatment values at the end of dialysis. The increase in plasma C5a$_{desArg}$ and SC5b-9 levels is typically less pronounced than C3a$_{desArg}$ (Bhakdi et al. 1988; Chenoweth et al. 1983a, b; Cheung et al. 1993; Deppisch et al. 1990). Although all dialysis membranes are associated with some degree of complement activation, generally, substituted cellulose membranes such as CA and Hemophan, are associated with lower C3a levels compared with unsubstituted cellulose such as cuprophan (Ivanovich et al. 1983). CTA and synthetic polymer membranes are associated with lower plasma C3a levels than CA (Chenoweth et al. 1983a; Deppisch et al. 1990; Hakim et al. 1984a; Smeby et al. 1986). Reduced temperature of the blood in the dialysis circuit leads to lower complement activation by cuprophan membranes (Maggiore et al. 1987). Complement activation can also be attenuated through magnesium chelation with citrate (MacDougall et al. 1985), or increased heparin dose (Cheung et al. 1994). Formaldehyde or peracetic acid reprocessing of cuprophan membranes also leads to lower complement activation and leukopenia compared with new, unprocessed membranes (Chenoweth et al. 1983b; Dumler et al. 1987; Hakim et al. 1984b), a phenomenon believed to be due to protein coating of the membrane surface (Cheung et al. 1989). If hypochlorite solutions are used in reprocessing of cuprophan dialyzers, presumably due to removal of the protein layer form the membrane surfaces (Cheung et al. 1989), complement activation and leukopenia return again to levels observed with new dialyzers (Dumler et al. 1987). However, since dialyzer reprocessing has declined significantly in clinical practice, these observations are more of historical importance.

9.4.1.3 In Vivo Consequences of Complement Activation

In animal models, findings of leukopenia, hypoxemia, pulmonary hypertension, increase in lung water, cardiac arrhythmias, decreased cardiac output and fluctuations in systemic arterial blood pressure have all been observed following injection of plasma exposed to cuprophan membranes (Cheung et al. 1986; Craddock et al. 1977; Walker et al. 1983). These phenomena are mediated by the anaphylatoxins C3a and C5a, which in turn induce neutrophil aggregation and attachment to pulmonary endothelial cells, resulting in peripheral leukopenia, pulmonary vasoconstriction and pulmonary hypertension. In addition, airway constriction and pulmonary interstitial edema induced by anaphylatoxins and arachidonic acid metabolites may result. Pulmonary leukosequestration or pulmonary hypertension per se does not lead to systemic hypoxemia but other, complement independent mechanisms may also play a role (Lemke et al. 1993; Lemke and Fink 1992; Schulman et al. 1993).

In the clinical context, the effects of intra-dialytic complement activation on patients are less well understood. For example in dialysis-induced peripheral leukopenia, C5a has been incriminated but non-complement factors, such as platelet-activating factors, may also pay a role. Further, anaphylatoxins may be involved in the development of acute pulmonary hypertension during hemodialysis (Schohn et al. 1986). In addition, anaphylatoxins may contribute to allergy-like symptoms during dialysis due to their ability to release histamine from mast cells. Depending on the rate of generation and subsequent inactivation and catabolism, as well as host susceptibility, anaphylatoxins may rarely be the cause of anaphylactoid reactions during dialysis. Other potential putative, subacute and chronic effects of complement activation during hemodialysis, which have been entertained, are neutrophil stimulation leading to the release of oxygen radicals (Sacks et al. 1978) and intra-granular proteases (Cheung et al. 1993; Goldstein et al. 1973; Wright and Gallin 1979) from the cells, which may result in catabolism of plasma proteins and injury of other tissues such as the kidneys and cardiovascular system. C5a has also been shown to promote the production of cytokines from monocytes (Schindler et al. 1990a) and the release of β_2-microglobulins from PBMC (Zaoui et al. 1990), which may contribute to the development of amyloidosis.

9.4.2 Bleeding and Clotting Abnormalities

Blood clotting complications are inherent to every hemodialysis treatment due to the close contact of blood with the membrane. Although clotting complications are usually not severe or even life threatening, they contribute to anemia in end-stage renal disease, reduce the effective surface area for solute transport across the dialyzer, and compromise the potential for dialyzer reuse.

9.4.2.1 Plasma Protein Mediated Coagulation

Plasma proteins are readily adsorbed onto extracorporeal surfaces once in contact with blood. Adhesion of platelets, leukocytes and to a lesser extent erythrocytes typically occurs subsequently (Kim 1987; Marshall et al. 1974). The physicochemical properties of the membrane determine the degree and types of proteins that are adsorbed. For instance, binding of the contact protein Hageman factor (factor XII) is enhanced by negatively charged surfaces, which in turn leads to activation of the intrinsic coagulation pathway (Salzman 1971; Vroman et al. 1971). Although activation of factor XII during hemodialysis could not be demonstrated in clinical studies (Vaziri et al. 1984b), it was demonstrated *in vitro* (Schulman et al. 1993).

The activation of contact proteins (Kozin and Cochrane 1988) facilitates the conversion of high molecular weight kininogen into kinins, for example bradykinin, which is a potent vascular permeability factor, vasodilator, and inflammatory mediator. For example, conversion of kininogen into bradykinin has been well described for the anionic sulfonate domain containing AN69 membrane (Colman et al. 1987; Kozin and Cochrane 1988; Lemke and Fink 1992; Salzman 1971; Vroman et al. 1971). Concomitant use of an angiotensin converting enzyme (ACE) inhibitor allows for the accumulation of bradykinin that is generated as a result of blood contact with the AN69 membrane. This phenomenon is due to the properties of ACE as a kininase, which inactivates bradykinin and is inhibited by use of an ACE inhibitor. Clinically, anaphylactoid reactions have been described during dialysis with the AN69 membrane, especially when ACE inhibitors are used (Colman et al. 1987; Tielemans et al. 1993). While significant activation of the coagulation cascade would lead to thrombosis and obstruction of the extracorporeal circuit, more subtle activation can be detected by increased consumption of fibrinogen or production of the fibrinopeptides A (FPA) and B (FPB), which are fragments cleaved off of fibrinogen during coagulation (Cheung et al. 1994; Gasparotto et al. 1984, Wilhelmson et al. 1981, 1983). Such an increase in plasma FPA levels can be prevented by adequate heparinization (Cheung et al. 1994; Wilhelmson et al. 1981, 1983). FPA, which is normally eliminated by the kidney, accumulates in kidney failure leading to elevated plasma levels in dialysis patients (Lane et al. 1984). Although plasma FPA levels have been used as markers of intra-dialytic clotting, their plasma levels are also affected by removal of these low molecular weight peptides (~1.5 kDa) by most dialysis membranes (Cheung et al. 1994), complicating the interpretation of FPA levels in dialysis.

In addition to coagulation, the fibrinolytic system, which counteracts coagulation under physiological conditions (Colman et al. 1987; Lindsay 1983) is also activated during dialysis through tissue plasminogen activator, which converts plasminogen to plasmin, an important fibrinolytic protein, especially when cellulose membranes are used (Speiser et al. 1987). Concomitantly, the plasma concentration of tissue plasminogen activator inhibitor decreases. Although the pulmonary vasculature has been entertained as a source of plasminogen activator, quasi as a response to injury by activated complement and granulocyte proteases, the stimuli for the release of the plasminogen activator in this setting are unknown.

9.4.2.2 Adhesion and Activation of Platelets

Activation of the coagulation pathways ultimately lead to conversion of prothrombin to thrombin, which in turn activates platelets (Mohammed et al. 1976). It can be assumed that platelets may play a central role in dialyzer thrombosis. Platelet adherence can be modulated by the type of protein primarily adsorbed onto the artificial dialyzer surfaces (Kim 1987). For example, whereas membrane coating with glycoproteins such as fibrinogen and γ-globulin, promotes platelet adhesion, albumin-coated surfaces are relatively resistant to platelet adhesion. After adhering to the surface, the platelets form pseudopods and spread over the foreign surface (Marshall et al. 1974; Sreeharan et al. 1982). In addition, a host of intracellular products including thromboxane A_2 (TXA_2) and adenosine diphosphate (ADP) can be released by the platelets in response to humoral or physical stimuli (Colman et al. 1987; Salzman 1971), and promote coagulation further by activating additional platelets. However, it should be noted that platelets are not the only source of TXA_2, since lung tissue may produce significant amounts of this substance in response to stimulation by the complement anaphylatoxins generated during hemodialysis with cuprophan dialyzers (Cheung et al. 1987). Platelet inhibitors, such as aspirin and dipyridamole can prevent these events (Lindsay et al. 1972; Salter et al. 1984). Prostacyclin (PGI_2), a potent stimulator of adenyl cyclase and inhibitor of platelet aggregation, has also been successfully used as the sole anticoagulant during hemodialysis, underscoring the importance of platelets in dialyzer clotting processes (Caruana et al. 1991; Smith et al. 1982; Zusman et al. 1981).

Activated platelets also release platelet factor 4 (PF4) and β-thromboglobulin (β–TG) (Dawes et al. 1978; Kaplan and Owen 1981; Nath et al. 1973) and their plasma levels can be used as markers of platelet activation. PF4 antagonizes heparin through binding and neutralization. Differences in PF4 release may partially account for the differences in heparin dosing requirements during hemodialysis between patients. However, plasma levels of these markers have to be interpreted with caution, since mechanisms independent of platelet activation may affect their values, for example release of endothelial cell-bound PF4 by administration of heparin during hemodialysis (Kaplan and Owen 1981). β–TG, which is normally eliminated by the kidney accumulates in renal failure, resulting in elevated circulating levels in dialysis patients (Dawes et al. 1978). Additional platelet activation, in that instance, can trigger an acute increase in plasma β–TG levels above the prior baseline. During dialysis, this can be prevented with adequate anticoagulation (Ireland et al. 1984). In addition to thrombin, platelets can be activated by mechanical disruption during hemodialysis (Green et al. 1980), probably caused by certain physicochemical properties of the dialyzer membrane surface and shear stresses during flow of the blood through the dialyzer. Platelet activation can also occur through neutrophil-derived platelet activating factor (PAF) (Camussi et al. 1984, 1978) and lung- or peripheral organ derived TXA_2 in response to complement activation (Cheung et al. 1987).

Platelet activation is not uniform among dialysis membrane types. For example, cuprophan dialyzers have been associated with increased thrombocytopenia compared with PMMA dialyzers (Hakim and Schafer 1985). Cuprophan is also associated with increased plasma β–TG levels when compared to polyacrylonitrile (Adler and Berlyne 1981; Sreeharan et al. 1982). Cuprophan has also been associated with a more profound adhesion and morphologic alteration of platelets when compared to polycarbonate (Sreeharan et al. 1982). Use of hemophan dialyzers has been associated with lower incremental increases in plasma PF4 compared with cuprophan (Spencer et al. 1985). Further, the use of cuprophan or AN-69 dialyzers was found to increase plasma PAF, which may contribute to dialysis-induced leukopenia and thrombocytopenia (Iatrou et al. 1995, 2002).

Finally, dialysis with PS membranes has been found to cause a significant increase in the level of platelet-bound GPIIb/IIIa, the receptor for fibrinogen on platelets that mediates platelet aggregation and adhesion. In comparison, CTA membrane use does not cause such an increase (Kuragano et al. 2003). This underscores that synthetic membranes are not automatically more biocompatible but that each biological response should be studied individually. Mixed platelet and leukocyte aggregates may also form during hemodialysis with both cuprophan and synthetic membranes (Lindsay et al. 1972; Silber and Moldow 1983). It is believed that this may facilitate cross-signaling and enhance the inflammatory response. Adhesion molecules, for example GMP140 on platelets and CD15s on leukocytes, may facilitate binding between these two cell groups during dialysis (Stuard et al. 1995). Various methods have been employed to assess the degree of platelet activation during hemodialysis. These include assessment of the degree of acute thrombocytopenia (Docci et al. 1984; Hakim and Schafer 1985; Sreeharan et al. 1982); electron microscopic evaluation of platelet morphology (Sreeharan et al. 1982); increases in plasma βTG and PF4 concentrations (Adler and Berlyne 1981; Spencer et al. 1985); and increases in plasma TXA_2 concentration (Hakim and Schafer 1985). Limitations of these measurement techniques are discussed above.

9.4.2.3 Clinical Correlates of Platelet Activation during Dialysis

In the discussion of dialyzer membrane associated coagulation disturbances, several additional factors other than the dialysis membrane itself can affect clotting in the dialyzer circuit and have to be considered. These include type and amount of anticoagulant employed, blood flow rate, blood path geometry in the entire dialysis blood circuit, ultrafiltration rate; as well as patient factors such as hematocrit, number and functional state of the platelets, coagulation protein levels, and fibrinolytic proteins.

Other elements in the blood and endothelium can also affect clotting in the dialysis circuit. Despite these limitations and although extremely rare, significant thrombocytopenia leading to hemorrhage has been reported following hemodialysis (Vicks et al. 1983). Acute platelet dysfunction following dialysis with cuprophan dialyzers, but not with other membranes, has been reported. Specifically resistance to collagen-induced aggregation, and prolonged bleeding times were reported in this context (Pavlopoulou et al. 1986; Sreeharan et al. 1982). Conversion of patients from cuprophan to polyacrylonitrile membranes leads to improvements in defective platelet adhesiveness and prolonged bleeding times (Mingardi et al. 1985). Retrospective data also demonstrate that dialysis with polyacrylonitrile membranes is associated with less arteriovenous fistula thrombosis, leg thrombosis, or fatal pulmonary embolism compared with cuprophan (Simon et al. 1987). A more recent modification of the AN69 membrane, the so-called AN69ST, which results from coating polyethyleneimine upon the polyacrylonitrile surface, produced a membrane that can bind circulating heparin and may therefore reduce the dose of systemically applied anticoagulant and thus the risk of bleeding (Chanard et al. 2008; Chanard et al. 2005). Importantly, the existing data are not definitive and do not allow final conclusions nor do they provide guidance for classification of dialysis membranes based on their thrombogenic potential. However, the existing data does support the conclusion that various classes of dialyzer membrane materials invoke differential thrombogenic effects in patients on hemodialysis.

9.4.3 Erythrocyte Abnormalities

Clinically important hemolysis events during hemodialysis are uncommon and often occur as acute hemolytic crises, often unrelated to the dialyzer membrane material employed. These events are often associated with dialysate problems such as contamination with chloramine, overheating of dialysate, and faulty proportioning of the electrolyte concentrate leading to severely hypotonic dialysate (Eschbach 1983). Mechanical injury of erythrocytes from roller pump function has also been reported (Blackshear et al. 1965). Theoretically, erythrocyte injury through shear stresses during flow along the dialyzer membrane surface or defective dialysis tubing may produce traumatic hemolysis (Gault et al. 1992; Sweet et al. 1996), but in practice, the dialyzer itself rarely causes hemolysis.

The appearance of anti-N antibodies, a type of cold agglutinin directed against the N antigen of erythrocytes (Fassbinder et al. 1976; Harrison et al. 1975; Salama et al. 1988) has been described. These antibodies, whose production has been associated with the use of formaldehyde in reuse processing techniques, can become clinically relevant by causing hemolysis at low temperatures. Therefore, thorough rinsing of the dialyzers following formaldehyde application or discontinuation of formaldehyde altogether both have markedly diminished the prevalence of anti-N antibodies (Lewis et al. 1981). Additional mechanisms of erythrocyte injury have been described through activation of the terminal components of the complement system leading to formation of the membrane attack complex. The latter can be demonstrated on erythrocyte fragments during cardiopulmonary bypass (Salama et al. 1988) and on neutrophils during hemodialysis (Deppisch et al. 1990). Whether these complexes are predisposing factors for or direct inducers of hemolysis in the context of hemodialysis is not known. In terms of clinical outcomes, one large observational study from Japan comparing substituted cellulose with synthetic membrane use, did not find an association between dialysis membrane choice and severity of anemia (Yokoyama et al. 2008).

9.4.4 Polymorphonuclear Leukocyte Abnormalities

9.4.4.1 Hemodialysis-Induced Leukopenia

Transient, hemodialysis-associated leukopenia, particularly neutropenia, is a well-described phenomenon related to membrane bioincompatibility. The onset during the hemodialysis treatment is early on, typically developing in the first 2-3 minutes and reaching its peak at 10-15 minutes (Chenoweth et al. 1983a, b; Kaplow and Goffinet 1968). Following discontinuation of dialysis, the leukocyte count usually returns to normal or may even exceed pre-dialysis values. This latter phenomenon, also called rebound leukocytosis, is felt to be due to increased levels of circulating granulocyte colony-stimulating factor (G-CSF) in this setting (Sato et al. 1994). The underlying pathophysiological mechanism consists of leukocyte sequestration in the pulmonary microcirculation (Dodd et al. 1983) due to binding of dialysis induced C5a and $C5a_{desArg}$ to their specific receptors, and the degree of complement activation correlates well with the development of leukopenia (Chenoweth et al. 1983a; Falkenhagen et al. 1987; Hakim et al. 1984b; Hakim and Schafer 1985; Ivanovich et al. 1983; MacDougall et al. 1985; Maggiore et al. 1987; Spencer et al. 1985). In addition, neutrophils attach to the dialyzer membrane surface (Cheung et al. 1991; Mason et al. 1976), but quantitatively this mechanism is of lesser importance. The action of various neutrophil surface receptors such as Mac-1 or CR3, LAM-1, CD15 may play a role in dialysis-induced leukopenia as well as neutrophil-derived signaling proteins such as PAF and leukotriene B_4 further promote cell aggregation. The clinical significance of transient neutropenia itself appears to be smaller than the pathophysiological mechanisms associated with this phenomenon, for example production of reactive oxygen species and dysfunction of circulating neutrophils. On the other hand, the severity of neutropenia may reflect and therefore serve as a marker for the associated noxious effects, which are discussed in the next sections.

9.4.4.2 Neutrophil Degranulation

As part of the neutrophil response to specific stimuli in host defense (Silber and Moldow 1983), a host of substances stored in the azurophilic and specific granules of neutrophils which possess proteolytic, antimicrobial, and/or cell modulating properties are released. Hemodialysis-associated neutrophil degranulation has been well described in the literature (Horl et al. 1986, 1985, 1988), but the pathophysiology of this process is not well understood. *In vitro* C3a and C5a can serve as mediators of neutrophil degranulation (Goldstein et al. 1973; Showell et al. 1982; Wright and Gallin 1979) and therefore have been incriminated in dialysis-induced neutrophil degranulation. The poor correlation of the plasma concentration of granular proteins with plasma C3a levels during dialysis is calling this mechanism into question. The lower plasma C3a levels induced by dialysis with PMMA membranes but higher plasma elastase levels if compared with cuprophan illustrates this discrepancy (Horl et al. 1986, 1985, 1988). Other mechanisms not related to complement activation have been incriminated in neutrophil degranulation (Cheung et al. 1993; Deppisch et al. 1992). There is a potential role of mechanical shearing of the cells supported by the observation that cuprophan plate dialyzers induce higher plasma levels of elastase and lactoferrin than comparable hollow fiber dialyzers (Schaefer et al. 1987). The release of proteolytic enzymes by neutrophils during dialysis may also contribute to a state of enhanced protein catabolism in dialysis patients (Heidland et al. 1983; Horl and Heidland 1984).

9.4.4.3 Release of Reactive Oxygen Species

In patients undergoing dialysis with cuprophan membranes, substantially greater levels of reactive oxygen species (ROS) are produced if compared with PMMA membranes (Himmelfarb et al. 1993), with C5a activation by cuprophan membranes being a possible mediator in this response. The release of ROS may contribute to injury of surrounding tissues, endothelial cells, plasma proteins and lipids (Maher et al. 1987; Schulman et al. 1991; Till et al. 1982). In keeping with this hypothesis, patients undergoing chronic dialysis with cuprophan membranes have been found to have significantly increased exhaled hydrogen peroxide concentrations compared with patients suffering from chronic kidney disease but who were not on dialysis (Rysz et al. 2007). The exhaled hydrogen peroxide may be a result of leukocyte activation and adherence in the pulmonary microvasculature. An increase in lipid-bound circulating hydroperoxides has also been observed among patients receiving dialysis with CU membrane but not with PS or PA membrane (Lucchi et al. 2005). These, albeit limited observations support the association of increased oxidative stress with bioincompatible membrane use in dialysis.

9.4.4.4 Neutrophil Dysfunction

In addition to a baseline degree of neutrophil function abnormalities observed in patients with uremia, neutrophils that are activated through contact with hemodialysis membrane surface temporarily lose their ability to respond to subsequent stimuli. Cell surface receptor alterations, reduced aggregation and adherence (Klempner et al. 1980; Spagnuolo et al. 1982), and defective oxidative metabolism and chemiluminescence (Cohen et al. 1982; Wissow et al. 1981) have all been observed. Contact with CA membranes has been shown to adversely affect neutrophil phagocytosis and motility *in vitro*, whereas this response could not be demonstrated with PS membranes (Henderson et al. 1975). In a clinical study of incident hemodialysis patients (Vanholder et al. 1991), deterioration in neutrophil function was greater if cuprophan compared with PS membrane dialyzers were used. In a more recent, prospective, cross-over study comparing CA with PS dialyzers serum levels of complement correlated negatively with neutrophil phagocytosis and peroxide production, and positively with neutrophil apoptosis indicating that complement activation may have modulated cell function and apoptosis following hemodialysis (Andreoli et al. 2007). Neutrophil dysfunction following dialysis may impair the host defense from infections and may therefore play an important role clinically contributing to impaired immunity in hemodialysis patients.

9.4.4.5 Modulation of Programmed Cell Death of Neutrophils

Alterations in programmed cell death or apoptosis of neutrophils may play a role in the pathophysiology of immune dysfunction in uremia (Jaber et al. 2001), but the effects of uremia itself, as well as hemodialysis-related humoral and cellular activation are complex. The effect of pro-inflammatory mediators such as C5a, IL-1β and TNF-α, for instance, (Colotta et al. 1992; Lee et al. 1993; Liles and Klebanoff 1995; Perianayagam et al. 2002), can extend the lifespan and functional activity of neutrophils to varying degrees, depending on membrane type, whereby modulating the apoptosis-inducing activity of uremic plasma on neutrophils (Jaber et al. 1999). Apoptotic activity could be significantly reduced in neutrophils exposed to plasma obtained from patients dialyzed with cuprophan, compared with CTA or PS dialyzers. In contrast, accelerated apoptosis is observed in leukocytes incubated directly with CU membranes (Carracedo et al. 1998). Where the balance between these pro- and anti- apoptotic effects of bioincompatible dialysis membranes on neutrophils lies remains to be further determined.

9.4.5 Lymphocytes and Natural Killer Cells

Compared to neutrophils, the effects of dialysis membranes on lymphocytes have been less extensively studied, potentially owing to the limited impact of dialysis on lymphocyte counts (Hobbs et al. 1981; Needleman et al. 1981). Some data however, is available on expression of interleukin-2 receptor (IL-2R) on T-lymphocytes during hemodialysis. Release of IL-2 and expression of IL-2R are increased when T-lymphocytes are activated by antigens and presence of IL-1. T-cell proliferation and maturation requires binding of IL-2 to IL-2R (Greene et al. 1989). One component of the IL-2R, the α chain is released into the plasma under certain conditions, and thus becomes soluble IL-2R. Plasma soluble IL-2R in turn can bind to plasma IL-2, thereby competitively inhibiting its effect at the T-cell bound IL-2R and down-regulating the effects of IL-2.

Clinical data suggests that hemodialysis with cuprophan may activate T-lymphocytes and subsequently cause dysfunction of these cells. For example, dialysis with cuprophan membranes was associated with greater expression of IL-2R on T-lymphocytes compared with PMMA membranes (Zaoui et al. 1991). Subsequent *in vitro* stimulation using phytohemagglutinin showed a poor response of the cuprophan-exposed T lymphocytes. The mechanism of T-cells activation by cuprophan membranes is not fully understood, but complement (Zaoui et al. 1991) and monocyte (Meuer et al. 1987) activation may play a role. Natural killer (NK) cells have a broad spectrum of cytotoxic activity against tumor cells, microorganisms, virus-infected cells, and foreign tissue transplants. Although NK cell counts have been shown to increase during dialysis with cuprophan membranes, their *in vitro* cytotoxic function was found to be reduced (Zaoui and Hakim 1993). By comparing different dialysis membrane types, cuprophan had more deleterious effects on NK cells than CA or polycarbonate membranes (Kay and Raij 1986, 1987). One may speculate if the higher incidence of malignancy among patients with chronic kidney failure (Lindner et al. 1981; Port et al. 1989) could be related to NK cells dysfunction.

Regarding B-lymphocyte activation, cuprophan, CA, or PS membranes alike, but not AN69, were all shown to cause B-cell activation (Descamps-Latscha et al. 1993). The molecular mechanisms that govern intra-dialytic B-cell activation have not been described in detail.

9.4.6 Monocyte Activation and Cytokine Release

Cytokines are polypeptides of middle molecular weight (10-45 kDa) that are synthesized by immunocompetent cells in response to infection, inflammation or trauma (Dinarello 1992a, 1991). While a large number of cytokines have been classified as interleukins (Vilcek and Le 1991), others, for example tumor necrosis factor-α (TNF-α), interferon, transforming growth factor and colony stimulating factors have not been included in this classification scheme (Vilcek and Le 1991). Interleukin-1, which appears in the circulation during hemodialysis, has been incriminated in the development of hypotension, fever and other acute phase responses observed (Henderson et al. 1983b). Subsequent *in vitro* models as well as clinical studies in patients on hemodialysis have confirmed increased production of pro-inflammatory cytokines including IL-1 and TNF-α in this setting (Dinarello 1992a, b; Pereira and Dinarello 1994).

9.4.6.1 Plasma Cytokine Levels

There is conflicting data on the effect of hemodialysis and the use of different types of membranes on the kinetics of IL-1 and TNF-α plasma levels. While several studies demonstrated an increase in plasma levels in response to hemodialysis using cellulose membranes (Bingel et al. 1988; Descamps-Latscha et al. 1986; Herbelin et al. 1990; Lonnemann et al. 1987; Luger et al. 1987; Pereira et al. 1994), others failed to confirm this finding (Davenport et al. 1991; Holmes et al. 1990; Powell et al. 1991).

Interestingly, non-dialyzed patients with chronic kidney failure did not show evidence of elevated IL-1 levels (Herbelin et al. 1990), leading to the conclusion that the hemodialysis procedure itself, rather than renal failure leads to increased IL-1 production. This hypothesis was further strengthened by the observation that hemodialysis with these "bioincompatible" cellulose membranes leads to a further rise in plasma levels of TNF-α (Canivet et al. 1994; Ghysen et al. 1990; Herbelin et al. 1990). In contrast, dialysis with "biocompatible" membranes such as PAN was not associated with a further rise in plasma levels of TNF-α (Canivet et al. 1994; Ghysen et al. 1990). In fact, in some studies, plasma levels of TNF-α declined during dialysis with PAN membranes (Canivet et al. 1994). However, others have failed to show elevated plasma levels of IL-1β or

TNF-α before, during or after a hemodialysis treatment. Conflicting data also exist on plasma levels of IL-1β and TNF-α in hemodialysis patients, which were elevated compared with healthy controls in one study (Pereira et al. 1994), but similarly elevated without differences between subgroups with chronic kidney disease (CKD) not on dialysis, on peritoneal dialysis and on hemodialysis (Herbelin et al. 1990; Herbelin et al. 1991). In addition to increased production, also decreased elimination caused by reduced renal function could be a cause of elevated plasma cytokine levels, underscoring the important role of the kidney in the clearance of these substances from the circulation (Descamps-Latscha et al. 1995; Pereira et al. 1994). While intermittent hemodialysis and peritoneal dialysis do not provide effective means of elimination of cytokines, studies in critically ill patients treated with continuous arteriovenous hemofiltration using a PAN membrane demonstrated removal of TNF-α by adsorption to the membrane and to a lesser degree by convection (Cottrell and Mehta 1992). Interleukin-1β is also present in PBMC harvested from patients on dialysis, in contrast to healthy subjects where it is not detectable (Blumenstein et al. 1988; Haeffner-Cavaillon et al. 1989; Lonnemann et al. 1990; Luger et al. 1987). Measurements of TNF-α and IL-6 parallel these results (Memoli et al. 1990; Oettinger et al. 1990; Ryan et al. 1991). In addition, a small study of four dialysis patients examined gene expression patterns of PBMC by comparing hemophan with PS membrane dialysis in a crossover design (Wilflingseder et al. 2008). Hemophan dialysis showed a comparative over-representation of genes involved in processes of immunity and defense, signal transduction, and apoptosis, whereby corroborating the previous results.

In vitro and *in vivo* studies have shown that when human blood is circulated through a hollow fiber cuprophan membrane, transcription of mRNA for IL-1β and TNF-α is apparent within 2 hours. However, once activated, these cells require a second stimulus, for example by infection or by dialysate contaminated with bacterial endotoxin (see Fig. 9.2) (Pereira and Dinarello 1995), to translate and synthesize the actual protein (Schindler et al. 1993; Schindler et al. 1990a, b; Urena et al. 1990). In contrast to cuprophan membranes, cytokine genes are not activated by membranes that are weak complement activators, during either *in vitro* or *in vivo* dialysis (Schindler et al. 1993; Schindler et al. 1990a, b).

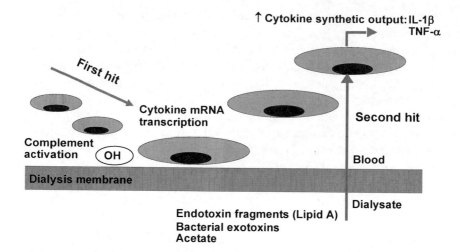

Fig. 9.2 Potential mechanisms for cytokine production during dialysis: The 'Double Hit Hypothesis'. Complement activation by dialysis membranes leads to transcription of mRNA for interleukin-1 beta (IL-1β) and tumor necrosis factor alpha (TNF-α) in monocytes. In the absence of a "second signal", the mRNA for those cytokines is not translated into protein. The second signal could potentially come from the dialysate, leading to synthesis of IL-1β and TNF-α. Concurrently, proteases cleave the extracellular fragment of the TNF receptors resulting in soluble TNF receptors (sTNFR). Thus, the hemodialysis procedure serves as a stimulus for cytokines such as IL-1β and TNF-α, as well as their specific antagonists. (Reproduced from Jaber BL, Pereira BJG (2005) Biocompatibility of Hemodialysis Membranes. In: Pereira BJG, Sayegh MH, Blake P (eds) Chronic Kidney Disease, Dialysis, & Transplantation. Companion to Brenner & Rector's the Kidney, 2nd edn. Elsevier Saunders, Philadelphia, (Jaber and Pereira 2005) with permission).

9.4.6.2 Cytokine Production and Dialysate-Born Pyrogen Reactions

The increasing use of high-flux and high-efficiency membranes carries with it the phenomenon of dialysate backfiltration. Although this phenomenon is welcomed from the perspective of optimizing dialyzer efficiency (see above section *Overview of Dialyzer Structure*), backfiltration also carries with it the risk of exposure to bacterial contaminants present in the dialysate (Baurmeister et al. 1989; Peterson et al. 1992; Tokars et al. 1990). Dialyzer reprocessing techniques that lead to increased membrane permeability may also potentially increase the risk of reverse passage of bacterial products from the dialysate to the blood (Donahue and Ahmad 1992; Graeber et al. 1993).

While bacterial endotoxins themselves, due to their high molecular weight ($\sim 10^6$ Da), cannot cross intact dialysis membranes, including high flux membranes, endotoxin molecule fragments and other, smaller cytokine-inducing products such as the lipid-A portion of endotoxins or muramyl peptides can cross dialysis membranes and stimulate PBMC. Presence of endotoxin can be detected by cytokine production by PBMC (Dinarello 1991) and can therefore be used to measure the permeability of different dialyzer membranes to bacterial products (Bingel et al. 1986; Evans and Holmes 1991; Lonnemann et al. 1992; Lonnemann et al. 1988a; Pereira et al. 1995). Results from studies using this technique have shown that high-flux synthetic membranes may be less prone to transfer of bacterial products from the dialysate than low-flux cellulose membrane types and that transmembrane passage of bacterial products can also occur in the absence of backfiltration, for example through diffusive processes (Lonnemann et al. 1992; Pereira et al. 1995; Urena et al. 1992). The hydrophobic properties of some synthetic membranes are believed to prevent translocation of bacterial toxins, which typically also carry hydrophobic domains, through avid adsorption of these toxins on the dialysate side of the membrane (Lonnemann et al. 1992). This supports the notion that, under the right preconditions, backfiltration may be used to enhance dialyzer performance and concomitantly avoid bioincompatible adverse effects.

9.4.6.3 Clinical Effects of Dialysis-Induced Monocyte Activation

Exogenous administration as well as extracorporeal generation, for example by dialysis, of inflammatory cytokines can mimic symptoms of systemic inflammatory diseases, infections, atherosclerotic vascular disease and malignancies. This observation also provides the basis to the so-called "Interleukin Hypothesis" (Henderson et al. 1983a), in which many of the acute and chronic complications of hemodialysis are partially attributed to the actions of cytokines activated during the dialysis treatments. For instance, administration of IL-1β in doses of 10-100 ng/kg has been shown to cause fever, sleepiness, anorexia, myalgia, arthralgia, headache and gastrointestinal disturbances, and in larger doses of over 300 ng/kg, hypotension in healthy subjects (Dinarello 1992a, b, 1991). TNF-α produces similar effects when administered at low doses of less than 1μg/kg, and the combination of both IL-1β and TNF-α function synergistically by precipitating circulatory shock (Okusawa et al. 1988). A more chronic exposure to cytokines may contribute to accelerated atherosclerosis and cardiovascular morbidity (Dinarello, 1992a, b, 1991). Chronic cytokine activation may also contribute to various bone, articular, and periarticular diseases (Raz et al. 1988; Cominelli et al. 1989; Schweizer et al. 1988) and β_2-microglobulin amyloidosis (Ohashi et al. 1992). In addition IL-1β, IL–6 and TNF-α may reduce appetite through peripheral effects affecting hepatic metabolism and may also stimulate hepatic acute phase proteins such as C-reactive protein, and suppress albumin synthesis, cause muscle breakdown and protein catabolism. It is important to note, however, that an association between dialysis-induced cytokine production and hard clinical endpoints has not been found to date.

9.5   CLINICAL IMPLICATIONS OF DIALYSIS MEMBRANE BIOCOMPATIBILITY

9.5.1 Hemodialysis-Induced Hypoxemia

Hemodialysis performed with cuprophan membrane and acetate dialysate is associated with a decline in systemic arterial partial oxygen tension (pO$_2$) of 10-15 mm Hg (Craddock et al. 1977; DeBacker et al. 1983; Hakim and Lowrie 1982). Although acetate dialysate is considered to be the major contributor to dialysis-induced hypoxemia (Dolan et al. 1981; Oh et al. 1985), membrane bioincompatibility may also contribute to this problem. This hypothesis is supported by clinical data of hypoxemia induced by hemodialysis in patients under controlled mechanical ventilation and unchanged settings (Jones et al. 1980). Sham hemodialysis without the use of dialysate was also shown to induce hypoxemia (Bergstrom et al. 1984). In addition, a decrease in pulmonary diffusion capacity (DLCO) (Craddock et al. 1977; Graf et al. 1980; Mahajan et al. 1977; Morrison et al. 1980) and transthoracic impedance (Graf et al. 1980), widening of alveolar-arterial oxygen tension gradient (DeBacker et al. 1983; Morrison et al. 1980), as well as in lung mechanics (Craddock et al. 1977; Dolan et al. 1981) have been demonstrated during hemodialysis. Further, the decrease in lung diffusion capacity is greater when using cuprophan compared with PAN membranes (Fawcett et al. 1987) and replacing unsubstituted cellulose with PMMA (Hakim and Lowrie 1982) or PAN (DeBacker et al. 1983; Vaziri et al. 1984a) membranes can improve dialysis associated hypoxemia. Finally, hypoxemia could be precipitated by infusion of blood plasma exposed to cuprophan membrane (Cheung et al. 1986; Graf H et al. 1980). This wealth of clinical data supports the notion that membrane bioincompatibility and not only dialysate incompatibility contributes to the development of dialysis-induced hypoxemia.

9.5.2 Pulmonary Hypertension

Increases in pulmonary arterial pressure that can be clinically significant (Agar et al. 1979), were demonstrated in patients receiving dialysis with cuprophan membranes, whereas dialysis with polycarbonate membranes did not show this phenomenon (Schohn et al. 1986). The actions of complement and other humoral factors are incriminated in the pathophysiology, as anaphylatoxins cause smooth muscle contraction *in vitro* (Cochrane and Muller-Eberhard 1968) and pulmonary hypertension in animals (Cheung et al., 1987). Complement can also induce airway constriction by way of thromboxane and leukotriene synthesis (Stimler-Gerard 1986). In addition, anaphylatoxins increase vascular permeability (Lepow et al. 1970) and pulmonary leukocyte sequestration, but the latter may not directly increase pulmonary arterial pressure.

9.5.3 Dialyzer Reactions

Reactions during hemodialysis of various kind, time of onset and severity, which can occasionally be life threatening, occur infrequently. These reactions called "dialyzer reactions" are identified after excluding or addressing symptoms due to volume removal, electrolyte shifts, improper composition of dialysate, and device malfunction. Manifestations may include single or multiple symptoms such as hypertension, hypotension, dyspnea, coughing, sneezing, wheezing, choking, rhinorrhea, conjunctival injection, headache, muscle cramps, back pain, abdominal pain, chest pain, nausea, vomiting, fever, chills, flushing, urticaria, and pruritus. These reactions can rarely be fatal (Caruana et al. 1985; Foley and Reeves 1985; Gutch et al. 1976; Hakim et al. 1984a; Henderson et al. 1983b; Ing et al. 1983; Key et al. 1983; Nicholls and Platts 1985; Ogden 1980; Poothullil et al. 1975; Popli et al. 1982; Rault and Silver 1985; Villarroel and Ciarkowski 1985). Causes of dialyzer reactions are diverse, with a multitude of potential causes and are not always the result of hypersensitivity to dialyzer components.

9.5.4 β_2-Microglobulin (β_2MG) and Amyloidosis

Amyloidosis due to deposition of β_2MG has been well described as a clinically relevant complication in patients receiving long term dialysis (Gejyo et al. 1985; Gorevic et al. 1985). The pathogenesis, although not completely settled, may be based on alterations of the β_2MG peptide in chronic kidney failure (Linke et al. 1989; Miyaya et al. 1993; Ogawa et al.

1988) facilitating tissue deposition. In addition, the substantially elevated plasma levels of β_2MG in patients with chronic kidney failure (30-60 fold) (Floege et al. 1991, 1988a, b; Jorstad et al. 1988; Ritz and Bommer 1988; Vincent et al. 1992) may also promote deposition. Cuprophan membrane activation induces more β_2MG release by PBMC than synthetic membranes *in vitro*. C5a or IL-1β may also stimulate mononuclear cells to release β_2MG (Zaoui et al. 1990). As β_2MG is also stored in neutrophil granules (Bjerrum et al. 1987), dialysis membrane induced neutrophil degranulation can also increase plasma β_2MG levels, although the quantity of released β_2MG through this mechanism may not be significant. These data, at least in principle, support the notion that not only lack of removal but also enhanced production of β_2MG may contribute to the related amyloidosis syndrome in hemodialysis (Ohashi et al. 1992). Although the data on enhanced β_2MG generation induced by cuprophan dialysis are inconclusive (Floege et al. 1988a, b, 1989; Ritz and Bommer 1988), they provide enough circumstantial evidence in support of a more enhanced β_2MG production due to cuprophan (Klinke et al. 1988) if compared with synthetic dialysis membranes (Floege et al. 1991; Vincent et al. 1992).

Removal of β_2MG by high-flux synthetic membranes is efficient and occurs probably through membrane adsorption and diffusion and convection alike (Jorstad et al. 1988). A reduced burden of β_2MG in tissues of patients dialyzed with synthetic compared with cuprophan membranes may be the result. Indeed, patients dialyzed with AN69 membrane tend to suffer from fewer bone cysts and carpal tunnel syndrome complications compared with those dialyzed with cuprophan membrane (Chanard et al. 1989; Miura et al. 1992; van Ypersele de Strihou et al. 1991). Although efficient removal of β_2MG by high-flux and high-efficiency dialyzer appears to be a more important aspect in amyloidosis prevention, inflammatory induction of β_2MG synthesis (Zaoui et al. 1990) as well as alteration of its structure by bioincompatible dialysis membrane exposure (Linke et al. 1989; Ogawa et al. 1988) may contribute to this syndrome as well, albeit the supporting data may not be considered definitive in this regard.

9.5.5 Susceptibility to Infection

Patients undergoing long-term hemodialysis are at risk for infections, and have a higher incidence of malignancy than the general population (Lindner et al. 1981; Port et al. 1989). These epidemiologic data point to renal disease or dialysis related immunodeficiency or both. The increased susceptibility of chronic hemodialysis patients to viral infections, their impaired immune response to vaccines, frequent cutaneous anergy and prolonged graft survival can be viewed as a dysfunction of the T lymphocyte cell line. The role of dialysis membrane bioincompatibility in this clinical problem it not fully understood. A prospective but small single center study in incident hemodialysis patients allocated to either cuprophan or PS based dialysis techniques, the cuprophan group displayed more significant neutrophil dysfunction (Vanholder et al. 1991). Sepsis episodes were also more common in the cuprophan group compared with the PS group, although definitive conclusions cannot be drawn from this preliminary study.

9.5.6 Protein Catabolism

Membrane bioincompatibility may play a contributing role in protein catabolism of dialysis patients. Two major pathophysiological mechanisms may conspire to result in enhanced protein breakdown, which are neutrophil degranulation with release of elastase (Silber and Moldow 1983), and activation of cytokines. Intra-granular proteins, such as elastase, are known proteolytic enzymes. Although elastase is typically bound and inhibited by plasma α_1-proteinase inhibitor, which limits its functional activity, concomitant activation of ROS (Himmelfarb et al. 1993) may potentiate the effect of proteases and elastase on protein degradation (Heidland et al. 1983; Horl and Heidland 1984; Horl et al. 1986, 1985, 1988; Weiss and Regiani 1984). The inflammatory cytokine IL-1β may also contribute to protein breakdown and catabolism in hemodialysis patients (Baracos et al. 1983). Clinical and *in vitro* data on amino acid turnover in cuprophan versus AN69 membrane hemodialysis have remained inconclusive in showing enhanced protein catabolism from bioincompatible dialysis techniques (Gutierrez et al. 1990; Haeffner-Cavaillon et al. 1989; Lim et al. 1993; Lonnemann et al. 1988a, b). Although theoretical considerations may support enhanced protein catabolism with dialysis using cellulose membrane such as cuprophan, compared with more biocompatible synthetic membranes, the available data on this question remains limited and unsettled at this time.

9.5.7 Membrane Biocompatibility and Clinical Outcomes in Patients with Acute Kidney Injury (AKI)

Experimental data in rats with ischemic AKI shows that exposure to blood plasma incubated with cuprophan membranes prolongs renal recovery and causes glomerular neutrophil infiltration if compared with rats exposed to PAN membrane-treated plasma (Schulman et al. 1991). These data support the notion that the use of bioincompatible membranes for dialysis in AKI may induce further kidney injury through inflammatory and oxidative actions of activated neutrophils. Since the 1990's several prospective studies have been undertaken to evaluate the clinical significance of these findings by comparing the effects of various dialyzer membranes on clinical outcomes of patients with AKI. In a meta-analysis of 10 trials totaling 1,100 patients, there was no demonstrable clinical advantage to the use of cellulose-derived versus synthetic membranes in patients with AKI who require intermittent hemodialysis (Alonso et al. 2008). Causes of heterogeneity among the trials were many including problems with randomization, blinding process, lack of *a priori* power analyses, use of substituted rather than unsubstituted cellulose membranes for comparison, use of membranes with various, not predetermined flux characteristics, missing or insufficient adjustment for disease severity or AKI etiology, failure to adjust for dialysis dose or center effect.

A series of small trials comparing cuprophan with synthetic (PMMA or PS) dialyzers for dialysis in kidney transplant recipients suffering from delayed graft function, presumably from ischemic acute graft injury, failed to show a difference in time to recovery or overall survival (Romao et al. 1998; Valeri 1994), or even longer time to recovery for the synthetic membrane group (Woo et al. 1998). Doubts over the definitive nature of the results of these relatively small studies remain, also since causes other than ischemic graft injury such as acute rejection or drug toxicity were not definitively ruled out. Although the question of dialyzer membrane selection in AKI remains unsettled pending better powered and better designed definitive studies, the use of substituted cellulose and synthetic membrane dialyzers in the management of AKI requiring dialysis is now well established, and the issue of unsubstituted cellulose membrane dialyzer use in AKI, despite the lack of evidence to the contrary, no longer appears to be a pertinent research question.

9.5.8   Membrane Biocompatibility and Clinical Outcomes in Patients with Chronic Kidney Failure

In retrospective analyses, a significantly lower mortality for patients with chronic kidney failure receiving hemodialysis with synthetic membranes compared with unsubstituted cellulose membranes has been consistently found (Hakim et al. 1996; Hornberger et al. 1992; Levin et al. 1991). In a small trial using a cross-over design, both high-flux CTA and PS were compared for their impact in blood lipid values (Wanner et al. 2004). Dialysis with PS membranes appeared to improve the profile of triglycerides, oxidized LDL and apolipoproteins better than dialysis with the CTA membranes, compared with a 6-week run-in phase using low-flux PS membranes used for all patients (Wanner et al. 2004), providing additional support for the afore-mentioned hypothesis. Outcome specific analyses from large observational studies have shown significant mortality risk reductions for infectious and cardiovascular outcomes (Bloembergen et al. 1999). Potential criticism for lack of adjustment for dialysis dose or membrane flux characteristics has been voiced, but the influence of imbalances in flux and solute removal should be relatively mild given the negative study results from the HEMO study (Eknoyan et al. 2002).

These clinical outcome results support theoretical, experimental data that identify advantages for biocompatible substituted cellulose or synthetic membrane types over unsubstituted cellulose in chronic hemodialysis. Certainly, other advances, such as improvement in dialyzer permeability for middle molecular weight solutes, other dialysis technology, improvements in dialysate composition and quality and an overall greater commitment of clinical and social resources to patients with chronic kidney failure may lead to improved outcomes. It is also important to emphasize that all synthetic membranes are not identical and may differ considerably in their biological impact on blood and blood components during dialysis. A study, for example, that evaluated arterial pulse wave velocities during dialysis found indications of reduced arterial compliance in PS compared with PA dialyzers (Mourad et al. 2004). These considerations, however should be viewed in light of the negative results of the so far largest and most well designed prospective randomized trial, the HEMO study, evaluating the impact of dialysis dose and use of high-flux dialyzers on clinical outcomes (Eknoyan et al. 2002).

9.6 CONCLUSION

In summary, this chapter provided an overview of recent advances in dialyzer structure and design, followed by a detailed discussion of the various biomaterials used for dialyzer membranes, with a focus on their physical, chemical and biological properties, as well as their biocompatibility. Particular attention was given to the clinical relevance of dialysis membrane biocompatibility including specific syndromes such as hemodialysis-induced hypoxemia, dialyzer reactions, β_2-microglobulin deposition, protein catabolism, susceptibility to infection as a result of immune dysfunction, and patient survival.

REFERENCES

Adler, A., Berlyne, G.: B-thromboglobulin and platelet factor-4 levels during hemodialysis with polyacrylonitrile. Am. Soc. Artif. Int. Organs 4, 100–102 (1981)

Agar, J.W., Hull, J.D., Kaplan, M., Pletka, P.G.: Acute cardiopulmonary decompensation and complement activation during hemodialysis. Ann. Int. Med. 90(5), 792–793 (1979)

Alonso, A., Lau, J., Jaber, B.L.: Biocompatible hemodialysis membranes for acute renal failure. Cochrane Database Syst. Rev. 23(1), CD005283 (2008)

Anderson, S., Garcia, D., Brenner, B.: Renal and systemic manifesta-tions of glomerular disease. In: Brenner, B., Rector, J.F. (eds.) The Kidney, 4th edn. Saunders, Philadelphia (1991)

Andreoli, M.C., Dalboni, M.A., Watanabe, R., et al.: Impact of dialyzer membrane on apoptosis and function of polymorphonuclear cells and cytokine synthesis by peripheral blood mononuclear cells in hemodialysis patients. Artif. Organs 31(12), 887–892 (2007)

Arnaout, M., Hakim, R.M., Todd, R.F., et al.: Increased expression of an adhesion-promoting surface glycoprotein in the granulocytopenia of hemodialysis. New England Journal of Medicine 312(8), 457–462 (1985)

Baracos, V., Rodemann, H.P., Dinarello, C.A., et al.: Stimulation of muscle protein degradation by leukocyte pyrogen (interleukin-1). N. Engl. J. Med. 308(10), 553–558 (1983)

Baurmeister, U., Vienken, J., Daum, V.: High-flux dialysis membranes: Endotoxin transfer by backfiltration can be a problem. Nephrol. Dial. Transplant. 4(suppl. 3), 89–93 (1989)

Bergstrom, J., Danielsson, S., Freychuss, U.: Dialysis, ultrafiltration and shamdialysis in normal subjects. Kidney Int. 27, 157(A) (1984)

Bhakdi, S., Fassbender, W., Hugo, F.: Relative efficiency of terminal complement activation. J. Immunol. 141(9), 3117–3122 (1988)

Bingel, M., Lonnemann, G., Shaldon, S., et al.: Human interleukin-1 production during hemodialysis. Nephron 43(3), 161–163 (1986)

Bingel, M., Lonnemann, G., Koch, K.M., et al.: Plasma interleukin-1 activity during hemodialysis: the influence of dialysis membranes. Nephron 50(4), 273–276 (1988)

Bjerrum, O., Bjerrum, O., Borregaard, N.: B2-microglobulin in neutrophils: an intragranular protein. J. Immunol. 138(11), 3913–3917 (1987)

Blackshear, P., Droman, F., Steinbach, J.: Some mechanical effects that influence hemodialysis. Trans. Am. Soc. Artif. Intern. Organs 11, 112–117 (1965)

Bloembergen, W.E., Hakim, R.M., Stannard, D.C., et al.: Relationship of dialysis membrane and cause-specific mortality. Am. J. Kidney Dis. 33(1), 1–10 (1999)

Blumenstein, M., Schmidt, B., Ward, R.A., et al.: Altered interleukin-1 production in patients undergoing hemodialysis. Nephron 50(4), 277–281 (1988)

Bokisch, V.A., Müller-Eberhard, H.J.: Anaphylatoxin inactivator of human plasma: its isolation and characterization as a carboxypeptidase. J. Clin. Invest. 49(12), 2427–2436 (1970)

Camussi, G., Segoloni, G., Rotunno, M., Vercellone, A.: Mechanisms involved in acute granolocytopenia in hemodialysis: cell-membrane direct interactions. Int. J. Art Organs 1(3), 123–127 (1978)

Camussi, G., Pacitti, A., Tetta, C., et al.: Mechanisms of neutropenia in hemodialysis. Trans. Am. Soc. Artif. Int. Organs 30, 364–368 (1984)

Canivet, E., Lavaud, S., Wong, T., et al.: Cuprophane but not synthetic membrane induces increases in serum tumor necrosis factor alpha. Am. J. Kid. Dis. 23(1), 41–46 (1994)

Carracedo, J., Ramirez, R., Martin-Malo, A., et al.: Nonbiocompatible hemodialysis membranes induce apoptosis in mononuclear cells: the role of G-proteins. J. Am. Soc. Nephrol. 9(1), 46–53 (1998)

Caruana, R., Hamilton, R., Pearson, F.: Dialyzer hypersensitivity syndrome: possible role of allergy to ethylene oxide. Am. J. Nephrol. 5(4), 271–274 (1985)

Caruana, R., Smith, M., Clyne, D., et al.: A controlled study of heparin versus epoprostenold sodium (prostacyclin) as the sole anticoagulant for chronic hemodialysis. Blood Purification 9(5-6), 296–304 (1991)

Chanard, J., Bindi, P., Lavaud, S., et al.: Carpal tunnel syndrome and type of dialysis membrane. BMJ 298(6677), 867–868 (1989)

Chanard, J., Lavaud, S., Paris, B., et al.: Assessment of heparin binding to the AN69 ST hemodialysis membrane: I. Preclinical studies. ASAIO J. 51(4), 342–347 (2005)

Chanard, J., Lavaud, S., Maheut, H., et al.: The clinical evaluation of low-dose heparin in haemodialysis: a prospective study using the heparin-coated AN69 ST membrane. Nephrol. Dial. Transplant. 23(6), 2003–2009 (2008)

Chenoweth, D.E., Cheung, A.K., Henderson, L.W.: Anaphylatoxin formation during hemodialysis: effects of different dialyzer membranes. Kidney Int. 24(6), 764–769 (1983a)

Chenoweth, D.E., Cheung, A.K., Ward, D.M., et al.: Anaphylatoxin formation during hemodialysis: a comparison of new and re-used dialyzers. Kidney Int. 24(6), 770–774 (1983b)

Cheung, A.K., LeWinter, M., Chenoweth, D.E., et al.: Cardiopulmonary effects of cuprophan-activated plasma in the swine: role of complement activation products. Kidney Int. 29(4), 799–806 (1986)

Cheung, A., Baranowski, R., Wayman, A.: The role of thromboxane in cuprophan-induced pulmonary hypertension. Kidney Int. 31(5), 1072–1079 (1987)

Cheung, A., Parker, C., Janatova, J.: Analysis of the complement C3 fragments associated with hemodialysis membranes. Kidney Int. 35(2), 576–588 (1989)

Cheung, A., Parker, C., Hohnholt, M.: B_2 integrins are required for neutrophil degranulation induced by hemodialysis membranes. Kidney Int. 43(3), 649–660 (1993)

Cheung, A., Faezi-Jenkin, B., Leypoldt, J.: Effect of thrombosis on complement activation and neutrophil degranulation during invitro hemodialysis. J. Am. Soc. Nephrol. 5(1), 110–115 (1994)

Cheung, A.K., Hohnholt, M., Gilson, J.: Adherence of neutrophils to hemodialysis membranes: role of complement receptors. Kidney Int. 40(6), 1123–1133 (1991)

Cochrane, C., Muller-Eberhard, H.: The derivation of two distinct anaphylatoxin activities from the third and fifth components of human complement. J. Exp. Med. 127(2), 371–386 (1968)

Cohen, M., Elliott, D., Chaplinski, T., et al.: A Defect in the Oxidative Metabolism of Human Polymorphonuclear Leukocytes that Remain in Circulation Early in Hemodialysis. Blood 60(6), 1283–1289 (1982)

Colman, R., Hirsh, J., Marder, V., et al.: Hemostasis and Thrombosis: Basic Principles and Clinical Practice. In: Colman, R., Hirsh, J., Marder, V., et al. (eds.) J.B. Lippincott, Philadelphia (1987)

Colotta, F., Re, F., Polentarutti, N., et al.: Modulation of granulocyte survival and programmed cell death by cytokines and bacterial products. Blood 80(8), 2012–2020 (1992)

Cominelli, F., Nast, C.C., Dinarello, C.A., et al.: Regulation of eicosanoid production in rabbit colon by interleukin-1. Gastroenterology 97(6), 1400–1405 (1989)

Cottrell, A.C., Mehta, R.L.: Cytokine kinetics in septic ARF patients on continuous veno-veno hemodialysis (CVVHD). J. Am. Soc. Nephrol. 3, 361 (1992)

Craddock, P.R., Fehr, J., Brigham, K.L., et al.: Complement and leukocyte-mediated pulmonary dysfunction in hemodialysis. N. Engl. J. Med. 296(14), 769–774 (1977)

Craddock, P.R., Fehr, J., Dalmasso, A.P., et al.: Hemodialysis leukopenia: pulmonary vascular leukostasis resulting from complement activation by dialyzer cellophane membranes. J. Clin. Invest. 59(5), 879–888 (1977a)

Craddock, P., Hammerschmidt, D., White, J.: Complement (C5a)-induced granulocyte aggregation in vitro. A possible mechanism of complement mediated leukostasis and leukopenia. J. Clin. Invest. 60(1), 260–264 (1977b)

Davenport, A., Crabtree, J., Androjna, C., et al.: Tumour necrosis factor does not increase during routine cuprophane haemodialysis in healthy. Nephrol. Dialysis Transplant. 6(6), 435–439 (1991)

Dawes, J., Smith, R., Pepper, D.: The release, distributions, and clearance of human B-thromboglobulin and platelet factor 4. Thromb. Res. 12(5), 851–861 (1978)

DeBacker, W.A., Verpooten, G.A., Borgonjon, D.J., et al.: Hypoxemia during hemodialysis: effects of different membranes and dialysate compositions. Kidney Int. 23(5), 738–743 (1983)

del Balzo, U., Levi, R., Polley, M.: Cardiac dysfunction caused by purified human C3a anaphylatoxin. Proc. Natl. Acad. Sci. U.S.A 82(3), 886–890 (1985)

Deppisch, R., Schmitt, V., Bommer, J., et al.: Fluid phase generation of terminal complement complex as a novel index of bioincompatibility. Kidney Int. 37(2), 696–706 (1990)

Deppisch, R., Betz, M., Hansch, G., et al.: Biocompatibility of the polyamide membranes. Contrib. Nephrol. 96, 26–46 (1992)

Descamps-Latscha, B., Herbelin, A., Nguyen, A.T., et al.: Haemodialysis-membrane induced phagocyte oxidative metabolism activation and interleukin-1 production. Life Supp. Sys. 4(4), 349–353 (1986)

Descamps-Latscha, B., Herbelin, A., Nguyen, A.T., et al.: Soluble CD23 as an effector of immune dysregulation in chronic uremia and dialysis. Kidney Int. 43(4), 878–884 (1993)

Descamps-Latscha, B., Herbelin, A., Nguyen, A.T., et al.: Balance between IL-1 beta, TNF-alpha, and their specific inhibitors in chronic renal failure and maintenance dialysis. Relationships with activation markers of T cells, B cells, and monocytes. J. Immunol. 154(2), 882–892 (1995)

Dinarello, C.: Cytokines: agents provocateurs in hemodialysis? Kidney Int. 41(3), 683–694 (1992a)

Dinarello, C.: Interleukin-1 and tumor necrosis factor and their naturally occurring antagonists during hemodialysis. Kidney Int. 42(supplement 38), S68–S77 (1992b)

Dinarello, C.A.: Interleukin-1 and interleukin-1 antagonism. Blood 77(8), 1627–1652 (1991)

Docci, D., Turci, F., Devl Vecchio, C., et al.: Hemodialysis-associated platelet loss: study of the relative contribution of dialyzer membrane composition and geometry. Int. J. Artif. Organs 7(6), 337–340 (1984)

Dodd, N., Gordge, M., Tarrant, J., et al.: A demonstration of neutrophil accumulation in the pulmonary vasculature during hemodialysis. Proc. Eur. Transpl. Assoc. 20, 186–189 (1983)

Dolan, M.J., Whipp, B.J., Davidson, W.D., et al.: Hypopnea associated with acetate hemodialysis: carbon-dioxide-flow dependent ventilation. N. Engl. J. Med. 305(2), 72–75 (1981)

Donahue, P.R., Ahmad, S.: Dialyzer permeability alteration by reuse (Abstract). J. Am. Soc. Nephrol. 3, 363 (1992)

Dumler, F., Zasuwa, G., Levin, N.: Effect of dialyzer reprocessing methods on complement activation and hemodialyzer-related symptoms. Artif. Organs 11(2), 128–131 (1987)

Eknoyan, G., Beck, G.J., Cheung, A.K., et al.: Effect of dialysis dose and membrane flux in maintenance hemodialysis. N. Engl. J. Med. 347(25), 2010–2019 (2002)

Eschbach, J.: Hematologic problems of dialysis patients. In: Drukker, W., Parsons, F., Maher, J. (eds.) Replacement of Renal Function by Dialysis. Martinus Nijhoff, Boston (1983)

Evans, R.C., Holmes, C.J.: In vitro study of the transfer of cytokine-inducing substances across selected high-flux hemodialysis membranes. Blood Purif. 9(2), 92–101 (1991)

Falkenhagen, D., Bosch, T., Brown, G., et al.: A clinical study on different cellulosic dialysis membranes. Nephrol. Dial. Transplant. 2(6), 537–545 (1987)

Falkenhagen, D., Mitzner, S., Stange, J., et al.: Biocompatibility: methodology and evaluation. Contrib. Nephrol. 103, 34–54 (1993)

Fassbinder, W., Pilar, J., Scheuermann, E., et al.: Formaldehyde and the occurence of anti-N-like cold agglutinins in RDT patients. Proc. Eur. Dial. Trans. Assoc. 13, 333–338 (1976)

Fawcett, S., Hoenich, N., Laker, M., et al.: Hemodialysis-induced respiratory changes. Nephrol. Dial. Transplant. 2(3), 161–168 (1987)

Fearon, D., Wong, W.: Complement ligand-receptor interactons that mediate biological responses. Ann. Rev. Immunol. 1, 243–271 (1983)

Floege, J., Granolleras, C., Koch, K.M., Shaldon, S.: Which membrane? Should beta-2 microglobulin decide on the choice of today's hemodialysis membrane? Nephron 50(3), 177–181 (1988a)

Floege, J., Wilks, M., Shaldon, S., et al.: Beta 2-microglobulin kinetics during haemofiltration. Nephrol. Dial. Transplant. 3(6), 784–789 (1988b)

Floege, J., Granolleras, C., Merscher, S., et al.: Is the rise in plasma beta-2-microglobulin seen during hemodialysis meaningful? Nephron 51(1), 6–12 (1989)

Floege, J., Bartsch, A., Schulze, M., et al.: Clearance and synthesis rates of B2-microglobulin in patients undergoing hemodialysis in normal subjects. J. Lab. Clin. Med. 118(2), 153–165 (1991)

Foley, R., Reeves, W.: Acute anaphylactoid reactions in hemodialysis. Am. J. Kid. Dis. 5(2), 132–135 (1985)

Fujimura, T., Uchi, Y., Fukuda, M., et al.: Development of a dialyzer with enhanced internal filtration to increase the clearance of low molecular weight proteins. J. Artif. Organs 7(3), 149–154 (2004)

Fukuda, M., Miyazaki, M., Uezumi, S., et al.: Design and assessment of the new APS dialyzer (APS-SA series). J. Artif. Organs 9(3), 192–198 (2006)

Galli, F., Rovidati, S., Chiarantini, L., et al.: Bioreactivity and biocompatibility of a vitamin Emodified multi-layer hemodialysis filter. Kidney Int. 54(2), 580–589 (1998)

Galli, F., Canestrari, F., Buoncristiani, U.: Biological effects of oxidant stress in haemodialysis: the possible roles of vitamin E. Blood Purif. 17(2-3), 79–94 (1999)

Gasparotto, M., Bertoli, M., Vertolli, U., et al.: Biocompatibility of various dialysis membranes as assessed by coagulation assay. Contrib. Nephrol. 37, 96–100 (1984)

Gault, M., Duffett, S., Purchase, L., et al.: Hemodialysis intravascular hemolysis and kinked blood lines. Nephron 62(3), 267–271 (1992)

Gejyo, F., Yamada, T., Odani, S., et al.: A new form of amyloid protein associated with hemodialysis was identified as ß2-microglobulin. Biochem. Biophys. Res. Commun. 129(3), 701–706 (1985)

Gerard, C., Hugli, T.: Identification of classical anaphylatoxin as the des-Arg form of the C5a molecule: evidence of a modulator role for the oligosaccharide unit in human des-Arg C5a. Proc. Natl. Acad. Sci. U.S.A 78(3), 1833–1837 (1981)

Ghysen, J., De Plaen, J.F., van Ypersele de Strihou, C.: The effect of membrane characteristics on tumour necrosis factor kinetics during haemodialysis. Nephrol. Dial. Transplant. 5(4), 270–274 (1990)

Girndt, M., Lengler, S., Kaul, H., et al.: Prospective crossover trial of the influence of vitamin E-coated dialyzer membranes on T-cell activation and cytokine induction. Am. J. Kidney Dis. 35(1), 95–104 (2000)

Göhl, H., Buck, R., Strathmann, H.: Basic features of the polyamide membranes. Contrib. Nephrol. 96, 1–25 (1992)

Goldstein, I.M., Brai, M., Osler, A.G., Weissmann, G.: Lysosomal enzyme release from human leukocytes: mediation by the alternative pathway of complement activation. J. Immunol. 111(1), 33–37 (1973)

Gorevic, P.D., Casey, T.T., Stone, W.J., et al.: Beta-2 microglobulin is an amyloidogenic protein in man. J. Clin. Invest. 76(6), 2425–2429 (1985)

Graeber, C.W., Halley, S.E., Lapkin, R.A., et al.: Protein Losses with Reused Dialyzers. J. Am. Soc. Nephrol. 4, 349 (1993)

Graf, H., Stummvoll, H.K., Haber, P., Kovarik, J.: Pathophysiology of dialysis related hypoxaemia. Proc. Eur. Dial. Transplant. Assoc. 17, 155–161 (1980)

Green, D., Santhanam, S., Krumlovsky, F.A., del Greco, F.: Elevated B-thromboglobulin in patients with chronic renal failure. J. Lab. Clin. Med. 95(5), 679–685 (1980)

Greene, W., Bohaleim, E., Siekavitz, M., et al.: Structure and regulation of the human IL-2 receptor. Adv. Exp. Med. Biol. 254, 55–60 (1989)

Gutch, C., Eskelson, C., Ziegler, E., et al.: 2-chloroethanol as a toxic residue in dialysis supplies sterilized with ethylene oxide. Dial. Transplant. 5, 21–25 (1976)

Gutierrez, A., Alvestrand, A., Wahren, J., Bergström, J.: Effect of in vivo contact between blood and dialysis membranes on protein catabolism in humans. Kidney Int. 38(3), 487–494 (1990)

Haeffner-Cavaillon, N., Cavaillon, J.M., Ciancioni, C., et al.: In vivo induction of interleukin-1 during hemodialysis. Kidney Int. 35(5), 1212–1218 (1989)

Hakim, R.M., Lowrie, E.G.: Hemodialysis-associated neutropenia and hypoxemia: the effect of dialyzer membrane materials. Nephron 32(1), 32–39 (1982)

Hakim, R.M., Breillatt, J., Lazarus, J.M., Port, F.K.: Complement activation and hypersensivity reactions to dialysis membranes. New Eng. J. Med. 311(14), 878–882 (1984a)

Hakim, R., Fearon, D., Lazarus, J.: Biocompatibility of dialysis membranes: effects of chronic complement activation. Kidney Int. 26(2), 194–200 (1984b)

Hakim, R.M., Schafer, A.I.: Hemodialysis-associated platelet activation and thrombocytopenia. American Journal of Medicine 78(4), 575–580 (1985)

Hakim, R.M., Held, P.J., Stannard, D.C., et al.: Effect of the dialysis membrane on mortality of chronic hemodialysis patients. Kidney Int. 50(2), 566–570 (1996)

Hammerschmidt, D., Harris, P., Wayland, J., et al.: Complement-induced granulocyte aggregation in vivo. Amer. Jour. Pathol. 102(2), 146–150 (1981)

Harrison, P., Jansson, K., Kronenberg, H., et al.: Cold agglutinin formation in patients undergoing hemodialysis: a possible relationship to dialyzer reuse. Aust. NZ J. Med. 5(3), 195–197 (1975)

Heidland, A., Horl, W., Heller, N., et al.: Proteolytic enzymes and catabolism: enhanced release of granulocyte proteinase in uremic intoxication and during hemodialysis. Kidney Int. Suppl. suppl. 16, S27–S36 (1983)

Henderson, L.W., Miller, M.E., Hamilton, R.W., Norman, M.E.: Hemodialysis leukopenia and polymorph random mobility - a possible correlation. J. Lab. Clin. Med. 85(2), 191–197 (1975)

Henderson, L., Cheung, A., Chenoweth, D.: Choosing a membrane. Am. J. Kid. Dis. 3(1), 5–20 (1983a)

Henderson, L.W., Koch, K.M., Dinarello, C.A., et al.: Hemodialysis hypotension: the interleukin-1 hypothesis. Blood Purif. 1, 3–8 (1983b)

Henne, W., Duenweg, G., Bandel, W.: A New Cellulose Membrane Generation for hemodialysis and hemofiltration. Artificial Organs 3, 466–469 (1979)

Herbelin, A., Nguyen, A.T., Zingraff, J., et al.: Influence of uremia and hemodialysis on circulating interleukin-1 and tumor necrosis factor alpha. Kidney Int. 37(1), 116–125 (1990)

Herbelin, A., Urena, P., Nguyen, A., et al.: Elevated circulating levels of interleukin-6 in patients with chronic renal failure. Kidney International 39(5), 954–960 (1991)

Himmelfarb, J., Ault, K., Holbrook, D., et al.: Intradialytic granulocyte reactive oxygen species production: a prospective, crossover trial. J. Am. Soc. Nephrol. 4(2), 178–186 (1993)

Hobbs, M.V., Feldbush, T.L., Needleman, B.W., Weiler, J.M.: Inhibition of secondary in vitro antibody responses by the third compoment of complement. J. Immunol. 128(3), 1470–1475 (1981)

Hoenich, N.A.: Membranes for dialysis: can we do without them? Int. J. Artif. Organs 30, 964–970 (2007)

Holmes, C., Evans, R., Ross, D., et al.: Plasma IL-1 and TNF levels during high-flux hemodialysis with cellulose triacetate membranes. Kidney Int. 37, 301 (1990)

Horl, W.H., Heidland, A.: Evidence for the participation of granulocyte proteinases on intradialytic catabolism. Clin. Nephrol. 21(6), 314–322 (1984)

Horl, W.H., Schaefer, R.M., Heidland, A.: Effect of different dialyzers on proteinases and proteinase inhibitors during hemodialysis. Am. J. Nephrol. 5(5), 320–326 (1985)

Horl, W.H., Riegel, W., Schollmeyer, P., et al.: Different complement and granulocyte activation in patients dialyzed with PMMA dialyzers. Clin. Nephrol. 25(6), 304–307 (1986)

Horl, W., Steinhauer, H., Riegel, W., et al.: Effect of different dialyzer membranes on plasma levels of granulocyte elastase. Kidney Int. suppl. 24, S90–S91 (1988)

Hornberger, J.C., Chernew, M., Petersen, J., Garber, A.M.: A multivariate analysis of mortality and hospital admissions with high-flux dialysis. J. Am. Soc. Nephrol. 3(6), 1227–1237 (1992)

Hugli, T.: The structural basis for anaphylatoxin and chemotactic functions of C3a, C4a, and C5a. Crit. Rev. Immunol. 1(4), 321–366 (1981)

Iatrou, C., Afentakis, N., Antonopoulou, S., et al.: The production of platelet-activating factor (PAF) during hemodialysis with cuprophane membrane. Does the calcium concentration in the dialysate play any role on it? Int. J. Artif. Organs 18(7), 355–361 (1995)

Iatrou, C., Afentakis, N., Nomikos, T., et al.: Is platelet-activating factor produced during hemodialysis with AN-69 polyacrylonitrile membrane? Nephron 91(1), 86–93 (2002)

Ing, T.S., Daugirdas, J.T., Popli, S., Gandhi, V.C.: First use syndrome with cuprammonium cellulose dialyzers. Int. J. Artif. Organs 6(5), 235–239 (1983)

Ireland, H., Lane, D., Curtis, J.: Objective assessment of heparin requirements for hemodialysis in human. J. Lab. Clin. Med. 103(4), 643–652 (1984)

Ivanovich, P., Chenoweth, D.E., Schmidt, R., et al.: Symptoms and activation of granulocytes and complement with two dialysis membranes. Kidney Int. 24(6), 758–763 (1983)

Jaber, B., Pereira, B.: Biocompatibility of Hemodialysis Membranes. In: Pereira, B., Sayegh, M., Blake, P. (eds.) Chronic Kidney Disease, Dialysis, & Transplantation. Companion to Brenner & Rector's the Kidney, 2nd edn. Elsevier Saunders, Philadelphia (2005)

Jaber, B.L., Balakrishnan, V.S., Cendoroglo, M.N., et al.: Apoptosis-inducing activity of uremic plasma during hemodialysis. Blood Purif. 16(6), 325–335 (1999)

Jaber, B.L., Cendoroglo, M., Balakrishnan, V.S., et al.: Apoptosis of leukocytes: basic concepts and implications in uremia. Kidney Int. suppl. 78, S197–S205 (2001)

Johnson, A., Hugli, T., Mulloer-Eberhard, H.: Release of histamine from mast cells by the complement peptides C3a and C5a. Immunology 28(6), 1067–1080 (1975)

Jones, R., Broadfield, J., Parsons, V.: Arterial hypoxemia during hemodialysis for acute renal failure in mechanically ventilated patients: observations and mechanisms. Clin. Nephrol. 14(1), 18–22 (1980)

Jorstad, S., Smeby, L.C., Balstad, T., Widerøe, T.E.: Removal, generation and adsorption of beta-2-microglobulin during hemofiltration with five different membranes. Blood Purif. 6(2), 96–105 (1988)

Kaplan, K., Owen, J.: Plasma levels of B-thromboglobulin and platelet factor 4 as indices of platelet activation in vivo. Blood 57(2), 199–202 (1981)

Kaplow, L., Goffinet, J.: Profound neutropenia during the early phase of hemodialysis. JAMA 203(13), 1135–1137 (1968)

Kay, N., Raij, L.: Immune abnormalities in renal failure in hemodialysis. Blood Purif. 4(1-3), 120–129 (1986)

Kay, N., Raij, L.: Differential effect of hemodialysis membranes on human lymphocyte natural killer function. Artif. Organs 11(2), 165–167 (1987)

Key, J., Nahmias, M., Acchiardo, S.: Hypersentivity reactions on first-time exposure to cucrophan hollow fiber dialyzer. Am. J. Kidney Dis. 2(6), 664–666 (1983)

Kim, S.: Platelet adhesion and prevention at blood polymer interface. Artificial Organs 11(3), 228–236 (1987)

Kjellstrand, P., Okmark, P., Odselius, R., et al.: Adherence of blood cells to dialyzer membranes as a measure of biocompatibility. Int. J. Artif. Organs 14(11), 698–702 (1991)

Klempner, M., Gallin, J., Balow, J., et al.: The effect of hemodialysis and C5ades arg on neutrophil subpopulations. Blood 55(5), 777–783 (1980)

Klinke, B., Rockel, A., Perschel, W., et al.: Beta-2-microglobulin adsorption and release in-vitro: influence of membrane material, osmolality and heparin. Int. J. Artif. Organs 11(5), 355–360 (1988)

Konstantin, P.: Newer membranes: cuprophane versus polysulfone versus polyacrylonitrile. In: Bosch, J., Stein, J. (eds.) Hemodialysis: High Efficiency Treatments. Churchill Livingstone, New York (1993)

Kozin, F., Cochrane, C.: The contact activation system of plasma: biochemistry and pathophysiology. In: Gallin, J., Goldstein, I., Snyderman, R. (eds.) Inflammation: Basic Principles and Clinical Correlates. Raven Press, New York (1988)

Kuragano, T., Kuno, T., Takahashi, Y., et al.: Comparison of the effects of cellulose triacetate and polysulfone membrane on GPIIb/IIIa and platelet activation. Blood Purif. 21(2), 176–182 (2003)

Lane, D., Ireland, H., Knight, I., et al.: The significance of fibrinogen derivatives in plasma in human renal failure. Br. J. Haematol. 56(2), 251–260 (1984)

Lee, A., Whyte, M.K.B., Haslett, C.: Inhibition of apoptosis and prolongation of neutrophil functional longevity by inflammatory mediators. J. Leukoc. Biol. 54(4), 283–288 (1993)

Lemke, H., Fink, E.: Accumulation of bradykinin generation formed by the AN69- or PAN 17DX-membrane is due to the presence of an ACE-inhibitor in vitro. J. Am. Soc. Nephrol. 3, 376(A) (1992)

Lemke, H., Eisenhauer, T., Krieter, D.: Generation of bradykinin, hypotension and anaphylactoid shock during hemodialysis. J. Am. Soc. Nephrol. 4, 362(A) (1993)

Lepow I, Willms-Kretschmer K, Patrick R, et al (1970) Gross and ultrastructural observations on lesions produced by intradermal injection of human C3a in man. Am J Pathol.; 61(1):13-24.

Levin, N.W., Zasuwa, G., Dumler, F.: Effect of membrane type on causes of death in hemodialysis patients. J. Am. Soc. Nephrol. 2, 335 (1991)

Lewis, K., Dewar, P., Ward, M.: Formation of anti-N-like antibodies in dialysis patients: effect of different methods of dialyzer rinsing remove formaldehyde. Clinical Nephrology 15(1), 39–43 (1981)

Liles, W.C., Klebanoff, S.J.: Regulation of apoptosis in neutrophils–Fas track to death? J. Immunol. 155(7), 3289–3291 (1995)

Lim, V., Bier, D., Flanigan, M., Sum-Ping, S.: The effect of hemodialysis on protein metabolism: a leucine kinetic study. J. Clin. Invest. 91(6), 2419–2436 (1993)

Lindner, A., Farewell, B., Sherrard, D.: High incidence of neoplasia in uremic patients receiving long term dialysis. Nephron 27(6), 292–296 (1981)

Lindsay, R.M., Ferguson, D., Prentice, C.R., et al.: Reduction of thrombus formation on dialyzer membranes by aspirin and RA 233. Lancet 300(7790), 1287–1290 (1972)

Lindsay, R.: Practical use of anticoagulant. In: Drukker, W., Parsons, F., Maher, J. (eds.) Replacement of Renal Function by Dialysis. Martinus Nijhoff, Boston (1983)

Linke, R., Hampl, H., Lobeck, H., et al.: Lysine-specific cleavage of B2-microglobulin in amyloid deposits associated with hemodialysis. Kidney Int. 36(4), 675–681 (1989)

Lonnemann, G., Bingel, M., Koch, K.M., et al.: Plasma interleukin-1 activity in humans undergoing hemodialysis with regenerated cellulosic membranes. Lymphokine Res. 6(2), 63–70 (1987)

Lonnemann, G., Binge, M., Floege, J., et al.: Detection of endotoxin-like interleukin-1-inducing activity during in vitro dialysis. Kidney Int. 33(1), 29–35 (1988a)

Lonnemann, G., Koch, K.M., Shaldon, S., Dinarello, C.A.: Studies on the ability of hemodialysis membranes to induce, bind, and clear human interleukin-1. J. Lab. Clin. Med. 112(1), 76–86 (1988b)

Lonnemann, G., Haubitz, M., Schindler, R.: Hemodialysis-associated induction of cytokines. Blood Purif. 8(4), 214–222 (1990)

Lonnemann, G., Behme, T.C., Lenzner, B., et al.: Permeability of dialyzer membranes to TNF alpha-inducing substances derived from water bacteria. Kidney Int. 42(1), 61–68 (1992)

Lonnemann, G., Mahiout, A., Schindler, R., et al.: Pyrogen retention by the polyamide membranes. In: Shaldon, S., Koch, K.M. (eds.) The Polyamide Membrane. Contr. Nephrol., vol. 96, pp. 47–63 (1992)

Lucchi, L., Iannone, A., Bergamini, S., et al.: Comparison between hydroperoxides and malondialdehyde as markers of acute oxidative injury during hemodialysis. Artif. Organs 29(10), 832–837 (2005)

Luger, A., Kovarik, J., Stummvoll, H.K., et al.: Blood-membrane interaction in hemodialysis leads to increased cytokine production. Kidney Int. 32(1), 84–88 (1987)

Lyman, D.: Membranes. In: Drukker, W., Parsons, F., Maher, J. (eds.) Replacement of Renal Function by Dialysis. Martinus Nijhoff, Boston (1983)

Lysaght, M.: Evolution of hemodialysis membranes. Contrib. Nephrol. 113, 1–10 (1995)

MacDougall, M., Diedrich, D., Wiegmann, T.: Dissociation of hemodialysis leukopenia and hypoxemia from complement changes during citrate anticoagulation. Kidney Int. 27, 166 (1985)

Macleod, A.M., Campbell, M., Cody, J.D., et al.: Cellulose, modified cellulose and synthetic membranes in the haemodialysis of patients with end-stage renal disease. Cochrane Database Syst. Rev. (3), Art. No.: CD003234 (2005), doi:10.1002/14651858.CD003234.pub2

Maggiore, Q., Enia, G., Catalano, C.: Effect of blood cooling on cucrophan induced anaphylatoxin generation. Kidney Int. 32, 908–911 (1987)

Mahajan, S., Gardiner, H., DeTar, B., et al.: Relationship between pulmonary functions and hemodialysis induced leukopenia. Trans. Am. Soc. Artif. Int. Organs 23, 411–415 (1977)

Maher, E., Wickens, D., Griffin, J., et al.: Increased free-radical activity during hemodialysis. Nephrol. Dial. Transplant. 2(3), 169–171 (1987)

Marshall, J.W., Ahearn, D.J., Nothum, R.J., et al.: Adherence of blood components to dialyzer membranes: Morphological studies. Nephron 12(3), 157–170 (1974)

Mason, R.G., Zucker, W.H., Bilinsky, R.T., et al.: Blood components deposited on used and reused dialysis membranes. Biomat. Med. Dev. Art. Org. 4(3-4), 333–358 (1976)

Memoli, B., Rampino, T., Libetta, C., et al.: Peripheral blood leukocytes interleukin-6 production in uremic hemodialyzed patients (Abstract). J. Am. Soc. Nephrol. 1, 369 (1990)

Meuer, S.C., Hauer, M., Kurz, P., et al.: Selective blockade of the antigen-receptor-mediated pathway of T cell activation in patients with impaired primary immune responses. J. Clin. Invest. 80(3), 743–749 (1987)

Mingardi, G., Vigano, G., Massazza, M.: Polyacrylonitrile membranes for hemodialysis: Long term effect on primary hemostatis. In: Smeby, L., Jorstad, S., Wideroe, T. (eds.) Immune and Metabolic Aspects of Therapeutic Blood Purification Systems. Karger, Basel (1985)

Miura, Y., Ishiyama, T., Inomata, A., et al.: Radiolucent bone cysts and the type of dialysis membrane used in patients undergoing long-term hemodialysis. Nephron 60(3), 268–273 (1992)

Miyaya, T., Oda, O., Inagi, R., et al.: B_2-microglobulin modified with advanced glycation end products is a major component of hemodialysis-associated amyloidosis. J. Clin. Invest. 92(3), 1243–1252 (1993)

Mohammed, S., Whitworth, C., Chuang, H., et al.: Multiple active forms of thrombin: Binding to platelets and effects on platelet function. Proc. Natl. Acad. Sci. USA 73(5), 1660–1663 (1976)

Morrison, J., Wilson, A., Vaziri, N., et al.: Determination of pulmonary tissue volume, pulmonary capillary blood flow and diffusing capacity lung before and after hemodialysis. Int. J. Artif. Organs 3(5), 259–262 (1980)

Mourad, A., Carney, S., Gillies, A., et al.: Acute effect of haemodialysis on arterial stiffness: membrane bioincompatibility? Nephrol. Dial. Transplant. 19(11), 2797–2802 (2004)

Muller-Eberhard, H.: Complement: Chemistry and pathways. In: Gallin, J., Goldstein, I., Snyderman, R. (eds.) Inflammation: Basic Principles and Clinical Correlates. Raven Press, New York (1988)

Nath, N., Niewiarowski, S., Joist, J.H.: Platelet factor 4: Antiheparin protein releasable from platelets: Purification and properties. J. Lab. Clin. Med. 82(5), 754–768 (1973)

Needleman, B.W., Weiler, J.M., Feldbush, T.L.: The third component of complement inhibits human lymphocyte blastogenesis. J. Immunol. 126(4), 1586–1591 (1981)

Nicholls, A.J., Platts, M.J.: Anaphylactoid reactions during hemodialysis are due to ethylene oxide hypersensitivity. Proc. Eur. Dial. Transplant. Assoc. Eur. Ren. Assoc. 21, 173–177 (1985)

Oettinger, C.W., Powell, A.C., Bland, L.A., et al.: Enhanced release of tumor necrosis factor alpha but not interleukin-1 beta by uremic blood stimulated with endotoxin (Abstract). J. Am. Soc. Nephrol. 1, 370 (1990)

Ogawa, H., Saito, A., Oda, O., et al.: Detection of novel beta 2-microglobulin in the serum of hemodialysis patients and its amyloidogenic predisposition. Clin. Nephrol. 30(3), 158–163 (1988)

Ogden, D.: New-dialyzer syndrome. New England J. Med. 302, 1262–1263 (1980)

Oh, M.S., Uribarri, J., Del Monte, M.L., et al.: A mechanism of hypoxemia during hemodialysis. Consumption of CO_2 in metabolism of acetate. Am. J. Nephrol. 5(5), 366–371 (1985)

Ohashi, K., Hara, M., Kawai, R., et al.: Cervical discs are most susceptible to beta 2-microglobulin amyloid deposition in the vertebral column. Kidney International 41(6), 1646–1652 (1992)

Okusawa, S., Gelfand, J.A., Ikejima, T., et al.: Interleukin 1 induces a shock-like state in rabbits: synergism with tumor necrosis factor and the effect of cyclooxygenase inhibiton. J. Clin. Invest. 81(4), 1162–1172 (1988)

Ouseph, R., Hutchison, C.A., Ward, R.A.: Differences in solute removal by two high-flux membranes of nominally similar synthetic polymers. Nephrol. Dial. Transplant. 23(5), 1704–1712 (2008)

Pavlopoulou, G., Perzanowski, C., Hakim, R.: Platelet aggregation studies during dialysis. Kidney Int. 29, 221(A) (1986)

Pereira, B.J., Dinarello, C.A.: Production of cytokines and cytokine inhibitory proteins in patients on dialysis. Nephrol. Dial. Transplant. 9(2), 60–71 (1994)

Pereira, B.J., Shapiro, L., King, A.J., et al.: Plasma levels of IL-1 beta, TNF alpha and their specific inhibitors in undialyzed chronic renal failure, CAPD and hemodialysis patients. Kidney Int. 45(3), 890–896 (1994)

Pereira BJ, Dinarello CA (1995) Role of cytokines in patients on dialysis [editorial]. Int J Artif Organs; 18(6):293-304.

Pereira, B.J.G., Snodgrass, B.R., Hogan, P.J., et al.: Diffusive and convective transfer of cytokine-inducing bacterial products across hemodialysis membranes. Kidney Int. 47(2), 603–610 (1995)

Perianayagam, M.C., Balakrishnan, V.S., King, A.J., et al.: C5a delays apoptosis of human neutrophils by a phosphatidyl inositol 3-kinase-signaling pathway. Kidney Int. 61(2), 456–463 (2002)

Pertosa, G., Grandaliano, G., Soccio, M., et al.: Vitamin E-modified filters modulate Jun N-terminal kinase activation in peripheral blood mononuclear cells. Kidney Int. 62(2), 602–610 (2002)

Peterson, J., Hyver, S., Cajias, J.: Backfiltration During Dialysis: A Critical Assessment. Seminars in Dialysis 5(1), 13–16 (1992)

Poothullil, J., Shimizu, A., Day, R.P., Dolovich, J.: Anaphylaxis from the product(s) of ethylene oxide gas. Ann. Intern. Med. 82(1), 58–60 (1975)

Popli, S., Ing, T., Daugirdas, J.: Severe reactions to cucrophan capillary dialyzers. Artif. Organs 6, 312–315 (1982)

Port, F.K., Ragheb, N.E., Schwartz, A.G., Hawthorne, V.M.: Neoplasms in dialysis patients: a population-based study. Am. J. Kidney Dis. 14(2), 119–123 (1989)

Powell, A., Bland, L., Oettinger, C., et al.: Lack of plasma interleukin-1 beta or tumor necrosis factor-alpha elevation during unfavorable hemodialysis conditions. J. Am. Soc. Nephrol. 2(5), 1007–1013 (1991)

Radovich, J.: Composition of polymer membranes for therapies of end-stage renal disease. Contrib. Nephrol. 113, 11–24 (1995)

Rault, R., Silver, M.R.: Severe reactions during hemodialysis. Am. J. Kidney Dis. 5(2), 128–131 (1985)

Raz, A., Wyche, A., Siegel, N., Needleman, P.: Regulation of fibroblast cyclooxygenase synthesis by interleukin-1. J. Biol. Chem. 263(6), 3022–3028 (1988)

Ritz, E., Bommer, J.: Beta-2-microglobulin derived amyloid–problems and perspectives. Blood Purif. 6(2), 61–68 (1988)

Romao, J.E.J., Abensur, H., Castro, M.C.M., et al.: Effect of biocompatibility on recovery from acute renal failure after cadaveric renal transplantation [abstract]. J. Am. Soc. Nephrol. 9, 181A (1998)

Ronco, C., Orlandini, G., Brendolan, A., et al.: Enhancement of convective transport by internal filtration in a modified experimental hemodialyzer: technical note. Kidney Int. 54(3), 979–985 (1998)

Ronco, C., Bowry, S.K., Brendolan, A., et al.: Hemodialyzer: from macrodesign to membrane nanostructure; the case of the FX-class of hemodialyzers. Kidney Int. suppl. 80, 126–142 (2002a)

Ronco, C., Brendolan, A., Crepaldi, C., et al.: Blood and dialysate flow distributions in hollowfiber hemodialyzers analyzed by computerized helical scanning technique. J. Am. Soc. Nephrol. 13(Suppl. 1), S53–S61 (2002b)

Ronco, C., Levin, N., Brendolan, A., et al.: Flow distribution analysis by helical scanning in polysulfone hemodialyzers: effects of fiber structure and design on flow patterns and solute clearances. Hemodial. Int. 10(4), 380–388 (2006)

Ryan, J., Beynon, H., Rees, A.J., et al.: Evaluation of the in vitro production of tumour necrosis factor by monocytes in dialysis patients. Blood Purif. 9(3), 142–147 (1991)

Rysz, J., Stolarek, R.A., Pedzik, A., et al.: Increased exhaled H_2O_2 and impaired lung function in patients undergoing bioincompatible hemodialysis. Int. J. Artif. Organs 30(10), 879–888 (2007)

Sacks, T., Moldow, C.F., Craddock, P.R., et al.: Oxygen radicals mediate endothelial cell damage by complement-stimulated granulocytes. J. Clin. Invest. 61(5), 1161–1167 (1978)

Salama, A., Hugo, F., Heinrick, D., et al.: Deposition of terminal C5b-9 complement complexes on erythrocytes and leukocytes during cardiopulmonary bypass. New Engl. J. Med. 318(7), 408–414 (1988)

Salter, M.C., Crow, M.J., Donaldson, D.R., et al.: Prevention of platelet deposition and thrombus formation on hemodialysis membranes: a double-blind randomized trial of aspirin and dipyridamole. Artif. Organs 8(1), 57–61 (1984)

Salzman, E.: Role of platelets in blood-surface interactions. Fed. Proc. 30(5), 1503–1508 (1971)

Sato, H., Ohkubo, M., Nagaoka, T.: Levels of serum colony-stimulating factors (CSFs) in patients on long-term haemodialysis. Cytokine 6(2), 187–194 (1994)

Schaefer, R., Heidland, A., Horl, W.: Effect of dialyzer geometry on granulocyte and complement activation. Am. J. Nephrol. 7(2), 121–126 (1987)

Schindler, R., Gelfand, J., Dinarello, C.: Recombitant C5a stimulates transcription rather than translation of IL-1 and TNF: priming of mononuclear cells with recombitant C5a enhances cytokine synthesis
induced by LPS, IL-1 or PMA. Blood 76, 1631–1635 (1990a)

Schindler, R., Lonnemann, G., Shaldon, S., et al.: Transcription, not synthesis, of interleukin-1 and tumor necrosis factor by complement.
Kidney Int. 37(1), 85–93 (1990b)

Schindler, R., Linnenweber, S., Shulze, M., et al.: Gene expression of in-
terleukin-1β during hemodialysis. Kidney Int. 43(3), 712–721
(1993)

Schohn, D.C., Jahn, H.A., Eber, M., Hauptmann, G.: Biocompatibility and
hemodynamic studies during polycarbonate versus cuprophan
membrane dialysis. Blood Purif. 4(1-3), 102–111 (1986)

Schulman, G., Fogo, A., Gung, A., et al.: Complement activation retards
resolution of acute ischemic renal failure in the rat. Kidney
Int. 40(6), 1069–1074 (1991)

Schulman, G., Hakim, R., Arias, R., et al.: Bradykinin generation by dialysis membranes: possible role in anaphylactic reaction. J. Am. Soc.
Nephrol. 3(9), 1563–1569 (1993)

Schweizer, A., Feige, U., Fontana, A., et al.: Interleukin-1 enhances pain
reflexes. Mediation through increased prostaglandin E2 levels.
Agents Actions 25(3-4), 246–251 (1988)

Showell, H., Glovsky, M., Ward, P.: Morphological changes in human polymorphonuclear leukocytes induced by Ca3 in the presence and
absence of cytochalasin. Int. Arch. Allergy Appl. Immunol. 69(1),
62–67 (1982)

Silber, R., Moldow, C.: Biochemistry and function of neutrophils, composition of neutrophils. In: Williams, W., Brutler, E., Erslev, A., et
al. (eds.) Hematology. McGraw-Hill, New York (1983)

Simon, P., Ang, K., Cam, G.: Enhanced platelet aggregation and membrane biocompatibility: possible influence on thrombosis and embolism in hemodialysis patients. Nephron 45(2), 172–173 (1987)

Smeby, L.C., Widerøe, T.E., Balstad, T., Jørstad, S.: Biocompatibility aspects of cellophane, cellulose acetate, polyacrylonitrile, polysulfone and polycarbonate hemodialyzers. Blood Purif. 4(1-3), 93–
101 (1986)

Smith, M.C., Danviriyasup, K., Crow, J.W., et al.: Prostacyclin substitution for heparin in long-term hemodialysis. Am. J. Med. 73(5),
669–678 (1982)

Sosa, M.A., Balk, E.M., Lau, J., et al.: A systematic review of the effect of
the Excebrane dialyser on biomarkers of lipid peroxidation. Nephrol. Dial. Transplant. 21(10), 2825–2833 (2006)

Spagnuolo, P.J., Bass, S.H., Smith, M.C., et al.: Neutrophil adhesiveness during prostacyclin and heparin hemodialysis. Blood 60(4), 924–929 (1982)

Speiser, W., Wojta, J., Korninger, C., et al.: Enhanced fibrinolysis caused by tissue plasminogen activator release in hemodialysis. Kidney Int. 32(2), 280–283 (1987)

Spencer, P., Schmidt, B., Samtleben, W., et al.: Ex vivo model of hemodialysis membrane biocompatibility. Trans. Am. Soc. Artif. Internal. Organs 31, 495–498 (1985)

Sreeharan, N., Crow, M.J., Salter, M.C., et al.: Membrane effect on platelet function during hemodialysis: a comparison of cuprophan and polycarbonate. Artif. Organs 6(3), 324–327 (1982)

Stimler, N.P., Bach, M.K., Bloor, C.M., Hugli, T.E.: Release of leukotrienes from guinea pig lung stimulated by $C5a_{des\ Arg}$ anaphylatoxin. J. Immunol. 128(5), 2247–2252 (1982)

Stimler-Gerard, N.: Immunopharmacology of anaphylatoxin-induced bronchoconstrictor responses. Complement 3, 137–151 (1986)

Streicher, E., Schneider, H.: The development of a polysulfone membrane. A new perspective in dialysis. Contrib. Nephrol. 46, 1–13 (1985)

Stuard, S., Carreno, M.P., Poignet, J.L., et al.: A major role for CD62P/CD15s interaction in leukocyte margination during hemodialysis. Kidney Int. 48(1), 93–102 (1995)

Sweet, S.J., McCarthy, S., Steingart, R., Callahan, T.: Hemolytic reactions mechanically induced by kinked hemodialysis lines. Am. J. Kidney Dis. 27(2), 262–266 (1996)

Tielemans, C., Goldman, M., Vanherweghem, J.: Immediate hypersensitivity reactions and hemodialysis. Adv. Nephrol. Necker Hosp. 22, 401–416 (1993)

Till, G.O., Johnson, K.J., Kunkel, R., Ward, P.A.: Intravascular activation of complement and acute lung injury. J. Clin. Invest. 69(5), 1126–1135 (1982)

Tokars, J.I., Alter, M.J., Favero, M.S., et al.: National surveillance of hemodialysis associated diseases in the United States. ASAIO J. 39(1), 71–80 (1990)

Urena, P., Gogusev, J., Valdovinos, R., et al.: Transcriptional induction of TNF-alpha in uremic patients undergoing hemodialysis (Abstract). J. Am. Soc. Nephrol. 1, 380 (1990)

Urena, P., Herbelin, A., Zingraff, J., et al.: Permeability of cellulosic and non-cellulosic membranes to endotoxins and cytokine production. Nephrol. Dial. Transplant. 7(1), 16–28 (1992)

United States Renal Data System (USRDS 2004) Annual Data Report: Atlas of End-Stage Renal Disease in the United States. National Institutes of Health, National Institute of Diabetes and Digestive and Kidney Diseases, Bethesda, MD (2004)

Valeri, A.: Biocompatible membranes in acute renal failure: a study in post-cadaveric renal ransplant acute tubular necrosis. J. Am. Soc. Nephrol. 3, 481 (1994)

van Ypersele de Strihou, C., Jadoul, M., Malghem, J., et al.: Effect of dialysis membrane and patient's age on signs of dialysis-related amyloidosis. The Working Party on Dialysis Amyloidosis. Kidney Int. 39(5), 1012–1019 (1991)

Vanholder, R., Ringoir, S., Dhondt, A., Hakim, R.: Phagocytosis in uremic and hemodialysis patients: a prospective and cross sectional study. Kidney Int. 39(2), 320–327 (1991)

Vaziri, N., Barton, C., Warner, A., et al.: Comparision of four dialyzer-dialysate combinations: effects on blood gases, cell counts, complement contact factors and fibrinolytic system. Contr. Nephrol. 37, 111–119 (1984a)

Vaziri, N., Toohey, J., Paule, P., et al.: Effect of hemodialysis on contact group of coagulation factors, platelets, and leukocytes. Am. J. Med. 77(3), 437–441 (1984b)

Vicks, S.L., Gross, M.L., Schmitt, G.W.: Massive hemorrhage due to hemodialysis-associated thrombocytopenia. Am. J. Nephrol. 3(1), 30–33 (1983)

Vienken, J., Diamantoglou, M., Hahn, C., et al.: Considerations on development aspects of biocompatible dialysis membranes. Artif. Organs 19(5), 398–406 (1995)

Vilcek, J., Le, J.: Immunology of cytokines: An introduction. In: Thomson, A. (ed.) The Cytokine Handbook. Academic Press, San Diego (1991)

Villarroel, F., Ciarkowski, A.: A survey on hypersensitivity reactions in hemodialysis. Artif. Organs 9(3), 231–238 (1985)

Vincent, C., Chanard, J., Caudwell, V., et al.: Kinetics of 125I-beta 2-microglobulin turnover in dialyzed patients. Kidney Int. 42(6), 1434–1443 (1992)

Vroman, L., Adams, A., Klings, M.: Interactions among human blood proteins at interfaces. Fed. Proc. 30(5), 1494–1502 (1971)

Walker, J., Lindsay, R., Peters, S., et al.: A sheep model to examine the cardiopulmonary manifestations of blood-dialyzer interactions. Am. Soc. Artif. Internal. Organs 6, 123–130 (1983)

Wanner, C., Bahner, U., Mattern, R., et al.: Effect of dialysis flux and membrane material on dyslipidaemia and inflammation in haemodialysis patients. Nephrol. Dial. Transplant. 19(10), 2570–2575 (2004)

Weiss, S., Regiani, S.: Neutrophils degrade subendothelial matrices in the present of alpha-1-proteinase inhibitor: cooperative use of lysosomal proteinases and oxygen metabolitews. Clin. Invest. 73(5), 1297–1303 (1984)

Wilflingseder, J., Perco, P., Kainz, A., et al.: Biocompatibility of haemodialysis membranes determined by gene expression of human leucocytes: a crossover study. Eur. J. Clin. Invest. 38(12), 918–924 (2008)

Wilhelmson, S., Asaba, H., Gunnarsson, B., et al.: Measurement of fibrinopeptide A in the evaluation of heparin activity and fibrin formation during hemodialysis. Clin. Nephrol. 15(5), 252–258 (1981)

Wilhelmson, S., Ivemark, C., Kudryk, B., et al.: Thrombin activity during hemodialysis: evaluated by the fibrinopeptide A assay: A comparison between a high and a low heparin dose regimen. Throm. Res. 31(5), 685–693 (1983)

Wissow, L., Covenberg, R., Burns, R.: Altered leukocyte chemiluminescence during dialysis. J. Clin. Immunol. 1(4), 262–265 (1981)

Woo, Y., King, B., Junor, B., et al.: Dialysis with biocompatible membranes may delay recovery of graft function following renal transplantation. J. Am. Soc. Nephrol. 9, 719 (1998)

Wright, D., Gallin, J.: Secretroy responses of human neutrophils: Exocytosis of specific (secondary) granules by human neutrophils during adherence in vitro and during exudation in vivo. J. Immunol. 123(1), 285–294 (1979)

Yamamoto, K., Matsuda, M., Hirano, A., et al.: Computational evaluation of dialysis fluid flow in dialyzers with variously designed jackets. Artif. Organs 33(6), 481–486 (2009)

Yancey, K., Hammer, C., Harvath, L., et al.: Studies of human C5a as a mediator of inflammation in normal human skin. J. Clin. Invest. 75(2), 486–495 (1985)

Yokoyama, H., Kawaguchi, T., Wada, T., et al.: Biocompatibility and permeability of dialyzer membranes do not affect anemia, erythropoietin dosage or mortality in japanese patients on chronic nonreuse hemodialysis: a prospective cohort study from the J-DOPPS II study. Nephron Clin. Pract. 109(2), c100–c108 (2008)

Zaoui, P.M., Stone, W.J., Hakim, R.M.: Effects of dialysis membranes on beta 2-microglobulin production and cellular expression. Kidney Int. 38(5), 962–968 (1990)

Zaoui, P., Green, W., Hakim, R.M.: Hemodialysis with cuprophane membrane modulates interleukin-2 receptor expression. Kidney Int. 39(5), 1020–1026 (1991)

Zaoui, P., Hakim, R.M.: Natural killer-cell function in hemodialysis patients: effect of the dialysis membrane. Kidney Int. 43(6), 1298–1305 (1993)

Zusman, R.M., Rubin, R.H., Cato, A.E., et al.: Hemodialysis using prostacyclin instead of heparin as the sole antithrombotic agent. N. Engl. J. Med. 304(16), 934–939 (1981)

ESSAY QUESTIONS

1. Classify hemodialysis membrane materials into three major categories according to their chemical structure; and name the most important pathophysiological responses of blood and blood components that come into contact with these membrane types.

2. Are there demonstrable biological effects that can be measured in terms of clinical outcomes in dialysis patients as a result of dialyzer membrane bioincompatibility? If yes, name some of these clinical effects and how they relate to dialyzer membrane bioincompatibility.

3. How is the flux of a hemodialyzer defined?

4. Explain the role that complement activation plays in hemodialyzer bioincompatibility.

5. What are the clinical effects of dialysis-induced monocyte activation?

6. Define the mechanism and possible clinical implications of dialyzer internal filtration and backfiltration.

7. What are the pathophysiologic mechanisms that may contribute to blood clotting in the dialyzer?

8. Explain the pathophysiologic mechanisms involved in transient hemodialysis-associated leukopenia, and its clinical relevance.

9. Is there a link between dialysis membrane bioincompatibility and β_2-microglobulin synthesis and deposition?

10. Is there scientific evidence from clinical trials to support the use of synthetic dialysis membranes in chronic renal failure in order to improve hard clinical outcomes?

MULTIPLE CHOICE QUESTIONS

Choose the best answer

1. A short jacket taper design of a dialyzer improves small solute clearance by...
   A. Enhancing dialysate flow
   B. Enhancing blood flow
   C. Providing the best dialysate and blood contact and least degree of channeling
   D. All of the above

2. Unsubstituted cellulose dialyzers are highly hydrophilic thereby contributing to...
   A. Increased biocompatibility
   B. Reduced biocompatibility
   C. Improved dialyzer performance
   D. Improved large molecule clearance

3. The AN69 dialyzer consists of a copolymer of acrylonitrile and methallyl sulfonate, rendering its membrane...
   A. Negatively charged
   B. Positively charged
   C. Electroneutral

4. Complement activation during hemodialysis does NOT cause...
   A. Neutrophil activation and chemotaxis
   B. Neutrophil endothelial adherence
   C. Vasospasm
   D. T-lymphocyte activation

5. Complement activation is greatest if dialysis is performed with...
   A. Polysulfone membranes
   B. Polycarbonate membranes
   C. Cellulose-acetate membranes
   D. Cuprohan membranes

6. Pulmonary effects of complement activation during hemodialyis do NOT include...
   A. Hypoxemia
   B. Bronchoconstriction (wheezing)
   C. Enhanced ventilaton and perfusion matching
   D. Pulmonary hypertension

7. Hemodialysis with the AN69 membrane induces bradykinin accumulation by...
   A. Facilitating conversion of high molecular weight kininogens into kinins
   B. Inhibiting enzymatic breakdown of bradykinin
   C. Activating angiontensin converting enzyme (ACE)
   D. None of the above

8. Hemodialysis-associated platelet activation may cause...
   A. Release of complement
   B. Induction of tumor necrosis factor-α
   C. Release of thromboxane A_2
   D. All of the above

9. Hemolysis during hemodialysis may be related to...
   A. Complement activation
   B. Pro-inflammatory cytokine release
   C. Circulating anti-N-antibodies
   D. All of the above

10. Hemodialysis-associated leukopenia is most pronounced...
    A. Toward the end of dialysis
    B. 10-15 minutes into the dialysis treatment
    C. Immediately at the end of the dialysis treatment
    D. 2-3 hours into the dialysis treatment

11. Hemodialysis-associated neutrophil degranulation...
    A. Is caused only by complement activation
    B. Does not occur during dialysis with synthetic membranes
    C. May contribute to protein catabolism in dialysis patients
    D. Correlates quantitatively with plasma concentrations of granular proteins

12. Reactive oxygen species during hemodialysis...
    A. Are not an important component of bioincomatibility in hemodialysis
    B. Can be measured in the exhaled alveolar gas mixture
    C. Are generated equally during dialysis with synthetic versus cuprophan membranes
    D. All of the above

13. Neutrophil activation following contact with hemodialysis membrane material...
    A. Improves neutrophil phagocytosis
    B. Reduces neutrophil phagocytosis
    C. Has no effect on neutrophil phagocytosis
    D. Is not associated with serum complement levels

14. Neutrophil apoptosis may be...
    A. Inhibited by hemodalysis with cuprophan membranes
    B. Accelerated by hemodalysis with cuprophan membranes
    C. All of the above
    D. None of the above

15. β_2-microglobulin is...
    A. Effectively removed by high flux dialysis membranes
    B. Effectively removed by high efficiency dialysis membranes
    C. Effectively removed by low-flux hemodialysis membranes
    D. None of the above

16. Dialyzer reactions are characterized by...
    A. Multiple symptoms including but not limited to hypotension, dyspnea, wheezing, nausea or vomiting
    B. Being exclusively associated with hypersensitivity reactions
    C. A usually mild and not life-threatening clinical course
    D. Their exclusive association with unsubstituted cellulose membranes.

17. Patients undergoing long-term hemodialysis...
    A. Are typically not at an increased risk for infectious complications
    B. May have an impaired T-lymphocyte and neutrophil function
    C. Typically show an adequate immune response to immunizations
    D. Display similar degrees of neutrophil dysfunction regardless of the hemodialysis membrane type used

18. Membrane bioincompatibility may...
    A. Contribute to protein catabolism in chronic hemodialysis patients
    B. Enhance protein breakdown through release of proteolytic enzymes from neutrophils activated during hemodialysis
    C. Activate protein catabolism through release of inflammatory cytokines, such as IL-1β
    D. All of the above

19. Membrane choice according to biocompatibility criteria for dialysis in the treatment of acute kidney injury...

    A. Has caused a measurable improvement in clinical outcomes of patients treated with hemodialysis for acute kidney injury

    B. Has been studied in large, well powered prospective randomized clinical trials

    C. Has been shown to impact renal inflammatory responses in animal models of acute kidney injury

    D. All of the above

20. Membrane biocompatibility...

    A. Plays no role in the clinical outcome of patients treated with hemodialysis for chronic renal failure

    B. May impact lipoprotein disorders in chronic hemodialysis patients

    C. Has been shown in a large clinical trial (the HEMO study) to be important for patient outcomes in chronic hemodialysis

    D. And its importance in cardiovascular disease progression in chronic hemodialysis patients is not supported by the evidence.

Chapter (10)

Dialyzer Reprocessing

Wayne Carlson, BS

CHAPTER OUTLINES

- History of dialyzer reprocessing
- Guidance and regulation of dialyzer reprocessing
- Process of dialyzer reprocessing
- Manual and automated reprocessing.
- Advantages and disadvantages of dialyzer reprocessing
- Water Quality
- Anti-N Antibodies
- Changes in ultrafiltration coefficient
- Current controversies
- Conclusion and future developments

CHAPTER OBJECTIVES

- Identify factors in the history of dialyzer reuse that influenced current practice.

- Describe the tasks associated with dialyzer reprocessing.

KEY TERMS

Efficacy
Endotoxin
Formaldehyde
Formalin
Hemodialyzer
High-flux
High-level Disinfectant
Peracetic Acid
Reproces
Reuse
Reverse Ultrafiltration
Sterilant

ABSTRACT

The practice of reprocessing and reusing hemodialyzers can be traced to the very origins of chronic hemodialysis. The basic process associated with the reuse of hemodialyzers remains the same after over 50 years of practice: upon completion of a dialysis treatment the used dialyzer is cleaned, tested for efficacy and integrity, high-level disinfected or sterilized, and stored in a controlled environment for subsequent use. Reprocessing can be performed manually or by automated reprocessing systems. Automated systems provide control and consistency to the process. Chemical cleaning agents associated with dialyzer reprocessing include bleach, hydrogen peroxide and peracetic acid. Commonly used chemical disinfectants and

A.T. Azar (Ed.): Modelling and Control of Dialysis Systems, SCI 404, pp. 481–517.
springerlink.com   © Springer-Verlag Berlin Heidelberg 2013

sterilants include formaldehyde, and peracetic acid. A processing substituting heated citric acid for chemical germicides has been used on a limited basis. Advantages associated with dialyzer reuse include economic, efficacy and environmental returns while disadvantages include possible increased infections, exposure to chemical agents, development of antibodies and changes in dialyzer performance. Current controversies associated with dialyzer reuse are linked to studies documenting switching from reusing dialyzers to using disposable dialyzers by a single provider in the United States. The future of dialyzer reprocessing is linked to the same economic factors that initially promoted the practice.

10.1 HISTORY OF DIALYZER REPROCESSING

The practice of reprocessing and reusing hemodialyzers can be traced back to the very origins of chronic renal replacement therapy. Actually, this statement is not quite accurate since one of the first comprehensive descriptions of the multiple use of hemodialyzers, by Stanley Shaldon at the Royal Free Hospital in London, did not involve reprocessing at all. The paper simply describes a technique for refrigerating and reusing a twin-coil dialyzer, (see Fig. 10.1), for subsequent use for the same patient. No attempt was made to clean or reprocess the dialyzer. The concerns raised in this early work were focused more on the ascetic condition of the dialysis circuit than the performance or efficacy of subsequent dialysis procedures (Shaldon et al. 1964).

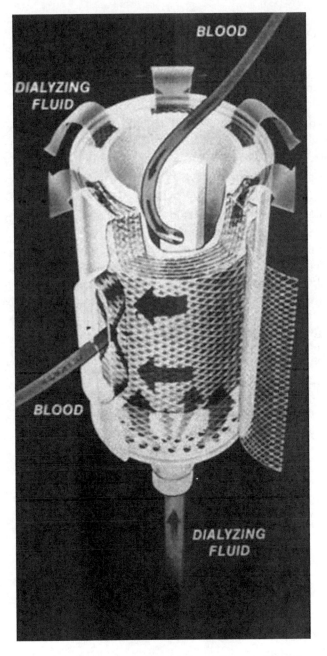

Fig. 10.1 Twin Coil Dialyzer. Adapted from Baxter Healthcare Corporation; with permission.

As used in current practice, the term "dialyzer reprocessing" is the cleaning, testing and disinfection/sterilization of a used hemodialyzer for subsequent use by the same patient. Reuse refers to using a dialyzer multiple times. The terms reprocessing and reuse are synonymous in current texts. Although dialyzer reprocessing is practiced worldwide the majority of information regarding the practice has been generated and published in the United States and Great Britain. This may be related to the rapid development and comparatively large scope of the chronic hemodialysis program in those countries compared to the rest of world. Dialyzer reprocessing was initially developed more as a time saving activity than as a process for conserving resources.

Initial citations reference the necessity of limiting post-dialysis technical activities associated with rebuilding Kiil dialyzers (see Fig.10.2). Early-on in the evolution of hemodialysis as a chronic therapy, home dialysis patients were required to disassemble, clean, rebuild, test and disinfect Kiil dialyzers after each treatment (Miach et al. 1976). This activity followed a 12 to 16 hour dialysis session and often took 1 to 2 hours to accomplish. To address the supplemental burden added by the rebuilding process, a technique for cleaning, testing and disinfecting the Kiil dialyzer was developed. This protocol, later adopted by many dialysis programs, used a variety of cleaning agents such as hydrogen peroxide and/or dilutes bleach solutions, to remove residual blood products from the flat-plate membrane surfaces of the Kiil dialyzer. The dialyzer was then pressure tested to ensure membrane integrity and filled with a formaldehyde solution. Although the Kiil reprocessing procedure required time and effort after a long dialysis session, the requirements were far less than those necessary to rebuild the Kiil after each use (Deane and Wineman 1989).

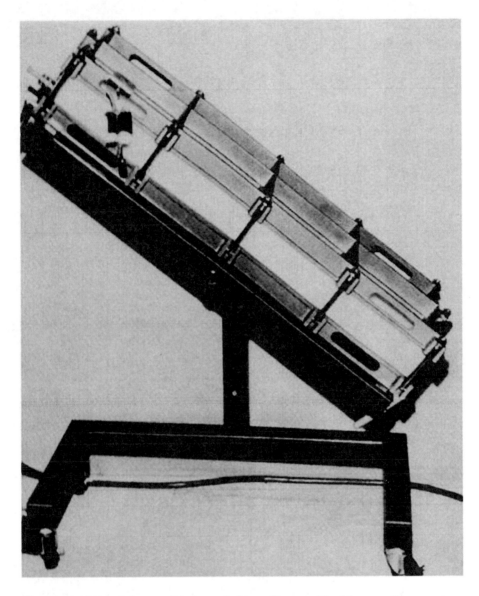

Fig.10.2 Kiil Dialyzer. [Adapted from Baxter Healthcare Corporation; with permission].

10.2   GUIDANCE AND REGULATION OF DIALYZER REPROCESSING

In the 1980's there was growing support for a consensus document detailing best practice in dialyzer reuse. This perceived need for standardization of method, with the accompanying rationale, was fueled by a rapid rise in the practice of dialyzer reprocessing and reuse. This escalation of the practice was based, in large part, on the change in funding for hemodialysis treatments in the United States. The funding mechanism was changed from a cost plus expenses model to a standardized composite rate, intended to cover the majority of dialysis-related expenses. In the United States, the percentage of chronic hemodialyzer centers practicing dialyzer reuse increased from 16% in 1976 to 60% in 1985. Although early studies validated that dialyzer reuse could be performed safely and effectively (Luehmann et al. 1982). There was concern in the community that the rapid adoption of reuse for reasons other than the immediate welfare of patients, may lead to abuse and negative outcomes.

The American Association of Medical Instrumentation convened a consensus development conference in 1983. From this conference came a recommended practice for dialyzer reuse. In 1984, after multiple drafts, the Recommended Practice for Reprocessing of Hemodialyzers, or ANSI/AAMI RD47 was released. The current revision, ANSI/AAMI RD47:2008 has been modified multiple times but the basic guidance remains unchanged. In 1987 the United States Centers for Medicare and Medicaid Services, (then the Healthcare Financing Agency or HCFA) adopted the recommended practiced as part of regulation to qualify for reimbursement by Medicare (AAMI 2008). The recommended practice has served as a model for other nations and compliance with the recommendations of RD47 has allowed the reprocessing of dialyzers to grow within the world dialysis community without affecting the efficacy of the therapy delivered. In the United States, as well as other countries, only dialyzer labeled for multiple-use are permitted to be reprocessed. The manufacturer of a dialyzer labeled for multiple-use must provide performance data through 15 uses and recommend at least one method of reprocessing (Nissenson and Fine 2005).

10.3 THE PROCESS OF DIALYZER REPROCESSING

Dialyzer cleaning protocols were developed for multiple dialyzer types, including coil, flat plate and hollow fiber dialyzers, but the basic steps of dialyzer reprocessing remains the same:

- Cleaning
- Testing
- Disinfection/Sterilization
- Storage

The methodology remains the same today even though the process is now accomplished, for the most part, using highly automated equipment.

10.3.1 Cleaning

The objective of the cleaning phase of dialyzer reprocessing is to remove residual blood product, deposited on the dialyzer membrane and within the confines of the dialyzer structure, during the dialysis treatment. Early work to identify the nature of membrane deposits, conducted on coil dialyzers, suggested that leukocytes constitute the principle blood component with only occasional deposits of platelets (Mason et al. 1976).

The deposits covered approximately 15 to 25% of the membrane surface area, as determined by visual examination, with the amount of material deposited on the membrane increasing only slightly after one or two uses and reprocessings. Although the area of the membrane covered by accumulated cellular deposits may not have been available for dialysis or ultrafiltration, this area was relatively small in comparison to the total membrane surface area. Flushing the used dialyzer membrane with water appeared to remove the accumulated protein debris. Additionally, Mason et al. observed that dialysis efficiency was not negatively affected even after multiple uses (Mason et al. 1976). This early work is quite important since the observations of Mason et al. that dialyzer performance is only minimally impacted by multiple use is critical for the validation of dialyzer reprocessing as an efficacious process. Early efforts to clean dialyzers employed untreated and minimally filtered tap water to rinse away residual blood products (Siemsen et al. 1974). Cleaning protocols were adjusted to use treated water for all reprocessing activities. Reprocessing procedures evolved to include procedures for flushing water through the blood compartment of the dialyzer (fiber flush) as well as reverse-ultrafiltration (RUF) of water across the dialyzer membrane (Varughese and Andrysiak 2000) (see Fig. 10.3). RUF involves pressurizing the dialysate compartment of a dialyzer with treated water and forcing water across the membrane into the blood compartment, where the water exits the blood ports (Varughese and Andrysiak 2000). RUF is especially effective in cleaning high-flux dialyzers (Ward and Ouseph 2003) and the pressure of the water used for reverse ultrafiltration must be monitored. Excess water pressure can collapse the

fibers within the dialyzer and may cause fiber failure, which, if not identified, lead to blood leaks upon initiation of dialysis during the subsequent
treatment.

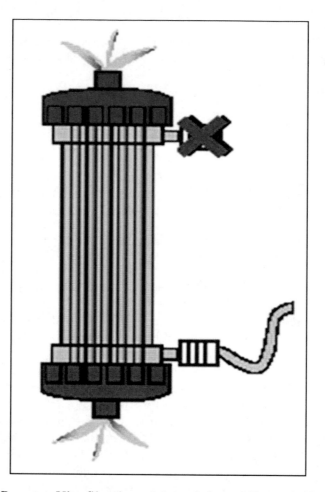

Fig. 10.3 Reverse Ultrafiltration. Adapted from Minntech Corporation;
with permission.

In an effort to increase the efficiency of dialyzer cleaning, adjunct
cleaning agents, such as dilute bleach solutions, sodium hydroxide, hydrogen peroxide and peracetic acid, were added to the cleaning solutions introduced into used dialyzers (Dennis et al. 1986). Bleach solutions were
especially popular since bleach was inexpensive, readily available and did
a reasonable job of removing proteins from dialyzer membranes and other

dialyzer surfaces. Early procedures called for the use of bleach solutions ranging in concentration from 0.5% to 4.3% with contact times ranging from 4 minutes to 7 minutes (Graeber et al. 1993). Dialyzers made from newly-developed synthetic membranes became commercially available in the late 1980's. When the dialyzer reprocessing cleaning protocols, developed for cleaning cellulosic membrane dialyzers, were applied to polysulfone dialyzer membranes, a significant increase in membrane ultrafiltration was noted. Not only did the bleach-cleaned polysulfone membrane become more porous to water, the bleach-treated membrane also became more porous to mid to large molecular weight blood components, such as albumin. The concentration of bleach used in the reprocessing cleaning phase and the bleach contact time became important factors since both concentration and exposure time facilitate the removal of polyvinylpyrrolidone (PVP) from the polysulfone membrane structure. This removal of PVP increases the membrane pore size and, thus, increases the ultrafiltration gradient and lowers the molecular cut-off for bleach-treated polysulfone membranes. This pore restructuring is associated with increased removal of large molecular weight proteins including albumin (Graeber et al. 1993).

Although alternative cleaning chemistries, such as sodium hydroxide and hydrogen peroxide, are documented in the literature, none have withstood the test of time and are no longer common practice (Luehmann et al. 1974). One issue associated with the cleaning agents and disinfectants/sterilants used in dialyzer reprocessing concerns the expression of concentration of these solutions, and is strictly semantic. The assumption is made that the beginning concentration of sodium hypochlorite and hydrogen peroxide, used to prepare dialyzer cleaning solutions, is 100%. Thus the solution commonly expressed as 0.5% bleach is actually a 1:199 dilution of a bleach to water that may have started as 5.25% sodium hypochlorite. In reality, the solution referred to as 0.5% bleach actually is a 0.026% sodium hypochlorite solution. This is further complicated by the fact that commercially-available bleach now contains sodium hypochlorite concentrations ranging from 5% to 10% (Clorox 2010).

For a cleaning agent to be effective the chemical must enhance the cleaning coefficient beyond that of water alone, without damaging the fragile dialyzer membrane. Additionally, the presence of cleaning agent in the dialyzer must be easily reduced to levels safe for clinical use and must not interfere with the efficacy of the disinfection/sterilization agent. The introduction of peracetic acid (PAA) as a dialyzer reprocessing agent changed the traditional approach of using separate cleaning and disinfection/sterilization agents, to using a single dialyzer reprocessing chemistry. A single-agent chemistry eliminated the necessity of testing a dialyzer, after the cleaning phase, to verify that the cleaning agent was reduced to acceptable levels, before the dialyzer was instilled with a different disinfecting agent (Berkseth et al. 1984). Peracetic acid solutions, sold under trade names such as Renalin, Pericidin, Peristeril, Peraldicide, Micro-X and Diolox are a mixture of peracetic acid, hydrogen peroxide and acetic acid. Peracetic acid solutions for dialyzer reprocessing are supplied in a stable, concentrated format. Once the solution is diluted to use-concentration the solutions become less stable and break down into acetic acid, oxygen and water. The more dilute the solution the less reversible the reaction. Once diluted with treated water, PAA solutions have a much shorter shelf life than concentrated PAA. As a dialyzer reprocessing agent, peracetic acid solutions provide safety, with relatively harmless breakdown products, and the efficacy of a high-level disinfectant/sterilant used for many years in Western Europe (Block 2001). Each dialyzer reprocessed with dilute peracetic acid solutions, however, must be tested to verify the chemical efficacy of the peracetic acid solution before each use (Minntech Corp 2004). This presence test validates that the reprocessed dialyzer was filled with an appropriate concentration of PAA solution and the solution dwelled in the dialyzer for an appropriate length of time.

10.3.2 Dialyzer Testing

Once the cleaning phase of reprocessing has been completed, the dialyzer in process must be tested to assure that two functional parameters have been met:

- Dialyzer Efficacy
- Membrane Integrity

10.3.2.1 Dialyzer Efficacy

One of the prime concerns associated with reusing hemodialyzers is that the ability of the dialyzer to perform the primary tasks associated with hemodialysis has not been diminished. The primary tasks are the balancing of electrolytes, the removal of small and mid-sized molecular waste products and the removal of water. Urea has long been used as the marker of efficacy for dialysis. The effectiveness of treatment is routinely measured as a function of urea reduction ratio (URR) or the urea index (K t/V). Both methods use urea reduction as a measure of adequacy of dialysis. Early work conducted by Dr. Frank Gotch indicated that a 20% decrease in the internal volume of a reprocessed dialyzer (referred to as Total Cell Volume (TCV) is equivalent to a 10% reduction in urea removal by the reprocessed dialyzer (Gotch 1980). The nephrology community agreed that a urea removal reduction of up to 10% was acceptable and fell within the variation associated with new dialyzers. This work has proven to be extremely important since Dr. Gotch provided a reliable method of validating efficacy of a reprocessed dialyzer simply by measuring the TCV. For this measurement to be meaningful, however, the TCV of the dialyzer must be determined before the first use. This "Preprocess" measurement provides the baseline against which all subsequent TCV measurements are compared. Since TCV is a simple and straight-forward concept, the methods for determining TCV are equally as simple. To make a manual determination of TCV, the contents of the blood compartment of the dialyzer is evacuated into a graduated cylinder. Generally this is accomplished by attaching an inflation bulb to one blood port of the dialyzer and the contents of the blood compartment are evacuated though the remaining open blood port and captured. Care must be taken when determining the TCV of high-flux dialyzers since the membrane is so porous that fluid can migrate from the dialysate compartment to the blood compartment of the dialyzer and artificially inflate or deflate the TCV. To prevent this inadvertent adjustment of the TCV, caps should be placed on the dialysate ports before the contents of the blood compartment are evacuated. Capping the dialysate ports creates a balanced pressure between the two dialyzer compartments. Automated reprocessing systems eliminate errors associated with manual determination of TCV and, in general, have safety systems that alert the operator if the TCV of a dialyzer falls below acceptable levels. Automated systems, in general, use either the weight of the evacuated solution or the change in pressure of a pressure-stabilized measurement cylinder to determine TCV.

10.3.2.2 Membrane Integrity

Testing membrane integrity verifies that the reprocessed dialyzer will not leak upon subsequent use. Pressurizing the blood compartment of a dialyzer in process with either positive or negative pressure, or monitoring pressure decay over a prescribed period will test the fiber integrity. The native pressure decay rate for specific membranes must be taken into account. Pressurized high-flux membranes can decay quickly and the monitoring period must be relatively short to accommodate the inherent pressure loss associated with the high permeability of the membrane.

10.3.3 High-Level Disinfection/Sterilization

Testing a dialyzer in process requires removing the fluid content of the dialyzer blood compartment and replacing it with air. Before the dialyzer can be instilled with either a high-level disinfectant or sterilant, the air must be completely flushed from the blood and dialysate compartments of the dialyzer. In both automated systems and manual reprocessing this is accomplished by first flushing the tested dialyzer with enough treated water to ensure that the entire dialyzer is air-free and fluid-filled. Flushing will make certain that air will not block the passage of fluid disinfectants/sterilants and all areas of the dialyzer will be exposed to chemical germicides.

Since the practice of reprocessing hemodialyzers began in the late 1960s, the variety of chemicals available to clean and disinfect dialyzers was somewhat limited. Formaldehyde, or more specifically, 37% formaldehyde stabilized with methanol (first marketed under the trade name Formalin), was inexpensive, effective and readily available in health care settings (Walker 1975). Formalin, however, has significant associated hazards, and environmental levels must be closely monitored to ensure staff safety. Formaldehyde is currently listed by the United States Environmental Protection Agency (EPA) as a suspected carcinogen (USEPA 1999). As the safety of handling formaldehyde solutions became a growing issue, replacement germicides for dialyzer reprocessing were investigated. Alternative germicides such as 27% saline solutions, sodium hydroxide, benzalkonium chloride and sodium hypochlorite are mentioned in the literature but the use of these agents never gained acceptance (Vercellone et al. 1978). One alternative, however, was adopted by a significant number of dialysis centers. During the early 1980's, peracetic acid (PAA) was introduced to the dialysis community as a chemical sterilant for use in dialyzer reprocessing. First introduced as a germicide for food production facilities, PAA was later adopted for use in water treatment and healthcare. PAA is relatively safe to use since the breakdown products are acetic acid, oxygen and water. In the concentrated form PAA is a strong oxidizer but is generally diluted to less than 4% by volume for use as a dialyzer reprocessing germicide. PAA also brought the advantage of being an effective cleaning agent as well as a germicide. During the reprocessing cycle, a dilute (2%) solution of PAA is first instilled into the dialyzer in process and used as a cleaner while a final-fill of 3.5% PAA solution is used as a terminal high-level disinfectant/sterilant. The language associated with the concentration of peracetic acid germicides can be confusing. In general, the concentrated form of peracetic acid germicides, such as Renalin, Peristeril and Perici-din, contain 20% - 26% hydrogen peroxide and 4% to 4.5% peracetic acid. A 3.5% dilution by volume of the concentrated PAA solution is used as a terminal germicide for dialyzer reprocessing. This solution is often referred to as 3.5% PAA. In reality, the solution contains 0.14% peracetic acid. Likewise, a 1% solution by volume is used to disinfectant the caps and connectors used with reprocessing and actually contains 0.04% peracetic acid. Both high-level disinfectants and sterilants are used for dialyzer reprocessing. The difference between the two classes of germicides is that a high-level disinfectant will kill all micro-organisms except for bacterial spores, while a sterilant will kill all micro-organisms including bacterial spores (CDC 2001; William and Weber 2008). Traditional germicides, such as formalin, are categorized as high-level disinfectants while currently popular germicides, such as peracetic acid, are categorized both as high-level disinfectants or sterilants, depending on the validation documentation provided by the manufacturer. This can be confusing since similar peracetic acid germicides from different manufacturers may be classified differently.

A critical factor associated with chemical germicides is the availability of test systems to validate the presence and the absence of the chemical. The presence test is necessary to establish that the chemical germicide is present in the reprocessed dialyzer at a level capable of rendering high-level disinfection or sterilization, as indicated by the germicide manufacturer. A test system for determining the absence of chemical germicide is necessary to validate that the reprocessed dialyzer has been rinsed free of chemical germicide and is safe for clinical use. Early test systems for formaldehyde involved adding a blue dye to the formalin solution to provide a visual indication that the formalin solution was present in the dialyzer. In reality, the only conclusion that can be drawn from this verification system is that the dialyzer contains blue dye. Test solutions, such as Schiff reagent, were used to demonstrate that the formalin had been rinsed from the reprocessed dialyzer. Peracetic acid disinfectants and sterilants are strong oxidants and cannot be used with color indicators. PAA users generally rely on test strips to indicate both presence and absence of the germicide.

A process, referred to as "germicide rebound" is associated with rinsing reprocessed dialyzers that have been filled with chemical germicide. A rebound in the level of germicide may occur if a dialyzer is allowed to sit without flow through the blood or dialysate compartments after rinsing and testing. The dialyzer materials that have been in contact with the chemical germicide while the dialyzer sat in storage may act as a "germicide sink" and slowly leach from into the solutions sitting in the dialyzer compartments (Luehmann 1990). To address this situation, dialyzer rinsing procedures usually include cautions to maintain flow in the dialysate and blood compartments of the dialyzer until dialysis is initiated. Likewise, dialyzers should be tested for the absence of chemical germicide as close to the time of initiation as practical.

10.3.3.1 Thermo-citric Reprocessing

An alternative process for cleaning, testing and sterilizing dialyzers was introduced to the dialysis community in the mid 1990s (Levin et al. 1995). Thermo-citric reprocessing relies on heat rather than a chemical germicide to sterilize the reprocessed dialyzer between uses. The original process involved cleaning the dialyzer with treated water alone, testing the performance and fiber integrity of the dialyzer and heating the water-filled dialyzer in an oven to 100° to 105° C for 20 hours. The process is limited to dialyzer membranes, such as polysulfone, which have demonstrated the capacity to withstand the elevated temperatures required by the process. Dialyzers contain a number of different materials, such as polycarbonate cases, polysulfone membranes and polyurethane potting material. The different materials included in a dialyzer have different coefficients of expansion; in other words the different materials expand at different rates when heated. The differences in the coefficients of expansion resulted in material failures during the 100°, 20 hour dwell period, required for terminal sterilization. The integrity of a dialyzer relies on a secure bond between the polycarbonate casing and the polyurethane potting material. The polycarbonate and polyurethane materials expand at different rates during the heat cycle, causing the urethane to separate from the polycarbonate dialyzer casing. This allows blood to leak into the dialyzer dialysate compartment upon subsequent use. Urethane separation was partially addressed by modifying the process to call for filling the dialyzer with 1.5% citric acid rather than water, before terminal sterilization. The use of 1.5% citric acid allowed the process temperature to be lowered to 95°C for 20 hours and still achieve demonstrate sterility. Since the process itself is the source of integrity failures, centers that use the thermo-citric process check for dialyzer leaks by pressure testing each re-processed dialyzer as part of the rinse procedure in preparation for clinical use (Levin et al. 1995).

10.3.4 Dwell and Storage

No disinfection or sterilization process is instantaneous. All disinfection/sterilization processes require a minimum contact time to assure microbial destruction. This applies to chemical disinfectants and sterilants, as well as thermo-citric reprocessing. The process dwell time will depend on the germicide or process in use, as well as environmental factors, such as storage temperature. Reprocessed dialyzers filled with 4% formalin routinely dwell at room temperature for 24 hours while dialyzers filled with 2% formalin dwell at 40°C for 24 hours. In general, PAA germicide manufacturers call for a dwell period of 11 hours at room temperature. Thermo-citric processing of dialyzers calls for filling the dialyzers with 1.5% citric acid and dwelling at 95°C for 20hours. Environmental factors may impact germicide dwell times and dialyzer storage conditions. Germicides, such as peracetic acid, have minimum and maximum temperature ranges; generally 15° to 24°C (Minntech Corp 2004). Additionally, PAA-filled dialyzers should not be stored in direct sunlight to minimize the breakdown of the PAA in the germicide solution. The temperature in the reprocessed dialyzer storage area and the position of the storage shelves or racks, with respect to windows, should comply with any conditions specific to the germicide or process and should comply with any guidance by the germicide manufacturer.

10.4 MANUAL AND AUTOMATED REPROCESSING

Dialyzers can be reprocessed quite effectively using manual processes. The first dialyzer reprocessing protocols were based on cleaning, testing and disinfecting the used dialyzer manually. Early in the development of dialyzer reprocessing, attempts were made to automate many of the repetitive steps that were a part of the process. Because the process is repetitive and routine, it is susceptible to mistakes and modification by the person performing the tasks. Dialysis centers developed large boards, containing multiple valves, on which the dialyzer was attached and, by opening and closing specific valves, the water, cleaning chemical and germicide flow to the dialyzer was regulated (see Fig. 10.4). Although these semi-automated systems partially address the routine activities incorporated into the reprocessing protocol, the timing and performance of the tasks are still dependent on the operator. When the workload increases, such as the accumulation of un-reprocessed dialyzers immediately following change of patient shifts, there is a tendency to speed-up the process by taking shortcuts and shaving time from the timed-steps incorporated into the process. Shortcuts and process modifications can lead to less than effective cleaning, testing and disinfection/sterilization of reprocessed dialyzers.

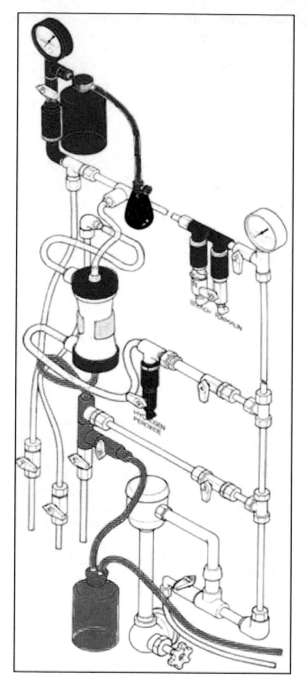

Fig.10.4 Manual Dialyzer Reprocessing Station. Adapted from Minntech Corporation; with permission.

Automated reprocessing systems were introduced to the dialysis market in the early 1980s. Reprocessing devices with names such as Lexivitron and Compudial were replaced by a few devices that grew to dominate the world dialyzer reprocessing market. The mid-1990s represented the highpoint for dialyzer reprocessing worldwide. Greater than 80% of the dialysis provided in the United States was delivered using reprocessed dialyzers and more than 50% of dialysis units that reprocessed dialyzers in the United States used automated systems. The predominant system in use was the Renatron II Dialyzer Reprocessing System, manufactured by Minntech Corporation. Additionally; the Seratronics DRS-4 System, manufactured by Fresenius and the ECHO System, manufactured by Mesa Medical, were also used by many dialysis units. Moreover, locally manufactured automated devices were available in many world dialysis markets. These automated reprocessing systems standardized the method by delivering a consistent process each time a dialyzer was reprocessed. Although automated reprocessing systems represent a capital investment, the expense is offset by a savings in labor. This savings in labor is realized because automated systems only require operators to connect and disconnect dialyzers and maintain the reprocessing records. The operator need not actively participate in all aspects of the process. In areas of the world where wages are relatively low, manual reprocessing continues to be an attractive method of reprocessing; even though manual reprocessing is labor intensive the practice can still reduce the cost of providing dialyzers. As wages rise, worldwide, manual reprocessing is becoming less at-tractive and is being replaced by the use of automated systems.

Automated dialyzer reprocessing systems, in general, incorporate a series of electrically operated valves to direct water, cleaning solutions and germicide flow through the blood and dialysate compartments of the dialyzer. The solution flow rate and pressures are controlled so that the resulting cleaning, testing and germicide-fill of the dialyzer is consistent. Dialyzer manufacturers often specify maximum flow rates and pressures for dialyzers and the automated reprocessing systems are configured to maintain these factors within the manufacturer's specifications. In addition to flushing dialyzers with water, automated systems also flush dialyzers with proportioned cleaning and germicide agents. Chemicals, such as bleach, formaldehyde, peracetic acid and citric acid are drawn from supply containers using dedicated mechanical pumps or, in the case of the Renatron System, solutions are moved using negative pressure created by a jet pump powered by the water supply. Regardless of the mechanism of transfer, the reprocessing chemicals are then diluted with purified water to create the final cleaning or germicidal solution. Automated systems, in general, use weight or pressure change within a fixed chamber to accurately proportion chemicals and water. A few automated systems require the user to attach fully-diluted cleaning and germicide solutions to the reprocessing system. These systems simply move solutions from the solution containers into the used dialyzer.

Most automated systems automate the labeling and recordkeeping functions associated with dialyzer reprocessing. Features such as searchable databases created for the management of reprocessing data, enabled dialysis staff to easily report on reprocessing outcomes. Variables such as patient name, dialyzer model, facility, time and staff can be used to filter the data. Easy access to reports permits dialysis staff to monitor and modify treatment parameters and modify treatment and reprocessing outcomes. Automated recordkeeping systems also provided an additional level of safety for patients by minimizing human error. Automated systems also provide modified processes for different dialyzer types, such as mid-level and high-flux dialyzers. The automated process adjusts to accommodate multiple ultrafiltration rates and variations in the size (volume) of dialyzers.

10.5   ADVANTAGES AND DISADVANTAGES OF DIALYZER REPROCESSING

10.5.1   Advantages of Reprocessing

The arguments for and against reprocessing dialyzers are based as much on emotion as on reason. There is an inherent perception in most cultures that "new is better". If an informed decision is to be made regarding the issue of dialyzer reuse, all relevant information must first be made available. The advantages afforded by using reprocessed dialyzers are often referred to as "The Three E's" and address a broad range of factors including economics, efficacy and the physical environment.

10.5.1.1   Economics

The principal advantage for reprocessing and reusing dialyzers is economic. A simplistic approach to determining dialyzer cost is to define the dialyzer cost as the sum of the cost of the dialyzer and the cost of disposal.

If a dialyzers costs $15 US and the cost of disposal is $1US the total dialyzer cost is $16 US. If the dialyzer is used 10 times the direct dialyzer cost per treatment is $1.60. This truly is a simplistic approach since dialyzer reprocessing requires an investment in time (labor), materials (disposables and solutions), capital equipment and generates overhead expenses. When implemented on the scale necessary to reprocess dialyzers from a typical dialysis center, the savings can be significant. Fig.10.5 represents a comparison between the cost of providing a disposable dialyzer and the total cost (labor + materials + capital + overhead) of providing a reprocessed dialyzer for a standard-sized dialysis facility.

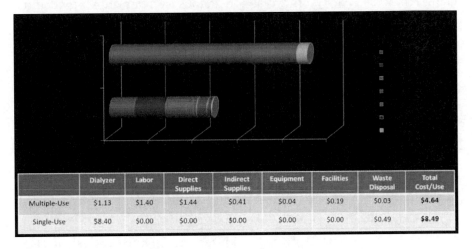

	Dialyzer	Labor	Direct Supplies	Indirect Supplies	Equipment	Facilities	Waste Disposal	Total Cost/Use
Multiple-Use	$1.13	$1.40	$1.44	$0.41	$0.04	$0.19	$0.03	$4.64
Single-Use	$8.40	$0.00	$0.00	$0.00	$0.00	$0.00	$0.49	$8.49

Fig. 10.5 Dialyzer Treatment Cost: Single-Use vs Multiple-Use. Adapted from Minntech Corporation; with permission.

The costs in Fig.10.5 are based on a single-use dialyzer cost of $8.40 and a multiple–use dialyzer used 16 times with a base cost of $18.00. Labor costs for reprocessing are based on an hourly labor rate with benefits of $18.75. The disposal costs used in figure X.5 are based on a used dialyzer weight of 2.35lbs (1.06kg) and a disposal cost of $.21/lb ($.46/kg). The economic benefit of reusing dialyzers, based on the size and scale represented in the example, is clearly evident.

10.5.1.2 Efficacy

This author speculates that no other single issue associated with chronic hemodialysis has been discussed for as long and has generated as much research and controversy as the efficacy of dialyzer reprocessing. As mentioned earlier, the first description of a protocol for preserving and reusing coil dialyzers was published in1962 (Shaldon et al. 1964). During the nearly 50 years since that first protocol was described at least eight large, multi-center studies have been conducted. The body of research represented by these studies indicates that treatments provided using reprocessed dialyzers are as efficacious as treatments provided using disposable dialyzers and leads the observer to conclude that factors other than reuse status have influence over the effectiveness of dialysis treatments (Fan et al. 2005).

10.5.1.3 First-Use Syndrome

Beginning in approximately 1980, a series of symptoms, referred to as "First-Use Syndrome" were identified in patients using new, unreprocessed dialyzers (Ogden 1980). The reactions were characterized by symptoms of anaphylacsis with the onset of symptoms early in the dialysis treatment. Speculation was made that the origins of First-Use Syndrome were multi-factorial and attributed to patient reactions to cellulose dialyzer membrane material and to the ethylene oxide sterilizing agent used in the manufacture of most dialyzers at the time (Marshall et al. 1984). Cellulosic membranes can be rendered less reactive by reprocessing. This is demonstrated by the decrease in neutrophil levels present in patients using reprocessed cellulosic membrane dialyzers compared to patients using new cellulosic dialyzers (Minntech Corp. 2004). Mitigation of first-use reactions was one of the reasons that dialysis centers that reprocess dialyzers began to pre-process reusable dialyzers before the first use. Pre-processing involves processing a dialyzer before the first clinical use. Pre-processing not only diminishes first use reaction but establishes a reliable dialyzer (cell) volume from which an accurate minimum (discard) volume can be calculated.

10.5.1.4 Environmental Advantage

A substantial case can be made that dialyzer reuse is justifiable solely because of the positive impact on the environment (Bond et al. 2011). Two distinctive aspects of dialyzer reuse can be noted: conservation of resources and minimization of waste. The conservation of resources applies to the raw materials required to manufacture and transport dialyzers for clinical use. Nearly 100% of the materials used in the fabrication of a synthetic hollow-fiber dialyzer are petroleum-based and, as such, a finite resource. In addition to limiting the raw materials required to manufacture dialyzers, reuse also minimizes the solid, chemical and airborne waste generated during the manufacturing process. Applying the same figures used to create the economic model for reuse (see Fig. 10.5), a center that reuses dialyzers 15 times will reduce the raw materials required to manufacture the dialyzers used by a dialysis center and dramatically reduce the resources necessary to transport and warehouse those dialyzers by a factor of 15.

The most obvious environmental impact associated with reusing dialyzers is the reduction in the biohazardous waste that must be discarded at the end of each dialysis treatment. In general, a used dialyzer weighs approximately 2.35 lbs (1.06 kg). This represents 2.35lbs (1.06 kg) of biohazardous waste that must be disposed of while satisfying the numerous requirements and prohibitions associated with local, regional and national guidance for the management of biohazardous materials. The proper disposal of used dialyzers can be quite expensive with reported costs ranging from $.21 US to $.50US/lb ($.46 - $1.10/kg) for blood-contaminated waste generated by a dialysis facility. To put this in perspective, the disposal of a used dialyzer can add more than $1 US to the cost of a treatment. Reprocessing a dialyzer 16 times, as used in our economic model, will reduce the cost of disposing of used dialyzers by a factor of 16. This represents a measureable and significant reduction in the cost of delivering dialysis (see Fig. 10.6).

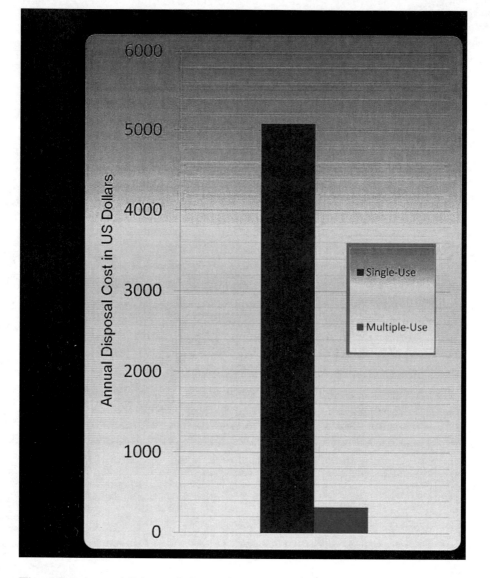

Fig. 10.6 Annual Disposal Cost of Single-Use Dialyzers vs Multiple-Use
Dialyzers (averaging 16 uses), based on a 66 patient clinic. Adapted from
Minntech Corporation; with permission.

10.5.2 Disadvantages of Reprocessing

An article published in 1994 called into question the efficacy of
dialyzer reprocessing using PAA (Held et al. 1994). The article claimed a

significant mortality advantage for dialyzers reprocessed using formaldehyde and for single-use when compared to mortality outcomes of patients
using dialyzers reprocessed with PAA (Held et al. 1994). Further analysis
of the data suggested that PAA may not have been a direct factor influencing the mortality outcomes but was associated with users who deviated
from the standard practice of using PAA with automated reprocessing
devices. This was supported by higher than average mortality rates in a
subset within the analysis, associated with manual reprocessing with PAA.
Further investigation revealed that a significant contributor to this manual
reprocessing subset was one small dialysis chain. When this chain was factored out of the analyzed data, the mortality advantage for formaldehyde
reprocessing or for single-use disappeared (Luehmann and Cosintino
1994). Additionally, the conclusion of higher mortality associated with
PAA reprocessing was questioned because a second subset of the data,
hospital-based dialysis units that reprocessed dialyzers using PAA, did not
demonstrate a mortality disadvantage. Factors such as this led to speculation that the mortality disadvantage, supported by the original data, was actually associated with un-identified factors (Collins et al. 1998). Subsequent retrospective analysis of large, multi-center and multi-organizational
renal patient data sets have supported the hypothesis that factors other than
dialyzer use influence morbidity and mortality outcomes of patients on
hemodialysis (Fan et al. 2005).

Since the efficacy of reusing dialyzers versus using disposable dialyzers
has been demonstrated to be virtually equivalent after years of analysis,
any disadvantages of using reprocessed dialyzers are primarily associated
with the additional surveillance and regulatory compliance that is linked
(rightly or wrongly) with reuse (Deane and Wineman 1989). Over the
course of dialyzer reprocessing history septic and pyrogenic events have
been linked to improper reprocessing protocols. In general, these events
involved using germicide concentrations that were less than effective
(Luehmann and Cosintino 1994), cleaning techniques that compromised
the ability of the reprocessing germicide to disinfect or sterilize the dialyzer or using water of unacceptable quality (Bland et al. 1989).

10.5.2.1 Improper Dilution

Improperly diluted reprocessing germicide is most often associated with
the manual reprocessing of hemodialyzers. Since the steps required to reprocess a dialyzer are repetitive by nature, shortcuts are often taken in the
manual process. Mixing germicide for manual reprocessing requires the
accurate proportioning of treated water and germicide as well as a means

of mixing the two components into a homogeneous solution. Abbreviating the process can result in a germicide solution that is not of uniform concentration within the germicide container and can result in a portion of reprocessed dialyzers filled with less than adequate germicide solutions. This practice may result in reprocessed dialyzers that have not been high-level disinfected, leading to septic events upon subsequent dialyzer use (Bland et al. 1989; Vanholder et al. 1990). Added care must be taken by the manual reprocessor to ensure proper mixing of germicide solutions.

Additionally, if a dialyzer is manually reprocessed care must be taken to assure that the water in the reprocessed dialyzer is completely replaced with reprocessing germicide. A common mistake, made by novice reprocessing personnel, is to assume that the volume of germicide required to fill the dialyzer is equivalent to the TCV, or volume of the dialyzer blood compartment. This is incorrect since the true germicide volume of the dialyzer also includes the volume of the dialysate compartment. The AAMI Recommended Practice for Dialyzer Reprocessing, (RD47) calls for the germicide concentration exiting the dialyzer to be at least 90% of the original germicide concentration (AAMI 2008). Testing the final germicide concentration can be difficult so a good surrogate is to fill the dialyzer with four compartment-volumes (both dialysate and blood compartments) of pre-diluted germicide (Arduino et al. 1993).

10.5.2.2 Header Sepsis

The United States Centers for Disease Control (CDC) reported on bacteremia associated with the contamination of the dialyzer header caps and header cap O-rings of high-flux dialyzers. The testing performed by the CDC confirmed that bacterial entrapment underneath and behind the O-rings of improperly reprocessed dialyzers was independent of the type of germicide (formaldehyde or PAA) and germicide concentration. The incidents were also associated with the practice of removing dialyzer header caps to clean bio-debris from the dialyzer header spaces (Beck-Sague et al. 1990; Bland et al. 1989). This makes perfect sense since the purpose of the O-ring in a dialyzer header cap is to prevent the passage of a solution from one side of the O-ring to the other. When header caps and O-rings are removed for cleaning, areas of the dialyzer header which had previously been sterile are exposed to microbial contamination. When the header caps are replaced back on the dialyzer, the areas behind and underneath the O-ring remain contaminated because the O-ring prevents germicide contact. When the dialyzer spaces are pressurized during subsequent treatments, the O-ring will be lifted slightly by the increased pressure created with each pulse of the blood pump. The blood in the extracorporeal circuit will then be exposed to the contaminated surfaces. The ensuing septic events are commonly referred to as "Header Sepsis" (see Fig. 10.7).

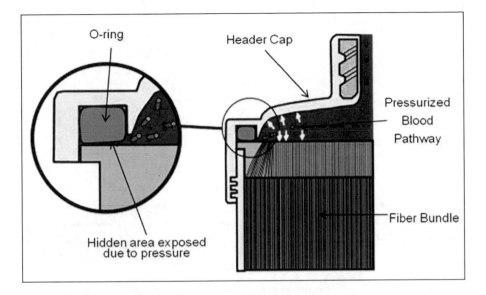

Fig. 10.7 Bacterial contamination under header o-ring. Adapted from Minntech Corporation; with permission.

One response that has successfully addressed header sepsis is to expose the header caps, O-rings and exposed dialyzer header spaces to germicide and to re-assemble the header components wet with germicide. This assures that all surfaces have been exposed to germicide and organisms cannot proliferate underneath and behind the header cap O-ring (AAMI 2008).

10.6 WATER QUALITY

As indicated in AAMI RD47, the water used to reprocess dialyzers should be of the same quality as water used for dialysis (AAMI 2008). This applies to the chemical impurities in the water as well as the microbiological content (see Fig. 10.8).

Contaminant	Maximum concentration (mg/l)[b]
Contaminants with documented toxicity in hemodialysis	
Aluminum	0.01
Total chlorine	0.1
Copper	0.1
Fluoride	0.2
Lead	0.005
Nitrate (as N)	2
Sulfate	100
Zinc	0.1
Electrolytes normally included in dialysis fluid	
Calcium	2 (0.05 mmol/l)
Magnesium	4 (0.15 mmol/l)
Potassium	8 (0.2 mmol/l)
Sodium	70 (3.0 mmol/l)

NOTE   This table is reproduced from ISO 13959.

[a]   The physician has the ultimate responsibility for ensuring the quality of water used for dialysis.

[b]   Unless otherwise noted.

Contaminant	Maximum concentration (mg/l)
Antimony	0.006
Arsenic	0.005
Barium	0.1
Beryllium	0.0004
Cadmium	0.001
Chromium	0.014
Mercury	0.0002
Selenium	0.09
Silver	0.005
Thallium	0.002

NOTE   This table is reproduced from ISO 13959.

Fig. 10.8 Maximum allowable chemical contaminant levels in water used to reprocess multiple-use dialyzers. ANSI/AAMI/ISO 11663:2009 Quality of dialysis fluid for hemodialysis and related therapies

The chemical content of the water used for reprocessing is important since certain impurities may interfere with the germicidal activity of the agent used for high-level disinfection or sterilization. Peracetic acid germicides are degraded by the heavy metals in the water used to dilute the germicide (Gotch 1980). The microbial water quality is equally important. Although microorganisms will be deactivated by the germicide instilled into a reprocessed dialyzer (or in the case of thermo-citric reprocessing, the 20 hour heat cycle), the killed bacteria will contribute to the endotoxin load within the dialyzer. Endotoxin is a lipid polysaccharide-polypeptide complex released from the cell walls of gram-negative organisms. When chemical germicides are diluted with water that contains gram negative organisms, the diluted germicide solution will contain endotoxin. Endotoxin reactions to tainted dialyzers are characterized by fever, chills, leucopenia and other symptoms (Gordon et al. 1988). Maximum allowable levels of endotoxin in water used to reprocess dialyzers are addressed in the AAMI Recommended Practice (AAMI 2008).

10.7   ANTI-N ANTIBODIES

As early as 1972, researchers identified a blood group referred to as NN red blood cell agglutination. The process was hypothesized to be associated with exposure to formalin and the antibody was called anti-N-like antibody. This choice of words differentiated the observed process from true anti-N antibody. Additional research confirmed the presence of anti-N-like antibodies and associated the process of these antibodies with patients who were treated using formalin-reprocessed dialyzers (Howell and Perkins 1972).

The formation and presence of anti-N-like antibodies was problematic for patients on hemodialysis since many of these patients were treated with dialyzers reprocessed using formaldehyde and were awaiting kidney transplantation (Kaehny et al. 1997). The presence of anti-N-like antibodies made the complex matching system associated with identifying a suitable graft for a patient even more difficult (Sharon 1981). The dialysis community initially responded by developing more robust rinsing procedures and more accurate testing for the presence of formaldehyde. Further research indicated that increasing the rigor of dialyzer rinsing did not completely eliminate the formation of anti-N-like antibodies. The formation of anti-N-like antibodies was not associated with the reprocessed dialyzers in general but specifically with dialyzers reprocessed using formaldehyde as a germicide (Deane and Wineman 1989).

10.8 REUSE-ASSOCIATED CHANGES IN ULTRAFILTRATION COEFFICIENT

The coefficient of ultrafiltration (K_{uf}) for a dialyzer describes the water permeability of the dialyzer membrane and is generally published for each dialyzer model marketed to the dialysis community. Dialyzer reprocessing techniques can increase or decrease the coefficient of ultrafiltration, depending on the chemical agents used during the process. When bleach is used as a reprocessing cleaning agent, the K_{uf} of the reprocessed dialyzer can increase. This process is associated with polysulfone dialyzer membranes and can be quite dramatic. Increased permeability of the membrane, upon repeated exposure to bleach solution, is also associated with an increase in molecular-weight cut-off. This process is attributed to polyvinyl-pyrrolidone removal from the polysulfone-membrane copolymer, causing an increase in membrane pore size (Graeber et al. 1993; Murthy et al. 1998). This increased pore size can result in unwanted removal of large molecular weight proteins, such as albumin, from the patient.

Interestingly enough, a small but measureable decrease in K_{uf} upon repeated reprocessing using PAA has also been documented (Fleming et al. 1991). Additionally, data generated during the HEMO study, a large prospective U.S. study that analyzed the outcomes of patients using high and low-flux dialyzers, indicated that the middle-molecular clearance of high-flux dialyzers, measured as Beta2 microglobulin removal, decreased significantly when high-flux dialyzers were reprocessed using PAA (Leypoldt et al. 1998). On closer scrutiny, an association can be made, not with all high-flux dialyzers and decreased Beta2 microglobulin clearance but rather with multiple uses of cellulosic membrane high-flux dialyzers. The ability of polysulfone membrane high-flux dialyzers to remove Beta2 microglobulin remains relatively stable through 15 uses (Leypoldt et al. 1998). Further analysis reveals logic to these findings. The mechanism for removal of middle-molecular substances by a cellulosic high-flux membrane is clearance and/or solute drag. The middle molecules pass through the pore structure and are sieved from the blood by the dialyzer cellulosic dialyzer membrane. Polysulfone high-flux membranes, in contrast, have an added mechanism of removal, termed by some as "entrapment" (Ward and Ouseph 2003).

The membrane structure of polysulfone is relatively thick (40 micron) and consists of tortuous pathways leading through the membrane wall. Speculation is that Beta2 microglobulin is trapped in the pore structure of polysulfone membranes rather than being cleared (sieved) into the dialysate solution. The entrapped Beta2 is flushed from the polysulfone membrane pore structure during reprocessing and the ability of the poly-sulfone high-flux dialyzer to remove Beta2 microglobulin is restored.

Cellulosic high flux membranes, on the other hand, achieve their high porosity because the membrane is relatively thin (15 micron) and the porous path between the blood and dialysate is somewhat short. It is speculated that deposition of protein on the internal cellulosic membrane wall limits access to the pore structure and decreases the membranes ability to remove larger molecular weight substances such as Beta2 microglobulin. In theory, the same mechanism that renders cellulosic membranes more biocompatible upon reuse with PAA also limits Beta2 microglobulin removal. The practical application of reuse with bleach, PAA, cellulosic and polysulfone membranes mediates the clinical implication; the vast majority of dialysis delivery systems incorporate ultrafiltration control and any change in the K_{uf} of a dialyzer upon reuse is compensated for by the delivery system. Similarly, the majority of high-flux dialyzers used worldwide has polysulfone, rather than cellulosic membranes.

10.9 CURRENT CONTROVERSIES

In 2000, the world's largest reprocessor of hemodialyzers, with 71,000 patients treated in 1078 dialysis clinics, announced a transition to using disposable dialyzers. Fresenius Medical Care of North America transitioned from primarily treating patients with formaldehyde-reprocessed dialyzers to using single-use, disposable dialyzers, over the following four years. Fresenius is also one of the world's largest manufacturers of hemodialyzers, producing nearly 45% of all hemodialyzers manufactured in 2009 (Fresenius Medical Care 2009). The change to single-use by Fresenius clinics in the United States was accompanied by a significant expansion of dialyzer manufacturing capacity by Fresenius in North America. A controversial paper, authored by Lowrie, Ofsthun and Lazarus, and published in 2004, detailing a decrease in mortality accompanying the transition from using reprocessed dialyzers to the use of disposable dialyzers in Fresenius clinics (Lowrie et al. 2004). The study was widely criticized for bias associated with data limited to one dialysis provider and the possibility of influence by other, unmeasured factors (Carlson 2004). Analysis of U.S. Medicare data, by the United States Renal Data Service did not find the mortality change indicated by the Lowrie et al. study. A second study by Lacson et al (2011) also affiliated with Fresenius North America, indicated a decrease in mortality when a smaller subset of clinics within the larger set of Fresenius clinics switched from reusing dialyzers to using disposable dialyzers. Again, the decrease in mortality identified in the Lacson et al article was not found in data analyzed and published by the United States Renal Data Service (USRDS 2006). This most recent analysis of the efficacy of dialyzer reprocessing again was inconclusive and raised questions regarding the effect of other, un-named factors on the morbidity and mortality of patients on hemodialysis.

10.10 CONCLUSION AND FUTURE DEVELOPMENTS

Since the primary driver of dialyzer reprocessing has been the economic benefit experienced by centers that reprocess dialyzers, the future of dialyzer reprocessing is also linked to continuing economic benefit. The continued growth of the ESRD population worldwide will require the dedication of an ever-growing percentage of healthcare resources. This escalation of the cost of providing dialysis may initiate a resurgence of the practice of reprocessing and reusing critical resources such as hemodialyzers.

ACKNOWLEDGEMENT

I would like to thank Kendall Larson for his valuable contribution to the assembly of this information.

REFERENCES

AAMI: Recommended Practice for Reuse of Hemodialyzers. Association for Advancement of Medical Instrumentation, Arlington (2008)

Arduino, M., McAllister, S., Bland, L.: Assuring Proper Germicide Concentrations in Reprocessed Hemodialyzers. Dial. Transplant. 22(11), 652–656 (1993)

Beck-Sague, C., Jarvis, W., Bland, L., et al.: Outbreak of gram-negative bacteremia and pyrogenic reactions in a hemodialysis center. Am. J. Nephrol. 10(5), 397–403 (1990)

Berkseth, R., Luehmann, D., McMichael, C., et al.: Peracetic acid for reuse of hemodialyzers, clinical studies. Trans. Am. Soc. Artif. Intern. Organs 30, 270–274 (1984)

Bland, L., Arduino, M., Aguero, et al.: Recovery of bacteria from reprocessed high flux dialyzers after bacterial contamination of the header spaces and o-rings. ASAIO Trans. 35(3), 314–316 (1989)

Block, S.S.: Disinfection, Sterilization and Preservation, 5th edn., p. 192. Lippincott, Williams and Wilkins, Philadelphia (2001)

Bond, T.C., Nissesnson, A.R., Krishnan, M., et al.: Dialyzer Reuse and Peracetic Acid and Patient Mortality. CJASN ePress (2011) (published on May 12, 2011), doi:10.2215/cjn.10391110

Carlson, W.G.: Reuse: what does the industry think? Nephrol. News Issues 18(11), 95, 97 (2004)

CDC: Recommendations for Preventing Transmission of Infections Among Chronic Hemodialysis Patients. MMWR Recomm Rep. 50(RR-5), 1–43 (2001), http://www.cdc.gov/mmwr/preview/mmwrhtml/rr5 005a1.html (accessed January 06, 2011)

Clorox Company: Clorox Regular-Bleach, Material Safety Data Sheet (2010), http://www.thecloroxcompany.com/products/msds /bleach/cloroxregularbleach0505_.pdf (accessed January 31, 2011)

Collins, A.J., Ma, J.Z., Constantini, E.G., Everson, S.E.: Dialysis Unit and Patient Characteristics Associates with Reuse Practices and Mortality: 1989 - 1993. J. Am. Soc. Nephrol. 9(11), 2108–2117 (1998)

Deane, N., Wineman, R.R.: Replacement of Renal Function by Dialysis: a textbook of Dialysis, 3rd edn., pp. 400–405. Kluwer, Dordrecht (1989)

Dennis Jr., M.B., Vizzo, J., Cole, J., et al.: Comparison of four methods of cleaning hollow-fiber dialyzers for reuse. Artif. Organs 10(6), 448–451 (1986)

Fan, Q., Liu, J., Ebben, J.P., et al.: Reuse-Associated Mortality in Incident Hemodialysis Patients in the United States, 2000 to 2001. Am. J. Kidney Dis. 46(4), 661–668 (2005)

Fleming, S., Foreman, K., Shanley, K., et al.: Dialyzer reprocessing with Renalin. Am. J. Nephrol. 11, 27–31 (1991)

Fresenius Medical Care, Annual Report (2009), http://www.fmc.com/portals/corp/sec/2009_FMC _Annual_Report.pdf (accessed January 31, 2011)

Gordon, S., Tipple, M., Bland, L., et al.: Pyrogenic reactions associated with the reuse of disposable hollow-fiber hemodialyzers. JAMA 260(14), 2077–2081 (1988)

Gotch, F.A.: Mass Transport in Reused Dialyzers. Proc. Clin. Dial. Transplant. Forum 10, 81–85 (1980)

Graeber, C.W., Halley, S., Lapkin, R., et al.: Protein losses with reused dialyzers. J. Amer. Soc. Nephrol. 4(3), 349 (1993)

Held, P., Wolfe, R., Gaylin, D., et al.: Analysis of the association of dialyzer reuse practices and patient outcomes. American Journal of Kidney Diseases 23(5), 692–708 (1994)

Howell, E.D., Perkins, H.A.: Anti-N-like antibodies in the sera of patients undergoing haemodialysis. Vox Sang 23, 291–299 (1972)

Kaehny, W.D., Miller, G.E., White, W.L.: Relationship between dialyzer reuse and the presence od anti-N-like antibodies in chronic hemodialysis patients. Kidney Int. 12, 59–65 (1997)

Lacson Jr, E., Wang, W., Monney, A., et al.: Abandoning Peracetic Acid-Based Dialyzer Reuse Is Associated with Improved Survival. Clin. J. Am. Soc. Nephrol. 6(2), 297–302 (2011)

Levin, N.W., Parnell, S.L., Prince, H.N., et al.: The use of heated citric acid for dialyzer reprocessing. J. Am. Soc. Nephrol. 6(6), 1578–1585 (1995)

Leypoldt, J.K., Cheung, A.K., Deeter, R.B.: Effect of Hemodialyzer Reuse: Dissociation Between Clearances and Small and Large Solutes. Am. J. Kidney Dis. 32(2), 295–301 (1998)

Lowrie, E.G., Zhensheng, L., Ofsthun, N., et al.: Reprocessing dialyzers for multiple uses: recent analysis of death risks for patients. Nephrol. Dial. Transplant. 19(11), 2823–2830 (2004)

Luehmann, D., Hirsch, D., Carlson, G., et al.: Dialyzer reuse in a large dialysis program. Trans. Am. Soc. Artif. Intern. Organs 28, 76–82 (1982)

Luehmann, D., Carlson, G., Keshaviah, P., et al.: Reuse of the model 4 Cordis Dow artificial kidney (CDAK-4). Proc. Clin. Dial. Transplant. Forum 4, 220–223 (1974)

Luehmann, D.A., Cosintino, L.C.: Safety of Dialyzer Reuse with Renalin: The Untold Story. Dial. Transplant. 23(5), 248–258 (1994)

Luehmann, D.: Dialyzer Reprocessing. Minntech Corporation, Minneapolis (1990)

Marshall, C., Shimizu, A., Smith, E.K., et al.: Ethylene oxide allergy in a dialysis center: prevalence in hemodialysis and peritoneal dialysis populations. Clin. Nephrol. 21(6), 346–349 (1984)

Mason, R.G., Zucker, W.H., Bilinsky, R.T., et al.: Blood Components Deposited On Used and Reused Dialysis Membranes. Biomat. Med. Dev., Art. Org. 4(3 & 4), 333–358 (1976)

Miach, P., Evans, S., Wilcox, A., et al.: Reuse of a disposable dialyzer for home dialysis. Med. J. 1(6), 146–147 (1976)

Minntech Corp., Renalin Directions for Use, p. 16 (2004)

Murthy, B.V., Sundaram, S., Jaber, B.L., et al.: Effect of formaldehyde/bleach reprocessing on in vivo performances of high-efficiency cellulose and high-flux polysulfone dialyzers. J. Am. Soc. Nephrol. 9(3), 464–472 (1998)

Nissenson, A.R., Fine, R.N.: Clinical Dialysis, 4th edn. Mcgraw-Hill, New York (2005)

Ogden, D.A.: New-dialyzer syndrome. N. Engl. J. Med. 302(22), 1262–1263 (1980)

Renalin® 100 Cold Sterilant Concentrate Instructions for Use, p. 11

Shaldon, S., Silva, H., Rosen, M.: Technique of refrigerated coil preservation haemidialysis with femoral venous catheritization. Br. Med. J. 2(5406), 411–413 (1964)

Sharon, R.: Relationship between formaldehyde-related antibodies and cross-reacting anti-N-like antibodies in patients undergoing chronic haemodialysis. J. Clin. Pathol. 34(1), 41–43 (1981)

Siemsen, A., Lumeng, J., Wong, E., et al.: Clinical and laboratory evaluation of coil reuse. Trans. Am. Soc. Artif. Organs 20, 589–594 (1974)

United States Environmental Protection Agency (USEPA), Integrated Risk Information system (IRIS) on Formaldehyde. National Center for Environmental Assessment, Office of research and Development, Washington, DC (1999)

US Renal Data System Annual Report (USRDS). National Institutes of Health/National Institute of Diabetes and Digestive and Kidney Diseases, Bethesda, Md (2006)

Vanholder, R., Vanhaecke, E., Ringoir, S.: Waterborne pseudomonas septicemia. ASAIO Trans. 36(3), M215–M216 (1990)

Varughese, P.M., Andrysiak, P.: Dialyzer Reuse. In: Curtis, J., Varrughese, P. (eds.) Dialysis Technology: A Manual for Dialysis Technicians, 2nd edn. National Association of Nephrology Technicians/Technologists, Dayton, OH (2000)

Vercellone, A., Piccolo, G., Aloatti, S., et al.: Reuse of hemodialyzers. Dial. and Transplant. 7, 350–359 (1978)

Walker, F.J.: Commercial Formaldehyde Soultions. In: Formaldehyde, 3rd edn. Kreiger, New York (1975)

Ward, R.A., Ouseph, R.: Impact of bleach cleaning on the performance of dialyzers with polysulfone membranes processed for reuse using peracetic acid. Artif. Organs 27(11), 1029–1034 (2003)

William, A.R., Weber, D.J.: Healthcare Infection Control Practices Advisory Committee (HICPAC). Guideline for Disinfection and Sterilization in Healthcare Facilities (2008), http://www.premierinc.com/safety/topics/guidelines/downloads/Disinfection_Nov_2008.pdf (accessed January 6, 2011)

ESSAY QUESTIONS

1. What is the difference between dialyzer reprocessing and dialyzer reuse?
2. List and describe "The Three Es" that make dialyzer reuse an attractive practice.
3. Outline the basic steps for reprocessing and subsequent reuse of a hemodialyzer.
4. What are the advantages and disadvantages of using reverse ultra-filtration as a dialyzer cleaning method?
5. What are the consequences of using bleach as a membrane cleaning agent?
6. Detail the process of thermo-citric reprocessing.
7. What is "Header Sepsis" and what actions can be taken to minimize this condition?
8. Describe the economic conditions that exist in a healthcare market in which automated dialyzer reuse is an attractive practice.
9. Explain the difference in the process of removing mid-molecular weight substances using a high-flux cellulosic membrane and a high-flux synthetic membrane.
10. What conditions in the healthcare market will promote the reuse of dialyzers moving into the future?

MULTIPLE CHOICE QUESTIONS

Choose the best answer

1. Dialyzer reprocessing was initially developed as a … activity
   A. Time saving
   B. Resource conservation
   C. Economic
   D. Aesthetic

2. … has served as a model for guidance and regulation for dialyzer reprocessing
   A. AAMI RD5
   B. AAMI RD47
   C. ISO 242
   D. The UN Healthcare Initiative

3. US manufacturers of dialyzers intended for multiple-use must provide dialyzer performance data through … uses

   A. 2
   B. 5
   C. 10
   D. 15

4. US manufacturers of dialyzers intended for multiple-use must recommend at least … method(s) of reprocessing

   A. 1
   B. 2
   C. 3
   D. 4

5. The objective of the cleaning phase of dialyzer reprocessing is …

   A. Remove residual blood products deposited on the dialyzer membrane
   B. Remove residual blood products within the confines of the dialyzer structure
   C. a and b
   D. None of the above

6. Early work indicated that the principle blood component deposited on a dialyzer membrane was …

   A. Platelets
   B. Red Cells
   C. Leukocytes
   D. Proteins

7. Reverse ultrafiltration involves pressuring the …

   A. Blood compartment
   B. Dialysate compartment
   C. Both blood and dialysate compartments
   D. Neither dialyzer compartment

8. Work by Dr. Gotch indicated that a 20% decrease in TCV is equivalent to a …

   A. 10% reduction in urea removal
   B. 20% reduction in urea removal
   C. 10% reduction in K_{uf}
   D. 20% reduction in K_{uf}

9. Dialyzers are tested for what two functional parameters…

    A. K_{uf} and F_{uf}

    B. Kt/V and URR

    C. TCV and membrane integrity

    D. Weight and dimension

10. Which two germicides are most commonly used in dialyzer reprocessing…

    A. Formalin and Formaldehyde

    B. Formalin and Gluteraldehyde

    C. Peracetic Acid and Citric Acid

    D. Peracetic Acid and Formalin

11. Germicides classified as high-level disinfectants kill all microorganisms except…

    A. Viruses

    B. Gram-Negative Bacteria

    C. Fungi

    D. Bacterial Spores

12. Germicide efficacy within a reprocessed dialyzer may be affected by…

    A. Direct Sunlight

    B. Germicide contact time

    C. Temperature

    D. All of the Above

13. Manual reprocessing is susceptible to…

    A. Short-cuts

    B. Process Modifications

    C. Mistakes

    D. All of the Above

14. First –use syndrome is associated with…

    A. Cellulosic membrane dialyzers

    B. Ethylene Oxide Sterilizing Agent

    C. a and b

    D. None of the above

15. Water used for dialyzer reprocessing should meet the same standards as water used for.....................

    A. Drinking
    B. Pharmaceutical manufacturing
    C. Dialysis
    D. Soft Drinks

16. The first comprehensive description of the multiple use of hemodialyzers referred to the reuse of what type of dialyzer?

    A. Flat Plate
    B. Hollow Fiber
    C. Coil
    D. Fiber Mesh

17. Reverse ultrafiltration involves pressurizing which compartment of the dialyzer with treated water?

    A. Blood
    B. Dialysate
    C. Both
    D. Neither

18. Reverse Ultrafiltration is especially effective in cleaning:

    A. Flat Plate Dialyzers
    B. Coil Dialyzers
    C. High-flux Dialyzers
    D. Spiral-Wound Dialyzers

19. What can degrade peracetic acid germicides?

    A. Heavy metals in the water
    B. AAMI-quality water
    C. Deionized water
    D. None of the above

20. The formation of anti-N-like antibodies is associated with:

    A. Reprocessing with formaldehyde
    B. Reprocessing with peracetic acid
    C. Reverse ultrafiltration
    D. Cleaning with bleach

Chapter (11)

Flow Modeling of Hollow Fiber Dialyzers

Manuel Prado-Velasco

CHAPTER OUTLINES

- General issues of dialyzer flows
- Flow modeling in a whole scenario
- 1D diffusive model of a hollow fiber dialyzer
- Lacks of 1D diffusive mathematical model
- A deeper insight in the mathematical flow modeling
- Flow modeling: progress and future
- Conclusion

CHAPTER OBJECTIVES

- Description of main physical mechanisms that govern the clearance of compounds in hollow dialyzers
- Modeling of a complete in-vivo and in-vitro scenario under ideal assumptions
- Knowledge of advanced analytical and mathematical methods to get down with more complex situations
- Knowledge of main lacks of current mathematical models of dialyzers
- Be able to distinguish inaccuracies due to numerical errors, internal assumptions and external variables

KEY TERMS

- Transport flows
- Dialyzer membranes
- Mathematical modeling
- Dialyzer clearance
- Urea kinetic
- Concentration Polarization
- Diffusion-convection-adsorption coupling
- Progress in hollow fiber flow modeling

ABSTRACT

Renal replacement therapies keep the same principles that guided the first dialysis session performed by Kolff in 1943 over a human patient. Despite the interest to build an artificial kidney that replicate better the complex dynamics of the human kidneys, this task is still very immature. However, therapies based on artificial kidneys could improve the clinical outcomes if professionals could predict better their performance. This chapter shows the state of the art concerning this subject, following a top-down approach.

A.T. Azar (Ed.): Modelling and Control of Dialysis Systems, SCI 404, pp. 519–562.
springerlink.com   © Springer-Verlag Berlin Heidelberg 2013

11.1 GENERAL ISSUES OF DIALYZER FLOWS

Hollow fiber dialyzers used in renal replacement therapies are designed to maximize the clearance of uremic toxins by a proper control of their transport across the fibers' porous membrane. The accuracy of mathematical models of dialyzer flows is therefore a critical objective for this task.

Figure 11.1 shows the major flows implicated in the clearance of uremic toxins in the renal system of a health subject(Guyton and Hall 2006), and in a hollow fiber dialyzer.

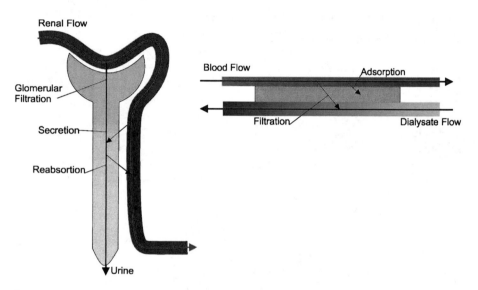

Fig. 11.1 Flows related to uremic toxins clearance in renal system vs. hollow fiber system

Both systems share the filtration (convective diffusion) as major mechanism of clearance. However, there are essential differences between them. Kidneys, via their minimal functional unit, the nephron, filters around 18 % of total renal flow, which in turn is about 22 % of cardiac output. This provides an average of 1100 ml/min of renal flow and 180 ml/min of glomerular filtration (GFR). Glomerular capillaries are impermeable to blood proteins; therefore the GFR is protein and cellular elements free. With the exception of compounds with high molecular weights or those partially bound to proteins, concentrations of compounds in GFR are similar to those in plasma.

Operating conditions and filtration on the hollow fiber dialyzer are very different. Blood flow rates (Q_b) are in 200 – 400 ml/min in standard dialysis sessions, and typical dialyzers work with net ultrafiltration (convection) rates around 20 ml/min, in such a way diffusion (and not convection) is the main transport mechanism implicated on the clearance. Recent efforts and research are claiming the importance to increase the weight of convective mechanism, what is supporting the interest for hemofiltration and hemodiafiltration techniques. However, filtration rates in these models are far away of the normal value of GFR. A simulation of the hemofiltration of human glomerulus by means of any type of hemofilter module was performed to evaluate the possibility to reach the value of GFR in renal system (Osada and Nakagawa 1992). Results suggested that this is not possible under current technology, even under the operating conditions of kidneys (with equal Q_b and filtration coefficient), due to differences in the design. It is remarkable to point that the capillary membrane in human glomerulus has $100 \cdot 10^6$ capillaries, against the $100 \cdot 10^3$ of a standard hollow filter. The differences of design are indeed much greater, as it can be noted analyzing the basic ultrastructure of glomerular capillaries.

But differences do not finish here. Urinary excretion is equal to filtration minus reabsorption rate plus secretion rate. Reabsorption and secretion are two active[1] transport mechanisms governed by cells of nephron tubules, whichallow an accurate regulation of excretion of compounds with variable rates as a function of internal homeostasis. In opposition to GFR, reabsorption and secretion are very selective. Table11.1 shows a comprehensive example of flow rates of cited mechanisms for several well-known compounds in a human being.

Table11.1 Filtration, Reabsorption, Secretion, and Final Excretion rates of several metabolites.

Compound	Filtered	Reabsorbed	Secreted	Excreted
Glucose (g/day)	180	180	0	0
Urea (g/day)	46.8	23.4	0	23.4
Creatinine (g/day)	1.8	0	0.5	2.3

In contrast, hollow fiber membrane adds the adsorption to the convection-diffusion mechanism of solute transport.

Therefore, the artificial kidney has important differences with respect to the human kidney, concerning transport flows and performance. These differences limit greatly the expected efficiency and selectivity of the artificial kidney and contribute to the reduction of life expectancy in chronic

---

[1] Although they can induce passive reabsorption and secretion mechanisms.

dialysis patients[2]. Despite these lacks, the artificial kidney allows homeostasis and life during many years in these patients, and many researchers point to the possibility of improve its performance.

One of the first barriers for this goal refers to the difficulty to model hollow fiber dialyzers that describe in an accurate manner the mass-transport mechanismsfor the many compounds involved. They are modulated by complex physicochemical mechanisms that depend on both solutes and membranes.

Compounds to be cleared from blood phase in renal patients are in general partially bounded to blood proteins, a small fraction of them are in turn adsorbed by membranes, building a coating layer during the hemodialysis session that modifies the transport of solutes.

Above phenomena together with the fact that blood shear is not proportional to the velocity gradient orthogonal to the streamline (nonnewtonian fluid), and therefore the viscosity coefficient μ is not constant, makes extremely complex the development of general structural mathematical models for the description of dialyzer flows dynamics.

The whole scenario has been overcome solving common situations of dialyzers easier to model and progressing from them. The same approach has been followed in this chapter for the sake of clarity.

In general, the mass transfer in a system with an interface (liquid – solid or liquid - gas) is given by a relationship of the general form:

$$\mathbf{J} = f(\mathbf{X}), \tag{11.1}$$

where J and X are conjugated flows and forces (vectors), respectively. Equation (11.1) governs general irreversible processes (Montero and Morán 1992). In absence of a surface adsorption, Equation (11.1) can be derived from Navier Stokes conservation equations plus Fick's law of diffusion (Nepomnyashchy et al. 2002). In addition, under common assumptions such as incompressibility of liquid (velocities much lower than speed of sound), and constancy of viscosity, this problem is isomorphic with that addressing the heat transfer of a system with an interface. Such isomorphism is achieved substituting Temperature by Concentration and thermal conductivity by diffusion coefficient.

This chapter is not focused to the general formulation of that interface-based system, since despite its complexity it does not address the inside of

---

[2] Renal system performs other key systemic functions that are not recovered by the artificial kidney that have also influence on this issue.

the porous membrane. However, much of the approach involved in that problem remains when the membrane is taken into account.

The flow (per unit of area) of a solute dissolved in a static solvent bulkacross a semipermeable membrane is as follows:

$$\mathbf{J}_S = -D_S \nabla c_s, \tag{11.2}$$

where subscript "s" refers to the particular solute, c_S is the solute concentration, and D_s is the associated diffusion coefficient. This equation is known as Fick's first law. It derives from the Teorell equation assuming that temperature is constant, pressure influence on chemical potential is negligible, and solution is ideal[3] (Friedman 1986). The Teorell equation is clarified below.

An interesting form of Eq.(11.2) appears in steady-state conditions with D_S constant. Continuity equation is then reduced to $\nabla \cdot \mathbf{J}_S = 0$ and Eq.(11.2) reduces to:

$$\nabla^2 c_S = 0 \tag{11.3}$$

Most of dialysis session with hollow fiber dialyzers can be considered working in quasi-steady state mode and then Eq.(11.3)would be valid (if separation would be governed only by diffusion).

Convection is a second contribution to solute flux across semipermeable membranes. It is due to the movement of fluid, which can be describedaccording to Euler method by the velocity in each spatial point, x, denoted as $v(x,t)$,. In this case $\mathbf{J}_s$is given (Chang and Lee 1988):

$$\mathbf{J}_S = -D_S \nabla c_s + S c_s \mathbf{v} \tag{11.4}$$

The variable S is the sieving coefficient, defined as the rate permeate / feed solute concentration, and it gives a measure of the ability of the membrane for rejecting the solute. It is related to the reflection coefficient,σ, through S = 1 - σ(Staverman 1951).Its value depends on the membrane, the operating conditions, and even the level of description, for each solute (Derjani-Bayeh and Rodgers 2002; Werynski et al. 1985).

Equation (11.4) governs the process of *convective diffusion* in a hollow fiber dialyzer, for non-electrolytes, and it is widely used for modeling the clearance of several uremic toxins during hemodialysis (HD). An

---

[3] Solution with thermodynamic properties similar to those of ideal gases.

important low molecular weight (MW) uremic toxin is urea. This one is used as marker for the adequacy of the HD and relevant clinical studies support its relationship with mortality, despite some controversies (Roa and Prado 2004). This is an important subject that pushesto develop accurate mathematical models of hollow fiber dialyzers. As a consequence, it will be slightly addressed in the following Section.

Equations (11.2) and (11.4) are also valid for non-ideal solutions. In such scenario, it is possible to consider an augmented diffusion coefficient, D^*_S, given by:

$$D_S^* = D_S \left(1 + \frac{d \ln \gamma_s}{d \ln c_s}\right), \tag{11.5}$$

where γ_s is the activity coefficient (Friedman 1986).

A third mechanism that governs also the clearance of solutes in artificial membranes used in hollow fiber filters is the adsorption (fouling). This process was defined by the IUPAC committee by the "depletion of one or more components in an interfacial layer". In the clinical membrane field it is associated with equilibrium interactions solute-surface, and it is usually related to proteins. Mathematical flow models in dialysis focus on the influence that fouling exerts on the other two mechanisms, diffusion and convection.

Several regions feature the boundary layer of the membrane. The concentration polarization (CP) layer retains the solutes accumulated near the membrane. CP can be divided in a gel layer, where molecules reach their critical solubility (concentration is assumed constant) and the final solute layer (cake) where solutes have been adsorbed by the membrane.

Kinetic processes involved in the developing and function of these layers include several irreversible steps. They depend on membrane fine structure, polymer's structure, molecular weight cut off and operating pressures. Dialyzers use ultrafiltration membranes, which are superficially characterized by a molecular weight cut off (MWCO) from 500 Da to 10^5 Da, with operating pressures being $0.5 - 5$ bar. Although there are interesting advances, the dynamics of fouling under in-vivo conditions are still not well known (Boerlage et al. 2002; Nilsson 1990). This is an important limitation for the accuracy of flow modeling.

Another challenging problem in flow modeling is due to the fact that many compounds in the blood phase, inside hollow fibers, and dialysate phase, are charged solutes. Diffusion, permeation and adsorption mechanisms of electrolytes are much more complex than in non-electrolytes because the electrochemical potential substitutes to chemical potential[4] as driving force. The addressing of this issue must also consider the influence of electrochemical interactions of the polymers constituents of the membrane.

The chemical potential of a solute "s" in a solution given by the following equation (considering the influence of pressure on μ negligible):

$$\mu_s = \mu_{s0} + RT \ln\left(\gamma_s c_s\right), \tag{11.6}$$

where R is the gas constant and T is the absolute temperature, must be extended to consider electrostatic forces if it is charged, as follows:

$$\tilde{\mu}_s = \mu_{s0} + RT \ln\left(\gamma_s c_s\right) + z_s F \psi \tag{11.7}$$

New terms in the latter equation are the valence of solute, z_S, the Faraday constant, F (around 96500 coul/mol), and the electrical potential, Ψ. The gradient of the electrochemical potential is now the driving force (generalized force) in Teorell equation, which gives the flow of solute as follows:

$$\mathbf{J}_S = -U_s c_S \nabla \tilde{\mu}_S \tag{11.8}$$

The term U_S is the solute mobility. Substituting (11.7) into (11.8) the electrodiffusion (Nerst-Plank) equation is obtained:

$$\mathbf{J}_S = -U_s c_S \left(RT\nabla(\gamma_S c_S) + z_S F \nabla \psi\right) \tag{11.9}$$

It can be extended, by adding the contribution of fluid movement (complete permeation):

$$\boxed{\mathbf{J}_S = -U_s c_S \left(RT\nabla(\gamma_S c_S) + z_S F \nabla \psi\right) + S c_s \mathbf{v}} \tag{11.10}$$

Therefore Eq.(11.10) is an extension of Eq.(11.4) for convective diffusion flows of charged solutes in a dialyzer.

Two mathematical conditions related to the electrical field are necessary to solve the convective form of Nerst-Plank equation. The first one states

---

[4] The chemical potential is the driving force of Teorell equation, from which the Fick's Law derives.

that the current density (amperes per unit of area), I_A, is given as the sum of contributions of each specie, i:

$$I_A = F \cdot \sum_i z_i J_i \qquad (11.11)$$

Second, a boundary condition of electroneutrality is needed. This states a relationship between positive and negative charges in the solution:

$$\sum z_i c_i + z_X X = 0, \qquad (11.12)$$

where X is the charge concentration associated with dissociated polar groups in the membrane matrix, and $z_X = \pm 1$. This boundary condition assumes that polar groups are uniformly distributed along the membrane.

The general solution to the Eq.(11.10) is very complex and there is not an analytical equation for it, excepting for some particular cases with additional restrictions. Numerical methods do not repair this issue, because one major problem arises from the bad knowledge above several key variables in the equation, as for instance the charge concentration in the membrane under in-vivo conditions.

Biomedical membranes used in hollow fiber dialyzers operate under conditions that exceed the scope of Eq. (11.10). The following paragraphs depict some key details that illustrate the complexity of this scenario.

Hemodialysis membranes have evolved from the dense cellophane membranes towards synthetic ones, based on polymers with enhanced properties for biofunctionality and biocompatibility.Membrane's synthetic polymers, such a Polyamid, used from Gambro^{TM}, are processed in such a way that cellular and protein interactions could be minimized and microinflammation and thrombogenic risks of patient reduced.

In addition, new membranes are designed and manufactured with larger pores, permeable even to small proteins such β_2-microglobulin (11800 D), with a proved role in amyloidosis on chronic hemodialysis patients. Several studies have shown that the increase of hemodialysis clearance of uremic toxins, in the middle and high molecular weight range, benefits patients' health. These membranes are known ashigh flux membranes. A formal classification can be found in (Daugirdas et al. 2007).

Concerning the MWCO range, hollow fiber membranes are considered of ultrafiltration type. They present different fine structures. There are asymmetric ones, with a fine structure characterized by a porous support side, and a dense thin layer of around 1 µm in thickness. More recent developments have achieving more homogeneous fine structures with even better diffusion.

The performance of the membrane is associated with the fine structure, the primary structure of polymers constituents, and other structural factors related to chemical interactions, such as cross-linking, presence of crystallites, or additives. The microphotography of a synthetic hollow fiber dialyzer is shown in Fig. 11.2. This one shows the cited thin layer at blood side.

Succinctly, these complex structures cannot be considered simple semipermeable barriers, because they interact with blood cellular elements and solutes, activating cellular membrane receptors, and therefore inducing the release of peptides and other compounds to the system, which in turn promote unwanted effects.

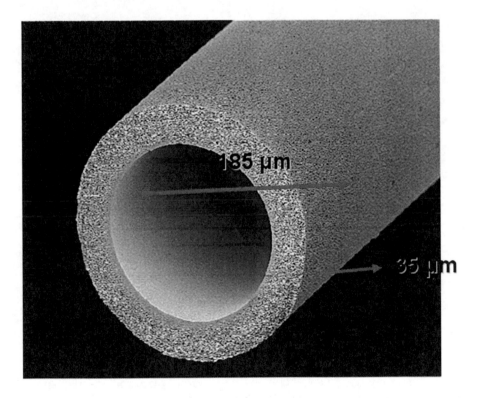

Fig. 11.2 Microphotography of hollow fiber dialyzer, which shows the difference between the fine structure at blood and dialysate side.

Moreover, Eq.(11.10) should be considered a simplification in presence of multiple solutes, due to interactions among them. In general, the flux of i-th component permeated across a polymer membrane could be formulated using Eq.(11.1) around the equilibrium point, which gives the following well-known equation(Groot and Mazur 1984; Osada and Nakagawa 1992):

$$J_i = \sum_j L_{ij} X_j,$$ (11.13)

where L_{ij} is the Jacobian of $f(X)$ in Eq.(11.1). These Jacobian entries are also known as phenomenological coefficients, which must be positive, and verify the following relationships(Montero and Morán 1992):

$$L_{ii} L_{jj} > L_{ij} L_{ji}$$
$$L_{ij} = L_{ji}$$ (11.14)

The second equation in (11.14) is known as Onsager relationships; having important implications in systems dynamics. Equation (11.13) is restricted around the equilibrium. However, in practice the range of application is wider.

Substituting the generalized forces by their known magnitudes, and adding the influence of pressure, p, in the electro-chemical potential, as well as temperature, the following generalization of the electro diffusion equation is obtained:

$$\mathbf{J}_i = -\sum_j L_{ij} (RT\nabla a_i + z_i F\nabla \psi + v_j \nabla p) + L_{it} \nabla T + S c_i \mathbf{v}$$ (11.15)

The term v_j is the specific volume (molar volume if J is molar flow) of specie j. It has been represented the activity of solute j as a_j, defined as:

$$a_i = \gamma_j c_j$$ (11.16)

Despite the extraordinary complexity of Eq.(11.15) the following Section will show the success that a very simplistic mathematical model of hollow fiber dialyzer can obtain; both under in-vitro and in-vivo conditions, for some relevant uremic toxins and ions. Subsequent Sections will present instruments and methods followed for increasing the accuracy of these models in more complex scenarios.

11.2 FLOW MODELING IN A WHOLE SCENARIO

According with the approach depicted above, this Section develops a first simplified mathematical model of transport flows for hollow fiber dialyzers in clinical scenario. A road of increasing complexity and accuracy has been followed.

The following figure shows an artificial kidney connected by means of an arteriovenous (AV) fistula to a patient. It shows one of the most used AV accesses for patients submitted to periodic hemodialysis(Daugirdas et al. 2007). Blood and dialysate circuits are presented together with their main medical devices, such as peristaltic pumps, air trap and heparin pump. Pressure and other monitors are not shown.

As seen in Fig. 11.3 blood and dialysate flows are in countercurrent, and adjustable inflow resistance is placed at the dialysate inlet, in such a way that average transmembrane pressure (blood outlet – dialysate outlet) could be positive, and therefore it could generate a convective flow from blood to dialysate (ultrafiltration).

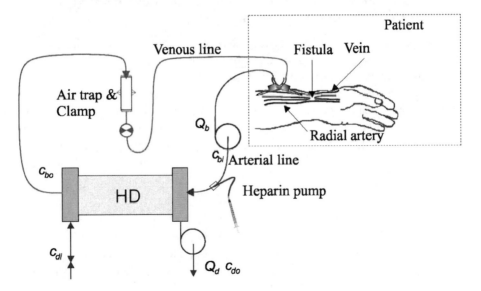

Fig. 11.3 Hollow fiber dialyzer connected to a renal patient through a radiocephalic arteriovenous (AV) fistula.

Nomenclature of flows (Q) and solute concentrations (c) are also indicated.Subscripts refer to the circuit and inlet or outlet of dialyzer.

The mathematical modeling of auxiliary devices in that whole system can be simplified, taking the magnitude values that they provide as boundary conditions. This manner, flow rates will be considered known and influence of heparin can be neglected.

Steady-state conditions can be assumed, by considering that the characteristic time of variation of blood solute concentrations in the accessible patient compartment is much greater than the residence time of blood along the artificial kidney. This is a common assumption in kinetic models used in hemodialysis (Prado et al. 2004; Sargent and Gotch 1980).

In order to build a first simplified model of the dialyzer, the renal clearance of a solute s, K_{KS}, could bedefined by the following equation(Guyton and Hall 2006):

$$K_{KS} = \frac{c_{uS} \cdot UFR}{c_{PS}},$$

(11.17)

where UFR is the urine flow rate, c_{uS} is the solute urine concentration, and c_{PS} is the plasma solute concentration.

Equation (11.17) can be rearranged to show that $K_{KS} \cdot c_{PS}$ is the urinary excretion rate of solute s. This equation suggests the possibility to model the total transport flow of solute s in the hollow fiber dialyzer of Fig. 11.3 by means of a dialyzer clearance, K_S. This is a technique widely extended, and dialyzers manufacturers provide clearances of several relevant compounds in dialysis, e.g. urea, for common operating conditions. Although it is a very simplistic model of dialyzer, this Section starts with it, fortesting subsequently how it is related to the electrodiffusion Eq.(11.10) and the derived equations.

A kinetic model of the human system is also neededto perform a numerical simulation of the whole system of Fig. 11.3. The complexity of this model depends on the dynamics of the required compounds within the human organism. The single pool kinetic model has been widely used for many relevant small molecular weight compounds, included urea, and several electrolytes (Prado et al. 2005a).

Selecting a single-pool kinetic model for the human organism, a first mathematical model of the whole system of Fig. 11.3, able to express the transport flows for a compound s, could be expressed as:

$$\frac{d(Vc_S)}{dt} + K_S c_S = G_S$$

(11.18)

The left term in Eq.(11.18) describes the total increase of mass of solute within a control volume defined by human subject, where V is the distribution volume of the solute s. The right term is the solute generation rate inside control volume, G_S. This equation can be rearranged, considering that the excreted flow rate Q_e is related to the derivative of volume as:

$$\dot{V} = \frac{dV}{dt} = -Q_e \tag{11.19}$$

And then Eq.(11.18) could be expressed:

$$\boxed{V\dot{c}_s = V\frac{dc_S}{dt} = G_S - K_S c_S - \dot{V}c_S = G_S - (K_S - Q_e)c_S} \tag{11.20}$$

Equation (11.20) is then a first model of transport flows and solute kinetics of the whole system of Fig. 11.3, under the claimed assumptions. It must be noted that the excreted flow rate, Q_e, of Eq.(11.19) is associated with a excreted solute rate $c_S Q_e$, in agreement with Eq.(11.18). Denoting Q_{UF} to the ultrafiltration flow rate, and considering that $Q_e = Q_{UF} + UFR$, this applies for small solutes with a membrane sieving coefficient, $S = 1$, and with renal filtration equal to renal excretion[5].

Equation (11.20) is certainly valid for an experimental system where the patient is substituted by a well-stirred pool. Accordingly, and before a deeper analysis of the hollow fiber dialyzer, this first model is applied in two classic situations, in-vivo and in-vitro, respectively.

Concerning the in-vivo analysis, the kinetics of urea of an End Renal Stage Disease (ESRD) anuric patient submitted to three session of HD per week, under stable conditions, will be simulated. The stability allows considering that urea pattern is approximately repeated every week. This is associated with the following mathematical condition(Depner and Cheer 1989):

$$c_s(t+p) = c(t), \tag{11.21}$$

for any time t, taking the period, p, equal to 1 week.

Figure 11.4 shows the source (Mathematica^{TM} language) of a comprehensive algorithm that identifies the dialyzer clearance, K_S (Kdial in the source code), and the generation of urea, G_S, of that patient. The code clarifies that G_S is obtained through the protein catabolic rate (PCR) of the patient, which is associated with G_S through an equation (Borah et al. 1978).

---

[5] It is also valid for anuric patients.

- **Integrated model equation**

```
c[t_, ci_, k_, beta_, G_, V0_] :=
   (ci - G / (k + beta)) / ((V0 + beta t) / V0) ^ (k / beta + 1.) + G / (k + beta);
```

- **Relationship protein catabolic rate - urea generation**

```
(* Urea Generation (mg/min) -PCR (g/dia) ,V(dl) *)
Gen[pcr_, V0_] := (pcr - 0.029 V0) / 4.3633;
```

- **Weekly pattern of uremic solute (urea) for an anuric end stage renal disease patient**

```
(* Inicialization *)
Tdial = 3.5 * 60; (* Dialysis duration, min *)
teta1 = (2 * 24 * 60 - Tdial); (* interdialysis time, min *)
teta2 = teta1;
teta3 = (3 * 24 * 60 - Tdial);
UF = 35; (* Ultrafiltration volume in dL*)
beta = -UF / Tdial; (* ultrafiltration flow, dl/min*)
c02 = 128; (*pre - dialysis urea blood concentration, mg/dl *)
c12 = 50; (*post - dialysis urea blood concentration, mg/dl *)
V0 = 70 * 0.58 * 10 (*Solute distribution volume, dL*)
(* Evolution of system during a week and identification of Kdial and G,
together with the computation of remaining solute concentrations *)
{c01, c11, c03, c13, pcr, Kdial} =
 {c01, c11, c03, c13, pcr, Kdial} /.
  FindRoot[{c[Tdial, c01, Kdial, beta, Gen[pcr, V0], V0 + UF] == c11,
    c[teta1, c11, 0, -beta * Tdial / teta1, Gen[pcr, V0], V0] == c02,
    c[Tdial, c02, Kdial, beta, Gen[pcr, V0], V0 + UF] == c12,
    c[teta2, c12, 0, -beta * Tdial / teta2, Gen[pcr, V0], V0] == c03,
    c[Tdial, c03, Kdial, beta, Gen[pcr, V0], V0 + UF] == c13,
    c[teta3, c13, 0, -beta * Tdial / teta3, Gen[pcr, V0], V0] == c01},
   {c03, 50}, {c13, 50}, {c01, 50}, {c11, 50}, {pcr, 50}, {Kdial, 1.}, MaxIterations → 50,
  AccuracyGoal → Infinity, WorkingPrecision → 16]
```

Fig. 11.4 MathematicaTM implementation of Equation (11.20) to obtain the urea pattern of an ESRD anuric patient submitted to three sessions of HD per week.

Other clinical details, such as the total ultrafiltration volume (UF), or the estimation of the urea distribution volume at the end of the session (V0 in source) from the patient weight (70 Kg), are also shown[6]. The algorithm uses an integrated form of Eq.(11.20), which is indicated in the first code line. Blood Urea Concentrations (BUC) at the second weekly session, namely c02 (pre-dialysis) and c12 (post-dialysis), are sampled and used as

---

[6] We use here a gross estimation based on the patient weight. There are more accurate methods for obtaining the urea distribution volume of a patient.

inputs to the mathematical model. Pre-dialysis and post-dialysis values in the first and third sessions are also computed as outputs by the algorithm.

The resulting urea kinetic pattern of this dialyzer + patient system has been plotted in Fig. 11.5, together with BUC values at the remaining weekly dialysis sessions.

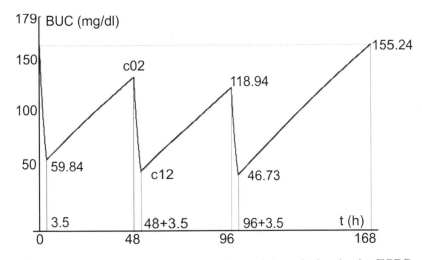

Fig. 11.5 Blood Urea Concentration (plasmatic) evolution in the ESRD patient of the study.

Despite the simplicity of the dialyzer and patient kinetic model, many studies have validated their good performance and accuracy in the description of the urea for patients submitted to dialysis(Roa and Prado 2004). There are several technical and clinical details that exceed the scope of this chapter.

With respect to the in-vitro scenario, the equation (11.20) has been used to describe the transport flow of LiCl in a system constituted by a hollow fiber (Gambro[TM] Polyflux 17 L) and a well-stirred volumetric flask. With that objective, sieving coefficients of Li^+ and Cl^- are considered equal to 1. This assumption is in agreement with other studies (Mercadal et al. 1998).

Experiments were performed with ultrapure water (Milli-Q, 15uS/cm). Concentrations were sampled by conductivity method in blood and dialysate circuits, and converted to concentrations after subtraction of bias. Dialysate flow rate (ultrapure water without LiCl), Q_d, was set to 500 ml/min, whereas blood flow rate (ultrapure water with LiCl), Q_b, was set to 100, 500, and 650 ml/min in consecutive series.

The whole system was primed with ultrapure water, and measurements started after blood from the well-stirred spinner flask with the initial LiCl concentration passed through dialyzer, for minimizing the influence of the system transient.

Plot experimental versus predicted salt concentration kinetics - Qb 100 ml/min

```
(* Data reading *)
Ts = Import["ResultadosAnaliticosCationes_Final.xls", {"Data", 1, Range[4, 16], 1}];
(* min *)
cSalt = Import["ResultadosAnaliticosCationes_Final.xls", {"Data", 1, Range[4, 16], 5}];
(* mg/ml *)
V0 = 258; (* ml *)
UF = -21; (* ml *) (* Positive reference flowing out single pool *)
Qb = 100; (* ml/min *)
c100[t_] := E^(-0.9628) * E^(-0.4216 t); (* exponential regression *)


(* IDENTIFICATION PROCESS *)
(* Compute AUCexp *)
itmax = Length[Ts];
AUCexp = Sum[(cSalt[[i + 1]] + cSalt[[i]]) / 2 * (Ts[[i + 1]] - Ts[[i]]),
    {i, 1, itmax - 1}]; (* mg/ml*min *)
(* Solve K such that AUCexp - AUCmodel is minimum *)
G = 0;
ci = cSalt[[1]];
Tdial = Ts[[itmax]]; (* Dialysis time *)
beta = -UF / Tdial; (* ultrafiltration flow, ml/min *)
(* Iterate *)
Kdial = k /. FindRoot[NIntegrate[c[t, ci, k, beta, G, V0], {t, 0, Tdial}] == AUCexp,
    {k, 0.42 * V0}, MaxIterations → 50]
```

Fig. 11.6 MathematicaTM source of the algorithm implemented to identify the dialyzer clearance under experimental conditions for $Q_b=100$ ml/min.

The value of dialyzer clearance for LiCl is identified by imposing the experimental measured values to the initial salt concentration, and to the Area under the Curve (AUC) of salt concentration. The algorithm is presented in Fig. 11.6, using as guess the value of the clearance obtained generating an exponential regression for data.

The ultrafiltration volume was negative, because dialysate pump impelled to the dialyzer inlet, in opposition to the position indicated in Fig. 11.3 (countercurrent is kept).

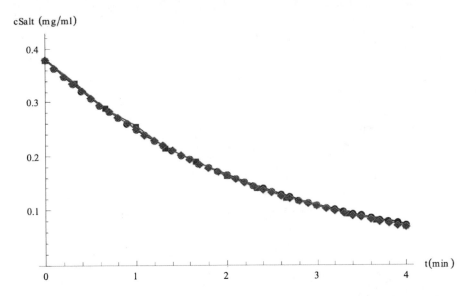

Fig. 11.7 Samples of LiCl from well-stirred volumetric flask (red-squares), together with exponential regression (purple-diamonds), and solution of Eq. (11.20) (blue - circles), for Q_b = 100 ml/min.

Figure 11.7 shows the agreement between in-vitro data, exponential regression and mathematical model expressed by Eq. (11.20), for the first dialysis session with Q_b = 100 ml/min. Differences among three trajectories and values are negligible, which suggest that the mathematical model is valid.

However, differences among experimental, regression, and mathematical model increase for Q_b = 500 ml/min, as presented in Fig. 11.8. This one clarifies also the difference between the exponential regression, and the solution of Eq. (11.20):

$$c_S(t) = \frac{G_S}{K_S + G_S} + (c_S(0) - \frac{G_S}{K_S + G_S})\left(\frac{V(0) - Q_e t}{V(0)}\right)^{\frac{K_S - Q_e}{Q_e}} \qquad (11.22)$$

The values of the identified clearances by the mathematical model were 104.46, 228.33, and 326.57 ml/min, for Q_b = 100, 500, and 650 ml/min, respectively. The homologues values from exponential regression were 108.77, 250.06, and 283.44 ml/min, respectively.

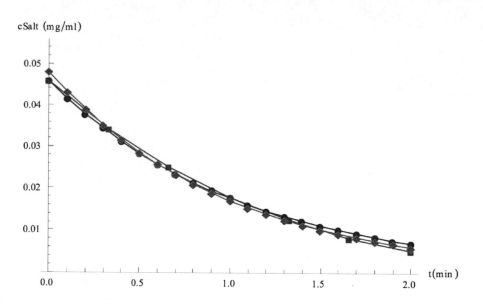

Fig. 11.8 Samples of LiCl from well-stirred volumetric flask (red-squares), together with exponential regression (purple-diamonds), and solution of Eq. (11.20) (blue - circles), for $Q_b = 500$ ml/min.

The deviation between dialyzer clearances identified through equation (11.20) and regression was highest in the third case, with 326 ml/min against 283.44 ml/min, respectively. This case is plotted in Fig. 11.9.

In summary, both in-vivo and in-vitro studies with low molecular weight compounds support the assumption that the hollow fiber membrane can be described by means of a constant clearance. This clearance should depend on flow rates in blood and dialysate circuits. Charged solutes and presence of several electrolytes in in-vitro experiments do not affect to this conclusion. Loss of accuracy in the third in-vitro series could be a consequence of the higher influence of starting transient of the experiment, due to the smaller residence time.

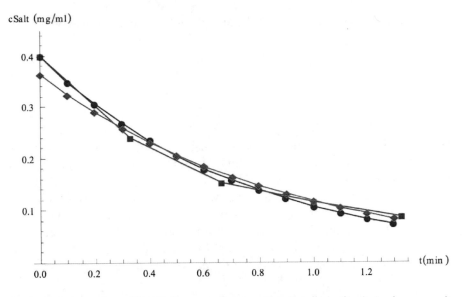

Fig. 11.9 Samples of LiCl from well-stirred volumetric flask (red-squares), together with exponential regression (purple-diamonds), and solution of equation (11.20) (blue - circles), for $Q_b = 650$ ml/min.

11.3 1D DIFFUSIVE MODEL OF A HOLLOW FIBER DIALYZER

The conditions to be fulfilled by the hollow fiber dialyzer for this extremely simplified mathematical modelare analyzed in this Section. It is necessary to integrate Eq.(11.10)under conditions of pure diffusion transport flow and assuming that there is no electrical field across the membrane. With these assumptions the cited equation transforms in the Fick's law, with the augmented diffusion coefficient.

$$U_s RT \left(1 + \frac{d \ln \gamma_s}{d \ln c_S} \right) = D_S^* \tag{11.23}$$

As we are interested in the component of solute flux normal to the membrane (x axis from blood to dialysate), then:

$$J_S dx = -D_S^* dc_S \tag{11.24}$$

And assuming steady-state conditions, it can be integrated to give:

$$J_S = \frac{D_S^*}{a}(c_{mbS} - c_{mdS}) = \frac{c_{mbS} - c_{mdS}}{\dfrac{a}{D_S^*}} \qquad (11.25)$$

The term D_S^*/a is the permeability of solute in that membrane, whereas c_{mbS} and c_{mdS} are solute concentrations in membrane phase over blood and dialysate sides, respectively. With the aim of obtaining J_S from solute concentrations in blood and dialysate phases, it can be assumed that solute concentrations are homogeneous for each coordinate value, z, in the streamline, excepting in a small non-stirred (diffusional layer) in the immediate vicinity of the membrane(Friedman 1986). Under such conditions, expressions similar to Eq.(11.25) in each layer can be obtained, which in turn can be reduced to the following equation:

$$J_S = \frac{c_{bS} - c_{dS}}{\dfrac{\delta^b}{D_S^b} + \dfrac{a}{D_S^*} + \dfrac{\delta^d}{D_S^d}} = K(z)(c_{bS} - c_{dS}) \qquad (11.26)$$

The term $K(z)$ is the apparent permeability of membrane for the solute s in the position$z$ of the streamline. The mass balance in the dialyzer can be completed using Eq.(11.26), as follows:

$$dW = K(z)(c_b - c_d)dA = Q_d dc_d = Q_b dc_b \qquad (11.27)$$

The subscript s of concentrations variables has been removed in the sake of clarity. The differential mass flow is written as a function of c_b-c_d in the right terms of equation, as follows:

$$(\frac{Q_b}{Q_d} - 1)dW = \frac{Q_b}{Q_d}Q_d dc_d - Q_b dc_b = Q_b dc_d - Q_b dc_b = Q_b d(c_b - c_d)$$

$$\Rightarrow dW = Q_b \frac{d(c_b - c_d)}{Q_b / Q_d - 1} \qquad (11.28)$$

Making it equal to left term of Eq.(11.27), gives:

$$Q_b \frac{d(c_b - c_d)}{Q_b / Q_d - 1} = K(r)(c_b - c_d) \Rightarrow$$

$$\frac{d(c_b - c_d)}{c_b - c_d} = K(r)\left(\frac{1}{Q_d} - \frac{1}{Q_b}\right) \tag{11.29}$$

And integrating along the streamline of hollow fiber dialyzer, z, the following relationship is obtained:

$$\ln \frac{c_{bi} - c_{do}}{c_{bo} - c_{di}} = \left(\frac{1}{Q_d} - \frac{1}{Q_b}\right)\int_0^A K(z)dA \tag{11.30}$$

$$\ln \frac{c_{bi} - c_{do}}{c_{bo} - c_{di}} = \left(\frac{1}{Q_d} - \frac{1}{Q_b}\right)K_o A \tag{11.31}$$

where K_o is defined as the average value of $K(z)$ along streamline, and A is the membrane area. Subscripts o and i refer to outlet and inlet, respectively. This manner, the total solute transport flow, $W = Q_b(c_{bi}-c_{bo}) = Q_d(c_{do}-c_{di})$, can be written as:

$$\ln \frac{c_{bi} - c_{do}}{c_{bo} - c_{di}} = \left(\frac{c_{bi} - c_{bo}}{W} - \frac{c_{do} - c_{di}}{W}\right)K_o A \Rightarrow$$

$$\boxed{W = K_o A \frac{(c_{bi} - c_{do}) - (c_{bo} - c_{di})}{\ln \dfrac{c_{bi} - c_{do}}{c_{bo} - c_{di}}} = K_o A \cdot LMCD} \tag{11.32}$$

The term that multiplies to $K_o A$ is the *Logarithmic Mean Concentration Difference* (LMCD) across membrane. This expression can be manipulated to give a model of the solute transport W, as a function of inlet solute concentrations and flow rates operating conditions.

The dialyzer diffusive efficiency is firstly defined as:

$$\varepsilon = \frac{c_{bi} - c_{bo}}{c_{bi} - c_{di}} \tag{11.33}$$

According to this nomenclature the maximum of term ε is 1[7]. Now, left term of Eq.(11.31) can be expressed in terms of ε and $R = Q_b/Q_d$, by means of solute mass balances in dialysate and blood circuits, as follows:

---

[7] It can be proved that maximum of ε is 1 if $Q_b < Q_d$ and $Q_d/Q_b < 1$ if $Q_d < Q_b$.

$$\frac{c_{bi} - c_{do}}{c_{bo} - c_{di}} = \frac{R - \frac{1}{\varepsilon}}{1 - \frac{1}{\varepsilon}}, \tag{11.34}$$

which can be substituted in Eq.(11.31) for solving ε in terms of operating conditions:

$$\varepsilon(R, NTU) = \frac{1 - e^{-NTU(1-R)}}{1 - Re^{-NTU(1-R)}} \tag{11.35}$$

The NTU (Number of Transfer Units) is defined as $K_o A / Q_b$. Therefore, the solute transport flow can be expressed:

$$\boxed{\begin{aligned} W &= Q_b(c_{bi} - c_{bo}) = \varepsilon(R, NTU) \cdot Q_b \cdot (c_{bi} - c_{di}) \Rightarrow \\ W &= d_S(R, NTU) \cdot (c_{bi} - c_{di}) \end{aligned}} \tag{11.36}$$

The term d_S is the solute dialysance (Wolf et al. 1951). Equation (11.36) describes the solute flow transport of a hollow fiber dialyzer under steady-state and pure diffusion. It is called 1D diffusion model of the hollow fiber dialyzer. Equally to the above problem of mass transfer in a system with an interface, the model given by Eq.(11.36) is isomorphic to the heat transfer in recuperative heaters (heat conduction)(Lienard-IV and Lienard-V 2001).

In the case of $c_{di} = 0$, as occurred in previous examples, the dialyzer can be described by means of a solute clearance parameter, K_S, that depends on operating flow rates and the apparent permeability of membrane for the solute:

$$W = K_S(R, NTU)c_{bi} \tag{11.37}$$

Therefore, the dialysance is equal to the clearance when $c_{di}=0$. In addition, if $c_{di}=0$, the efficiency coincides with the dialyzer extraction coefficient, E, commonly used both in renal physiology (Guyton and Hall 2006) and artificial kidneys (MacKay Valera et al. 1995):

$$E = \frac{c_{bi} - c_{bo}}{c_{bi}} \tag{11.38}$$

With the aim of validating the mathematical model (11.37), the product K_oA for LiCl in the above in-vitro study has been identified.

The equations of the 1D diffusive model have been implemented in Mathcad^{TM}, as shown in Fig. 11.10. It shows the equation of efficiency of the dialyzer in agreement with the general expression(11.35), as well as in the degenerated case that appears when $R = 1$.

Number of transfer units, NTU, as a function of R and efficiency

$NTU := 5.$ **Guess**

Given

$$\varepsilon b = \frac{1 - e^{NTU \cdot (1-R)}}{R - e^{NTU \cdot (1-R)}}$$

$NTransfUnit(R, \varepsilon b) := Find(NTU)$

Asymptotic case (when R = 1)

Given

$$\varepsilon b = \frac{NTU}{1 + NTU}$$

$NTransfUnitAsym(\varepsilon b) := Find(NTU)$

Efficiency as a funcion of K and Quf

$$efi(K, Quf, Qb) := \frac{K - Quf}{Qb - Quf}$$

Fig. 11.10 MathcadTM source of the methods implemented to identify the NTU from dialyzer clearance under experimental conditions described in text.

An additional issue that arises when it is required to obtain the efficiency from the experimental dialyzer clearance is due to the ultrafiltration flow rate. The 1D diffusivemodel assumes that there is not fluid movement.

However, it is necessary to take into account a small net ultrafiltration from dialysate towards blood circuit.

The following mass balance for the target solute passing through the dialyzer blood circuit can be written:

$$W = Q_b c_{bi} - (Q_b - Q_{UF})c_{bo} = Q_b(c_{bi} - c_{bo}) + Q_{UF}(c_{bi} - (c_{bi} - c_{bo})) \quad (11.39)$$

Introducing the definition of efficiency [Eq.(11.33)] as well as the condition $c_{di} = 0$, the expression could be rearranged as follows:

$$W = c_{bi}(\varepsilon Q_b + (1-\varepsilon)Q_{UF}) \quad (11.40)$$

Therefore, the term between brackets could be considered the clearance of the dialyzer working under diffusive and convective transport mechanisms:

$$K_S = \varepsilon Q_b + (1-\varepsilon)Q_{UF} \quad (11.41)$$

Equation (11.41) is a misleading expression, because equation (11.35) is not valid under convection mechanism, according to the assumptions taken to reach it. Several authors have proposed different strategies to separate or disconnect diffusion from convection mechanisms. A comprehensive review can be read in(Jaffrin 1995). However, those mechanisms are really linked and those strategies are not very effective. A well-known expression that illustrates the sought separation is as follows (Clark 2001; Jaffrin 1995; Werynski and Waniewski 1995):

$$K_S = K_{dS} + T_r Q_{UF} \quad (11.42)$$

where K_{dS} is the diffusive clearance of the dialyzer when $Q_{UF} = 0$, and T_r is the transmission coefficient of the membrane. Although K_{dS} can be obtained from the theoretical 1D model previously developed, the T_r term is an empirical variable that depends on the diffusive mechanism. A proposed equation for T_r was (Clark 2001):

$$T_r = S \cdot \left(1 - \frac{K_d}{Q_b}\right) \quad (11.43)$$

The term S is the sieving coefficient defined in Eq.(11.4).

According to the low value of the net ultrafiltration rate in our experiments and in agreement with other authors, we have used the function $\varepsilon(R,NTU)$ given in Eq.(11.35) for the efficiency of Eq.(11.41). This method has been widely used provided the convective term is small. This manner, the experimental value of ε in our LiCl series can be extracted by the final equation of Fig. 11.10.

The algorithm for identifying the value of K_oA has been codified in Mathcad^{TM}, as shown in Fig. 11.11 for the first dialysis of LiCl. It is composed by three stages. The first one is devoted to compute K_oA from the

Case 1 - LCl

$$Qb := 100 \qquad Quf := \frac{-21}{4} = -5.25 \qquad Kdial := 0.40488 \cdot 258 = 104.459 \qquad Qd := 500$$

$$\varepsilon b := efi(Kdial, Quf, Qb) = 1.042 \qquad \text{Blood efficiency}$$

$$\varepsilon b := min(1, \varepsilon b) = 1$$

$$R := \frac{Qb}{Qd} = 0.2$$

$$NTU := NTransfUnit(R, \varepsilon b) = 29.259$$

$$KA := NTU \cdot Qb = 2.926 \times 10^3 \qquad \text{ml/min}$$

Sensitivity (Delta KA per unit of variation of blood efficiency) in operation point

$$S := \frac{(NTransfUnit(R, \varepsilon b) - NTransfUnit(R, \varepsilon b - 0.1)) \cdot Qb}{0.1} = 2.663 \times 10^4$$

$$\left(ErrEstKA := S \cdot 0.1 = 2.663 \times 10^3 \right) \qquad \text{Delta KA (ml/min) for 10 \% of Delta effficiency}$$

Prediction for KA 400 ml/min

$$NTU := \frac{400}{Qb} = 4$$

- -

$$Kpred := \frac{1 - e^{NTU \cdot (1-R)}}{R - e^{NTU \cdot (1-R)}} \cdot (Qb - Quf) + Quf = 96.54 \qquad \text{ml/min}$$

Fig. 11.11 MathcadTM codification of the KoA identification for the first in-vitro dialysis session with LiCl ($Q_b = 100$ ml/min).

NTU dimensionless group, which in turn is solved from ε. The sensitivity of K_oA to errors in ε is computed in the second stage. The last stage performs a prediction of the dialyzer clearance for a value of K_oA equal for the three in-vitro dialysis sessions.

The values of K_oA identified according to this procedure for the three in-vitro dialysis sessions are shown in Table 11.2.

Table 11.2 Values of KoA, together with dimensionless variables and other relevant data from in-vitro experiments.

Q_b(ml/min)	Q_{UF}(ml/min)	ε	NTU	K_oA (ml/min)	S_n
100	-5.25	1	29.26	$2.92 \cdot 10^3$	9.1
500	-4.5	0.462	0.857	428.5	4.1
650	-8.27	0.509	1.239	805.6	5.0

The difference among the K_oA values obtained could seem unexpected, because the experiment accomplished properly the assumptions of the 1D diffusive model of the hollow fiber dialyzer. However, the high normalized sensitivity $(S_n = S/K_oA)$ to errors in ε suggests a plausible reason for that divergence in a parameter that should be unique for that membrane. This phenomenon is forgotten most of times by physicians, who use to consider that the major source of K_oA differences is the lack of knowledge and variability of variables on in-vivo conditions.

As shown in Table 11.2, sensitivity is directly related to NTU dimensionless group. The efficiency of a dialyzer increases with NTU, in such a way that ε reaches values around 0.5 for NTU values about 1. The slope ε-NTU is reducedwhen NTU grows, in such a way that it is not cost-effective to operate with NTU values much greater than 1 -2.

It has been set a value of K_oA approximately equal to that of the session with smaller sensitivity, and compared the associated predicted dialyzer clearances with the experimental dialyzer clearances identified previously. Taken K_oA = 400 ml/min, differences predicted - experimental clearances were 96.5 vs. 104.46, 219.72 vs. 228.331, and 228.55 vs. 326.537, for Q_b = 100, 500, and 650 ml/min, respectively. That is, predicted dialyzer clearances were good for Q_b = 100, and 500 ml/min, but fail for Q_b = 650 ml/min.

The bad behavior of the session for Q_b = 650 ml/min, agrees with the greater deviations of LiCl concentrations of Fig. 11.9, and it could be associated with the higher influence of starting transient (steady-state condition), and the higher value of convection (Table 11.2).

11.4 SUCCINCT REVIEW OF LACKS OF 1D DIFFUSIVE FLOW MODELING OF HOLLOW FIBER DIALYZERS

With the aim of motivating the development of new mathematical models of hollow fiber dialyzers, this Section reviews several of the limits associated with the previous diffusive flow modeling.

The scope of the described 1D diffusive model is limited to steady-state conditions with diluted solutions, Newtonian fluids, without convection,with highly diffused compounds that do not interact with membrane either other compounds, and with fiber arrangements highly symmetrical inside the dialysate compartment of the dialyzer. In addition, the assumption of independence of K_oA with the operating flow rates compel to has a design of the dialysate compartment that guarantees the fully development of turbulence and the adherence and steady-state condition of the limit-layer external to fibers.

These assumptions are not fulfilled in practice. However, it is frequent the use of the 1D diffusive model for low molecular weight solutes, like urea. This justifies divergences between the delivered and expected clearance. Unfortunately these divergences are not well understood, and sometimes are due to other factors, like the sensitivity previously analyzed and even to variables external to the dialyzer.

The dynamics of patient as well as the presence of vascular access recirculation pertain to the last type of variables. For instance, the distribution of urea in patients has been modeled by means of a single pool compartment in the Second Section, but many studies confirm that urea kinetics in humans follows a two-pool distribution. Most compounds require even more compartments, and the identification of these ones is complex, with properties dependent on each human.

Moreover, the vascular access recirculation is still not well monitored, and some of the clinical methods used to estimate it have a performance worse than clinical could expect.

The complexity of the problem was justified in previous Sections, and the addressing of cited limitations exceeds the scope of this chapter. Notwithstanding, two internal phenomena that cause important divergence between expected and delivered clearance in urea must be cited.

The first of them is called polarization of concentration, which causes an increase of the coupling between convection and diffusion mechanisms. It is due to the appearance of a higher concentration layer in the vicinity of blood side wall of membrane caused by its fouling along dialysis session. It will be better studied in the following Section.

A second phenomenon is the modulation of K_oA with the dialysate flow rate, due to the modification of the fluid regime and solute transport characteristic at the dialysate side (Allen et al. 1995). This behavior is the base of a new methodology of non-regenerated dialysate recirculation for enhance the diffusive clearance of dialyzers (Prado and Roa 2007; Prado et al. 2005b; Prado et al. 2005c).

11.5   A DEEPER INSIGHT IN THE FLOW MODELING OF DIALYZERS

The above review concerning the lacks of the 1D diffusive mathematical model of hollow fiber dialyzer shows a very complex scenario. Despite the intensive research in this area, accurate models are very limited in scope, particularly under in-vivo conditions.

Because the scarce knowledge in the local interactions compounds - membrane matrix under on-line conditions, empiric approaches are many times used. These ones allow filling the gap of physics-based approaches.

Due to the difficulty to present a complete picture of models and recent advances, this Section presents an interesting mathematical model that joins empiric equations with physics laws. It was presented in (Paris et al. 2002) for modeling the ultrafiltration in a tubular membrane that retains completely the solute. Authors tested that model with dextran T500 and distilled water (solvent).

The model takes into account diffusion and convection mechanisms in a single cylindrical geometry, under conditions that induce the fouling of the membrane, associated with the adsorption and chemical interaction with solute. Accordingly, the model has the potential to address the mechanism of concentration polarization under controlled conditions.

That mathematical model provides an easy framework that help to deep in the three transport mechanisms that appear under in-vivo conditions.

The equations that describe the physics of flow transport in a fluid are known as Navier-Stokes conservation equations. Flow transport can be addressed here using conservation of mass (continuity) and momentum equations. The conservation of energy will not be addressed here despite its relevance, because the physicochemical mechanisms where this law has influence are modeled with empirical equations. A sketch of the membrane is presented in Fig. 11.12.

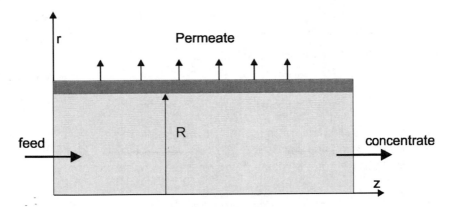

Fig. 11.12 Diagram of the tubular membrane, taking advantage of its symmetry.

The equation of continuity for an incompressible solvent has the following general form:

$$\nabla \bullet \mathbf{v} = 0 \tag{11.44}$$

Adopting cylindrical coordinates, and assuming that motion does not depend on θ, and that the axial velocity (v_z) variation along z can be neglected, the Eq.(11.44) remains as:

$$\boxed{\frac{1}{r}\frac{\partial(rv_r)}{\partial r} = 0} \tag{11.45}$$

where r is the radial coordinate, and $\partial v_z / \partial z = 0$.

The equation of continuity for a solute with concentration c, without internal generation and assuming that Fick's law is valid, is given as follows:

$$\frac{\partial c}{\partial t} + \mathbf{v} \cdot \nabla c = \nabla \cdot (D \nabla c) \tag{11.46}$$

Under steady-state conditions and the geometry of the tubular membrane, the equation can be simplified as follows:

$$v_z \frac{\partial c}{\partial z} + v_r \frac{\partial c}{\partial r} = \frac{1}{r} \frac{\partial}{\partial r}\left(D r \frac{\partial c}{\partial r} \right)$$

(11.47)

It is assumed a parabolic profile in the axial velocity (laminar regime), therefore v_z does not vary with z and verifies:

$$v_z(r) = 2u_0 \left(1 - \left(\frac{r}{R} \right)^2 \right)$$

(11.48)

The term R is the radio of the tubular membrane (from center to the feed fluid side of membrane), and u_0 is the feed axial velocity. The following boundary conditions are associated with classical conditions of symmetry:

$$v_r(z,0) = 0$$
$$\frac{\partial c(z,0)}{\partial r} = 0$$

(11.49)

Whereas at the inlet of feed fluid, it is verified (c_0 is the feed concentration):

$$v_r(0,r) = 0$$
$$c(0,r) = c_0$$

(11.50)

Boundary conditions (11.49) and (11.50) are necessary to solve the Eqs.(11.45) and (11.47), using the profile given by Eq.(11.48), but the problem is still not closed, because boundary conditions at $r = R$ are necessary.These conditions must address the permeation flux across the membrane, which is governed by more complex mechanisms.

A usual approach to this problem is to consider the membrane region as a porous medium where Darcy's law is valid. This one states the momentum conservation equation, describing the local apparent velocity as follows:

$$\mathbf{v} = -\frac{K}{\mu}(\nabla p + \rho \nabla U)$$

(11.51)

The term p is the fluid pressure, and it has been assumed that mass forces derive from the potential U. The Darcy coefficient K does not depend on the fluid, but on the porous medium. It has a value proportional to a^2, where a is the porous dimension. The Darcy's law is really a phenomenological equation based on the laminar movement of fluid in the region, that is, it assumes that $\rho \cdot a \cdot v_c / \mu \ll 1$, where v_c is the local velocity in the porous medium.

Because the small radial dimension of the membrane, it is usual to neglect U variation. It can be integrated then the equation that results from (11.51), taking into account the technique of permeability resistances in series used in (11.26), which gives the following expression for the local permeation flux (apparent velocity across the membrane):

$$v_m = \frac{1}{\mu(R_F + R_P(z))}(p(z) - p_p)$$
(11.52)

The terms R_F and $R_p(z)$ are the hydraulic fouled membrane resistance and the hydraulic resistance due to polarization concentration. The latter depends on the position in the axial line, z. The term p_p is the pressure at the permeate side of membrane.

The value of $p(z)$ is known according to the laminar motion inside the tubular membrane, which was assumed with the Eq.(11.48), therefore:

$$p_0 - p(z) = \frac{16}{Re} \frac{\rho u_0^2}{R} z$$
(11.53)

Where the Reynolds number in the tubular channel is $Re = 2\rho u_0 R / \mu$, and p_o is the pressure at $z=0$(feed).

The value of $R_p(z)$ in Eq.(11.52)can be found by empirical equations. There is not enough knowledge to perform a solid physicochemical foundation of this variable, despite intensive research has been received.

The model proposed in (Paris et al. 2002) suggested the use of the modified resistance-in-series model for this purpose. This one uses a dead-end filtration approximation to calculate R_p as follows:

$$R_p = \alpha \frac{N}{S}$$
(11.54)

where α is the specific resistance of the fouling layer, and N is the numbers of moles adsorbed over the area S. If mean concentration in the concentration boundary layer, c_m, is approximated using plane geometry, then:

$$c_m = \frac{N}{S\delta}$$

(11.55)

The term δ is the width of the concentration boundary layer. Accordingly, the equation (11.54) can be expressed as follows:

$$R_p = \alpha\delta c_m$$

(11.56)

The value of c_m can be obtained performing a mass balance for the solute retained over the concentration boundary layer. Integrating Eq. (11.2) where J_S can be written as cJ_p, with J_p is the permeate flow at the interface membrane - fluid, the following equation follows for the concentration inside the concentration boundary layer:

$$cJ_p = D\frac{\partial c}{\partial r} \Rightarrow c(z,r) = c(z,R)e^{J_p r/D}$$

(11.57)

Therefore, c_m remains as:

$$c_m(z) = \frac{1}{\delta}\int_R^{R+\delta} c(r,z)dr \Rightarrow$$

$$c_m(z) = \frac{c(z,R)}{Pe}\left(e^{Pe} - 1\right)$$

(11.58)

The term Pe is the Pecklet number ($J_p / (D/\delta)$), which relates convective to diffusive flow of solute.

Finally, the specific resistance has been related experimentally with the pressure increase across it. Then:

$$\alpha = \alpha_0\Delta p$$

(11.59)

Substituting Eq.(11.59) and Eq. (11.58) into Eq. (11.56)the expression for R_p remains as follows:

$$R_p(z) = \frac{\alpha_0 c(z,R)\delta}{Pe}(e^{Pe}-1)(p(z)-p_p)$$ (11.60)

Equations (11.60) and (11.53) provide the terms $R_p(z)$ and $p(z)$ for the Eq.(11.52).

It is now possible to set the boundary conditions for $r = R$, as follows:

$$v_r(z,R) = v_m$$
$$c(z,R)v_m = D\frac{\partial c(z,R)}{\partial r}$$ (11.61)

The mathematical model for flow transport in this tubular membrane is given by Eqs.(11.45), (11.47), (11.48), (11.49), (11.50), (11.52), (11.53), (11.60), and (11.61). All these equation have been boxed.

This model was solved in (Paris et al, 2002) applying a finite volume analysis with a mesh more refined near the boundary layer than the remaining tubular space, and the results were tested with an experimental controlled setup.

The model predicted with success the influence of feed axial velocity, u_0, on the permeate flux, J_p, and the relationship between J_p and transmembrane pressure at high feed concentrations ($u_0 = 0.216$ ms^{-1}, $c_0 = 8$g l^{-1}). In this case J_p shows the characteristic limiting flux behavior for high transmembrane pressures, due to the polarization of concentration. However, at low concentration ($c_0 = 1$g l^{-1}) the limiting flow is not reached by the model, in opposition to the experimental system. An interesting suggestion of the model was that the decrease in the permeate flux along the membrane length is due to the increase of δ, rather than the increase of c_m.

This model seems providing much accurate and solid results than well-known models concerning the polarization of concentration, like the gel-polarization model and the osmotic pressure model. The gel-polarization model is not able to describe the independence of limiting flux with pressure, together with the dependence with feed velocity. The osmotic pressure model fails completely when tries to explain the limiting flow by means of the increase of osmotic concentration of the rejected solute.

However, and despite this model provides a more accurate prediction, it is still unable to explain the behavior of the limiting flow under low concentrations. This is remarkable, considering that the tubular membrane could be taken as a simplistic hollow fiber dialyzer with a single fiber, that this membrane retains completely the solute and then the diffusion is limited to the fluid phase, the high symmetry (inside and outside the fiber), and the absence of interactions with other solutes and biological mechanisms.

This example should help to understand the complexity of this area.

11.6   FLOW MODELING OF DIALYZERS: PROGRESS AND FUTURE

The development of mathematical models of hollow fiber dialyzers able to predict accurately the clearance of uremic toxins under in-vivo conditions faces with huge barriers. Convection and diffusion mechanisms are well known but the coefficients that modulate the generalized forces must be identified experimentally yet, and multiple interactions affect them. Worst, the adsorption mechanism is associated with a fouling layer that affects to global permeability and induces the phenomenon known as concentration polarization, above managed. The latter promotes a limit of the permeate flow due to the building of a high concentration boundary layer.

Most of the mathematical models used for clinical conditions do not consider the distributed nature of the flow transport and therefore are unable to give accurate predictions when the diffusion is combined with other flow transport mechanism. Classical formulae used to manage ultrafiltration perfusion show clearly this simplification.

Advances in mathematical models oriented to renal dialysis try to correct this situation, starting with the 1D diffusive model of hollow fiber dialyzer. For instance, the mathematical model presented in (Stiller and Mann 1999)improved the description of the distributed nature of ultrafiltration flow along the streamline for hemodiafilters (HDF). However, that model does not address properly the polarization of the concentration. An approach to the latter problem for clinical hemodialysis was presented in (Wupper et al. 1997; Wupper et al. 1996).

Plasma proteins add complexity to the dynamics of these systems. Blood phase is not a Newtonian fluid, and different strategies must be applied to simplify this issue. A mathematical model that adds a more accurate treatment to plasma viscosity and oncotic pressure than others mathematical models used in renal dialysis was presented in (Legallais et al. 2000), with successful outcomes under controlled in-vitro conditions. However, and in spite of the consideration of distributed nature of permeation along the streamline and the concentration polarization, the accuracy achieved in plasma solution for several molecular weights compounds did not surpass 20 %.

Cited contributions provide mathematical models based on conservation laws, with empirical equations restricted to the estimation of variables associated with no well-known mechanisms. Other approaches are completely empirical. As an example, the model presented in (Vaussenat et al. 1997)gives an empiric equation to estimate the variation of hydraulic permeability with time during a session of hemodiafiltration.

Important advances are also developing in the ability to monitor the dynamics of processes in hollow fiber dialyzers, which are providing clues about causes of inaccuracies. For example, it is now possible to obtain the solute concentration field by means of computerized tomography in-vitro (Frank et al.2000), or even to measure the local permeate flow through magnetic resonance (Hardy et al. 2002).

An additional issue that emerges under in-vivo conditions is related to the flow transport across barriers of cell components in blood. This effect can be addressed by means of the partition coefficient of solute cell / plasma, P, and the time constant, τ, related to the diffusion of the solute across cell barriers. It is possible to define a blood water flow rate, Q_{bw}, that is used to calculate the dialyzer clearance under in-vivo conditions. The following equation was presented in (Lim et al. 1990):

$$Q_{bw} = 0.93 Q_b \left(1 - HTO + P(1 - e^{-t_r/\tau})HTO\right) \tag{11.62}$$

The hematocrit, HTO, is given in p.u. (per unit) and t_r is the residence time of dialyzer. The factor 0.93 corrects the volume of proteins and lipids. Other authors have proposed slight variants of Eq.(11.62), but all of them are indeed gross approximations that allow neglecting the presence of blood cell components. A more accurate prediction of flow transport in this system compels to perform a mathematical modeling of blood cell barriers, considering even active transport.

11.7 CONCLUSION

A comprehensive review of the state of the art in flow modeling of hollow fiber dialyzers has been presented. A top-down approach has been followed, starting from general concepts associated with flows and irreversible processes and the mathematical modeling of a whole clinical scenario. The scenario has been described with very simplistic mathematical models, which have been completed in a subsequent step, showing the advantages and limitations of the approach. An experimental in-vitro study performed in our laboratory has also been used for analyzing the accuracy of the mathematical model under controlled conditions.

Subsequent sections have presented a more complex mathematical model based on Navier Stokes conservation equations, together with several phenomenological expressions. This model has been analyzed to give a clear idea about the general approach currently used in this research area.

The chapter has finished with a succinct review of the progress and future in this domain.

ACKNOWLEDGMENTS

I am grateful to Prof. Manuel Valera and Dr. Joaquín Jimenez for their experimental support with in-vitro experiments.

REFERENCES

Allen, R., Frost, T.H., Hoenich, N.: The influence of the dialysate flow rate on hollow fiber hemodialyzer performance. Artificial Organs 19(11), 1176–1180 (1995)

Boerlage, S.F.E., Kennedy, M.D., Dickson, M.R., et al.: The modified fouling index using ultrafiltration membranes (MFI-UF): characterisation, filtration mechanisms and proposed reference membrane. Journal of Membrane Science 197(1-2), 1–21 (2002)

Borah, M.F., Shoenfeld, P.Y., Gotch, F.A., et al.: Nitrogen balance during intermittent dialysis therapy of uremia. Kidney Int. 14(5), 491–500 (1978)

Clark, W.R.: Quantitative characterization of hemodialyzer solute and water transport. Seminars in Dialysis 14(1), 32–36 (2001)

Chang, Y.-L., Lee, C.-J.: Solute transport characteristics in hemodiafiltration. Journal of Membrane Science 39(2), 99–111 (1988)

Daugirdas, J.T., Blake, P.G., Ing, T.S. (eds.): Handbook of Dialysis. Lippincott Williams & Wilkins, Philadelphia (2007)

Depner, T.A., Cheer, A.: Modeling urea kinetics with two vs. three BUN measurements. ASAIO J. 35(3), 499–502 (1989)

Derjani-Bayeh, S., Rodgers, V.G.J.: Sieving variations due to the choice in pore size distribution model. Journal of Membrane Science 209(1), 1–17 (2002)

Frank, A., Lipscomb, G.G., Dennis, M.: Visualization of concentration fields in hemodialyzers by computed tomography. Journal of Membrane Science 175(2), 239–251 (2000)

Friedman, M.H.: Principles and Models of Biological Transport. Springer, Heidelberg (1986)

de Groot, S.R., Mazur, P.: Non-equilibrium thermodynamics. Dover Publications, Inc., New York (1984)

Guyton, A.C., Hall, J.E.: Textbook of Medical Physiology, 11th edn. Elsevier, Saunders (2006)

Hardy, P.A., Poh, C.K., Liao, Z., et al.: The use of magnetic resonance imaging to measure the local ultrafiltration rate in hemodialyzers. Journal of Membrane Science 204(1-2), 195–205 (2002)

Jaffrin, M.: Convective mass transfer in hemodialysis. Artif. Organs 19(11), 1162–1171 (1995)

Legallais, C., Catapano, G., von Harten, B., Baurmeister, U.: A theoretical model to predict the in vitro performance of hemodiafilters. Journal of Membrane Science 168(1-2), 3–15 (2000)

Lienard IV, J.H., Lienard V, J.H.: A heat transfer textbook, 3rd edn. Phlogiston Press, Cambridge (2001)

Lim, V., Flanigan, M., Fangman, J.: Effect of hematocrit on solute removal during high efficiency hemodialysis. Kidney Int. 37(6), 1557–1562 (1990)

MacKay Valera, V., Fernandez, I.P., Herrera Carranza, J., Sancez Burson, J.: An in vitro study of the influence of a drug's molecular weight on its overall (Clt), diffusive (Cld) and convective (Clc) clearance through dialysers. Biopharm Drug Dispos. 16(1), 23–35 (1995)

Mercadal, L., Petitclerc, T., Jaudon, M.C., et al.: Is ionic dialysance a valid parameter for quantification of dialysis efficiency? Artificial Organs 22(12), 1005–1009 (1998)

Montero, F., Morán, F.: Biofísica: procesos de autoorganización en Biología, primera edición edn. Eudema, Salamanca (1992)

Nepomnyashchy, A.A., Velarde, M.G., Colinet, P.: Interfacial Phenomena and Convection. CRC Press (2002)

Nilsson, J.L.: Protein fouling of uf membranes: Causes and consequences. Journal of Membrane Science 52(2), 121–142 (1990)

Osada, Y., Nakagawa, T. (eds.): Membrane Science and Technology. Marcel Dekker, Inc. (1992)

Paris, J., Guichardon, P., Charbit, F.: Transport phenomena in ultrafiltration: a new two-dimensional model compared with classical models. Journal of Membrane Science 207(1), 43–58 (2002)

Prado, M., Roa, L., Palma, A., Milán, J.A.: A novel mathematical method based on urea kinetic modeling for computing the dialysis dose. Computer Methods and Programs in Biomedicine 74(2), 109–128 (2004)

Prado, M., Roa, L.M.: Combining dialysate and blood recirculation to boost uremic toxin removal: theory and simulation study. Artificial Organs 31(12), 895–901 (2007)

Prado, M., Roa, L.M., Palma, A., Milán, J.A.: Double target comparison of blood-side methods for measuring the hemodialysis dose. Kidney International 68(6), 2863–2876 (2005a)

Prado, M., Roa, L.M., Palma, A., Milán, J.A.: Improving hollow fiber dialyzer efficiency with a recirculating dialysate system I: Theory and applicability. Ann. Biomed. Eng. 33(5), 642–655 (2005b)

Prado, M., Roa, L.M., Palma, A., Milán, J.A.: Improving hollow fiber dialyzer efficiency with a recirculating dialysate system II: Comparison against two-chamber dialysis systems. Ann. Biomed. Eng. 33(11), 1595–1606 (2005c)

Roa, L.M., Prado, M.: The role of urea kinetic modeling in assessing the adequacy of dialysis. Crit. Rev. Biomed. Eng. 32(5-6), 461–539 (2004)

Sargent, J., Gotch, F.: Mathematic modeling of dialysis therapy. Kidney Int. suppl. 10, S2–S10 (1980)

Staverman, A.J.: The theory of measurement of osmotic pressure. Rec. Trav. Chim. 70(4), 344–352 (1951)

Stiller, S., Mann, H.: A model of solute transport through the dialyzer membrane in hemodiafiltration. Seminars in Dialysis 12(1), S76–S80 (1999)

Vaussenat, F., Bosc, J.Y., LeBlanc, M., Canaud, B.: Data acquisition system for dialysis machines. A model for membrane hydraulic permeability. Asaio Journal 43(6), 910–915 (1997)

Werynski, A., Malchesky, P., Lewandowski, J., et al.: Theoretical formulation of sieving coefficient evaluation for membrane plasma separation. Artif. Organs 9(3), 250–254 (1985)

Werynski, A., Waniewski, J.: Theoretical description of mass transport in medical membrane devices. Artif. Organs 19(5), 420–427 (1995)

Wolf, A.V., Laird, N.M., Henry, R.R.: Artificial kidney function: Kinetics of hemodialysis. J. Clin. Invest. 30(10), 1062–1070 (1951)

Wupper, A., Dellanna, F., Baldamus, C.A., Woermann, D.: Local transport processes in high-flux hollow fiber dialyzers. Journal of Membrane Science 131(1-2), 181–193 (1997)

Wupper, A., Woermann, D., Dellanna, F., Baldamus, C.A.: Retrofiltration rates in high-flux hollow fiber hemodialyzers: analysis of clinical data. Journal of Membrane Science 121(1), 109–116 (1996)

ESSAY QUESTIONS

1. Calculate the expression of LMCD for a concurrent flow dialyzer.
2. Analyze the influence of the access recirculation on the effective dialyzer clearance. Figure 11.13 shows the recirculation flow rate over a simplified diagram of the vascular access.

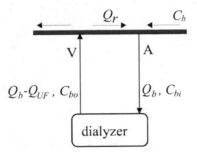

Fig. 11.13 Recirculation flow rate in the vascular access

3. Describe a method to measure the GFR assuming that one can select a compound with null secretion and reabsorption.
4. Solve and analyze using any mathematical package the urea kinetic profile for a patient submitted to daily dialysis. Consider the same assumptions and blood urea concentrations samples taken with patient of Section 11.2.
5. Proof that the diffusive dialyzer clearance is lesser or equal to $\min(Q_b, Q_d)$.
6. Use the electrodiffusion equation to determine the expression for the electrical mobility of an ion across a uniform membrane.
7. The electrodiffusion equation can be integrated for a bi-ionic system constituted by only a couple cation – anion with equal charge, without external potential either convection. The solution gives the following equation for the membrane potential:

$$\Delta\Psi = \frac{RT}{F} \cdot \frac{U_C - U_A}{U_C + U_A} \ln\frac{c_b}{c_d} \tag{11.63}$$

Terms U_A and U_C are mobility of anion and cation, whereas c_b and c_d are concentration of electrolyte at blood and dialysate side of the membrane.
Analyze the implications of this equation on the in-vitro experiment presented in Section 11.2.

8. Analyze the sensitivity of convection and diffusion to the porous size, *a*, under the assumptions described in chapter.
9. Analyze qualitatively the identification'serror of the dialyzer clearance associated with the assumption of 1-pool kinetic modeling for a human.
10. Obtain the equation that describes the diffusive efficiency for an array of two dialyzers connected as indicated in Fig. 11.14.

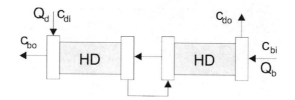

Fig. 11.14 Array of serial dialyzers with sequential flows

MULTIPLE CHOICE QUESTIONS

Choose the best answer

1. Renal replacement therapies refer to...
   A. Hormonal therapies to keep health without kidneys
   B. The use of dialyzers to clear urea and creatinine
   C. The clearance of uremic toxins by means of semipermeable membranes that could be artificial (hemodialysis) or natural (peritoneal dialysis)
   D. Kidney transplant

2. The first dialysis session was performed over a human in...
   A. 1800
   B. 1930
   C. 1980
   D. 1943

3. Which of the following transport mechanisms of nephrons are not present in kidneys?
   A. Filtration
   B. Secretion
   C. Diffusion
   D. Adsorption

4. Which is the main transport mechanism involved in urinary excretion?

    A. Reabsorption
    B. Filtration
    C. Secretion
    D. Adsorption

5. Which of the following equations refer to the Fick law under non ideal solutions?

    A. $\mathbf{J}_S = -D_S \nabla c_s$

    B. $\mathbf{J}_S = -D_S \nabla c_s + S c_s \mathbf{v}$

    C. $\mathbf{J}_S = -D_S \left(1 + \dfrac{d \ln \gamma_s}{d \ln c_s} \right) \nabla c_s$

    D. $\mathbf{J}_S = -U_S c_S \nabla \tilde{\mu}_S$

6. Which is the electrical term that must be added to the driven force to give the electrochemical potential of solute?

    A. $RT \ln (\gamma_s c_s)$

    B. $z_S F \psi$

    C. $U_S c_S \nabla \tilde{\mu}_S$

    D. $RT \nabla (\gamma_s c_s) + z_S F \nabla \psi$

7. Which is the characteristic dimension of thin layer of asymmetric dialysis membranes?

    A. 1 mm
    B. 10μm
    C. 1 nm
    D. 1 μm

8. Where do phenomenological coefficients of force – flow come from?

    A. Empirical studies
    B. Eigenvalues of the Jacobian of the $\mathbf{X} - \mathbf{J}$ relationship
    C. Onsager relationships
    D. Prigonine's dissipative structures

9. Which of the following equations match the dialyzer clearance of a compound?

A. $\dfrac{W}{c_{bi}}$

B. $\dfrac{Kt}{V}$

C. $\dfrac{W}{c_{di}}$

D. $\varepsilon \cdot Q_d$

10. Which condition must verify the glomerular renal filtration of a compound whose dynamics is given by Eq.(11.20)?
   A. Null secretion
   B. GFR = UFR
   C. Null reabsorption
   D. Secretion = Reabsorption

11. Is it necessary to compute the protein catabolic rate as an intermediate step to obtain Gs for the in-vivo study of Section 11.2?
   A. Yes, as shows the implemented algorithm
   B. No, it is only a related variable
   C. Yes, it is necessary because the solution of concentration depends on it
   D. Yes, because the catabolic rate is the base that originates Gs

12. Why is it necessary the steady state condition to integrateEq.(11.24)?
   A. Because J_s must be null
   B. Due to the independency of J_s with respect x under that condition
   C. Because the diffusive coefficient is then constant
   D. It is not necessary

13. Which is the meaning of each addend in the denominator of Eq. (11.26)?
   A. In-series hydraulic permeabilities
   B. In-series hydraulic resistances
   C. In-series diffusive permeabilities
   D. In-series diffusive resistances

14. The expression of LMCD given by Eq.(11.32) is valid for...
    A. Countercurrent dialyzers
    B. Concurrent dialyzers
    C. For any steady-state dialyzer
    D. Countercurrent array of dialyzers

15. The expression of the dialyzer efficiency is given by Eq.(11.33) provided...
    A. That the unique transport solute mechanism is diffusion.
    B. It is a general definition of the efficiency from the blood side.
    C. It is a definition of the efficiency for steady-state dialyzers.
    D. $C_{di} = 0$.

16. The solute flow rate transported from blood to dialysate can be written as the product clearance x blood inlet concentration, provided...
    A. Blood concentration is greater than dialysate concentration.
    B. Solute concentration at dialysate inlet is null.
    C. Solute concentration at the dialysate outlet is null.
    D. Concentrations are in steady-state.

17. The Eq.(11.41) for the clearance shows...
    A. The uncoupling between diffusion and convection mechanisms in the dialyzer.
    B. It is a misleading equation because the efficiency does not verifyEq.(11.33).
    C. It is a misleading equation because the efficiency does not verify Eq.(11.35).
    D. The coupling between diffusion and convection mechanisms in the dialyzer.

18. When K_oA was identified from the in-vitro study, it was expected that...
    A. The values of K_oA from the three series were equal
    B. The values of K_oA from the three series depend on blood flow rate
    C. The values of K_oA from the three series depend on dialysate flow rate
    D. The values of K_oA from the three series increased with NTU

19. The NTU dimensionless group should be...
    A. Low if one expect to reach high efficiencies
    B. Very high if one expect to reach high efficiencies
    C. Near 1 – 2 if one expect to achieve a good efficiency without excessive values of operating flow rates
    D. High if one seeks saving dialysate fluid

20. The sensitivity of K_oA to errors in the efficiency...
    A. It is always low
    B. It is high if NTU is high
    C. It is always high
    D. It depends on many variables

Chapter (12)

Single Pool Urea Kinetic Modeling

Alicja E. Grzegorzewska; Ahmad Taher Azar; Laura M. Roa; J. Sergio Oliva;
José A. Milán; Alfonso Palma

CHAPTER OUTLINES

- Compartment effects in hemodialysis
- Historical review of urea kinetics
- Single pool Urea Kinetic model (SPUKM)
- Mathematical models for hemodialysis dose calculation
- Optimum single pool hemodialysis dose
- Residual renal function and dialysis dose
- Normalized protein catabolic rate (protein nitrogen appearance) and dialysis dose
- Dynamic approach to Kt/V: the time constant in hemodialysis
- Final remarks and conclusions

CHAPTER OBJECTIVES

- Discuss the historical review of dialysis quantification
- To show development of urea kinetic modeling
- To compare advantages and disadvantages of SPFV and SPVV models
- Describe the mathematical models for calculating hemodialysis dose.
- Discuss the optimum dose for hemodialysis.
- To provide examples for practical use of SPUKM
- Discuss the relationship between single pool urea kinetic model and nutritional status of dialysis patients

KEY TERMS

- Diffusion
- Convection
- Hemodialysis adequacy
- Kt/V
- Total body water
- Ultrafiltration
- Urea clearance
- Urea distribution volume
- Urea generation rate
- Urea kinetics
- Urea rebound
- Urea reduction rat

ABSTRACT

   Hemodialysis (HD) is one of the treatments included in what is called the Renal Replacement Therapy (RRT). As every treatment, hemodialysis

A.T. Azar (Ed.): Modeling and Control of Dialysis Systems, SCI 404, pp. 563–626.
springerlink.com   © Springer-Verlag Berlin Heidelberg 2013

has its dose. How quantify this hemodialysis dosage was one of the results of the National Dialysis Cooperative Study (NCDS) published in 1983. A formula based in the Urea Kinetic Modeling (UKM) was developed. This formula was the dimensionless equation Kt/V where K is the dialyzer clearance rate of urea (or volume of plasma cleared), t is the duration of the dialysis session and V is the urea distribution volume (the total body water volume). Because of the complexity of urea kinetic modeling, a number of shortcut methods of estimating Kt/V have been proposed. The aims of this chapter are twofold: 1) to give an overview of single pool urea kinetic modeling and 2) to introduce concepts and methods needed to manage the approaches available to estimate the single pool Kt/V.

12.1 COMPARTMENT EFFECTS IN HEMODIALYSIS

Most of the toxins to be removed do not reside solely in the blood, but they are distributed in several 'compartments'. Compartmentalization of solutes during hemodialysis is ultimately important because it results in a reduced amount of solute removal during dialysis (Schneditz and Daugirdas 2001). The system may be modeled so that the distribution of these toxins has three such compartments. The first is the blood itself, called the extracellular compartment. The second is the interstitial compartment, which is comprised of the fluid that bathes the cells of the body. The final compartment is the intracellular compartment, which is made up of all the fluid inside the cells. When blood passes through the dialyzer, the extracellular compartment is cleaned at a fast rate. The blood then re-enters the body, and picks up more toxins via exchange with the interstitial fluid compartment. This also occurs at a relatively fast rate, though it is slower than the extracellular/dialysate exchange. The interstitial compartment also exchanges toxins with the intracellular compartment. This exchange is by far the slowest of the three, and limits the rate at which dialysis may be performed. The slowness of the exchange is a function of how much passive diffusion of the molecule is impeded by its size or electrical charge when traversing the cellular membrane. The exchange of toxins between these three compartments is necessary in order to remove the toxins that have built up in the body. When these models are used, a major assumption is made. The assumption is that there is instantaneous uniform distribution between compartments. That is, as a substance diffuses between compartments, it is assumed to be completely mixed throughout the compartment immediately. This is obviously impossible in reality, but is a necessary approximation that is required to maintain a linear mathematical model. Figure 12.1 shows a diagram of the exchanges that go on among these three compartments (Kupcinskas 2000).

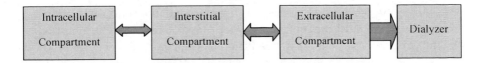

Fig. 12.1 Exchange of toxins occurs between various fluid compartments during dialysis as a function of concentration and potential gradients. The relative speed of exchange is represented by the width of the arrow (Kupcinskas 2000).

12.2 HISTORICAL REVIEW OF UREA KINETIC MODELING

Kolff et al (1944) wrote "urea" is at the utmost only partly co-responsible for the clinical symptoms of uremia, but nevertheless we chose it as a measure for the results of the dialyses. This choice was very successful. Urea is used up today in evaluation of dialysis adequacy, because this solute is already present in the body (no injection or ingestion is needed), the effects of absorption, hepatic and enteric circulation, and binding to proteins can be ignored. Diffusion of urea as a small solute (molecular weight 60.1 daltons) is so rapid among body compartments that a simple single compartment model should be adequate for most applications (Vanholder 1992; Vanholder et al. 2003). Urea distribution volume (V) is equated to total body water. Additionally, urea is easily and inexpensively measured, accumulates in uremia, is easily removed by the dialyzer, and the clearance (K) of urea can be used to gauge the effectiveness of hemodialysis (HD), since clearances of all toxins correlate to some extend with K of urea (Depner 1999a; Depner 2005). Serum urea concentration correlates well with symptoms and signs of renal failure (Giovannetti and Maggiore 1964), but urea levels do not correlate well with outcome. Patient outcome appears to depend more on why the serum urea concentration rises or falls. If it rises because of poor dialysis, the outcome is poor but if it rises because of an increase in protein intake, the outcome may be improved (Laird et al. 1983; Lowrie et al. 1981).

Wolf et al. (1951) introduced a term "dialysance", defined as "the rate of excretion per unit concentration gradient between plasma and bath fluid". In dialysance calculations, the concentration gradient of a solute across the dialysis membrane was used, because the solute dialysate concentration rose during the HD session until the dialysate was replaced with a fresh supply.

$$\text{Dialysance} = \frac{\text{Removal Rate}}{C - D} \qquad (12.1)$$

where C is blood, plasma or serum solute (urea) concentration and D is dialysate solute (urea) concentration. Dialysance is a more robust expression of dialyzer potential than clearance because it accounts for accumulation of solute in the dialysate compartment (Depner 2005). For single-pass dialysis, clearance and dialysance are equal, so clinicians tend to use the more familiar term "clearance". In a stagnant solution of serum allowed to equilibrate with dialysate across a semipermeable membrane, the clearance of a permeable solute falls with time, approaching zero as the concentrations equalize. Dialysance, however, remains constant, equal to the initial clearance when the dialysate concentration was zero. To assess the potential of a dialyzer to remove a solute found on both sides of the membrane, for example, sodium, dialysance is a more appropriate measure (Depner 2005).

Babb et al (1971) formulated "the square meter - hour hypothesis", indicating that the most important determinants of solute removal rate during HD were the dialysis membrane surface area and the time spent on dialysis. Other studies have shown a non-linear relationship between length of the dialysis treatment and survival rates, but did not show a clear threshold level for inadequate dialysis. The results of the National Cooperative Dialysis Study (NCDS) showed the relationship between the urea kinetics and the clinical outcome of patients on hemodialysis (Lowrie et al. 1981). The NCDS design was based on the assumption that blood urea nitrogen (BUN) could be used as a surrogate for uremic toxins and that the dose of dialysis could be defined by the level of BUN achieved. A total of 160 patients from nine American centers were prospectively randomized into one of four treatment groups. The groups were based on combinations of low and high time-averaged urea concentrations (TAC), and short and long dialysis time. The time averaged urea concentration is the mean BUN during a full dialysis cycle which is a thrice weekly schedule and can be calculated as follows:

$$\text{TAC urea} = \frac{\left(C_{pre1} + C_{post}\right) + \left(C_{post} + C_{pre2}\right)Id}{2\left(I_d + T_d\right)} \qquad (12.2)$$

where C_{pre1} is the pre-dialysis blood urea concentration, C_{post} is the post dialysis urea concentration, C_{pre2} is the pre-dialysis urea concentration of the next dialysis session, I_d is the interdialytic interval (in minutes) and T_d is the duration of dialysis (minutes).

Groups I and III had low BUN (expressed as either midweek predialysis BUN or time-averaged urea concentrations), with long treatment time (t) in I and short t in III; groups II and IV had high BUN, with long t in II and short t in IV. The target dialysis time in this study was either 3 h or 4.5 h, and the target midweek predialysis BUN was 70 and 120 mg/dL as shown in Fig. 12.2, the study was designed to hold BUN constant at two levels over a wide range of normalized protein catabolic rate (nPCR) which is a direct measure of the rate of urea generation (G) normalized to V (Gotch, 2000). The hypothesis was that the high BUN group II and IV patients would have a higher probability of failure than the low BUN group I and III patients (Gotch, 2001).

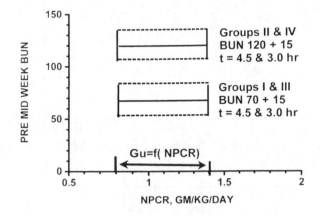

Fig. 12.2 The NCDS was designed to examine the effect of low or high BUN on clinical outcome. Adapted from Gotch FA (2000) Kt/V is the best dialysis dose parameter. Blood Purif 18(4):276-285, with permission from Karger Publisher.

Results of statistical analysis of the probability of clinical outcome failure as a continuous function of TAC and nPCR done by Laird et al. (1983) are shown in Fig. 12.3. The results shown in Fig. 12.4 confirmed the hypothesis for patients with nPCR ≥ 0.8, the lower bound targeted for the study. The high BUN groups II and IV had a probability of failure (PF) of 52%, while the low BUN groups I and III had a much lower PF (13%). The group V of patients as shown in Fig. 12.4 had a low nPCR (0.60 to 0.80 g/kg/day). In this group, there was a very high incidence of failure (75%), irrespectively of the BUN. It was suggested that this group might have failed for nutritional reasons, but the clinical symptoms were similar to those in groups II and IV with symptoms of uremia (Gotch 2001). The conclusions from the statistical analysis were 'therapy should be prescribed to reduce the BUN to the level for groups I and III (about 70 mg/dL) and low protein intake is associated with greater morbidity' and 'measure or select a PCR and prescribe adequate protein intake' (Lowrie et al. 1981; Sargent 1983; Lowrie and Teehan 1983; Lowrie et al. 1983).

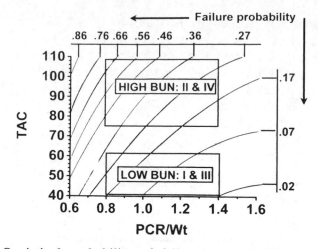

Fig. 12.3 Statistical probability of failure in the NCDS reported as a function of TAC and PCR/Wt. Adapted from Gotch FA (2000) Kt/V is the best dialysis dose parameter. Blood Purif 18(4):276-285, with permission from Karger Publisher.

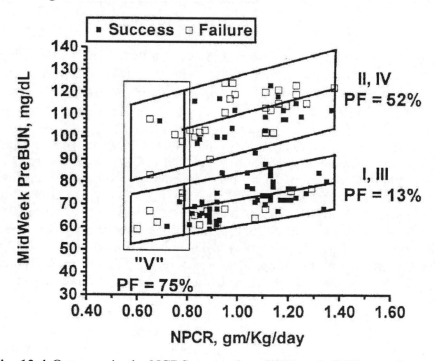

Fig. 12.4 Outcome in the NCDS mapped on BUN and nPCR coordinates. Adapted from Gotch F.A (2001) Evolution of the Single-Pool Urea Kinetic Model, Semin Dial.; 14(4): 252-256, with permission.

Since the early 1970's, there has been a flurry of activity in the renal therapy research community aimed at finding the optimal way to dialyze a patient. Most notably, the search has focused on finding a universal parameter that tells whether or not the patient is receiving adequate therapy. A landmark study completed in 1985 by Gotch and Sargent showed that a parameter known as the Kt/V index or dialysis dose is used to describe the effectiveness of a single HD session and to predict long-term effects of HD treatment (Gotch and Sargent 1985). The dialysis index Kt/V means the urea clearance (K, ml/min) times the length of the dialysis treatment (t, min) divided by the patients' volume of urea distribution (V, l) presumed to the same as total body water. To calculate this complex, interdependent relationship, a modeling program was devised by Gotch and his colleagues, and called urea kinetic modeling (UKM). UKM is simply a method for describing and modeling the combined effects of urea removal and urea generation, while taking into account the total distribution of urea within the body, and hence providing a measure both of solute clearance and nutrition (Levy et al. 2004). In Gotch's model, the probability of dialysis failure was a constant step function of Kt/V: it was higher when Kt/V was ≤ 0.8 and abruptly decreased when it was > 0.9 as shown in Figs. 12.5 and 12.6 (Gotch and Sargent 1985; Locatelli et al. 2005). Thus the BUN and nPCR plot of the NCDS study design in Fig. 12.2 could also be represented by a family of Kt/V lines with slopes of BUN vs nPCR decreasing as Kt/V increased. The step function was used to construct the modeling line for adequate dialysis. As a consequence, Kt/V >1.0 per HD treatment was considered of no apparent clinical value. Initial reports using UKM from the NCDS suggested that, for a protein intake of > 0.8 g/kg/day, a Kt/V value of 0.8 should provide adequate dialysis (Lowrie et al. 1981). Gotch and Sargent found that if a patient's Kt/V index was greater than 1, the patients were generally being adequately dialyzed (Gotch and Sargent 1985). However, a subsequent analysis of the same NCDS data by Keshaviah (1993) concluded that there was an exponential decrease in the probability of failure as Kt/V increased and also suggested the benefit of a Kt/V >1.2. This was determined by comparing the number of hospitalization days for a multicenter dialysis patient population with the patient Kt/V index. This ratio can be approximated to the natural logarithm of the initial urea concentration divided by the final urea concentration. Solving this equation for the final concentration of urea results in finding that the final urea concentration should be less than 36% of the initial concentration. In this way, it is related to the percent removal Eq. (12.3). Therefore, Kt/V can be expressed as (Gotch and Sargent 1985):

$$\frac{Kt}{V} = \ln\left[\frac{C_o}{C_f}\right] > 1; \quad C_f < 0.36\,C_o \qquad (12.3)$$

where C_o is the pre-dialysis BUN and C_f is post- dialysis BUN.

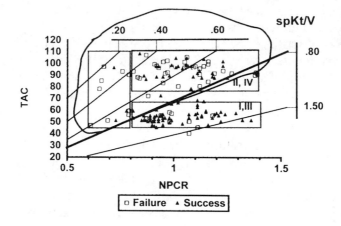

Fig. 12.5 The failure rate was high for all patients with spKt/V < 0.8 irrespective of the BUN. Adapted from Gotch FA (2000) Kt/V is the best dialysis dose parameter. Blood Purif 18(4):276-285, with permission from Karger Publisher.

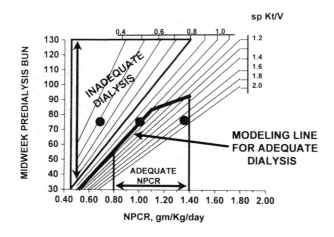

Fig. 12.6 The mechanistic analysis showed BUN was virtually irrelevant to adequacy of dialysis. A BUN of 75 mg/dL could represent low nPCR and low Kt/V or very high NPCR and high Kt/V. Adapted from Gotch FA (2000) Kt/V is the best dialysis dose parameter. Blood Purif 18(4):276-285, with permission Karger Publisher.

UKM seems to be the best tool available at present for improving outcomes and evaluating dialysis adequacy. Although it is necessary to further define UKM standards and/or develop other tools, Kt/V represents important tool for dietitians. Because dialysis adequacy may have a direct effect on morbidity and mortality, it continues to be of crucial importance to study its effects. The rigor of formal UKM supports the prescription of an appropriate dose of hemodialysis and allows errors in the delivered dose of dialysis to be easily recognized. Furthermore, formal UKM facilitates the identification of the variable(s) in the delivery of the hemodialysis prescription that were problematic, if the delivered dose was not the prescribed dose. Therefore, the HD Adequacy Work Group recommends that formal UKM should be implemented as a component of a complete Continuous Quality Improvement Program (CQI) program for end-stage renal disease (ESRD) care.

12.3 SINGLE POOL UREA KINETIC MODEL (SPUKM)

There are many models that can be used to predict the performance of the dialysis process. These models generally fall into two distinct categories: one pool models and two pool models. The single pool model is discussed in this chapter while the double pool model will be discussed in details in Chapter 13.

12.3.1 Single Pool Fixed Volume (SPFV) Urea Kinetic Model

Clinical use of SPFV urea kinetic model was first reported by Gotch et al. (1974). The SPFV assumes that total body water is a single and fixed pool (no urea generation) (Depner 2005). This compartment is containing a fixed amount of urea equal to the concentration (C) multiplied by the compartment volume (V_{urea}), which is equated to total body water. The blood concentration of solute at any time is considered to be a function of urea generation rate (G), solute distribution volume (V), dialysis time (t_d), the patient` residual urea clearance (K_r) and the dialyzer clearance (K_d) (Sargent and Gotch 1975).

Urea enters the compartment only from the liver where it is generated from amino acid catabolism (G) as shown in Fig. 12.7. Removal occurs constantly through the patient's native kidneys with clearance K_r and intermittently through the dialyzer with clearance K_d. Total clearance (K) is the sum of K_r and K_d during dialysis and equal to K_r alone between dialysis procedures. The rate of change in the compartment's urea content, $d(V_{urea}C)/dt$, is the difference between the generation rate (G) and the removal rate (−KC) (Depner 2005). Thus, applying the urea mass balance we obtain the next equation (Lowrie and Teehan 1983):

$$\frac{d(U)}{dt} = G - KC \qquad (12.4)$$

where G is the urea generation rate (in milligrams per minute, mg/min), K is the clearance of urea (in decilitres per minute, dL/min), C is the urea concentration (in milligrams per dL, mg/dL), t is time (in minutes, min), U is total body urea content in mg (is the product of urea distribution volume and urea concentration), V is the volume of distribution for urea (dL). The product of K and C is urea removed in the time t.

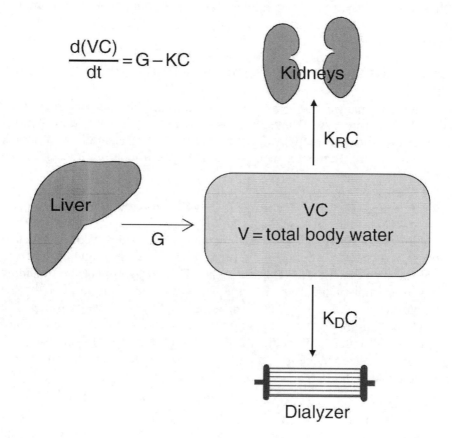

Fig. 12.7 The single-compartment model of urea mass balance. Adapted from Depner TA (2005) Hemodialysis adequacy: basic essentials and practical points for the nephrologist in training. Hemodial Int; 9(3):241-54, with permission.

Equation 12.4 describes changes in BUN both during and between dialyses. If the time interval between dialyses is made uniform, the change in BUN is identical for intra and inter-dialysis periods and the average pre and post- dialysis values can then be calculated knowing only values for G & V. A time-averaged BUN is then obtained by averaging pre- and post-dialysis values (Depner 1990). Equation (12.4) can be expanded also as follows:

$$V\frac{dC}{dt} + C\frac{dV}{dt} = G - (K_R + K_d)C \tag{12.5}$$

Assuming a fixed distribution volume (zero ultrafiltration), the second term of the left hand side of Eq. (12.5) is negligible (dV/dt = 0) (Sargent and Gotch 1974):

$$V\frac{dC}{dt} = G - (K_R + K_d)C \tag{12.6}$$

Dividing both sides of Eq. (12.6) by V yields:

$$\frac{dC}{dt} = \frac{G}{V} - \frac{(K_R + K_d)}{V}C \tag{12.7}$$

Solving Eq. (12.7) yields the following equation that allowed calculation of serum urea concentration during and between hemodialysis (Sargent and Gotch 1974):

$$C = C_o e^{-\frac{(K_r + K_d)t}{V}} + \frac{G}{K_r + K_d}\left(1 - e^{-\frac{(K_r + K_d)t}{V}}\right) \tag{12.8}$$

Equation 12.8 quantifies the fundamental mechanisms by which solute removal is achieved by either dialyzer clearance or renal clearance and the concentration of solute is a function of both Kt/V and the urea generation rate, G. Serum urea concentration (C) changes during each HD session (falls exponentially during dialysis, not linearly) and between consecutive HD sessions (increases due to urea generation). Writing Eq. (12.6) for BUN build up over the interdialytic interval θ yields:

$$\frac{dC}{d\theta} = \frac{G}{V} - \frac{K_R}{V}C \tag{12.9}$$

Solving Eq. (12. 9) for C_o yields (Gotch 1995):

$$C_o = C_t e^{-\frac{K_r\theta}{V}} + \frac{G}{K_r}\left(1 - e^{-\frac{(K_r\theta)}{V}}\right) \tag{12.10}$$

Eq. (12.10) can be applied only if K_r are greater than zero. If $K_r = 0$, then the pre-dialysis BUN for the next dialysis session can be calculated as follows (Gotch, 1995):

$$C_o = C_t + \frac{G \times \theta}{V} \qquad (12.11)$$

where V is the post-dialysis urea distribution volume in dL and θ is the interdialytic period in minutes and can be calculated as follows:

$$\theta = \text{days} \times 24 \times 60 - t \qquad (12.12)$$

Thus the rise in BUN between dialysis is determined by G, V and θ. In the steady state when the body inventory or mass of solute is constant and when the dialysis is not required, there will be no accumulation of urea or water and the left hand side of Eq. (12.5) can be neglected as follows (Sargent and Gotch 1974):

$$0 = G - K_r C \qquad (12.13)$$

Solving Eq. (12.12) for C yields:

$$C = \frac{G}{K_r} \qquad (12.14)$$

When the patient departs from steady state, such as is the case with intermittent dialysis therapy, the mass balance statement becomes a little more complex since the body inventory or content of solute is changing. In this case, the left hand side of Eq. (12.13) is no longer zero and must be written as in Eq. (12.6) (Sargent and Gotch 1996). If we assume that the loss of fluid during dialysis is negligible compared to total body water (what is not actually true during the dialysis session) and that urea generation during dialysis is also negligible, Eq. (12.5) can be expressed as:

$$V \frac{dC}{dt} = -K C \qquad (12.15)$$

This means that the variation of the urea concentration depends on both the urea concentration at any given time and the urea clearance. A solution for the Eq. (12.15) can be formulated as follows:

$$C(t) = C_o \, e^{-Kt/V} \qquad (12.16)$$

Equation (12.16) expresses the time dependence of the concentration of urea during the hemodialysis and at the end of the HD session ($t = T_d$). The logarithmic expression of this equation is Lowrie's formula (Lowrie and Teehan 1983) (see Appendix for MATLAB calculation of Kt/V using Lowrie formula):

$$\frac{Kt}{V} = \ln\left[\frac{C_o}{C_t}\right] = -\ln\left[\frac{C_t}{C_o}\right] \tag{12.17}$$

where ln = the natural logarithm.

Analogously the half-life of urea can be introduced with $C_t = C_0/2$:

$$\ln\left(\frac{C_{pre}}{C_{post}}\right) = \ln 2 = \frac{Kt_{half\ time}}{V} \tag{12.18}$$

Thus, the half-life of urea can be expressed as:

$$t_{half\ time} = \frac{V}{K}\ln 2 \tag{12.19}$$

When assuming dialysis will reduce the urea concentration to 10% of its initial value, we can compare $t_{half\ life}$ to $t_{10\%}$ and will find the ratio:

$$\frac{t_{10\%}}{t_{half\ life}} = \frac{\ln 10}{\ln 2} = 3.32 \tag{12.20}$$

A calculated result means that about 50% of urea is removed after approximately 30% of dialysis time.

The outstanding attractiveness of the SPFV model is its simplicity. There are only two urea plasma measurements necessary to calculate the dose parameter Kt/V. With only few additional considerations the model and its accuracy can be enhanced. Based on SPFV model, Gotch developed a new model of HD solute kinetics called "standard clearance" (standard Kt/V) which can be used uniformly to measure and thus explicitly compare the doses of dialysis provided by any combination of intermittent and continuous dialysis treatments (Gotch 1998).

Example 12.1

The analyses of blood samples from a real patient before and after a four hour dialysis session have resulted in the following values: 112 mg/dL and 28 mg/dL, respectively. Calculate the Kt/V using the Lowrie's formula.

Solution

Kt/V using Lowrie's formula can be calculated as:

$$\frac{Kt}{V} = \ln\left[\frac{C_o}{C_t}\right] = \ln\left[\frac{112}{28}\right] = 1.39$$

Example 12.2

Calculate the post-dialysis BUN concentration using SPFV urea kinetic model if the pre-dialysis BUN of a female patient is 105 mg/dL, post-dialysis urea distribution volume is 41.6 L, effective dialyzer clearance is 210 ml/min, residual renal clearance is 5 ml/min, the urea generation rate is 7.08 mg/min and the dialysis time is 4 h.

Solution

The post-dialysis BUN concentration can be calculated based on SPFV model as follows:

$$C = C_0 e^{-\frac{(K_r + K_d)\,t}{V}} + \frac{G}{K_r + K_d}\left(1 - e^{-\frac{(K_r + K_d)\,t}{V}}\right)$$

$$= 105 \times e^{-\frac{(0.05 + 2.1) \times 240}{416}} + \frac{7.08}{0.05 + 2.1}\left(1 - e^{-\frac{(0.05 + 2.1)\,240}{416}}\right) \approx 33\,\text{mg/dl}$$

Example 12.3

If the post-dialysis BUN concentration for a female patient is 58 mg/dL, and the post-dialysis urea distribution volume is 46.3 L, residual renal clearance of the patient is 0 mL/min. Estimate the pre-dialysis BUN for the next dialysis session based on SPFV model if the urea generation rate is 5.7 mg/min.

Solution

The estimated pre-dialysis BUN for the next dialysis session can be calculated based on SPFV model as follows:

$$C_0 = C_t + \frac{G \times \theta}{V} = 58 + \frac{5.7 \times 2640}{463} \approx 91\,\text{mg/dl}$$

12.3.1.1 Urea Reduction Ratio (URR)

Another method for assessing an adequate dialysis is the urea reduction ratio (URR) that is related to the Kt/V. In 1991 the urea reduction ratio (URR) was introduced by Lowrie and Lew (1991). The URR is the fractional reduction in urea during a dialysis session and is expressed as a percentage.

$$URR = \left(1 - \frac{C_t}{C_o}\right) \times 100 \tag{12.21}$$

Another form of Eq. (12.21) can be written as:

$$URR = (1 - R) \times 100 \tag{12.22}$$

where $R = C_t/C_o$ is the called the urea reduction fraction. The mathematical relationship between Kt/V and URR can be defined as:

$$URR = \left(1 - e^{-Kt/V}\right) \times 100 \tag{12.23}$$

where e is a mathematical constant of approximately 2.72. By rearranging and solving for Kt/V, URR can be used to predict SPFV Kt/V as follows:

$$\frac{Kt}{V} = -\ln[1 - R] \tag{12.24}$$

The linear correlation between URR and Kt/V ($0.93 < r < 1.0$) was shown in the range of commonly observed Kt/V values ($0.6 - 1.3$) (Basile et al, 1990; Grzegorzewska and Banachowicz, 2006) but URR and Kt/V association becomes exponential for Kt/V >1.3 (Basile et al, 1990). As a result of the latter fact, a broad range of Kt/V values may be observed at each URR value, and differences become even broader with increasing URR values $>65\%$ (De Oreo and Hamburger, 1995; Sherman et al., 1995). In 1992 the Health Care Financing Administration (HCFA) introduced standards for dialysis adequacy initially as URR > 60 or Kt/V > 1.0, and shortly thereafter upgraded to 65 or 1.2, respectively (HCFA, 1994). The URR does not include any modifications for ultrafiltration or T_d. It should be noted that all quantifiers which use R (C_t/C_o) in the equation are highly sensitive to the blood sample draw technique, especially the conditions and timing of the post-dialysis blood draw.

Example 12.4

If a patient has a pre-dialysis BUN of 130 mg/dL and post-dialysis BUN of 35 mg/dL, calculate the URR.

Solution

$$\text{URR} = \left(1 - \frac{35}{130}\right) \times 100 = 73\%$$

12.3.2 Single Pool Variable Volume (SPVV) Model

The classical SPVV method of urea kinetic modeling as proposed by Sargent and Gotch (1985) is based on three measurements of plasma UN concentrations (pre- and post-HD blood urea for the first session of the week and pre-HD blood urea for the second session of the week) and measurements of dialyzer and residual renal urea clearances (three-point SPVV) (see Fig. 12.8). Once the urea distribution volume (V) has been determined, the urea generation rate (G) can be calculated from the increase in the plasma UN value over the interdialytic interval plus the amount of urea excreted in the urine. Because urea generation during the dialysis session will have an effect (albeit a minor one) on the computation of V, simple algebra cannot be used to solve for V and G. These are derived by the iterative solution that takes into account the decrease in urea distribution volume that occurs during dialysis because of ultrafiltration and the subsequent increase in V during the interdialytic period.

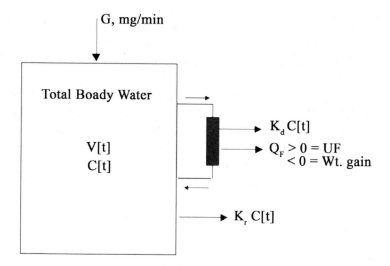

Fig. 12.8 Single pool urea kinetic model.

Since the single pool urea kinetic model with variable volume assumes the patient's body to be consisting of a single internal urea distribution compartment of the non-constant volume $V(t)$ and urea concentration $C(t)$ (Smye et al. 1993; Gotch 2001) (see Fig. 12.8), the initial dialysis conditions are assigned to V_0 and C_0. The urea distribution volume changes due to fluid retention between HD sessions and ultrafiltration during dialysis. Therefore, V can be represented as a function of time as follows (Sargent and Gotch 1980):

During Dialysis

$$\frac{dV}{dt} = -Q_f \tag{12.24}$$

and

$$V_t = V_0 - Q_f t \tag{12.25}$$

where V is the postdialysis V, V_0 is pre-dialysis V and Q_f is the rate of fluid removal.

After Dialysis

$$\frac{dV}{d\theta} = \alpha \tag{12.26}$$

and

$$V_0 = V_t + \alpha \times \theta \tag{12.27}$$

where the interdialytic fluid accumulation is considered to be constant at rate of α which is the rate of interdialytic volume expansion and can be calculated as follows:

$$\alpha = \frac{\text{weight gain (dl)}}{\text{interdialytic period (min)}} \tag{12.28}$$

The mass flux balance again can be described by a differential equation similar to the previous in Eq. (12.4) but now enhanced with a variable volume and G. Combining Eqs. (12.5) and (12.25) yields:

$$\left(V_0 - Q_f t\right)\frac{dC}{dt} + C\frac{d\left(V_0 - Q_f t\right)}{dt} = G - KC \tag{12.29}$$

$$\Rightarrow \left(V_0 - Q_f t\right)\frac{dC}{dt} = G - KC - CQ_f \tag{12.30}$$

$$\frac{dC}{G-\left(K+Q_f\right)C}=\frac{dt}{V_0-Q_f t} \quad (12.31)$$

This means that the momentary change of urea mass content ($V(t)\,C(t)$) of the single pool is determined by the gain of urea from (virtual) generation and the loss of urea by dialysis activity. These simple mathematical relationships and the easiness of measurement explain why Kt/V, an otherwise complex measure of the mean clearance during dialysis, has become so popular as a measure of dialysis and a benchmark for the current standards of dialysis adequacy (Depner 1999b). The analytical solution of Eq. (12.31) is straightforward and results in the formula (Gotch 1995):

$$C(t)=C_0\left(\frac{V_0-Q_f t}{V_0}\right)^{\frac{K-Q_f}{Q_f}}+\frac{G}{K-Q_f}\left[1-\left(\frac{V_0-Q_f t}{V_0}\right)^{\frac{K-Q_f}{Q_f}}\right] \quad (12.32)$$

The pre-dialysis BUN for the next dialysis session can be estimated as follows (Gotch 1995):

$$C_0(t)=C_t\left(\left(\frac{V_t+\alpha\times\theta}{V_t}\right)^{\frac{-K_r+\alpha}{\alpha}}\right)+\frac{G}{K_r+\alpha}\left[1-\left(\frac{V_t+\alpha\times\theta}{V_t}\right)^{\frac{-K_r+\alpha}{\alpha}}\right] \quad (12.33)$$

Eq. (12.33) can be applied only if K_r are greater than zero. If $K_r = 0$, then the pre-dialysis BUN for the next dialysis session can be calculated as follows (Gotch 1995):

$$C_0=C_t\times\frac{V_0}{V_t}+\frac{G\times\theta}{V_0} \quad (12.34)$$

where Ct is the post-dialysis BUN concentration in mg/dL, Vo and Vt are the pre- and post-dialysis urea distribution volumes (dL), respectively, θ is the interdialytic period in minutes. A theoretical plot of Eqns. (12.30) and (12.32) is shown in Fig. 12.9.

The modeling process begins with measured values of C and C_0 and requires fitting of V and G to Eq. (12.32). The volume of urea distribution (V) is calculated using computational software. The kinetic determination of V is based on the assumption of a single pool of urea that is coextensive with total body water and that expands during the interdialytic interval from fluid retention and contracts during hemodialysis by ultrafiltration.

Assuming a thrice weekly hemodialysis schedule, the computational software reiterates the following two formulae until unique values are found to satisfy both expressions (NKF-K/DOQI 2001).

$$V_t = Q_f \times t \left[\left[1 - \left[\frac{G - C_t(K + K_r - Q_f)}{G - C_0(K + K_r - Q_f)} \right]^{\frac{Q_f}{K + K_r - Q_f}} \right]^{-1} - 1 \right]$$ (12.35)

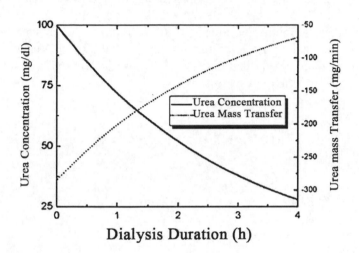

Fig. 12.9 Typical shape of a single pool modeled urea concentration and urea mass transfer rate curves during hemodialysis.

Urea generation rate can be determined from the interdialysis interval when K_d is zero while V is primarily derived from the ratio of the change in C from beginning to end of dialysis and the supplied value for K_d (NKF-K/DOQI 2001).

$$G = \frac{(K_r + \alpha) \left[C_0 - C_t \left(\frac{V_t + \alpha\theta}{V_t} \right)^{-\frac{K_r + \alpha}{\alpha}} \right]}{1 - \left(\frac{V_t + \alpha\theta}{V_t} \right)^{-\frac{K_r + \alpha}{\alpha}}}$$ (12.36)

where V_t is the post-dialysis urea distribution volume in dL; Q_f is the rate of volume contraction during dialysis in dL/min that is calculated from total weight loss during dialysis divided by the length of dialysis, t; G is the interdialytic urea generation rate in mg/min; K_r is the kidney urea clearance in dL/min; and C_t and C_{pre} are the BUN concentrations at the end and beginning of a dialysis treatment in mg/dL, α is the rate of interdialytic volume expansion and is calculated by the total interdialytic weight gain divided by the length of the interdialytic interval, θ.

Example 12.5

Calculate the post-dialysis BUN using SPVV urea kinetic model if the pre- and pre-dialysis BUN of a male patient is 129 mg/dL. The pre-and post-dialysis urea distribution volume is 40.65 L and 37.27 L, respectively, the ultrafiltration rate is 9.53 ml/min, effective dialyzer clearance is 206.4 mL/min, residual renal clearance is 3 ml/min, the urea generation rate is 7.95 mg/min and the dialysis time is 4 h.

Solution

The post-dialysis BUN can be calculated based on SPVV model as follows:

$$C(t)=C_o\left(\frac{V_o-Q_f t}{V_0}\right)^{\frac{K_d+K_r-Q_f}{Q_f}}+\frac{G}{K_d+K_r-Q_f}\left[1-\left(\frac{V_o-Q_f t}{V_0}\right)^{\frac{K_d+K_r-Q_f}{Q_f}}\right]$$

$$= 38.93 + (4.04 \times 0.6983) = 41.75 \cong 42 \text{ mg/dL}$$

Example 12.6

The post-dialysis BUN concentration for a female patient is 36 mg/dL. The pre- and post-dialysis urea distribution volume is 35.45 L and 31.48 L, respectively, residual renal clearance of the patient is 0 ml/min. Estimate the pre-dialysis BUN for the next dialysis session based on SPVV model if the urea generation rate is 7.79 mg/min.

Solution

The estimated pre-dialysis BUN for the next dialysis session can be calculated based on SPVV model as follows:

$$C_o = C_t \times \frac{V_o}{V_t} + \frac{G \times \theta}{V_o} = 36 \times \frac{354.5}{314.8} + \frac{7.79 \times 2640}{354.5} = 98.55 \cong 99 \text{ mg/dL}$$

Example 12.7

For a male-patient who received dialysis three times weekly, the pre-BUN was 171 mg/dL, the post-dialysis urea distribution volume after 4 hours dialysis was 37.35 L and the post-dialysis BUN was 56 mg/dL. The residual urea clearance of the patient is 0 ml/min and the interdialytic weight gain is 1.5 kg. Calculate the urea generation rate (G).

Solution

The interdialytic period in minutes can be calculated using Eq. (12.12) as follows:

$$\theta = days \times 24 \times 60 - t = 2640 \text{ min}$$

The rate of interdialytic volume expansion can be calculated as follows:

$$\alpha = \frac{\text{weight gain (dL)}}{\text{interdialytic period (min)}} = \frac{15}{2640} = 0.00568 \text{ dL/min}$$

Urea generation rate (G) can be determined using Eq. (12.36) as follows:

$$G = \frac{(K_r + \alpha) \left[C_o - C_t \left(\dfrac{V_t + \alpha\theta}{V_t} \right)^{\frac{K_r + \alpha}{\alpha}} \right]}{1 - \left(\dfrac{V_t + \alpha\theta}{V_t} \right)^{-\frac{K_r + \alpha}{\alpha}}}$$

$$G = \frac{(0.00568) \left[171 - 56 \left(\dfrac{373.5 + 0.00568 \times 2640}{373.5} \right)^{-1} \right]}{1 - \left(\dfrac{373.5 + 0.00568 \times 2640}{373.5} \right)^{-1}}$$

$$= 17.24 \text{ mg/min}$$

12.4   MATHEMATICAL MODELS FOR HEMODIALYSIS DOSE CALCULATION

A mathematical model is a set of mathematical expressions that are sufficient to explain the behavior of a given system for a particular purpose. Once a mathematical model is built, if it is simple enough, it may be possible to get an exact "analytical" solution. But this is almost impossible in many cases and then it is necessary to study the model by simulation (numerically exercising the model and studying how input variations affect outputs). However, the need for some time to be spent using a computer program has led to attempts to use various mathematical models to calculate Kt/V, which can be used by nephrologists as they evaluate patients clinically. These models all make use of the relationship between pre- and post-dialysis BUN. Unfortunately, as was observed by Movilli (1996), these simplifications rely on various assumptions, which, depending on the extent to which they are valid, can lead to very marked, and highly clinically relevant, differences in calculated Kt/V. The accuracy of such techniques has been questioned. Different mathematical models for single pool Kt/V calculation are summarized in Table 12.1.

Table 12.1 Different mathematical models for single pool Kt/V calculation

Model	Formula
Lowrie Model (Lowrie and Teehan 1983)	$Kt/V = \ln\left[C_o/C_t\right]$
Jindal Model (Jindal et al. 1987)	$Kt/V = \left[0.04\times\left(\dfrac{C_o-C_t}{C_o}\right)\times100\right]-1.2$
Keshaviah Model (Keshaviah et al. 1988)	$Kt/V = 1.62\times\ln\left[C_o/C_t\right]$
Barth Model (Barth 1988)	$Kt/V = \left[0.031\times\left(\dfrac{C_o-C_t}{C_o}\right)\times100\right]-0.66$
Calzavara Model (Calzavara et al. 1988)	$Kt/V = \dfrac{2\times(C_o-C_t)}{C_o+C_t}$
Daugirdas First Generation Model (Daugirdas 1989a, b)	$Kt/V = -\ln\left(R-0.008\times t - f\times\dfrac{UF}{W}\right)$
Basile Model (Basile et al. 1990)	$Kt/V = \left[0.023\times\left(\dfrac{C_o-C_t}{C_o}\right)\times100\right]-0.284$

Table 12.1 (*continued*)

Ijely Model (Jelly and Raja 1991)	$Kt/V = \left[0.018 \times \left(\dfrac{C_o - C_t}{C_o}\right) \times 100\right]$
Daugirdas Second Generation Model (Daugirdas 1993)	$\dfrac{Kt}{V} = -\ln\left(R - 0.008 \times t\right) + \left(4 - 3.5R\right)\dfrac{UF}{W}$
Kerr Model (Kerr et al. 1993)	$Kt/V = \left[0.042 \times \left(\dfrac{C_o - C_t}{C_o}\right) \times 100\right] - 1.48$
Azar Model (Azar 2008)	$Kt/V = -0.081 + 1.082 \times \ln(C_o) - 1.053 \times \ln(C$

C_o = Predialysis blood urea concentration; C_t = Postdialysis blood urea concentration; ln = natural log; t = dialysis duration (hours); R is the ratio of the postdialysis to predialysis BUN, f = a fudge factor, UF = ultrafiltration volume per dialysis (L); Wt = postdialysis body weight of the patient (kg)

12.4.1 Estimation of Single Pool Hemodialysis Dose: Daugirdas Kt/V Formula

In 1995, Daugirdas has introduced an empirical formula of clinical relevance that is very easy to use and widely accepted, even though it is partially based on statistical analysis and not purely on individual measurements. Two blood samples are needed, an arbitrary value for V is assumed and renal clearance is not included. An estimation of Kt/V also accounts for the effects of time and intradialytic body weight loss on the amount of solute convected by ultrafiltration. In the first-generation formula of Daugirdas, SPVV Kt/V was originally predicted as follows (Daugirdas 1989a, b):

$$_{sp}(Kt/V) = -\ln\left(R - 0.008 \times t - f \times \dfrac{UF}{W}\right) \qquad (12.37)$$

where R is the ratio of the post-dialysis to pre-dialysis BUN, t is the length of the dialysis session in hours, f is a fudge factor, UF is the ultrafiltration volume in liters, W is the post-dialysis weight in kg. The term 0.008 * t represented the ΔR value during the dialysis session as the result of urea generation, and the term f * UF/W represented the ΔR as the result of the additional urea removed due to volume contraction (Daugirdas 1989a, b). It was recognized that the correction factor f for UF/W varied as function of Kt/V. It was proposed that f be set to 1.0 in the usual clinical Kt/V range of 0.7 to 1.3, to 1.25 when Kt/V was less than 0.7, and to 0.75 when Kt/V was more than 1.3 (Daugirdas 1989a, b). In the Kt/V range of 0.7 to 1.3 (f = 1.0), the first-generation formula of Daugirdas corresponds very well with the Kt/V value computed from three-point SPVV modeling (Daugirdas 1989a, b), but it tends to overestimate this Kt/V as the Kt/V increases above 1.3. Because higher Kt/V values are now commonly delivered, a second-generation formula was developed (Daugirdas 1993): (see Appendix for MATLAB calculation of Kt/V using Daugirdas formula of 1993):

$$_{sp}(Kt/V) = -\ln(R - 0.008 \times t) + (4 - 3.5R) \times 0.55 \times \frac{UF}{V} \qquad (12.38)$$

where V is the post-dialysis urea distribution volume (liters) and can be assumed to be 55% of the post-dialysis weight (W) in kg (Daugirdas 1995). Using the latter assumption, the equation becomes:

$$_{sp}(Kt/V) = -\ln(R - 0.008 \times t) + (4 - 3.5R) \times \frac{UF}{W} \qquad (12.39)$$

V can be also calculated from the anthropometric formulae. The most widely used is the Watson et al. formulae (Watson 1980):

Male: V = 2.447 - 0.09156 × age (years)
$$ \qquad (12.40)$$
+ 0.1074 × height (cm) + 0.3362 × post-dialysis weight (kg)

Female: V = -2.097 + 0.1069 × height (cm)
$$ \qquad (12.41)$$
+ 0.2466 × post-dialysis weight (kg)

The modeled volume should be within about 25% of the anthropometric value for V. A more powerful use of V is to follow the modeled value over time. Although values for V have a substantial variation from treatment to treatment, a large change in V may reflect an error in blood sampling technique, an unrecorded change in the amount of dialysis (K × t) given, or the presence of access recirculation (AR) (Daugirdas et al. 2007).

Correlations between URR and Kt/V obtained in 3-month interval evaluations in the same patients yielded values of r about 0.5 (Grzegorzewska and Banachowicz 2006: URR (r = 0.541), -ln(R) (r = 0.545), Daugirdas first-generation formula (r = 0.528), Daugirdas second-generation formula (r = 0.524). Although URR is highly correlated with Kt/V in population studies, it fails to reflect the actual dose received by an individual patient as shown in Fig. 12.10. Convective losses of solute during dialysis contribute to the overall effect of the treatment but are not reflected in URR because they are not accompanied by a change in urea concentration. For patients undergoing intermittent HD, it is possible to receive adequate treatment when the URR is below the standard or conversely, to receive inadequate treatment when URR is above the standard. For a patient with a Kt/V of 1.3 and no fluid loss during dialysis,

URR is 0.71; whereas if fluid loss is 10% of body weight, URR is 0.63 as shown in Fig. 12.10. In contrast to Kt/V, URR does not provide a measure of protein catabolism or residual clearance and offers no logical method for correcting a prescription that is inadequate. For these reasons, URR was not considered acceptable by the National Kidney Foundation Kidney Disease Outcomes Quality Initiative (NKF-K/DOQI) Hemodialysis Adequacy Work Group as a measure of, or as a standard for, dialysis. Therefore URR is less of a practical simplification than a mathematical simplification.

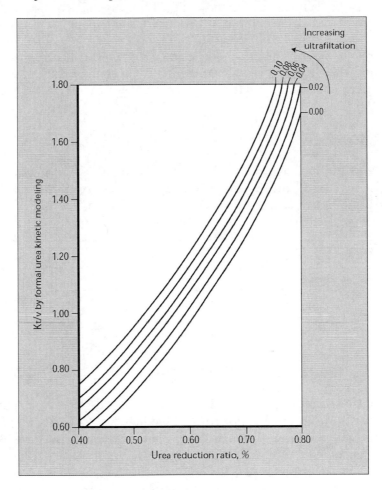

Fig. 12.10 A nomogram based on Daugirdas second generation formula showing the actual relationship between Kt/V and urea reduction ratio (URR). Adapted from Palmer BF (1998) The Dialysis Prescription and Urea Modeling. In Schrier RW, editor. Atlas of diseases of the kidney, Vol. 5; pp. 6.1-6.8; Current Medicine, Philadelphia: Blackwell Science; with permission.

URR and SPFV Kt/V include changes in BUN during HD session, but they do not account for the change in V because of ultrafiltration that occurs during nearly all HD sessions (adding 10% - 30% more to clearance), and to a lesser extent they do not account for the generation of solute that occurs during a 3- to 5-hr HD treatment (Depner 2005). Because of urea generation during dialysis and because of urea removal in the course of ultrafiltration, which contributes to the urea clearance (K), but does not affect R, Kt/V computed as -ln(R) differs from the Kt/V derived from the classical three-point SPVV by an average of 18% (Daugirdas 1989a, b). Additionally, the fixed, single-pool formulations do not account for post-HD urea rebound due to recirculation and re-equilibration, and for the effects of residual renal clearance. A method of correcting URR for post-HD urea rebound by using the equilibrated end-session urea concentration has been suggested (Kerr et al. 1993; Maduell et al. 1998).

Example 12.8

A 54-years old male patient has a pre-dialysis BUN of 106 mg/dL, post-dialysis BUN of 39 mg/dL and post-dialysis weight of 57 kg. Calculate $_{sp}Kt/V$ using Daugirdas formula if the ultrafiltration volume is 2 L and the dialysis time is 4 hours.

Solution

$$\frac{Kt}{V} = -\ln\left(R - 0.008 \times t\right) + \left(4 - 3.5R\right) \times \frac{UF}{W}$$

$$\frac{Kt}{V} = -\ln\left(\frac{39}{106} - 0.008 \times 4\right) + \left(4 - 3.5 \times \frac{39}{106}\right) \times \frac{2}{57}$$

$$= -(-1.091) + 0.095 = 1.186$$

An analysis of error showed that this second-generation formula eliminated the overestimation of Kt/V in the high ranges (1.4 – 2.1) found with the first-generation formula. Also, total error was reduced with the second-generation formula, being within 5% across the entire tested Kt/V (0.7 – 2.1) (Daugirdas 1993). Use of V in the denominator of the urea clearance expression had to be analogous to correcting glomerular filtration rate (GFR) for body surface area (BSA). BSA can be derived from Haycock et al (1978) formula:

$$\text{BSA (m}^2) = \text{post-HD body weight}^{0.5378} \text{ (Kg)}$$
$$\times \text{ height}^{0.3964} \text{ (cm)} \times 0.024265 \tag{12.42}$$

or the equations of Dubois and Dubois (1989):

$$\text{BSA (m}^2) = 0.007184 \times \text{post-HD body weight}^{0.425} \text{ (Kg)}$$
$$\times \text{ height}^{0.725} \text{ (cm)} \tag{12.43}$$

Normalizing GFR to BSA compensates for the association of GFR with BSA: GFR/BSA values were similar in men and women, but GFR/V values were substantially different (Daugirdas et al. 2009; Lowrie 2000). The decline of BUN concentration during dialysis is the same for all patient sizes when K is indexed to V. In clinical studies, overweight HD patients (with higher V) were shown to receive less dialysis as measured by SPVV urea Kt/V, and conversely, those with lower body mass index (BMI) were shown to receive higher SPVV urea Kt/V (Salahudeen et al.1999). On the other hand, with the same Kt/V, women and small men received lower dialysis dose (lower Kt) (Spalding et al. 2008). BMI can be calculated as follows:

$$\text{BMI (kg/m}^2) = \text{weight (kg)/height}^2 \text{ (m)} \tag{12.44}$$

Dry body weight and BMI were progressively lower with values of SPVV urea Kt/V increasing from < 1.23 to > 1.68 (Salahudeen et al. 2003). SPVV Kt/V was also shown to be inversely correlated with dry body mass and height. Such negative correlations occurred despite longer dialysis sessions (may be not sufficiently longer) provided to patients with greater dry body mass and height [positive correlations were shown between patients' height ($r = 0.428$, $p = 0.026$) and dry body mass ($r = 0.547$, $p = 0.000$) and duration of HD session] (Grzegorzewska and Banachowicz 2008). Lowrie et al. (2002) postulated no scaling Kt values. Because the use of V_{urea} as a normalizing factor has been questioned, alternative parameters were evaluated or proposed for scaling dialysis dose. Among them there were body weight (Spalding et al. 2008; Suri et al. 2007), BSA (Daugirdas et al. 2008a, b; Lowrie et al. 2005; Spalding et al. 2008), resting energy expenditure, high metabolic rate organ mass, liver size (Daugirdas et al. 2008b) and bioelectrical resistance (Basile et al. 2010). When scaling to BSA, the assumption is that a man and a woman of the same height and weight will require the same GFR or Kt. Rescaling to surface area would obligate more dialysis for smaller patients, more dialysis for women, and potentially, less dialysis for larger, male patients (Daugirdas et al. 2008a). Values of Kt normalized to bioelectrical resistance were significant outcome predictor (Basile et al. 2010). The problem of scaling dialysis dose is still not solved.

12.4.2 Comparison of Adequacy Models

The National Kidney Foundation's Kidney Disease Outcomes Quality Initiative (K/DOQI) recommends use of the Daugirdas second-generation formula for delivered dialysis dose (Kt/V) calculation. Differences between Kt/V calculated using SPFV and SPVV models are shown on Fig. 12.11. Kt/V, calculated using SPFV model as –ln (R), yielded values approximately 15% lower than those shown using SPVV models, which include ultrafiltration volume contributing to urea clearance. Kt/V, calculated using the first-generation and second-generation formulae of Daugirdas, were not significantly different in this study, because the Kt/V ranges were not very high and the overestimation error shown for the first-generation formula could not be expressed (Grzegorzewska and Banachowicz 2006).

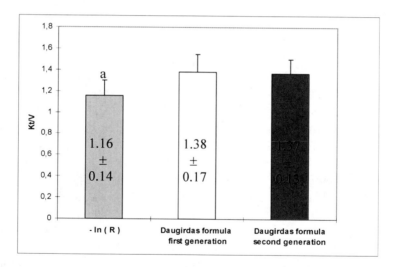

Fig. 12.11 Comparison of Kt/V values (mean ± SD) obtained using SPFV model [Kt/V = -ln(R)] and SPVV model (Kt/V calculated using first-generation and second-generation formulae of Daugirdas) in the study of Grzegorzewska and Banachowicz (2006).

Nonlogarithmic formulae were also developed and compared to Daugirdas second-generation formula like Barth formula (see Fig. 12.12), Jindal, Basile, and Kerr formulae (see Table 12.1). Despite the fact that no one formula can replace the Daugirdas second-generation formula, the studies advise using Barth's formula as a nonlogarithmic counterpart to the Daugirdas formula. Barth's formula is simple and can be obtained using a simple pocket calculator in routine clinical practice. Every calculated Kt/V value should have bookmarks with regard to how the formula was calculated, including the postdialysis blood sampling method (Kovacic et al. 2003).

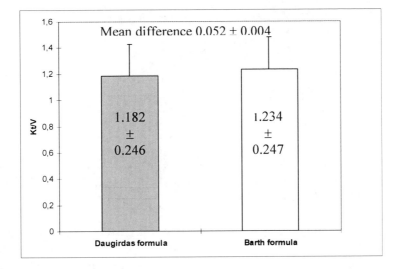

Fig. 12.12 Comparison of Kt/V values (mean ± SD) obtained using second generation of Daugirdas formula (Daugirdas, 1993) and Barth formula (Barth, 1988) in the study of Kovavic et al (2003).

Azar (2008) recommended using Ijely's formula as a nonlogarithmic counterpart to the Daugirdas second-generation formula and using Azar Kt/V formula as a logarithmic formula (see Fig. 12.13). Azar and Daugirdas second-generation formulae are more accurate than the other models. Ijely's formula is simple, does not use an expression of a natural logarithm, and can be obtained with a simple pocket calculator in routine clinical practice. Azar has demonstrated the least mean of the absolute values of the differences between Azar Kt/V values and Daugirdas second-generation Kt/V values for single pool Kt/V (see Fig. 12.13). Grouping models containing ln(Co/Ct) terms (Azar, Daugirdas, Kesheviah, Lowrie) and those incorporating the (Co–Ct)/Co ratio (i.e. the urea reduction) (Barth, Basile, Calzavara, Ijely, Jindal, Kerr) there was a better correlation for all models employing the logarithmic transformation (R^2 = 0.949– 0.947 cf. R^2 = 0.937– 0.939). Also, there was a better correlation for all models employing the nonlogarithmic transformation (R^2 = 0.995–0.997).

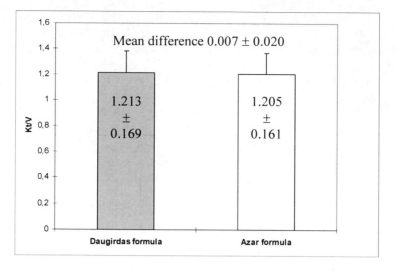

Fig. 12.13 Comparison of Kt/V values (mean ± SD) obtained using second-generation of Daugirdas formula (Daugirdas 1993) and Azar formula in the study of Azar (2008).

In conclusion, mathematical formulae are not perfect, but some are less imperfect than others. Logarithmic methods are to be preferred. Common sense dictates that 'bedside' analyses should never supplant the routine application of more comprehensive analyses, unless prospective studies supply evidence of comparable reliability (Kovacic et al. 2003).

12.5 OPTIMUM SINGLE POOL HEMODIALYSIS DOSE

Minimal value of the second-generation VVSP Kt/V accepted in 1997 by National Kidney Foundation's Kidney Disease Outcomes Quality Initiative (NKF-K/DOQI 1997) and the Renal Association in London (The Renal Association, 1997), in 1999 by Canadian Society of Nephrology (Deziel C et al. 1999) and maintained by NKF-K/DOQI (2001) was 1.2 for single HD session, performed three times a week in adult patient. The Kt/V target value of 1.3 for adequate HD session was suggested by NKF-K/DOQI guidelines (2001) and of 1.35 – 1.40 by the Renal Association (1997). For four HD sessions per week, the target Kt/V was 1.0; the minimum Kt/V was 0.9 per dialysis (Depner 2005). According to European Best Practice Guidelines (EBPG for hemodialysis 2002, 2007) the minimum prescribed HD dose per session for a thrice-weekly schedule should be 1.4 for SPVV Kt/V in anuric patients. When the HD schedule deviates from three HD sessions per week, the standard HD dose no longer applies (Depner 2005).

Current NKF-K/DOQI guidelines and clinical practice recommendations suggest using SPVV Kt/V calculated monthly via urea kinetic modeling or Daugirdas' second-generation natural logarithm formula for monitoring the delivered HD dose (NKF-K/DOQI 2006). For patients receiving thrice-weekly HD, NKF-K/DOQI recommends prescribing a target dose of ≥ 1.4 to ensure delivery of SPVV Kt/V ≥ 1.2 per session (NKF-K/DOQI 2006). To be truthful, we really do not know what is the exact optimal HD dose for individual dialysis patient. Thus, a question arises how dialysis dose expressed as URR or Kt/V is associated with patient's outcome (survival, hospitalization rate). McClellan et al (1998) reported a 'reversed J shape' to the URR risk profile among patients treated in one US End-Stage Renal Disease network. The relative risks of death in URR groups 50–54%, 55–59%, 60–64%, 65–69% (reference), 70–74%, and 75–79% were 1.56, 1.51, 1.38, 1.00 (reference), 1.45, and 1.49. Chertow et al (1999) also described a 'reversed J shape' to the URR death risk profile. Risk was higher at the extremes of the URR distribution than at its middle. The relative risk of death was 1.27, 1.10, 1.00 (reference group), 1.04, and 1.19 in the quintiles of URR (URR < 60.0%, 60.0 – 64.1%, 64.1 – 67.4% (reference), 67.4 – 71.0% and > 71.0%). Hospitalization risk profiles also show dependence on URR. The Fresenius Medical Care (NA) data system revealed hospitalization odds ratios of 1.42, 1.16, 1.10, 1.01, 1.06, 1.00 (reference), and 1.19 for URR $\leq$ 45%, 45–50%, 50–55%, 55–60%, 60–65%, 65–70% (reference), and >70% (Lowrie et al. 1998a).

Assuming optimal URR between 65% and 69%, it is reasonable that low URR (< 65%), indicating underdialysis, is associated with higher morbidity and mortality. But why higher URR (> 69%) was also related to worse outcome, although BUN even after HD session frequently was not in the normal range? Interestingly, adjusting URR for height and weight as well as the case mix measures suggested that outcome continued to improve even when URR exceeds 75% (Li et al. 2000). According to Lowrie (2000) finding higher morbidity and mortality at high URR or Kt/V may not indicate toxic overdialysis, because persons with high URR or Kt/V tend to have low V that contributes to higher Kt/V. The low V also reflects malnourishment that contributes to greater death risk (Chertow et al. 1999; Kopple et al. 1999). Black patients are treated a lower URR than whites but enjoy better survival on dialysis than whites (Owen et al. 1998) because blacks tend toward greater body mass than whites (Kopple et al.,1999; Lowrie et al.,

1999; Owen et al., 1998), and greater body mass contributes to better survival (Kopple et al. 1999). On the other hand, high dialysis dose in small patients, not sufficiently nourished, may lead to further deterioration of nutritional status, and increased risk of morbidity and death (Lowrie 2000).

Minimal value of URR accepted in 1997 by the Renal Association, in 1999 by Canadian Society of Nephrology (CSN 1999) and in 2001 by NKF-K/DOQI was 65% for single HD session, performed three times a week in adult patient. The URR target value of 70% for adequate HD session is suggested by NKF-K/DOQI guidelines in 2001. According to European Best Practice Guidelines (EBPG 2002) URR is an unacceptable index to prescribe and monitor HD therapy.

Similarly like URR, mortality as a function of Kt/V tends to show a J-shaped curve (Owen et al. 1998). Lowrie et al (1999) have been proposed (urea clearance * time) product (Kt) as a more rigorous index of HD dose. A gender-dependent minimum mortality risk, computed in cross-sectional analysis, showed that no additional benefit above a Kt of 40–45 and 45–50 l/HD session for females and males, respectively, may be expected irrespective of size and volume of the patient (Lowrie et al. 1999). However, HD dose estimated in terms of Kt/V has been related to morbidity and mortality in large database studies (Acchiardo et al., 1992; Bloembergen et al. 1996; Collins et al. 1994; Hakim et al. 1994; Held et al. 1996; Lowrie et al. 1998b; Parker et al. 1994; Shinzato et al. 1997). Held et al (1996) demonstrated that mortality risk was lower by 7% with each 0.1 higher level of delivered Kt/V. The cross-sectional database analyses showed that minimum mortality expressed as the standard mortality ratio requires $_{sp}$Kt/V of 1.4 to 1.6 (Hakim et al. 1994; Parker et al. 1994). The relative risk of death did not decrease further beyond values of Kt/V > 1.3 or URR >70%, either adjusting (Eknoyan et al. 2002; Held et al. 1996) or not for co-morbid conditions (Owen et al. 1993). However, there are also studies showing further benefit in term of reduced mortality with increased doses of HD therapy (Collins et al. 1994; Hakim et al. 1994; Parker et al. 1994; Shinzato et al. 1997), especially in diabetic patients (Collins et al. 1994). According to Collins et al (1994) a diabetic patient should receive Kt/V of ≥ 1.4 (mean 1.6). When the relative risk of death was adjusted for the length of the HD sessions, Cox model confirmed the independent predictive effect on outcome of single pool Kt/V shown in over 50 000 HD Japanese patients (Shinzato et al. 1997; Maeda 1999).

HD dose influences important laboratory parameters, disturbed by loss of renal function and accumulation of uremic toxins (Grzegorzewska et al. 2005; Harter 1983; Ifudu et al. 1996; Movilli et al. 2001). Already, in

1983, Harter has found that reducing dialysis dose significantly decreased hematocrit and hemoglobin and increased the transfusion requirements. Ifudu et al (1996) showed positive effect of higher URR (72%) compared to their standard URR (61%) on hematocrit in patients treated with a fixed dose of erythropoietin. In 2001, it was shown that adequate HD diminished requirement for recombinant erythropoietin, even in cases in which cellulose dialysis membranes were used (Movilli et al. 2001). In mentioned study, hematocrit did not correlate with Kt/V, whereas erythropoietin dose and Kt/V were inversely correlated.

Dialysis dose may be modified during dialysis due to intentional changes in dialysis duration, blood or dialysate flow, the choice of hemodialyzer (Hauk et al. 2000; Leypoldt et al. 1997) or to unintentional loss of membrane surface area from clotting or coating of the membrane. Cumulative solute removal is greater when HD session is longer, but solute removal rate falls exponentially during an extended dialysis (Depner 1999a). The delivered dose of HD should be checked monthly in stable HD patients, because the session-to-session variation in Kt/V is small in such patients (NKF-K/DOQI 2001).

12.6 RESIDUAL RENAL FUNCTION AND DIALYSIS DOSE

Residual renal function (RRF) is often used as a synonym for glomerular filtration rate (GFR), considered as the gold standard measurement of kidney function. Preserved RRF enhances solute and water removal from the patient` body and increases effectiveness of dialysis treatment. The contribution of RRF to total solute and water clearance may be significant, especially in the first year of dialysis and often facilitates to attain targets of Kt/V. Adding renal clearance (K_r) and dialysis clearance (K_d) provides more information on magnitude of patients` purification from uremic metabolites. When K_r is zero, the interdialytic rise in the BUN concentration is linear; if $K_r > 0$, the rise in BUN will be more shallow and curvilinear resulting from continuous kidney urea excretion (NKF-K/DOQI 2001). To add urea K_r to urea K_d, one must take into consideration the different durations of their effects, which is usually 3 to 5 hr, thrice weekly for K_d and 168 hr per week for K_r (Depner 2005):

$$Kt / V = \frac{\left[\left(K_d \times T_d \right) + \left(K_r \times T_r \right) \right]}{V} \qquad (12.45)$$

where T_d is time on dialysis and T_r is the mean time interval between two dialysis procedures. However, it is worthy to remember that kidney function and the clearances of artificial kidney membranes are not biologically equivalent processes. Having preserved RRF, usually means to have better hormonal and metabolic renal status, what showed to be important for clinical outcome. The available methods for measurement RRF and the advantages and disadvantages are discussed in the Chapter 3. One of the indicators of RRF in dialysis patients is the daily or weekly urine volume. Measurement of urine volume is relatively readily available and inexpensive. A major limitation of this measure in using it as an outcome variable is its imprecision.

The residual renal clearance of urea nitrogen (K_{ru}) can be calculated as follows (Jindal and Goldstein 1988; Gotch 1995):

$$K_{ru}\,(mL/min) = \frac{UUN \times V_{urine}}{BUN \times \theta} \qquad (12.46)$$

where UUN is the urine urea nitrogen concentration in mg/dL, BUN is the average blood urea nitrogen concentration during interdialytic interval in mg/dL, Vurine is the urine volume collected over interdialytic interval (mL) and θ is the interdialytic interval in min. The units for the UUN and BUN must be the same, as they cancel each other. The estimated average blood urea nitrogen concentration during interdialytic interval can be calculated as follows (Jindal and Goldstein 1988; Gotch, 1995):

$$BUN = 0.25 \times C_o + 0.75 \times C_t \qquad (12.47)$$

where C_o is the pre-dialysis BUN concentration and C_t is the post-dialysis BUN concentration.

Example 12.9

A 39-year old male patient has a pre-dialysis BUN of 105 mg/dL and post-dialysis BUN of 24 mg/dL. Calculate the residual renal clearance if the urine volume is 1200 mL, urine urea nitrogen is 180 mg/dL and the interdialytic interval is 2640 min.

Solution

The residual renal clearance can be calculated as follows:

$$BUN_{Blood} = 0.25 \times 105 + 0.75 \times 24 = 44.25 \text{ mg/dL}$$

$$K_{ru} = \frac{UUN \times V_{urine}}{BUN \times \theta} = \frac{180 \times 1200}{44.25 \times 2640} = 1.5 \text{ mL/min}$$

Once K_{ru} is calculated, it can be used to calculate total K't/V (corrected for K_{ru}), using the following formula (Gotch 1995):

For thrice-weekly dialysis:

$$K't / V(\text{corrected}) = Kt / V + (5.5 \times K_{ru} / V) \qquad (12.48)$$

For twice-weekly dialysis:

$$K't / V(\text{corrected}) = Kt / V + (9.5 \times K_{ru} / V) \qquad (12.49)$$

where V is the volume of distribution of urea in L. However, the trend has been to ignore the residual renal function in the dialysis prescription, given that residual renal function is time consuming to measure and may deteriorate rapidly in hemodialysis patients. If dialysis therapy is reduced based on the presence of residual renal function and then a fall in renal function occurs which is not detected promptly, underestimation of dialysis dose may result (Blake and Daugirdas 1996).

Taking into account the K_r, the guidelines of K/DOQI 2006 for the minimal haemodialysis dose (Kt/V) in a 3 times per week program are: 1.2 for patients with $K_r < 2.0$ ml/min/1.73 m^2 BSA and 0.9 for patients who have $K_r > 2.0$ ml/min/1.73 m^2 BSA as shown in Table 12.2 (NKF-K/DOQI, 2006). The recommended target value of spKt/V was set 15% higher from the lowest value, thus target spKt/V in a 3 times per week program is 1.4 and 1.15 in patients without and with residual renal function, respectively.

Table 12.2 K/DOQI recommendation for the calculation of Kt/V in patients with and without K_{ru} (NKF-K/DOQI 2006)

Dialysis Frequency	Minimum (target) $_{sp}$Kt/V	
	$K_{ru} < 2.0$ ml/min/1.73 m^2	$K_{ru} >$ ml/min/1.73 m^2
2 times / week	Not recommended	2.0 (2.3)
3 times / week	1.2 (1.4)	0.9 (1.15)
4 times / week	0.8 (0.9)	0.6 (0.7)
$K_{ru} < 2.0$ ml/min/1.73m^2 → No reduction in Kt/V target (1.4, 15% higher than the minimum of 1.2) $K_{ru} > 2.0$ ml/min/1.73 m^2, reduce the minimum Kt/V by 20%		

Casino and Lopez (1996) developed a new parameter of the standard urea model which is the equivalent renal urea clearance (eK_{ru} or originally EKR) that provides a kinetic estimate of the time averaged Kt. A value of eK_{ru} represents both dialytic and interdialytic periods whereas Kt/V and URR reflects only the dialytic time. This disparity would underscore the superiority of eK_{ru} and, hence, could provide an opportunity to use eK_{ru} to compare the amount of dialysis among different dialysis regimens. The eK_{ru} is computed as the ratio of net urea generation rate (G, mg/min) to time-averaged urea concentration (TAC, mg/mL) (Casino and Lopez 1996):

$$eK_{ru} = \frac{G}{TAC} \qquad (12.50)$$

For example, for a dialysis patient with G = 6 mg/min and TAC = 40 mg/dL, eK_{ru} is 15 mL/min, independently from type and schedule of treatment. If the above patient had some residual renal function and was not yet on dialysis, a G of 6 mg/min and a steady state BUN of 40 mg/dL would correspond to K_{ru} = 15 mL/min: thus, eK_{ru} for a dialysis patient is equivalent to K_{ru} for an identical patient not being on dialysis (Casino and Lopez 1996). The relationship between Kt/V and eK_{ru} is shown in Fig. 12.14 and can be calculated as follows (Casino and Lopez 1996):

For thrice-weekly dialysis:

$$eK_{ru} = 1 + 10 \times Kt / V \qquad (12.51)$$

For twice-weekly dialysis:

$$eK_{ru} = 1 + 6.2 \times Kt / V \qquad (12.52)$$

For once-weekly dialysis

$$eK_{ru} = 0.7 + 3 \times Kt / V \qquad (12.53)$$

The value of eK_{ru} can be added to the measured residual renal urea clearance and can be expressed either in milliliters per minute or in liters per week. When expressed as liters per week, eKru, which is now equivalent to (K × t), or volume of plasma cleared during the week, can be further divided by V to arrive at a weekly Kt/V-urea (Daugirdas et al. 2007).

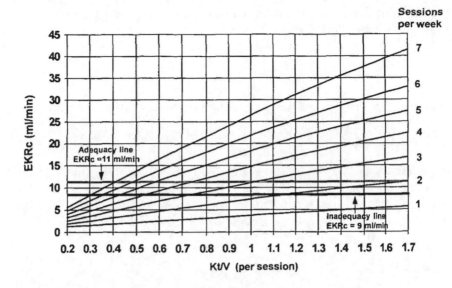

Fig. 12.14 The equivalent renal urea clearance corrected for urea volume (EKRc) as a function of Kt/V per session in anuric HD patients. Data points were obtained from computer simulation for HD sessions per week varying from 1 to 7. The fixed input values were: V = 40 L, t_d = 240 min, ultrafiltration volume (UFV) = 3 L, nPCR = 1 g/kg/day; for any given schedule Kt/V was changed from 0.2 to 1.7, step 0.1. The EKRc lines of 9 and 11 ml/min respectively establish equivalency to Kt/V of 0.8 (Inadequacy line) and 1.0 (Adequacy line) on 3 HD/week. The daily dialysis line for 7 HD/week can also be used to establish kinetic equivalence between HD and peritoneal dialysis. Adapted from Casino and Lopez (1996), with permission.

The Casino-Lopez-derived eK_{ru} does not appear to be equivalent to either peritoneal dialysis (PD) Kt/V-urea or to residual renal urea clearance in terms of outcome (Daugirdas et al. 2007). The resulting effective renal urea clearance by Casino-Lopez is significantly higher than a consensus-derived continuous equivalent clearance for PD because the reasonable minimum target level of PD weekly Kt/V-urea (derived as the sum of residual renal and peritoneal urea clearance) is about 2.0-2.2.

Gotch (1998) has developed a new adjusted equation for eK_{ru} for hemodialysis regimens to correct the problem of Casino-Lopez. Gotch computes an adjusted eK_{ru} as being equal to net urea generation rate

(G, mg/min) divided by the mean weekly pre-dialysis plasma urea level as follows (Gotch 1998):

$$eK_r = \frac{G}{C_{avg}}$$ (12.54)

Where C_{avg} is the average weekly pre-dialysis plasma urea concentration.

Example 12.10

If a person has a urea generation rate of 7.5 mg/min and the time averaged urea concentration (TAC) of 40 mg/dL, calculate the equivalent renal urea clearance (eK_{ru}) using Casino-Lopez formula and adjusted Gotch formula if the peak BUN for this person during thrice-weekly hemodialysis schedule is 90, 85, 80 mg/dL.

Solution

a) The equivalent renal urea clearance (eK_{ru}) using Casino-Lopez formula can be calculated as:

$$eK_{ru} = \frac{G}{TAC} = \frac{7.5}{40} = 0.1875 \text{ dL/min} = 18.75 \text{ mL/min}$$

b) The equivalent renal urea clearance (eK_{ru}) using adjusted Gotch formula can be calculated as:

$$eK_{ru} = \frac{7.5}{(90+85+80)/3} = 0.088 \text{ dL/min} = 8.8 \text{ mL/min}$$

12.7 NORMALIZED PROTEIN CATABOLIC RATE (PROTEIN NITROGEN APPEARANCE) AND DIALYSIS DOSE

Since urea is quantitatively the only significant end product of protein metabolism, the urea generation rate can be directly converted to a rate of protein catabolism (or protein intake when there is no net catabolism or anabolism). The following equation (Borah Method) takes into consideration the non-urea nitrogen and non-urinary losses which comprise a minor but significant fraction of total protein catabolism (Borah et al. 1978):

$$PCR (PNA) = 9.35 \times G + 0.294 \times V$$ (12.55)

where PCR is protein catabolic rate (g/day), PNA is protein nitrogen appearance, G is the urea generation rate (mg/min), V is the pot-dialysis urea distribution volume (L). Borah et al (1978) also derived a formula to calculate urea generation rate directly from PCR as follows:

$$G = 0.154 \times PCR - 1.7 \tag{12.56}$$

The term protein nitrogen appearance (PNA) is mathematically identical to the protein catabolic rate (PCR) (NKF-K/DOQI 2000). In the clinically stable patient, PNA can be used to estimate protein intake but there are several limitations to PNA as an estimate of dietary protein intake (DPI) as stated by NKF-K/DOQI (2000):

1. "PNA approximates protein intake only when the patient is in nitrogen equilibrium (steady-state). In the catabolic patient, PNA will exceed protein intake to the extent that there is net degradation and metabolism of endogenous protein pools to form urea. Conversely, when the patient is anabolic (eg, growth in children, recovering from an intercurrent illness, or during the last trimester of pregnancy) dietary protein is utilized for accrual of new body protein pools, and PNA will underestimate actual protein intake."

2. "PNA changes rapidly following variations in protein intake. Hence, PNA may fluctuate from day to day as a function of protein intake, and a single PNA measurement may not reflect usual protein intakes."

3. "When DPI is high, PNA underestimates protein intake (ie, nitrogen balance is unrealistically positive). This is probably caused by increased nitrogen losses through unmeasured pathways of excretion (eg, respiration and skin)."

4. "PNA may overestimate DPI when the protein intake is less than 1 g/kg/d (possibly due to endogenous protein catabolism)."

5. "Normalizing PNA to body weight can be misleading in obese, malnourished, and edematous patients. Therefore, it is recommended that for individuals who are less than 90% or greater than 115% of SBW, the adjusted edema-free body weight (aBWef) be used when normalizing PNA to body weight."

SBW - Standard Body Weight
TNA - Total Nitrogen Appearance

PNA may be normalized (nPNA) to allow comparison among patients over a wide range of body sizes. The most convenient index of size is the urea distribution volume (V), because it is calculated from urea modeling, is equivalent to body water volume, and is highly correlated with fat free or lean body mass. Total body weight is a poor index of PNA because nitrogen appearance is not affected by body fat. However, because V is an index that is less familiar to clinicians and not readily available, it is customary to convert V to a normalized body weight by dividing by 0.58, its average fraction of total body weight. The resulting nPNA is expressed as the equivalent number of grams of protein per kilogram of body weight per day, but it is important to note that body weight in the denominator is not the patient's actual body weight but instead is an idealized or normalized weight calculated from V/0.58 (Depner and Daugirdas 1996):

$$nPCR = PCR \times \frac{V}{0.58} \tag{12.57}$$

where nPCR is the normalized protein catabolic rate (g/kg/day). The nPCR can be used to identify patients who might benefit from counseling about their dietary protein intake. Furthermore, it can be used to determine whether the hemodialysis dose needs to be escalated because of sustained high protein intake.

The formulas used to calculate the single-pool Kt/V ($_{sp}$Kt/V) and PNA (PCR) can be divided into two separate groupings (NKF-K/DOQI 2000): those that depend on a three-BUN measurement SPVVM and those that depend on a two-BUN measurement SPVVM. The two-BUN method is more complex than the three-BUN method, because it requires computer iteration over an entire week of dialysis to arrive at G (urea generation rate). In the two-BUN method, a pre-dialysis and post-dialysis BUN only are obtained. There is no third BUN sample taken during the interdialytic interval prior to the next dialysis. The two-BUN method calculates G from the absolute value of the pre-dialysis BUN (C_0) and Kt/V. Because

C_0 is determined both by G and by Kt/V, if Kt/V is known (calculated from the fall in BUN during dialysis), then G can be determined from the absolute value of C_0 (by the complicated iteration scheme over an entire week). Note that the absolute value of C_0 is not used to calculate Kt/V, which is determined by the log ratio of C_0/C_t.

In the three-BUN method, three BUN measurements are needed which are the BUN before dialysis, after dialysis, and at some third point during the interdialytic interval. This method calculates the urea generation rate (G) from the end of the first dialysis to the beginning of the second dialysis and is primarily determined by the difference between the two-BUN values (post- to pre-). It also requires iteration and a computer but only over the time span of a single dialysis and a single interdialysis interval (NKF-K/DOQI 2000). Although the three-BUN method is mathematically simpler, it is actually more difficult to do because it requires waiting 48 to 72 hours before the third BUN can be drawn. It is also a more narrow measure of G because it is constrained to the single interdialysis period and can be manipulated by the patient who becomes aware that the measurement will be done when the first two blood samples are drawn. A graphical nomograms have been developed and validated that allow the calculation of PCR based on pre-dialysis and post-dialysis BUN samples from the same dialysis session (Sargent et al. 1978). The relationship between normalized PCR (nPCR), the first-of-week pre-dialysis serum urea nitrogen, and Kt/V for patients undergoing dialysis three times per week is shown in Fig. 12.15 (Daugirdas and Depner 1994). Figure 12.16. shows the aforementioned estimation with the use of the midweek pre-dialysis serum urea nitrogen. As mentioned previously, K't/V = Kt/V when K_{ru} is negligible. Otherwise, use Eq. (12.48) and Eq. (12.49) to compute K't/V from Kt/V and K_{ru}.

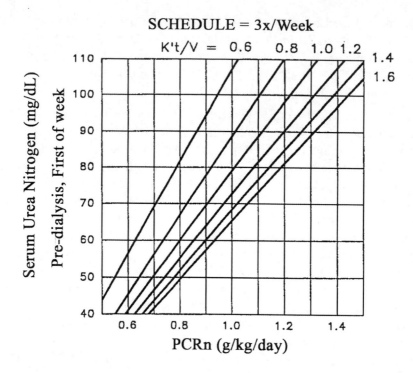

Fig. 12.15 Estimating the normalized protein catabolic rate (PCRn) from K't/V and the pre-dialysis serum urea nitrogen. Use this nomogram only for a 3x/week schedule, when serum urea nitrogen values are obtained prior to the first session of the week. To use, first estimate K't/V. Begin with the pre-dialysis serum urea nitrogen on the y-axis. Proceed horizontally to the proper K't/V line. Drop perpendidular to the x-axis to fond the PCRn. Adapted from Daugirdas JT, Depner TA (1994) A nomogram approach to hemodialysis urea modeling. Am J Kidney Dis.; 23(1):33-40, with permission from Elsevier.

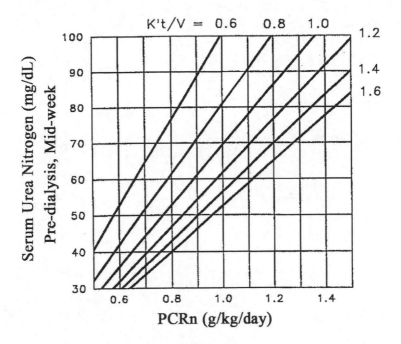

Fig. 12.16 Estimating the normalized protein catabolic rate (PCRn) from Kt/V and the pre-dialysis serum urea nitrogen for a thrice weekly schedule using the midweek serum urea nitrogen value. Adapted from Daugirdas JT, Depner TA (1994) A nomogram approach to hemodialysis urea modeling. Am J Kidney Dis.; 23(1):33-40, with permission from Elsevier.

In patients receiving intermittent hemodialysis values of nPCR can also be calculated from pre-dialysis and post-dialysis BUN measurements using Garred (1995) formula or Depner and Daugirdas (1996) formulas as follows:

Garred formula (Garred 1995):

$$nPCR = \left[(0.0076 \times Kt / V) \times (C_o + C_t)\right] + 0.17 \qquad (12.58)$$

Depner and Daugirdas formulas (Depner and Daugirdas 1996):

For thrice-weekly dialysis:

- Beginning of a week:

$$nPCR = \left[\frac{C_o}{36.3 + 5.48 \times Kt / V + 53.5/Kt / V}\right] + 0.168 \qquad (12.59)$$

- Midweek:

$$nPCR = \left[\frac{C_0}{25.8 + 1.15 \times Kt/V + 56.4/Kt/V}\right] + 0.168 \quad (12.60)$$

- End of a week:

$$nPCR = \left[\frac{C_0}{16.3 + 4.3 \times Kt/V + 56.6/Kt/V}\right] + 0.168 \quad (12.61)$$

For twice-weekly dialysis:

- Beginning of a week:

$$nPCR = \left[\frac{C_0}{48 + 5.14 \times Kt/V + 79/Kt/V}\right] + 0.168 \quad (12.62)$$

- End of a week:

$$nPCR = \left[\frac{C_0}{33 + 3.6 \times Kt/V + 88.2/Kt/V}\right] + 0.168 \quad (12.63)$$

For patients with significant residual renal function, C_0 was adjusted upward according to the following empirically derived equations:

For thrice-weekly dialysis:

$$C_0' = C_0\left[1 + \left(0.7 + \frac{3.08}{Kt/V}\right) \times \frac{K_r}{V}\right] \quad (12.64)$$

For twice-weekly dialysis:

$$C_0' = C_0\left[1 + \left(1.15 + \frac{4.56}{Kt/V}\right) \times \frac{K_r}{V}\right] \quad (12.65)$$

where C_0' and C_0 are expressed in mg/dL, K_r in mL/min, and V in L.

The Kt/V (based on the Urea Kinetic Modeling) is now the preferred method for quantifying the delivered dose of hemodialysis. Nephrologists can control two elements of the dialysis prescription, the dialyzer clearance K and the session time (manipulated variables). When we multiply these two variables, the result is the volume cleared Kt. Kt/V provides a measure of the dose of dialysis given during a single treatment or of the amount of urea that has been removed from the patient. Although usually dose refers to "amount given" in this case is the contrary, as the Kt/V is a measure of "amount withdrawn from circulation" or "urea removal". In spite of that, many nephrologists calculate the delivered dose of dialysis using the Kt/V based on the urea kinetics. Delivered Kt/V should be measured several times in the year in every patient in all the dialysis units. The dialysis dose measured by the Kt/V, although widely discussed, continues to be an obligated part of the target "adequacy of dialysis" (Vanholder and Ringoir 1992).

Example 12.11

A 62-years old male patient has a pre-dialysis BUN of 116 mg/dL, post-dialysis BUN of 34 mg/dL and post dialysis weight of 90 kg.
a) Calculate $_{sp}$Kt/V using Daugirdas formula if the ultrafiltration volume is 4 l and the dialysis time is 4 hours.
b) Using the calculated Kt/V in part (a), calculate nPCR by Garred formula and Depner-Daugirdas formulas if all blood samples were obtained at the midweek HD session.

Solution

a) The $_{sp}$Kt/V can be calculated according to Daugirdas formula as follows:

$$_{sp}(Kt/V) = -In\left(\frac{34}{116} - 0.008 \times 4\right) + \left(4 - 3.5\frac{34}{116}\right) \times \frac{4}{90}$$

$$= -(-1.3428) + 0.132 = 1.47$$

b) The nPCR can be calculated according to Garred formula [Eq. (12.58)] as follows:

$$nPCR = \left[(0.0076 \times Kt/V) \times (C_o + C_t)\right] + 0.17$$

$$= \left[(0.0076 \times 1.47) \times (116 + 34)\right] + 0.17 = 1.85 \text{ g/Kg/day}$$

According to Depner-Daugirdas formula [Eq. (12. 60)]:

$$nPCR = \left[\frac{C_o}{25.8 + 1.15 \times Kt/V + 56.4/Kt/V}\right] + 0.168$$

$$= \frac{116}{25.8 + 1.15 \times 1.47 + 56.4/1.47} + 0.168 = 1.76 + 0.168$$

$$= 1.93 \text{ g/kg/day}$$

It is noted that the difference between the two formulas is very small.

12.8   DYNAMIC APPROACH TO Kt/V: THE TIME CONSTANT IN HEMODIALYSIS

If instead of studying the Kt/V, an approach is discussed from system dynamics perspective (where the system would be formed by the patient, the dialyzer and the connection interface between them), then an explanation of what is happening in this system will be given. So, the reasons for the relationship between these parameters and survival can be extracted. To provide a dynamic approach of Kt/V, the formulation established by Lowrie in 1983 is taken as a starting point, since this is the basis for other mathematical formulations on the Kt/V that have been made. The dynamic model described by Lowrie for the intradialytic behavior of urea is a first-order differential equation and it is stable, so their dynamic behavior is governed by its time constant.

Defining the time constant: In engineering, the time constant (usually denoted by the Greek letter τ, tau) is the rise time characterizing the response to a time-varying input of a first-order, linear time-invariant system. The time constant is the main characteristic of a first-order system. This constant represents the time it takes the system's step response to reach $1 - 1/e \approx 63.2\%$ of its final (asymptotic) value. In our case this would correspond to a decrease up to 36.8% of the total urea.

Once known the limitations of the urea kinetic model in their approach to the value of the total body volume, which also considered negligible the fluid loss during the session, the possible influences on the clearance constant (K) has the type of vascular access, dialyzer membrane and changes in blood flow during HD session, the two main components of Kt/V can be separated: one of them is V/K (min) or time constant ( ) and the other is the time of HD session (t, min). Both components from Eq. (12.16) can be related as follows as follows:

$$\tau \, (\text{min}) = \frac{V}{K} = t \ln \left[\frac{C_o}{C_t} \right] \qquad (12.66)$$

Thus, the time constant ($\tau = V/K$) can be defined as a measure of the dynamics of the urea clearance rate on dialysis since it expresses the minutes required to remove a given concentration of urea according to both the patient's total body volume and the clearance rate (K).

The time constant is a dimensional parameter, expressed in minutes. It represents the dynamics of the interface between the patient and the dialysis machine as shown in Fig. 12.17. For example, in an electrical circuit RC (a first order system) the time constant is the time required for a capacitor to charge to 63.2% of the total charge or for an inductor to be crossed by that percentage of the total current. The time constant of the circuit RC is the product of R and C, i.e. the value of the elements of the circuit. So, the time constant depends on the resistor and the capacitor, which are the physical elements of the circuit. In the present case, and by analogy, the time constant in hemodialysis represents the time in which urea concentration had fallen by 63.2%. These data are obtained by equating the session time to the time constant.

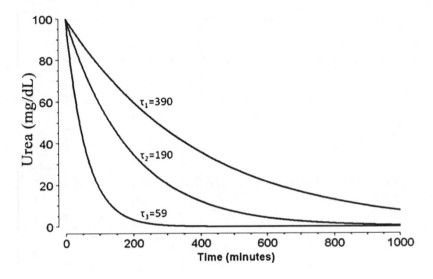

Fig. 12.17 Dynamics of urea clearance versus time of HD session, for different values of the time constant (τ): 59, 190 and 390 minutes.

Then, for $t = \tau$, yields:

$$C(t)=C_o\,e^{-Kt/V}=C_o\,e^{-t/\tau}=C_o\,e^{-1}=0.368\,C_o \qquad (12.67)$$

That is, if the pre-dialysis BUN is 100 mg/dL, the post-dialysis BUN will be 36.8 mg/dL. This dynamics will be faster if the time constant is low, and will be slower if V/K is high. A faster dynamic (low time constant, 59 minutes for example) means that the patient will reach normal values of urea concentration (about 20 mg/dL) in a period of time shorter. Slow dynamics (represented by a high time constant, e.g. 390 minutes) will result in a longer time to reach normal levels of urea. In Fig. 12.17 real values of time constants of patients found in clinical practice are shown. In particular, the values chosen to illustrate this figure have been the maximum time constant of a patient (from over 2200 patients), the minimum value and average value.

12.9 FINAL REMARKS AND CONCLUSIONS

An assessment of the dialysis dose is essential for dialysis patients. The Kt/V is a very useful tool although is not the only parameter used by nephrologists in planning the HD treatment of patients. UKM uses mathematical models to measure the movement of urea within the patient's body during dialysis and provides a quantitative method for developing a treatment prescription for a specific patient. Any mathematical model to compute Kt/V is valid and the international guidelines are very useful for this purpose. However, in 2009 there was a lively debate among several renowned authors that Kt/V is clinically illogical parameter (Jenkins PG 2009; Lowrie 2009; Spalding et al. 2009). Evidence to date indicates that UKM is beneficial because it assists clinicians in individualizing dialysis prescriptions and provides the hemodialysis care team with guidance about which specific parameters of the prescription to modify to achieve the target hemodialysis dose. It provides a mechanism to check for errors in the delivered dose of hemodialysis and it provides the greatest support for continuous quality improvement (CQI) efforts in the delivery of hemodialysis (NKF-K/DOQI 2000). It also permits calculation of the normalized protein nitrogen appearance (nPNA), formerly normalized protein catabolic rate (nPCR), which represents an indirect measure of protein intake by calculating the amount of urea generated by the patient. Thus, UKM which does provide an estimate of protein intake is more useful than URR.

A drawback of UKM is the complexity of the calculations that requires the use of computational devices and software. Although the cost of the computers and software is low, it is a factor for some dialysis centers (NKF-K/DOQI 2000). The estimated nPNA by UKM does not correlate well with reported dietary protein intake if patients are in a catabolic state as a result of illness, stress, or undernutrition, as they often are, or if loss of urea via residual renal function is not taken into account. Also, the PNA may be inaccurate when Kt/V is extremely high or low (> 1.8 or < 0.9), because both are derived from similar variables. Other drawbacks of UKM are that the calculations make assumptions pertaining to dialyzer clearance, patient size, and predictability of urea movement that may not be accurate for some patients and may skew the value. Also, UKM is fairly expensive and time consuming. UKM is better for patients who are unstable in their dietary habits or health status because these patients' urea clearances and dose of dialysis needed may fluctuate widely (NKF-K/DOQI 2000).

In the last decade of the twentieth century dialysis machines providing online assessment of Kt/V were introduced and became increasingly used. Online clearance methods do not need blood samples. The equipment (online clearance monitor) is build-in to dialysis machine and calculates HD dose from measurements of dialysate conductivity using sodium flux as a surrogate for urea (Petitclerc et al. 1993; Polaschegg 1993) or dialysate urea (Hernandez–Herrera et al. 2001). Online Kt/V measured by the conductivity method was shown to be lower by approximately 15% than SPVV Kt/V obtained using Daugirdas second generation formula (Grzegorzewska and Banachowicz 2008). Mean difference between SPVV Kt/V and online Kt/V was 0.21 ± 0.14. The agreement measurement performed using the Bland and Altman method (Bland and Altman 1986) indicated that online Kt/V may be 0.48 below or 0.07 above SPVV Kt/V (Grzegorzewska and Banachowicz 2008). A correlation coefficient between Kt/V obtained online and calculated as SPVV Kt/V with urea measurement in blood probes varied between 0.5 (Grzegorzewska and Banachowicz 2008; Vlatković and Stojimirović 2006) and 0.956 (Maduell et al., 2005). Value of V for online Kt/V calculation was obtained using anthropometric data by Watson equations (Watson et al. 1980). It was shown, that estimates of urea distribution volume which based on patient weight, height, age and sex are overestimated, causing underestimated online Kt/V (Manzoni et al. 1996; Wuepper et al. 2003). Underestimation accounts for 22% for V of 55% of dry body mass and 23% for V derived from anthropometric equations. The difference between SPVV Kt/V and online Kt/V was explained by both overestimation of V (+17%) and underestimation of urea clearance (-11%) (Manzoni et al. 1996). According to the European Best Practice Guidelines on HD, online clearance should not substitute for monthly measurements but it is an acceptable method for calculating HD on a treatment-by-treatment basis (EBPG for Hemodialysis 2002). Today the on line measurement of Kt (and consequently Kt/V) using biosensors or ionic dialysance is coming more and more common. The reader will find a study of the on line Kt/V in another chapter in this book.

It has been also shown in this chapter how an approximation to the dynamics of hemodialysis can be made, separating the dimensionless parameter Kt/V in its two dimensional components: V/K (which would be the time constant of the system) and the session time. When dialysis dynamics of urea is known in a stable patient we can know the time necessary to get our target for blood urea. V/K has been established as an independent significant risk factor for mortality. However, a week point of this predictor is non-linear relationship with mortality rate. Thus, V/K is not superior to Kt/V in this respect. It has been shown that, depending on the dynamics (given by the time constant) and on the dialysis time, post-dialysis blood urea levels vary considerably from one patient to another. This is why dialysis treatments should be individualized as much as possible, not only controlling the session time but perhaps also the number of weekly sessions. From here there are two possibilities: one option could be to identify treatments adapted to the time constant of each patient and the other to analyze the modification of the parameters that influence the time constant and its relationship to mortality. We could also consider merging these two paths. Further analysis should be performed with the aim of checking the influence of V/K on other parameters related to the health of the patient.

APPENDIX A: CALCULATION OF Kt/V WITH MATLAB

A.1 Program to get the Kt/V by Lowrie's formula of 1983:

```
% Program that calculates the Kt/V by Lowrie's formula of 1983

home;
clear all;
clc;

%%%%%%%% Data input %%%%%%%%

% ts = input(Session time = ');
Cpre = input('Urea pre = ');
Cpost = input('Urea post = ');
% K = input('K = ');
% V = input('V = ');


%%%%%%%% Calculation %%%%%%%%

KTV = log (Cpre) - log (Cpost);

% Another way for calculating it: Kt/V = log (Cpre/Cpost)

%%%%%%%% Showing results %%%%%%%%

disp('The Kt/V calculated by Lowrie is: ');
disp(KTV);

%%%%%%%% FIN %%%%%%%%
```

A.2 Program to get the Kt/V by Daugirdas' formula of 1993:

```
% Program to calculate the Kt/V by Daugirdas of 1993

home;
clear all;
clc;

%%%%%%%% Data input %%%%%%%%

Cpre = input('Urea pre = ');
Cpost = input('Urea post = ');
K = input('K = ');
ts = input('Session time (in minutes) ts = ');
V = input('Volume V = ');
UF = input('UF = ');
W = input('Post HD weight (Kg) = ');

%%%%%%%% Calculations %%%%%%%%

% Daugirdas-93 (7)  Kt/V = -ln (R - 0.008T) +(4 - 3.5R) x UF/W
R = Cpost / Cpre;
KTV = - log (R – 0.008 * (ts/60)) + (4 - 3.5 * R) * UF/W;

%%%%%%%% Showing results %%%%%%%%

disp('The Kt/V calculated by Daugirdas-1993 is: ');
disp(KTV);

%%%%%%%% FIN %%%%%%%%
```

REFERENCES

Acchiardo, S.R., Hatten, K.W., Ruvinsky, M.J., et al.: Inadequate dialysis increases gross mortality rate. ASAIO J. 38(3), M282–M285 (1992)

Azar, A.T.: Estimation of accurate and new method for hemodialysis dose calculation. Clinical Medicine: Urology 1, 15–21 (2008)

Babb, A.L., Popovich, R.P., Christopher, T.G., et al.: The genesis of the square meter-hour hypothesis. Trans. Am. Soc. Artif. Intern. Organs 17, 81–91 (1971)

Barth, R.H.: Direct calculation of Kt/V: A simplified approach to monitoring of hemodialysis. Nephron 50(3), 191–195 (1988)

Basile, C., Casino, F., Lopez, T.: Percent reduction in blood urea concentration during dialysis estimates KtV in a simple and accurate way. Am. J. Kidney Dis. 15(1), 40–45 (1990)

Basile, C., Vernaglione, L., Lomonte, C., et al.: Comparison of alternative methods for scaling dialysis dose. Nephrol. Dial. Transplant. 25(4), 1232–1239 (2010)

Blake, P., Daugirdas, J.: Quantification and prescription, general principles. In: Jacobs, C., Kjellstrand, K.M., Koch, K.M., Winchester, J.F. (eds.) Replacement of Renal Function by Dialysis, pp. 619–656. Kluver Academic Publishers, Dordrecht (1996)

Bland, J.M., Altman, D.G.: Statistical methods for assessing agreement between two methods of clinical measurement. Lancet 1(8476), 307–310 (1986)

Bloembergen, W.E., Stannard, D.C., Port, F.K., et al.: Relationship of dose of haemodialysis and cause-specific mortality. Kidney Int. 50(2), 557–565 (1996)

Borah, M.F., Schoenfeld, P.Y., Gotch, F.A., et al.: Nitrogen Balance during Intermittent Dialysis Therapy of Uremia. Kidney Int. 14(5), 491–500 (1978)

Calzavara, P., Vianello, A., Da Porto, A., et al.: Comparison Between Three Mathematical Models of Kt/V. Int. J. Artif. Organs 11(2), 107–110 (1988)

Canadian Society of Nephrology (CSN) Clinical practice guidelines the delivery of haemodialysis. J. Am. Soc. Nephrol. 10, S306–S310 (1999)

Casino, F.G., Lopez, T.: The equivalent renal urea clearance. A new parameter to assess dialysis dose. Nephrol. Dial. Transplant. 11, 1574–1581 (1996)

Chertow, G.M., Owen, W.F., Lazarus, J.M., et al.: Exploring the reverse J-shaped curve between urea reduction ratio and mortality. Kidney Int. 56(5), 1872–1878 (1999)

Collins, A.J., Ma, J.Z., Umen, A., et al.: Urea index and other predictors of haemodialysis patient survival. Am. J. Kidney Dis. 23(2), 272–282 (1994)

Daugirdas, J.T., Blake, P.G., Ing, T.S. (eds.): Handbook of Dialysis, 4th edn. Lippincott, Williams and Wilkins, Philadelphia (2007)

Daugirdas, J.T.: The post: pre-dialysis plasma urea nitrogen ratio to estimate Kt/V and NPCR: Mathematical modeling. Int. J. Artif. Organs 12(7), 411–419 (1989a)

Daugirdas, J.T.: The post:pre-dialysis plasma urea nitrogen ratio to estimate Kt/V and NPCR: Validation. Int. J. Artif. Organs 12(7), 420–427 (1989b)

Daugirdas, J.T.: Second generation logarithmic estimates of single-pool variable volume Kt/V: an analysis of error. J. Am. Soc. Nephrol. 4(5), 1205–1213 (1993)

Daugirdas, J.T., Depner, T.A.: A nomogram approach to hemodialysis urea modeling. Am. J. Kidney Dis. 23(1), 33–40 (1994)

Daugirdas, J.T.: Simplified equations for monitoring Kt/V, PCRn, eKt/V, and ePCRn. Adv. Ren. Replace Ther. 2(4), 295–304 (1995)

Daugirdas, J.T., Depner, T.A., Greene, T., et al.: Surface-area normalized Kt/V: a method of rescaling dialysis dose to body surface area – implications for different-size patients by gender. Semin. Dial. 21(5), 415–421 (2008a)

Daugirdas, J.T., Levin, N.W., Kotanko, P., et al.: Comparison of proposed alternative methods for rescaling dialysis dose: resting energy expenditure, high metabolic rate organ mass, liver size, and body surface area. Semin. Dial. 21(5), 377–384 (2008b)

Daugirdas, J.T., Meyer, K., Greene, T., et al.: Scaling of measured glomerular filtration rate in kidney donor candidates by anthropometric estimates of body surface area, body water, metabolic rate, or liver size. Clin. Am. Soc. Nephrol. 4(10), 1575–1583 (2009)

De Oreo, P., Hamburger, R.: Urea reduction ratio is not a consistent predictor of Kt/V. J. Am. Soc. Nephrol. 6, 597 (1995)

Depner, T.A.: Prescribing Hemodialysis: A Guide to Urea Modeling, 2nd edn. Springer, Heidelberg (1990)

Depner, T.A.: History of dialysis quantitation. Semin. Dial. 12(suppl.1), S14–S19 (1999a)

Depner, T.A.: Why Daily hemodialysis is better: solute kinetics. Semin. Dial. 12(6), 462–471 (1999b)

Depner, T.A., Daugirdas, J.T.: Equations for normalized protein catabolic rate based on two-point modeling of hemodialysis urea kinetics. J. Am. Soc. Nephrol. 7, 780–785 (1996)

Depner, T.A.: Hemodialysis adequacy: Basic essentials and practical points for the nephrologist in training. Hemodialysis Int. 9(3), 241–254 (2005)

Deziel, C., Hirsch, D.J., Hoult, P.: The Canadian Society of Nephrology. Clinical practice guidelines the delivery of haemodialysis. J. Am. Soc. Nephrol. 10(suppl. 13), 306–310 (1999)

Dubois, D., Dubois, E.F.: A formula to estimate the approximate surface area if height and weight be known. Nutrition 5(5), 303–311 (1989)

Eknoyan, G., Beck, G.J., Cheung, A.K., et al.: Effect of dialysis dose and membrane flux in maintenance hemodialysis. N. Engl J. Med. 347(25), 2010–2019 (2002)

European Best Practice Guidelines (EBPG) for hemodialysis; section II: hemodialysis adequacy. Nephrol. Dial. Transplant. 17(suppl. 7), 16–31 (2002)

European Best Practice Guidelines (EBPG) on hemodialysis. Nephrol. Dial. Transplant. 22(supp. 2), ii16–ii21 (2007)

Garred, L.J., Barichello, D.L., Canaud, B., McCready, W.G.: Simple Equations For Protein Catabolic Rate Determination From Pre And Post Dialysis Blood Urea Nitrogen. ASAIO J. 41(4), 889–895 (1995)

Giovannetti, S., Maggiore, Q.: A low-nitrogen diet with proteins of high biological value for severe chronic uraemia. Lancet 1(7341), 1000–1003 (1964)

Gotch, F.A.: Kinetic modeling in hemodialysis. In: Nissenson, A.R., Fine, R.N., Gentile, D.E. (eds.) Clinical Dialysis, 3rd edn., pp. 156–189. Appleton & Lange, East Norwalk (1995)

Gotch, F.A.: The current place of urea kinetic modeling with respect to different dialysis modalities. Nephrol. Dial. Transplant. 13(suppl. 6), 10–14 (1998)

Gotch, F.A.: Kt/V is the best dialysis dose parameter. Blood Purif. 18(4), 276–285 (2000)

Gotch, F., Sargent, J.: A mechanistic analysis of the National Cooperative Dialysis Study (NCDS). Kidney Int. 28(3), 526–534 (1985)

Gotch, F., Sargent, J., Keen, M., et al.: Individualized quantified dialysis therapy of uremia. Proc. Clin. Dial. Transplant. Forum 4(4), 27–35 (1974)

Gotch, F.A.: Evolution of the Single-Pool Urea Kinetic Model. Semin. Dial. 14(4), 252–256 (2001)

Grzegorzewska, A.E., Banachowicz, W.: Comparisons of Kt/V evaluated using an online method and calculated from urea measurements in patients on intermittent hemodialysis. Hemodial Int. 10(suppl. 2), S5–S9 (2006)

Grzegorzewska, A.E., Banachowicz, W.: Evaluation of hemodialysis adequacy using online Kt/V and single-pool variable-volume urea Kt/V. Int. Urol. Nephrol. 40(3), 771–778 (2008)

Grzegorzewska, A.E., Banachowicz, W., Leander, M.: Results of improvement in adequacy of intermittent hemodialysis in uremic patients. Rocz. Akad. Med. Bialymst. 50, 314–318 (2005)

Hakim, R.M., Breyer, J., Ismail, N., et al.: Effects of dose of dialysis on morbidity and mortality. Am. J. Kidney Dis. 23(5), 661–669 (1994)

Harter, H.R.: Review of significant findings from the National Co-operative Dialysis Study and recommendations. Kidney Int. Suppl. 13, S107–S112 (1983)

Hauk, M., Kuhlmann, M.K., Riegel, W., et al.: In vivo effects of dialysate flow rate on KtV in maintenance haemodialysis patients. Am. J. Kidney Dis. 35(1), 105–111 (2000)

Haycock, G.B., Schwartz, G.J., Wisotsky, D.H.: Geometric method for measuring body surface area: a height-weight formula validated in infants, children and adults. J. Pediatr. 93(1), 62–66 (1978)

Health Care Financing Administration (HCFA), Core Indicators Project Initial Results, Opportunities to Improve Care for Adult In-Center Hemodialysis Patients. Baltimore, Department of Health and Human Services, Health Care Financing Administration, Health Standards and Quality, Bureau (1994)

Held, P.J., Port, F.K., Wolfe, R.A., et al.: The dose of haemodialysis and patient mortality. Kidney Int. 50(2), 550–556 (1996)

Hernandez-Herrera, G., Martin-Malo, A., Rodriguez, M., et al.: Assessment of the length of each hemodialysis session by online dialysate urea monitoring. Nephron 89(1), 37–42 (2001)

Ifudu, O., Feldman, J., Friedman, E.A.: The intensity of hemodialysis and the response to erythropoietin in patients with end-stage renal disease. N. Engl. J. Med. 334(7), 420–425 (1996)

Jely, G.K., Raja, R.M.: Simplified calculation of PCR and Kt/V. Abstr. In: 24th Annual JASN Meeting, p. 329 (1991)

Jindal, K.K., Goldstein, M.B.: Urea kinetic modelling in chronic hemodialysis: Benefits, problems, and practical solutions. Seminars in Dialysis 1, 82–85 (1988)

Jindal, K.K., Manuel, A., Goldstein, M.B.: Percent Reduction Of The Blood Urea Concentration During Dialysis (PRU), A Simple And Accurate Method To Estimate Kt/V_{urea}. ASAIO Trans. 33(3), 286–288 (1978)

Jenkins, P.G.: The illogic of Kt/V. Kidney Int. 75, 337 (2009)

Kaufman, A.M., Schneditz, D., Smye, S., et al.: Solute disequilibrium and multicompartment modeling. Adv. Ren. Replace Ther. 2(4), 319–329 (1995)

Kerr, P.G., Argiles, A., Canaud, et al.: Accuracy of Kt/V estimations in high-flux haemodiafiltration using percent reduction of urea: incorporation of urea rebound. Nephrol. Dial. Transplant. 8(2), 149–153 (1993)

Kesheviah, P.R., Hanson, G.I., Berkseth, R.O., et al.: A Simplified Approach To Monitoring In Vivo Therapy Prescription. ASAIO Trans. 34(3), 620–622 (1988)

Keshaviah, P.: Urea kinetic and middle molecule approaches to assessing the adequacy of hemodialysis and CAPD. Kidney Int. 43(suppl. 40), S28–S38 (1993)

Kolff, W., Berk, H., Welle, N., et al.: The artificial kidney: a dialyzer with great area. Acta Med. Scand. 117, 121–134 (1944)

Kopple, J.D., Zhu, X., Lew, N.L., et al.: Body weight-for-height relationships predict mortality in maintenance hemodialysis patients. Kidney Int. 56(3), 1136–1148 (1999)

Kovacic, V., Roguljic, L., Jukic, I., et al.: Comparison of methods for hemodialysis dose calculation. Dial. Transplant. 32(4), 170–175 (2003)

Kupcinskas, R.: A Method for Optical Measurement of Urea in Effluent Hemodialysate. PhD. Worcester Polytechnic Institute (2000)

Laird, N.M., Berkey, C.S., Lowrie, E.G.: Modeling success or failure of dialysis therapy: the National Cooperative Dialysis Study. Kidney Int. 23(suppl. 13), 101–106 (1983)

Leypoldt, J.K., Cheung, A.K., Agodoa, L.Y., et al.: Hemodialyzer mass transfer-area coefficients for urea increase at high dialysate flow rates. The Haemodialysis (HEMO) Study. Kidney Int. 51(6), 2013–2017 (1997)

Levy, J., Morgan, J., Brown, E.: Oxford Handbook of Dialysis, 2nd edn. Oxford University Press, USA (2004)

Li, Z., Lew, N.L., Lazarus, J.M., et al.: Comparing the urea reduction ratio (URR) and the {urea clearance / dialysis time} product (Kt) as outcome based measures of hemodialysis dose. Am. J. Kidney Dis. 35(4), 598–605 (2000)

Locatelli, F., Buoncristiani, U., Canaud, B., et al.: Dialysis dose and frequency. Nephrol. Dial. Transplant. 20(2), 285–296 (2005)

Lowrie, E.G.: The normalized treatment ratio (Kt/V) is not the best dialysis dose parameter. Blood Purif. 18(4), 286–294 (2000)

Lowrie, E., Laird, N., Parker, T.F., et al.: Cooperative dialysis study. Kidney Int. 23(suppl. 13), S1–S122 (1983)

Lowrie, E., Teehan, B.: Principles of prescribing dialysis therapy: Implementing recommendations from the National Cooperative Dialysis Study. Kidney Int. 23(suppl. 13), S113–S122 (1983)

Lowrie, E.G., Lew, N.L.: The urea reducton ratio (URR): a simple method for evaluating haemodialysis treatment. Contemp. Dial. Nephrol. 12, 11–20 (1991)

Lowrie, E.G., Laird, N.M., Parker, T.F., et al.: Effect of the hemodialysis prescription on patient morbidity: Report from the National Cooperative Dialysis Study. N. Engl. J. Med. 305(20), 1176–1181 (1981)

Lowrie, E.G., Zhu, X., Lew, N.L., et al.: Predictors of hospitalization among hemodialysis patients. Memorandum to FMC(NA) medical directors. Fresenius Medical Care (NA) Ref. No. 98-08-07 (August 7, 1998a)

Lowrie, E.G., Zhu, X., Lew, N.L.: Primary associates of mortality urea reduction ratio as outcome-based measures of dialysis dose. Am. J. Kidney Dis. 32(6 suppl. 4), S16–S31 (1998b)

Lowrie, E.G., Chertow, G.M., Lew, N.L., et al.: The {clearance / time} product (Kt) as an outcome based measure of dialysis dose. Kidney Int. 56, 729–737 (1999)

Lowrie, E.G., Li, Z., Ofsthun, N., et al.: Body size, dialysis dose and death risk relationships among hemodialys is patients. Kidney Int. 62(2), 1891–1897 (2002)

Lowrie, E.G.: Response to 'The illogic of Kt/V'. Kidney Int. 75, 337 (2009)

Lowrie, E.G., Li, Z., Ofsthun, N., et al.: The online measurement of hemodialysis dose (Kt): clinical outcome as a function of body surface area. Kidney Int. 68(5), 1344–1354 (2005)

Maduell, F., Garcia-Valdecasas, J., Garcia, H., et al.: Urea reduction ratio considering urea rebound. Nephron 78(2), 143–147 (1998)

Maduell, F., Puchades, M.J., Navarro, V., et al.: Monitoring hemodialysis dose with ionic dialisance in on-line hemodiafiltration [Article in Spanish]. Nefrologia 25(5), 521–526 (2005)

Manzoni, C., Di Filippo, S., Corti, M., et al.: Ionic dialysance as a method for the on-line monitoring of delivered dialysis without blood sampling. Nephrol. Dial. Transplant. 11(10), 2023–2030 (1996)

Maeda, K.: An overview of dialysis treatment in Japan (as of December 31, 1997). Journal of Japanese Society for Dialysis Therapy 32(1), 1–17 (1999)

McClellan, W.M., Soucie, J.M., Flanders, D.W.: Mortality in end-stage renal disease is associated with facility-to-facility differences in adequacy of hemodialysis. J. Am. Soc. Nephrol. 9(10), 1940–1947 (1998)

Movilli, E., Cancarini, G.C., Zani, R., et al.: Adequacy of dialysis reduces the doses of recombinant erythropoietin independently from the use of biocompatible membranes in haemodialysis patients. Nephrol. Dial. Transplant. 16(1), 111–114 (2001)

NKF-K/DOQI: Clinical Practice Guidelines and Clinical Practice Recommendations, Updates: Hemodialysis Adequacy, Peritoneal Dialysis Adequacy, Vascular Access. Am. J. Kidney Dis. 48(suppl. 1), S28–S58 (2006)

NKF-K/DOQI: Clinical practice guidelines for hemodialysis adequacy: Update. Am. J. Kidney Dis. 37(1 suppl. 1), S7–S64 (2001)

NKF-K/DOQI: Clinical Practice Guidelines for Nutrition in Chronic Renal Failure. Am. J. Kidney Dis. 35(6 suppl. 2), S1–S140 (2000)

NKF-K/DOQI: Clinical Practice Guidelines for hemodialysis adequacy. Am. J. Kidney Dis. 30(3 suppl. 2), S15–S136 (1997)

Oliva Gómez, J.S., Roa Romero, L.M., et al.: Dynamical approach to the dimensionless expression Kt/V. A retrospective study on the Andalusian population on treatment with hemodialysis. In: Proceedings of the XXVII Annual Congress of the Spanish Society of Biomedical Engineering, Cadiz, pp. 243–246 (2009); ISBN: 978-84-608-0990-6

Owen Jr., W.F., Lew, N.L., Liu, Y., et al.: The urea reduction ratio and serum albumin concentration as predictors of mortality in patients undergoing haemodialysis. N. Engl. J. Med. 329(14), 1001–1006 (1993)

Owen, W.F., Chertow, G.M., Lazarus, J.M., et al.: Dose of hemodialysis and survival: Differences by race and sex. J. Am. Med. Assoc. 280(20), 1764–1768 (1998)

Parker III, T.F., Husni, L., Huang, W., et al.: Survival of hemodialysis patients in the United States is improved with a greater quantity of dialysis. Am. J. Kidney Dis. 23(5), 670–680 (1994)

Petitclerc, T., Goux, N., Reynier, A.L., et al.: A model for non-invasive estimation of in-vivo dialyzer performances and patient's conductivity during hemodialysis. Int. J. Artif. Organs 16(8), 585–591 (1993)

Polaschegg, H.D.: Automatic non-invasive intradialytic clearance measurements. Int. J. Artif. Organs 16(4), 185–191 (1993)

Salahudeen, A.K., Fleischmann, E.H., Bower, J.D.: Impact of lower delivered Kt/V on the survival of overweight patients on hemodialysis. Kidney Int. 56(6), 2254–2259 (1999)

Salahudeen, A.K., Dykes, P., May, W.: Risk factors for higher mortality at the highest levels of spKt/V in haemodialysis patients. Nephrol. Dial. Transplant. 18(7), 1339–1344 (2003)

Sargent, J.: Control of dialysis by a single-pool urea model: The National Cooperative Dialysis Study. Kidney Int. 23(suppl. 13), S19–S26 (1983)

Sargent, J., Gotch, F., Borah, M., et al.: Urea kinetics: A guide to nutritional management of renal failure. Am. J. Clin. Nutr. 31, 1696–1702 (1978)

Sargent, J.A., Gotch, F.A.: The study of uremia by manipulation of blood concentrations using combinations of hollow fiber devices. Trans. Am. Soc. Artif. Intern. Organs 20A, 395–401 (1974)

Sargent, J.A., Gotch, F.A.: The analysis of concentration dependence of uremic lesions in clinical studies. Kidney Int. suppl. 2(2), S35–S44 (1975)

Sargent, J.A., Gotch, F.A.: Mathematic modeling of dialysis therapy. Kidney Int. Suppl. 10, S2–S10 (1980)

Sargent, J.A., Gotch, F.A.: Mathematic modeling of dialysis therapy. Kidney Int. 18, 2–10 (1980)

Sargent, J., Gotch, F.: Principles and biophysics of dialysis. In: Drukkcr, W., Parsons, F., Maher, J. (eds.) Replacement of Renal Function by Dialysis, 2nd edn. Martinues Nijhoff, Hague (1985)

Schneditz, D., Daugirdas, J.T.: Compartment effects in hemodialysis. Semin. Dial. 14(4), 271–277 (2001)

Sherman, R.A., Cody, R.P., Rogers, M.E., et al.: Accuracy of the urea reduction ratio in predicting dialysis delivery. Kidney Int. 47(1), 319–321 (1995)

Shinzato, T., Nakai, S., Akiba, T., et al.: Survival in long-term haemodialysis patients: results from the annual survey of the Japanese Society for Dialysis Therapy. Nephrol. Dial. Transplant. 12(5), 884–888 (1997)

Smye, S.W., Hydon, P.E., Will, E.: An Analysis of the Single-Pool Urea Kinetic Model and Estimation of Errors. Phys. Med. Biol. 38(1), 115–122 (1993)

Spalding, E.M., Chandna, S.M., Davenport, A., et al.: Kt/V underestimates the hemodialysis dose in women and small men. Kidney Int. 74(3), 348–355 (2008)

Spalding, E.M., Chandna, S.M., Davenport, A., Farrington, K.: Response to the illogic of Kt/V. Kidney Int. 75, 337 (2009)

Suri, R.S., Garg, A.X., Chertow, G.M., et al.: For the Frequent Hemodialysis Network (FHN) Trial Group: Frequent Hemodialysis Network (FHN) randomized trials: study design. Kidney Int. 71, 349–359 (2007)

The Renal Association, Recommended standards for haemodialysis. Royal College of Physicians of London. Treatment of adult patients with renal failure. Recommended Standards and Audit Measure 29(3), 190–191 (1997)

Vanholder, R.C.: Assessment of Urea and Other Uremic Markers for Quantification of Dialysis Efficiency. Clin. Chem. 38(8), 1429–1436 (1992)

Vanholder, R., De Smet, R., Glorieux, G., et al.: Review on uremic toxins: classification, concentration, and interindividual variability. Kidney Int. 63(5), 1934–1943 (2003)

Vlatković, V., Stojimirović, B.: Determination of the delivered hemodialysis dose using standard methods and on-line clearance monitoring. Vojnosanit. Pregl. 63(8), 743–747 (2006)

Watson, P.E., Watson, I.D., Batt, R.D.: Total body water volumes for adult males and females estimated from simple anthropometric measurements. Am. J. Clin. Nutr. 33(1), 27–39 (1980)

Wolf, A.V., Remp, D.G., Kiley, J.E., et al.: Artificial kidney function; kinetics of hemodialysis. J. Clin. Invest. 30(10), 1062–1070 (1951)

Wuepper, A., Tattersall, J., Kraemer, M., et al.: Determination of urea distribution volume for Kt/V assessed by conductivity monitoring. Kidney Int. 64(6), 2262–2271 (2003)

ESSAY QUESTIONS

1. List the main compartments of solute distribution during hemodialysis.
2. Why urea is used up today in the evaluation of dialysis adequacy?
3. What does URR stand for? And what is the Kt/V used for?
4. List the two main categories of UKM and state the main difference between them.
5. What is the main difference between SPFVM and SPVVM?
6. Describe the advantages and disadvantages of UKM
7. State the main limitations to PNA as an estimate of dietary protein intake (DPI) as recommended by NKF-K/DOQI.
8. Differentiate between the two main measurements used to calculate the single-pool Kt/V ($_{sp}$Kt/V) and PNA (PCR).
9. Using the following Table:

Parameter	Patient A.B.	Patient A.C.
Pre-HD urea (mg/dL)	120	90
Post-HD urea (mg/dL)	40	30
Post-HD V (L)	40	38
UF (L)	2	3

   Which patient urea removal was greater during HD session? Comment on your results.
10. Write a matlab program to calculate the Daugirdas Kt/V using the one-compartment method of Daugirdas (1993).

MULTIPLE CHOICE QUESTIONS

Choose the best answer

1. If a patient has a pre-dialysis BUN of 142 mg/dL and post-dialysis BUN of 40 mg/dL, the URR is...
   A. 74.8 %
   B. 71.8 %
   C. 75.5 %
   D. 77.6 %

2. If a patient dialysed three times a week has a pre-dialysis BUN of 125 mg/dL, post-dialysis BUN of 42 mg/dL, dialysis time of 4 h and the second pre-dialysis BUN of 113 mg/dL, then the TAC of this patient is...
   A. 71 mg/dL
   B. 66 mg/dL
   C. 75 mg/dL
   D. 55 mg/dL

3. The post-dialysis BUN concentration for a male patient is 44 mg/dL, the post-dialysis urea distribution volume is 46.5 L, residual renal clearance of the patient is 0 mL/min. The estimated the pre-dialysis BUN for the next dialysis session based on SPFV model if the urea generation rate is 11 mg/min is...
   A. 115.5 mg/dL
   B. 120.5 mg/dL
   C. 106.5 mg/dL
   D. 125.5 mg/dL

4. The post-dialysis BUN concentration for a female patient is 61 mg/dL. The pre- and post-dialysis urea distribution volume is 33 L and 30 L, respectively, residual renal clearance of the patient is 0 mL/min. Estimate the pre-dialysis BUN for the next dialysis session based on SPVV model if the urea generation rate is 7.56 mg/min.
   A. 125.58 mg/dL
   B. 127.58 mg/dL
   C. 130.58 mg/dL
   D. 135.58 mg/dL

5. For a male-patient who received dialysis three times weekly, the pre-BUN was 153 mg/dL, the post-dialysis urea distribution volume after 4 hours dialysis was 34.09 L and the post-dialysis BUN was 45 mg/dL. The residual urea clearance of the patient is 0 ml/min and the interdialytic weight gain is 3 kg. The urea generation rate is...

    A. 11.6 mg/min
    B. 17.8 mg/min
    C. 18.5 mg/min
    D. 15.7 mg/min

6. A patient has urea concentrations of 150 and 60 mg/dL before and after 4 hour dialysis session, respectively, UF of 2.5 L, post-dialysis weight of 70 kg. Calculate the dialysis dose using Azar and Daugirdas second generation formula.

    A. 1.03 and 1.09
    B. 1.13 and 1.19
    C. 1.22 and 1.28
    D. 1.26 and 1.32

7. We have the following data from a patient: $C_o = 143$ mg/dL, $C_t = 37$ mg/dL, K = 176 mL/min, session time = 232 min, V = 40 L, UFV = 2 L, post-dialysis weight = 87 kg. The Kt/V of the patient using the Lowrie's one-compartment method (1983) is...

    A. 1.21
    B. 1.52
    C. 1.12
    D. 1.35

8. For the patient in question 1, the Daugirdas Kt/V using the one-compartment method of Daugirdas (1993) is...

    A. 1.55
    B. 0.93
    C. 1.18
    D. 1.34

9. What elements of the dialysis prescription (Kt/V) can be controlled by the nephrologists?

    A. The urea distribution volume (V) and the time of dialysis session (t).
    B. The dialyzer clearance (K) and the time of dialysis session (t).
    C. Only the dialyzer clearance (K).
    D. Only the time of dialysis session (t).

10. If a patient has URR of 68%, then its Kt/V by Lowrie (1983) is…
    A. 1.1456
    B. It cannot be calculated. Missing data.
    C. 1.1394.
    D. All answers are incorrect.

11. Which is the minimum $_{sp}$Kt/V recommended by DOQI guidelines for a schedule of three hemodialysis sessions per week?
    A. 0.8
    B. 1.1
    C. 1.3
    D. 1.2

12. Due to the variability in measuring Kt/V which are the targets values recommended by DOQI guidelines for spKt/V?
    A. 1.4
    B. 1.1
    C. 1.2
    D. 1.3

13. The measurement methods to calculate the single-pool Kt/V ($_{sp}$Kt/V) and PNA (PCR) are…
    A. Two Measurement method
    B. Three Measurement method
    C. A and B

14. A dialysis patient has a pre-dialysis BUN of 108 mg/dL and post-dialysis BUN of 35 mg/dl. The residual renal clearance if the urine volume is 1500 mL and urine urea nitrogen is 150 mg/dL is…
    A. 1.4 mL/min
    B. 1.6 mL/min
    C. 2.0 mL/min
    D. 1.8 mL/min

15. If a patient has a urea generation rate of 10.5 mg/min, the time averaged urea concentration of 75 mg/dL, the peak BUN for this person during thrice-weekly hemodialysis schedule is 110, 120, 115 mg/dL, the equivalent renal urea clearance (eK_{ru}) using Casino-Lopez formula is…
    A. 18 mL/min
    B. 15 mL/min
    C. 13 mL/min
    D. 14 mL/min

16. Using the data of question 15, the equivalent renal urea clearance (eK_{ru}) using adjusted Gotch formula is...

    A. 10.15 mL/min
    B. 9.13 mL/min
    C. 12.25 mL/min
    D. 13.18 mL/min

17. A male dialysis patient has Kt/V of 1.33 when the pre- and post-dialysis BUN concentrations are 159 mg/dL and 61 mg/dL, respectively. All blood samples were obtained at the midweek HD session. The nPCR according to Garred formula will be...

    A. 2.4 g/kg/day
    B. 1.8 g/kg/day
    C. 2.1 g/kg/day
    D. 1.5 g/kg/day

18. Using the data of question 17, the nPCR according to Depner-Daugirdas formula will be...

    A. 2.1 g/kg/day
    B. 1.8 g/kg/day
    C. 2.7 g/kg/day
    D. 2.45 g/kg/day

19. We have the following data from a patient...
C_o = 100 mg/dL, C_t = 30 mg/dL, session time = 240 min.
The time constant of this patient is...

    A. τ = 210 min
    B. τ = 289 min
    C. τ = 240 min
    D. All the previous answers are wrong.

20. If the urea generation rate is 9.5 mg/min and post-dialysis urea distribution is 39 L, then PCR (PNA) using Borah method is...

    A. 88.4 g/day
    B. 95.4 g/day
    C. 100.3 g/day
    D. 105.6 g/day

Chapter 13

Double Pool Urea Kinetic Modeling

Ahmad Taher Azar, Masatomo Yashiro, Daniel Schneditz, and Laura M. Roa

CHAPTER OUTLINES

- Single pool model versus double pool model.
- Mathematical analysis of double pool urea kinetic models.
- Estimation of equilibrated post-dialysis blood urea concentration.
- Estimation of post-dialysis urea rebound.
- Estimation of equilibrated dialysis dose.
- Regional blood flow model
- Conclusion

CHAPTER OBJECTIVES

- Introduce the difference between single and double pool urea kinetic models.
- Discuss the concept of urea rebound.
- Explain the mathematical analysis of double pool urea kinetic models.

- Describe the different methods of estimating equilibrated urea concentration and urea rebound.
- Describe the different methods of calculating the double pool Kt/V.
- Discuss the concept of regional blood flow models.
- Explain the mathematical analysis of regional blood flow model.

KEY TERMS

- Single pool urea kinetic models
- Double pool urea kinetic models
- Intracellular compartment
- Extracellular compartment
- Urea rebound
- Equilibrated urea concentration
- Equilibrated dialysis dose Kt/V
- Access recirculation
- Cardiopulmonary recirculation
- High-efficiency dialysis
- Regional blood flow model

ABSTRACT

Urea kinetic modelling (UKM) has been generally accepted as a method for quantifying hemodialysis (HD) treatment. During hemodialysis, reduction in the urea concentration in the intracellular fluid (ICF) compartment will lag behind that in the extra cellular fluid (ECF) compartment, and

A.T. Azar (Ed.): Modelling and Control of Dialysis Systems, SCI 404, pp. 627–687.
springerlink.com   © Springer-Verlag Berlin Heidelberg 2013

following the end of dialysis, a "rebound" in the blood level of urea will occur where it continues to rise due to diffusion of urea from the ICF to ECF to establish an equilibrium state. Because of compartment effects, the dose of dialysis with regard to urea removal is significantly overestimated from immediate post-dialysis urea concentrations, because 30 to 60 min are required for concentration gradients to dissipate and for urea concentrations to equilibrate across body water spaces during the post-dialysis period. To avoid the delay of waiting for an equilibrated post-dialysis sample, it became necessary to describe and to quantitate effects causing the urea compartmentalization during dialysis; two-pool modeling approaches have been developed that more accurately reflect the amount of urea removed. This in turn gives more adequate measures not only of dialysis adequacy, but also of the protein catabolic rate, an important nutritional measure that is clinically monitored in dialysis patients. This chapter discusses the double pool urea kinetic models and regional blood flow models in order to understand the concept of urea rebound.

13.1 SINGLE POOL MODEL VERSUS DOUBLE POOL MODEL

A single pool model can only describe the urea kinetics correctly if the patient is in complete equilibrium. This is fairly correct within the intermediate phases of two dialyses. During dialysis this is completely incorrect because the patient from this aspect can be regarded as composed of two fractional urea distribution volumes: The intracellular fluid (ICF) and the interstitial and intravascular plasma fluid, both forming the extracellular fluid (ECF). The urea concentration within both of these aqueous distribution spaces of the body of the ESRD patient is inhomogeneous during dialysis. This is due to strong concentration gradients generated by dialysis. Dialysis has only access to the ECF, because the patient is connected via the cannula positioned within his arterio-venous fistula or graft. Urea once removed by dialysis from extracellular space will be refilled by a concentration gradient across the cell membrane. This is a non-instantaneous process. Typically it takes 30 min to equilibrate 95% of an initial urea gradient over the hypothetical cell membrane if the gradient is not perpetuated by further dialysis. This effect, usually referred as *rebound*, is the measurable trace of the delayed urea mass transfer across the cell membrane (Schneditz et al. 1993; Spiegel et al. 1995; Leblanc et al. 1996; Garred et al. 1997; Jean et al. 1998, 1999; Alloatti et al. 1998; Yashiro et al. 2004). The rebound phenomenon indicates that urea behaves as if it distributed between two distinct compartments (intracellular and extracellular) (Matthews and Downey 1984), and causes that the simple single pool urea model fails to accurately predict urea concentrations during and after HD session. Two types of urea disequilibrium have been demonstrated: classic diffusion (membrane) - limited disequilibrium and flow-related disequilibrium (Depner et al. 1991; Kaufman et al. 1995; Schneditz et al. 1992a). The membrane-dependent disequilibrium results from restrictive movement of a solute between the patient's tissue compartments, causing concentration gradients to develop especially during rapid solute removal. Flow-dependent disequilibrium causes solute gradients to develop between areas of different specific perfusion.

Single-pool urea kinetic model neither accounts for the different rates of urea transfer between fluid compartments (NKF-K/DOQI 2001; Schneditz et al. 1995; Schneditz and Daugirdas 2001), nor for recirculation through the vascular access (Tattersall et al. 1996c; Leblanc et al. 1996; Daugirdas et al. 1996a). With increased dialyzer efficiency, urea removal from the extracellular compartment can exceed its apparent diffusive transfer rate from the intracellular compartment to the extracellular compartment (K_{ei}), which is estimated at 800 ml/ min (Heineken et al. 1987; Metry et al. 1993; Sharma et al. 2000). Although higher K_{ei} values have been observed, the relative resistance of urea movement from the cells to the interstitium and blood effectively render the intracellular compartment an unequilibrated reservoir of urea that is not accounted for by single-pool models of urea kinetics (NKF-K/DOQI 2001; Vanholder et al. 1996; Star et al. 1992; Flanigan et al. 1991). According to the double pool model, the release of sequestered urea continues for 30 to 60 min after completion of the hemodialysis session. Thus, the effective delivered dose of hemodialysis will be overestimated if this sequestered urea pool is large and is not considered (kinetic underestimation of true V) (Daugirdas et al. 1999; Tattersall et al. 1996a; Abramson et al. 1994). The use of dialyzers with high K, especially in patients with a small V that permit short dialysis times such as pediatric patients (increased K/V), increases the risk of significant double-pool effects (Smye et al. 1994, 1992).

13.1.1 The Concept Of Urea Rebound

Post-dialysis urea rebound (PDUR) has three components: access recirculation, cardiopulmonary recirculation (CpR), and entry of urea from poorly accessible tissue compartments that were not well depurated during the dialysis treatment (Daugirdas et al. 2004; Kooman et al. 2001). The effects of access recirculation on the post-dialysis blood sample are normally obviated by obtaining this sample using a slow-flow technique (at 50 to 100 mL/min of extracorporeal blood flow) for sampling the post-dialysis blood approximately 15s after dialysis (NKF-K/DOQI 2001; Kapoian et al.

1997). CpR is due to rapid partial closure of the arteriovenous (AV) urea gradient after cessation of dialysis, as cleared blood is no longer returned to the heart. If the blood is sampled from an arterial site, then an early rise in urea concentration will be noted as early as 10 to 15 s after dialysis has ceased, as a result of this blood pool re-equilibration effect. Approximately 1 min after the end of dialysis, the effect of CpR should have largely dissipated (Schneditz et al. 1992b). The third component of post-dialysis rebound is due to release of urea from sites where it had been sequestered during dialysis, as a result of a low rate of perfusion relative either to urea stores or to some tissue barrier (e.g., the cell membrane) (Daugirdas et al. 2004). Third-phase rebound theoretically depends on the size of the sequestered urea pool (thought to include skeletal muscle) and the extent to which urea removal from this tissue pool has been impeded during dialysis by virtue of reduced blood flow (Yashiro et al. 2004; Daugirdas and Schneditz 1995; Schneditz and Daugirdas 1994; Schneditz et al. 1993).

The rebound phenomenon is less important for the assessment of HD adequacy in long-duration low-flux dialysis because the two compartments have time to equilibrate (Jean et al. 1998). The magnitude of post-HD urea rebound, measured as the percent increase in urea concentration from the end-HD to the equilibrated value, varies between 10 and 22% in standard HD sessions (Maduell et al. 1998; Pedrini et al. 1988). In a high-flux HD session (urea clearance 500 mL/min), underestimation of the post-dialysis urea concentration in the blood sample taken immediately after HD end can results in the overestimation of Kt/V by up to 25% (Abramson et al. 1994; Vanholder et al. 1996). Among predictive factors for urea rebound the efficiency of the session (high K_d, high Kt/V) influences directly the magnitude of urea rebound (Abramson et al. 1994; Flanigan et al., 1991; Tattersall et al. 1996a, b). Also, short-time HD sessions (<3 h), HD sessions in small V patients (Evans et al. 1992; Smye et al. 1992) or complicated by hemodynamic instability (Ronco et al. 1992) are followed by greater rebound.

PDUR is a critical problem, which influences the calculation of equilibrated post-dialysis blood urea concentration C_{eq} thus increasing the risk of malestimation of the true dose of dialysis $_{eq}(Kt/V)$.

13.2 DOUBLE POOL UREA KINETIC MODEL

Both the cell membrane two-pool model (Sargent and Gotch 1989) and the regional blood flow two-pool model (Schneditz et al. 1993) provide a more physiological description of urea (and other solutes) kinetics (Schneditz et al. 1995). In the cell model, concentration disequilibrium between intracellular and extracellular spaces during HD is attributed to a limited solute permeability of the cell membrane. The regional blood flow model theorizes delayed solute diffusion from poorly perfused to highly perfused organ systems. In both cases PDUR is the effect of the intercompartmental re-equilibration occurring at the end of HD (Schneditz et al. 1993; Pedrini et al. 1988). Clinical application of multicompartmental models for Kt/V estimates requires too many input parameters (Burgelman et al. 1997; Cappello et al. 1998), some of which (i.e. the intercompartmental solute clearance) cannot be obtained in the individual case. Thus, the use of these models is restricted to experimental studies.

To make it accessible to mathematical considerations the urea mass kinetics must be simplified to an interaction of the urea generating component, which is the liver, both the intra- and extracellular pool each with a given buffer volume and the urea eliminating processes like a residual clearance of the native kidneys and the urea removal performed by the dialysis machine as shown in Fig. 13.1 (Goldau 2002). The liver excretes urea with a time dependent generation rate $G(t)$ to the ECF space of volume $V_e(t)$ and concentration $C_e(t)$. The extracellular volume connects with the intracellular volume by the intercompartmental urea mass transfer area coefficient K_{ei} (Pedrini et al. 1988). K_{ei} can be thought of as a clearance term, giving the movement of urea across the cell membrane in response to a concentration gradient (units are mL/min). In adults, K_{ei} is approximately

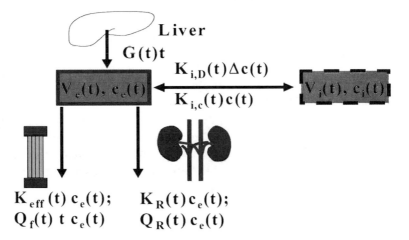

Fig. 13.1 A simplified representation of the participating constituents of the two pool urea kinetic model of an ESRD patient (Goldau 2002).

800 mL/min, assumed to scale for surface area, while pediatric data puts this figure at ~ 8.0 ± 1.1 ml/kg/min (Sharma et al. 2000; Sharma 2001). Urea generation G is assumed to occur in the ECF compartment. Some ESRD patients may have retained a fraction of residual clearance and filtration, expressed by K_r and Q_r that is only effecting ECF. Dialysis as the life-preserving treatment of the ESRD patient is the only path a substantial amount of urea can leave the body via the extracellular space (Goldau 2002).

13.2.1 Mathematical Description of Double Pool Urea Kinetic Model

With constant dialyzer clearance K_d the single-pool urea kinetic model predicts a logarithmic decline in urea concentrations, even if effects of concomitant urea generation, residual renal clearance, and ultrafiltration are taken into account. And after the end of dialysis without continuing K_d there is a slow but steady increase in urea concentrations until the next treatment. Thus, blood urea concentrations sampled during dialysis are expected to show a linear decline when the logarithms of the concentrations are plotted versus time (see Fig. 13.2). Mechanistically, and as the effects of urea generation, residual clearance, and ultrafiltration are of smaller magnitude, the slope of the linear decrease k refers to the ratio of clearance to distribution volume, K/V which describes the speed or rate of dialysis in units of 1/time. If the rate of dialysis is maintained for a treatment duration t, the dose of dialysis is given as the product of rate times duration, or Kt/V. As the decrease of solute concentration is linear on a semi-logarithmic plot, it is sufficient to sample the pre- and end-dialysis urea concentrations for the determination of K/V and Kt/V, respectively.

Experimental blood urea concentrations sampled during dialysis under stable treatment conditions, however, show a systematic deviation from the expected single-exponential (or linear, after logarithmic transformation) decline of intra-dialytic blood urea concentrations (see Fig. 13.2). The concentrations are significantly smaller than those predicted from the single-pool behavior. In the semi-logarithmic plot the discrepancy between experimental concentrations and the single-pool prediction increases within the first 30 to 60 min of treatment and stabilizes thereafter. After approximately 30 min the logarithmic decline of experimental concentrations

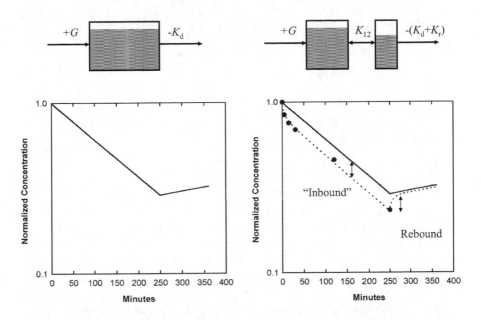

Fig. 13.2 Change in solute concentration C_t relative to initial concentration C_0 in the single-compartment case (left panel) where solute is always equilibrated, and in the two-compartment case (right panel) where solute concentration in the peripheral compartment lags behind the solute concentration in the central, accessible compartment. The decrease in solute concentration is linear in the semi-logarithmic plot for the single-compartment situation (left panel) but falls below the equilibrated concentration in the two-compartment situation (experimental data shown as full symbols, right panel). Abbreviations: dialyzer clearance K_d, residual renal clearance K_r, intercompartment clearance K_{12}, solute generation rate G

essentially follows a parallel to the single-pool model. The concentration at the end-of dialysis is much lower than the single-pool estimate. The two curves represent the theoretical equilibrated decrease in comparison to the experimental and non-equilibrated decrease. The difference between both represents a concentration gradient between equilibrated and experimental concentrations which develops during dialysis (as solute "inbound") and dissipates after dialysis as solute rebound.

The concentration gradient clearly shows that the single-pool assumption is not supported by experimental data. One approach to account for the deviation is to add a second compartment. One of these compartments is easily accessible to extracorporeal clearance and is therefore referred to as central compartment (Depner 1991; Sargent and Gotch 1989). The other compartment where solute appears to be sequestrated is not as accessible and therefore it is referred to as peripheral compartment (Depner 1991; Sargent and Gotch 1989). Central and peripheral compartments are usually linked allowing for solute exchange. The processes of solute generation, volume change, and residual clearance are then incorporated under more or less strict mechanistic and/or physiological considerations. With these assumptions, there are two possibilities to arrange two compartments relative to extracorporeal clearance.

13.2.1.1 Serial Two-Compartment Model

The classic two-compartment model is easily adapted to correct for gradients within the blood compartment (Sharma et al. 2000; Sharma 2001; Burgelman et al. 1997; Smye and Will 1995; Schneditz et al. 1995). In the standard pharmacokinetic approach central and peripheral compartments are connected in series (see Fig. 13.3). The kinetics can be derived from the mass balance equations for both central (index 1) and peripheral (index 2) compartments. For the central compartment the change in solute mass m is given by the sum of processes removing and/or adding solute as

$$\frac{dm_1}{dt} = -K_d C_1 - K_r C_1 + K_{12}(C_2 - C_1) + G \qquad (13.1)$$

where solute removal by the dialyzer and by residual kidney function is determined by the sum of dialyzer clearance K_d and residual renal clearance (if any) K_r times solute concentration in the central compartment C_1; solute exchange between compartments is assumed to occur by diffusion which is modeled as a first-order process and proportional to the concentration gradient C_2-C_1, and where the proportionality constant K_{12} is termed intercompartement clearance; and, finally solute influx because of constant solute generation rate G.

For the peripheral compartment the change in solute mass m is given by the exchange between compartments and given as

$$\frac{dm_2}{dt} = -K_{12}(C_2 - C_1) \qquad (13.2)$$

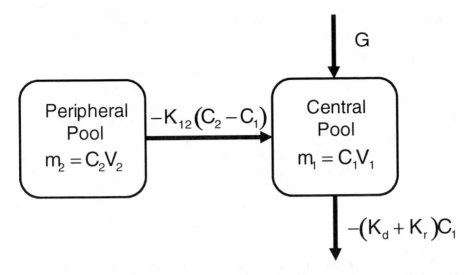

Fig. 13.3 Serial two-compartment model with accessible central (index 1) and directly inaccessible peripheral compartment (index 2). Abbreviations: dialyzer clearance K_d, residual renal clearance K_r, intercompartment clearance K_{12}, solute generation rate G, solute concentration C, distribution volume V

Notice that in this description which is applicable for both constant and variable volume models, K_d, K_r, and K_{12} refer to the sum of both diffusive and convective clearance. K_d, K_r, K_{12}, and G are usually assumed as constant. K_d and K_r can be measured, G can be calculated (estimated) from the increase in solute concentrations measured between dialysis treatments. K_{12} must be identified from experimental data or taken from literature. In this model solute transport from peripheral to central parts of the body is assumed to be controlled by diffusion only.

With $m=CV$ and assuming constant compartment volumes these two equations can be simplified to the following set of inhomogeneous ordinary differential equations with constant coefficients and which can be solved by standard mathematical methods (Gotch and Keen 2005).

$$\frac{dC_1}{dt} = -\left(\frac{K_d + K_r + K_{12}}{V_1}\right)C_1 + \left(\frac{K_{12}}{V_1}\right)C_2 + G \qquad (13.3)$$

$$\frac{dC_2}{dt} = \left(\frac{K_{12}}{V_2}\right)C_1 - \left(\frac{K_{12}}{V_2}\right)C_2 \qquad (13.4)$$

Removal of excess fluid volume by ultrafiltration during hemodialysis is in the range of 5% of total body water. Ultrafiltration importantly contributes to increased solute removal because of convective solute flux and it also increases the efficiency of dialysis as the ratio K/V increases as V decreases. Therefore, the effects of convective solute transport and changing distribution volumes must be accounted for in hemodialysis urea kinetic modeling. Still, exact analytical solutions can be obtained under the assumption of constant ultrafiltration rates and proportional fluid removal from both central and peripheral compartments (Grandi et al. 1995, Schneditz and Daugirdas 1994). The details are beyond the scope of the description in this chapter and the reader is referred to specialized literature.

The benefit of exact analytical solutions to various urea kinetic models is given by considerable simplification of subsequent calculations. For example, fitting the two-compartment urea kinetic model to experimental data for the purpose of identifying important model parameters such as K_{12} is considerably simplified if numerical techniques and iterative recalculations can be avoided.

As compartment volumes are interpreted as water volumes, and as the distribution volume plays an important role for prescription and control of dose of dialysis, the sum of both compartment volumes should be equal to the single-compartment volume.

When the serial two-compartment urea kinetic model is fitted to experimental data, the peripheral volume is about two times larger than the central volume ($V_2=2*V_1$), and the intercompartment urea clearance K_{12} is in the range of 0.8 L/min. Since total body water is distributed between extra- and intracellular compartments in a similar ratio, central and peripheral compartments have been interpreted as extra- and intracellular spaces, respectively, and the intercompartment clearance as measure for permeability of the cell membrane. While these interpretations must be questioned (Schneditz et al. 2009) because urea is known for its extremely high permeability across cell membranes due to special urea transporters (Brahm 1983; Duchesne et al. 2001; Smith 2009; Timmer et al. 2001; Wagner et al. 2002; Zhao et al. 2007), the serial two-compartment model is well suited to describe the time course of urea concentrations within and also between dialysis treatments.

Not only is the urea concentration measured at the end of dialysis lower than predicted for the equilibrated concentration because of compartment effects so that dose of dialysis is erroneously overestimated, the downward deviation of urea concentrations within dialysis also leads to a reduction of effective solute removal which is proportional to C_1 and not to the equilibrated concentration C_{eq}. This reduction can be accounted for by defining an effective clearance. The small compartment is more efficiently cleared while the large peripheral compartment considerably lags behind extracorporeal clearance.

13.2.1.2 Parallel Two-Compartment Model

Transport of solutes by diffusion is very efficient over short distances up to the range of millimeters, but for distances beyond that range efficient transport relies on convection such as blood flow through different organ systems – and through dialyzers (Dedrick and Bischoff 1968; Dedrick et al. 1968; Renkin 1955). The mass balance for an organ with defined in-and outflows is given as

$$\frac{dm_1}{dt} = Q_{in} C_{in} - Q_{out} C_{out} \tag{13.5}$$

where Q is blood flow and where subscripts in and out refer to in- and outflow, respectively (see Fig. 13.4). Volume in- and outflows are not identical in the variable volume models because of ultrafiltration Q_u so that with:

$$Q_{out} = Q_{in} - Q_u \tag{13.6}$$

$$\frac{dm_1}{dt} = Q_{in} \left(C_{in} - C_{out} \right) + Q_u C_{out} \tag{13.7}$$

With the familiar expression for (dialyzer) clearance:

$$K = Q_{in} \frac{C_{in} - C_{out}}{C_{in}} + Q_u \frac{C_{out}}{C_{in}} \tag{13.8}$$

and considering that removal of solute from the organ refers to an accumulation of solute in blood which requires a change in signs Eq. (13.5) can be rewritten as:

$$\frac{dm_1}{dt} = -K_1 C_{in} \tag{13.9}$$

In this equation K_1 is the organ clearance. Notice, that the inflow concentration C_{in} is different from the organ concentration C_1.

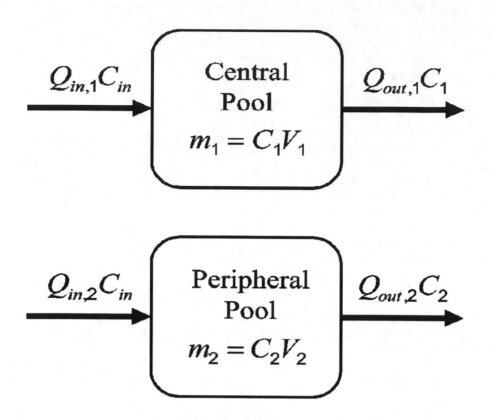

Fig. 13.4 Parallel two-compartment model where both compartments (index 1, 2) are accessible. Abbreviations: blood inflow Q_{in}, blood outflow Q_{out}, solute concentration in the inflow C_{in}, solute mass m, solute concentration C, and solute distribution volume V

As the cardiovascular system is organized in parallel loops (Fig. 13.4, Fig. 13.5) the inflow concentration to organ #2 is also given by C_{in} and the mass balance for that organ is therefore given as:

$$\frac{dm_2}{dt} = -K_2 C_{in} \qquad (13.10)$$

For a two-compartment system it is recognized that by combining Eq. (13.9) and Eq. (13.10):

$$dm_1 = \frac{K_1}{K_2} dm_2 \qquad (13.11)$$

And for the constant volume model:

$$dC_1 = \frac{K_1}{V_1} \frac{V_2}{K_2} dC_2 \qquad (13.12)$$

It thus follows from Eq. (13.12) that the two-compartment system reduces to the single compartment case when clearances and distribution volumes of both organ systems are equal ($K_1=K_2$, and $V_1=V_2$) or when efficiencies K/V are equal for each organ, such as providing a small clearance for the small organ and a large clearance for a large organ. In other words, when regional flows are scaled to distribution volumes, no compartment

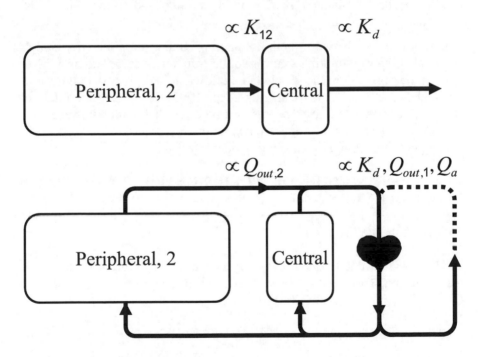

Fig. 13.5 Comparison of serial and parallel two-compartment models. Intercompartment transport varies with intercompartment clearance K_{12} in the serial model and with peripheral blood flow $Q_{out,2}$ in the parallel model. Extracorporeal clearance varies with dialyzer clearance K_d in the serial and with K_d, central blood flow $Q_{out,1}$, and access blood flow Q_a in the parallel two-compartment model

effect is expected. On the other hand, if specific blood flows Q/V and efficiencies or rates of removal are different between organs, a two-compartment effect is expected, as then $dC_1 \neq dC_2$ [Eq. (13.12)]. This is indeed the case for the large muscle skin and bone compartment with a small urea clearance and the small internal organ compartment with a high urea clearance.

The solution of a parallel two-compartment model requires expressing the inflow concentration C_{in} in Eq. (13.9) and Eq. (13.10) in terms of compartment concentrations C_1 and C_2. Then, the model can be rewritten as a system of inhomogeneous ODEs and solved (Schneditz and Daugirdas 1994). During hemodialysis, the inflow concentration C_{in} is perturbed because of extracorporeal solute removal which affects mixed venous blood concentration and, as a consequence, inflow concentration to the parallel organ systems. For a more detailed discussion the interested reader is referred to the specialized literature (Schneditz and Daugirdas 1994, Schneditz et al. 2009).

A comparison between both two-compartment urea kinetic models shows that the rate-limiting step for solute transfer is described as a diffusion-limited process in the serial, and as flow-limited process in the parallel model (see Fig. 13.5) (Schneditz et al. 1995). The algebraic relationships are more difficult to be expressed in the parallel model, however, the flow-limited transport is a more physiologic representation of solute exchange between compartments during hemodialysis.

13.3   ESTIMATION OF EQUILIBRATED POST-DIALYSIS BLOOD UREA CONCENTRATION

13.3.1 Standard Method

The standard equilibrated post-dialysis blood urea concentration is the measured urea from a blood sample taken at 30 or 60 min after the end of HD (Chirananthavat et al. 2006).

13.3.2 Smye Method

The measurement of equilibrated post-dialysis blood urea concentration requires a sample taken 30 min post- HD and this is often impractical in the conventional outpatient hemodialysis setting. In an attempt to overcome this practical problem, Smye et al. have suggested a third early intra-dialytic blood sample for urea (70 to 90 min from the beginning) that may be used to calculate equilibrated post-dialysis urea concentration (Smye et al. 1992). Smye et al. (1994) proposed that intradialytic blood sample should be obtained more than 60 min after dialysis (but at least 20 min before the end of dialysis. The Smye method of drawing the intradialytic and postdialysis blood samples was not specified in its original description. If these samples are both drawn at full blood flow rate, or after stopping the blood pump and not clearing the dead space in the arterial line, then the urea concentration in the samples will reflect the urea levels actually processed by the dialyzer (Pflederer et al. 1995). In the presence of access recirculation, the urea concentration of both the intradialytic and postdialysis urea samples drawn in this manner may be markedly lower that the urea level present in the arterial blood. The degree of reduction will be proportional for both as long as the dialyzer urea clearance and the degree of access recirculation are similar when the two samples are drawn (Pflederer et al. 1995). Another method of performing the Smye technique is to obtain the intradialytic and postdialysis samples 20 s after slowing the blood flow rate to 50 mL/min. When the pump is slowed to 50 mL/min, access recirculation ceases, and the dialyzer inlet blood reflects the arterial BUN concentration (when an A-V access is used) during dialysis. A third method is to obtain the intradialytic and post-dialysis samples two minutes after slowing the blood flow rate to 50 mL/min. After the pump is slowed or stopped, the dialyzer no longer returns cleared blood to the heart and the arteriovenous gradient largely dissipates within two minutes; in patients with an arteriovenous access, the mixed venous post-dialysis urea concentration can be estimated from a sample obtained from the dialyzer inlet line two minutes after having slowed the blood flow rate to 50 mL/min (Schneditz et al. 1992; Pflederer et al. 1995).

Indeed, the Smye model has proven accurate in the prediction of equilibrated urea (Pflederer et al. 1995; Garred et al. 1997). However, the requirements of this approach (a third blood sample and mathematical calculation) may limit its clinical application. The Smye method is based on the notion that compartment disequilibrium during dialysis produces a deviation from the expected monoexponential fall in the serum BUN, and the extent of this deviation can be used to predict the equilibrated post-dialysis BUN value. According to Smye, the equilibrated post-dialysis BUN (C_{eq}) is defined as:

$$C_{eqSmye} = C_o \exp\left[\frac{-t_d}{t_s} \ln \frac{C_s}{C_t}\right] \qquad (13.13)$$

where C_{eq} is the equilibrated post-dialysis BUN; C_o the pre-dialysis BUN; C_s is the mid-dialysis BUN concentration (usually obtained after 70 min of hemodialysis); C_t is the BUN concentration at the end of hemodialysis; t_d is the duration of hemodialysis; and t_s is the time at which C_s is drawn.

The resulting concentration C_{eq} is used to calculate the equilibrated dialysis dose $_{eq}(Kt/V)$. Small errors in the intradialytic sample result in larger errors in C_{eq} estimate (Smye et al. 1999), and wide limits of agreement with the kinetic $_{eq}(Kt/V)$ have been demonstrated with the application of this method (Maduell et al. 1997). In a small study using this formula to generate a calculated equilibrated Kt/V, the average error was only 13%, in comparison to a measured equilibrated value (Smye et al. 1994). Double-pool effects of urea removal can substantially reduce the accuracy of single-pool urea kinetic calculations. Thus, some patients whose dialysis dose is measured by the single pool model alone may be at risk for unappreciated under-delivery of hemodialysis. For this reason, the HD Adequacy Work Group encourages the use of equilibrated Kt/V measurements, especially in patients with high efficiency dialysis (Spiegel et al. 1995).

Other methods have been used to predict $_{eq}$BUN using intradialytic BUN sampling (Pflederer et al. 1995; Garred et al. 1997; Canaud et al. 1997, 2000; Bhaskaran et al. 1997; Jean et al. 1999). While these methods avoid blood sampling after HD without detaining the patient beyond the treatment time, the accuracy of these methods is influenced by the method and timing of taking the intradialytic blood sample (Pflederer et al. 1995; Daugirdas et al. 1996b). If severe vascular access recirculation is present, and if the blood sample is taken at full blood flow without slowing or stopping it to prevent sample dilution with recirculated blood, the intradialytic BUN will be artificially low and will result in significant overestimation of the true $_{eq}$BUN, and as a consequence a significant underestimation of the true Kt/V-value. Thus, it is necessary to pay careful attention to the method of intradialytic blood sampling. Furthermore, the accuracy was also affected by not taking a BUN sample after HD, and it was also reported that BUN measured 30 min before the end of HD was significantly lower than that measured 30 min after HD (Castro et al. 2001).

Another method for the prediction of $_{eq}$BUN, which uses BUN samples from the early part of the post-dialysis rebound, has also been reported. Goldstein and Brewer (2000) examined the time course of urea rebound and reported that a logarithmic curve generated from sampling the BUN value at 0.5 and 15 min post-HD might be used to determine a reliable estimate of $_{eq}$BUN at 50 min post-HD. Daugirdas et al (2004) found that the use of the blood drawn immediately or 20 s post-dialysis caused a lowering in the slope coefficient for rate of dialysis (K/V) from 0.6 to 0.39. As such, for the vigorous measurement, the equilibrated BUN should be used to yield the accurate $_{eq}(Kt/V)$.

Example 13.1

Calculate the equilibrated post-dialysis urea concentration using the Smye method if the pre-dialysis BUN is 105 mg/dL; intradialytic urea concentration after 120 min of hemodialysis is 57 mg/dL; post-dialysis urea concentration is 37 mg/dL The time of dialysis is 240 min.

Solution

The equilibrated post-dialysis urea concentration using the Smye method can be calculated as:

$$C_{eq} = C_o \times \exp\left[\frac{-t_d}{t_s} \ln \frac{C_s}{C_t}\right] = 105 \times \exp\left[\frac{-240}{120} \ln \frac{57}{37}\right] = 44.2 \text{ mg/dL}.$$

13.3.3 Soft Computing Methods

Different neural networks were applied to predict the equilibrated Urea (Guh et al. 1998; Fernandez et al. 2001), to provide equilibrated indexes (Goldfarb-Rumyantzev et al. 2003; Gabutti et al. 2004) or to estimate urea rebound (Azar et al. 2010, Azar and Wahba 2011). Artificial Neural Network (ANN) applications in dialysis are described in detail in chapter 22.

A novel hybrid system combining different soft computing paradigms such as neural networks and fuzzy systems has been developed by Azar (2011) for predictive modeling of dialysis variables in order to estimate the equilibrated dialysis dose ($_{eq}Kt/V$), without waiting for 30 to 60 min post-dialysis to obtain the equilibrated urea sample which is inconvenient for patients and costly to the dialysis unit. The results are highly promising, and a comparative analysis suggests that the proposed modeling approach outperforms other traditional urea kinetic models (UKM). The description of this hybrid system is described in detail in chapter 26.

13.4 ESTIMATION OF POST-DIALYSIS UREA REBOUND

13.4.1 Standard Method

The standard equilibrated post-dialysis blood urea concentration (True C_{eq}) using 30 min or 60 min post dialysis urea sample is used to calculate the true PDUR as the simple ratio (Alloatti et al. 1998):

$$PDUR = \frac{C_{eq} - C_t}{C_t} \times 100\% \qquad (13.14)$$

Where C_{eq} is the equilibrated post-dialysis BUN and C_t is the BUN concentration at the end of hemodialysis;

13.4.2 Smye Method

The calculated equilibrated post-dialysis BUN concentration (C_{eq}) using the Smye method [Eq. (13.13)] is used to calculate the $PDUR_{Smye}$ as follows:

$$PDUR_{Smye} = \frac{C_{eqSmye} - C_t}{C_t} \times 100\% \qquad (13.15)$$

Example 13.2

Using the same patient data as in Example 13.1, calculate the percentage of urea rebound using the Smye method.

Solution

Post-dialysis urea rebound using the Smye method is calculated as:

$$PDUR_{Smye} = \frac{C_{eqSmye} - C_t}{C_t} \times 100\% = \frac{44.2 - 37}{37} \times 100\% = 19.6\%$$

13.4.3 Rate Adjustment Method

The amount of urea rebound depends on the intensity or rate of dialysis delivered to the patient (Daugirdas et al. 2004; Spiegel et al. 1995; Leblanc et al. 1996). The rate of dialysis can be expressed as the number of Kt/V units per hour, or (Kt/V) divided by t in hours. A formula has been designed and validated that can predict the amount of rebound based on the rate of dialysis (Daugirdas et al. 2007). The so-called rate equation is based on a regional blood flow model and avoids the requirement of having to draw a post-dialysis BUN level 30–60 min after the completion of dialysis. PDUR can be calculated using the rate equation as follows (Daugirdas and Schneditz 1995):

For Arterial Access

$$PDUR = 0.6 \times \text{rate of dialysis} + 0.03 \qquad (13.16)$$

For Venous Access

$$PDUR = 0.47 \times \text{rate of dialysis} + 0.02 \qquad (13.17)$$

Example 13.3

Calculate the percentage of urea rebound using the rate equation if the delivered single pool Kt/V for a patient using arterial access is 1.312 and the dialysis time is 240 min.

Solution

Post-dialysis urea rebound using the rate equation method is calculated as:

$$PDUR = 0.6 \times \frac{_{sp}(Kt/V)}{t_{hours}} + 0.03 = \left(0.6 \times \frac{1.312}{4} \right) + 0.03 = 0.2268$$

Thus, the percentage of urea rebound is 22.7 %

13.5 ESTIMATION OF EQUILIBRATED DIALYSIS DOSE $_{eq}(Kt/V)$

The single pool Kt/V {$_{sp}(Kt/V)$} actually measures the dialyzer removal of urea, not the actual patient clearance of urea (Beige et al. 1999). As dialysis time is shortened and the intensity of dialysis increases, the error in the estimation of the delivered dose of dialysis increases, because the effects of urea equilibrium are accentuated (NKF-K/DOQI 2001; Jean et al. 1999; Leblanc et al. 1996). Urea disequilibrium may occur because of diffusion disequilibrium between body water compartments (membrane dependent), flow disequilibrium because of differences of blood flow in various tissues and organs, and disequilibrium caused by cardio-pulmonary recirculation of blood. The latter type of disequilibrium is only seen in patients undergoing arterio-venous hemodialysis and not those undergoing veno-venous (VV) HD (Sherman and Kapoian 1997). Membrane, flow, and recirculation disequilibrium errors are magnified as dialysis time is shortened and the intensity of the session increased (e.g., increasing Q_B) (NKF-K/DOQI 2001). For these reasons, a more accurate description of the delivered dose of dialysis has been developed that uses the equilibrated post-dialysis BUN and bypasses the necessity of keeping the patient in the dialysis unit for an hour to obtain the true equilibrated post-dialysis BUN sample. The error associated with the VVDP model was smaller than the single pool estimate because the close agreement between the results of the VVDP model and the rate equation estimate of equilibrated Kt/V, an alternative formulation of Kt/V based on kinetic models which adjust for the disequilibrium of urea during dialysis.

The magnitude of PDUR, measured as the percent increase in urea concentration from the end-HD to the equilibrated value, varies between 10 and 17% in standard HD sessions and 24% after high efficiency treatments, up to values of as much as 45% in some patients. Among the relatively few predictive factors for PDUR the efficiency of the session (high dialyzer K, or high K/V) influences directly the magnitude of urea rebound (Abramson et al. 1994). Also, short-time sessions (<3 h), HD sessions in small V patients, or complicated by hemodynamic instability are followed by greater rebound (Jean et al. 1998; Leblanc et al. 1996). A difference of about 0.2 between $_{sp}(Kt/V)$ and $_{eq}(Kt/V)$ was found in standard HD. This difference increases unpredictably in high efficiency treatments (Abramson et al. 1994). Several methods have been developed to calculate $_{eq}(Kt/V)$ and can be described in the following sections (Daugirdas et al. 1997).

13.5.1 Standard Method

The standard $_{eq}(Kt/V)$ is calculated by using the true equilibrated urea (C_{eq}) taken 30 or 60 min after the end of HD using the following equation (Daugirdas et al. 1999):

$$_{eq}(Kt/V) = \frac{_{sp}(Kt/V)}{\ln\left(\dfrac{C_o}{C_t}\right)} \ln\left(\frac{C_o}{True\ C_{eq}}\right) \tag{13.18}$$

Daugirdas et al (1999) estimated the relationship between single-pool and true double-pool urea distribution volume as follows:

$$V_{dp} = \frac{V_{sp}}{V_{sp}/V_{dp}} \tag{13.19}$$

Where V_{sp}/V_{dp} ratio is calculated as follows (Daugirdas et al. 1999):

$$\frac{V_{sp}}{V_{dp}} = \frac{\ln\left[F_{dp}\dfrac{C_o}{C_t}\right]}{F_{dp}\ln\left(\dfrac{C_o}{C_t}\right)}$$

(13.20)

where F_{dp} is the ratio of the post-dialysis to equilibrated urea nitrogen concentration (C_t/C_{eq}). Daugirdas et al (1999) demonstrated that "F_{dp} is related to dialysis efficiency and was found to be approximately 0.82 when dialysis was delivered at 0.4 single-pool Kt/V units/hr. Regardless of dialysis efficiency and the value for F_{dp}, the V_{sp}/V_{dp} ratio was found to approach unity at a URR of approximately 0.67, corresponding to a single-pool Kt/V value of approximately 1.3. When Kt/V is lower than this value, the analysis predicts that V_{sp} will be lower than V_{dp}. When Kt/V is greater than 1.3, the analysis predicts that V_{sp}/V_{dp} will be greater than unity".

Example 13.4

Calculate the double pool Kt/V using the standard method if the delivered single pool Kt/V is 1.23, pre-dialysis and post-dialysis urea concentrations are 143 mg/dL and 51 mg/dL respectively. The equilibrated urea concentration measured 30 min after HD 58 mg/dL.

Solution

The standard double pool Kt/V can be calculated as follows (Daugirdas et al. 1999):

$$_{eq}(Kt/V) = \frac{sp(Kt/V)}{\ln\left(\dfrac{C_o}{C_t}\right)}\ln\left(\frac{C_o}{True\ C_{eq}}\right) = \frac{1.23}{\ln\left(\dfrac{143}{51}\right)}\ln\left(\frac{143}{58}\right) = 1.076$$

Thus, the difference between single pool Kt/V and double pool Kt/V is:

$$\Delta Kt/V = 1.23 - 1.076 = 0.154$$

13.5.2 Smye Method

The $_{eq}(Kt/V)$ using Smye method is derived by applying the Daugirdas second generation formula (Daugirdas 1993) and replacing the ratio R by the following ratio (Smye et al. 1992, 1994):

Smye ratio for $_{eq}(Kt/V)_{Smye}$:

$$_{eq}R_{Smye} = \frac{C_{eqSmye}}{C_o} \qquad (13.21)$$

Where C_{eqSmye} is the equilibrated post-dialysis BUN calculated by Smye method [Eq. (13.13)] using the intradialytic blood sample for urea. Therefore:

$$_{eq}(Kt/V)_{Smye} = -\ln\left(_{eq}R_{Smye} - 0.008 \times t\right) + \left(4 - 3.5 \times {}_{eq}R_{Smye}\right) \times \frac{UF}{W} \qquad (13.22)$$

Example 13.5

Using the same data in example 13.1, calculate the double pool Kt/V using the Smye method. The post-dialysis weight is 63 kg and the ultrafiltration volume is 4 L.

Solution

Smye ratio for $_{eq}(Kt/V)_{Smye}$ is: $_{eq}R_{Smye} = \dfrac{44.2}{105} = 0.421$

The equilibrated Kt/V is calculated according to Smye method as follows:

$$_{eq}(Kt/V)_{Smye} = -\ln\left(0.421 - 0.008 \times 4\right) + \left(4 - 3.5 \times 0.421\right) \times \frac{4}{63} = 1.1$$

13.5.3 Original Tattersall Method

The equilibrated dialysis dose $_{eq}(Kt/V)$ can be calculated using the Tattersall method as follows (Tattersall et al. 1996b):

$$_{eq}(Kt/V)_{Tatt} = sp(Kt/V)\left[\frac{t}{t+B}\right] \qquad (13.23)$$

where t is the time of dialysis in minutes and B is Tattersall's time constant which is 35 min.

Example 13.6

In example 13.4, the standard $_{eq}(Kt/V)$ is calculated. Using the same delivrd single pool Kt/V value of 1.23 and the dialysis time of 240 min, calculate the double pool Kt/V using the Tattersall method and obtain the difference between the measured and calculated method.

Solution

The equilibrated Kt/V according to the Tattersall method is calculated as follows:

$$_{eq}(Kt/V)_{Tatt} = 1.23 \left[\frac{240}{240+35} \right] = 1.073$$

The difference between the standard method and the Tattersall method is 0.003 which is very small.

13.5.4 Maduell Method

Maduell et al (1997) stated that rebound urea was inversely correlated to urea distribution volume (V), not influenced by dialysis time and directly related to the dialysis efficiency. Through linear regression analysis he developed a formula to calculate Kt/V considering urea rebound according Kt/V, V and K as follows:.

$$_{eq}(Kt/V)_{Mad} = \left[0.906 \times {}_{sp}(Kt/V) \right] - \left[0.26 \times (K/V) \right] + 0.007 \quad (13.24)$$

Where K/V is the hourly Kt/V (rate of dialysis)

Example 13.7

Calculate the equilibrated Kt/V according to the Maduell formula using the same date in Example 13.4.

Solution

First, the rate of dialysis is calculated as:

$$\frac{K}{V} = \frac{Kt/V}{t} = \frac{1.23}{4} = 0.31 \, hr^{-1}$$

Then, the double pool Kt/V according to Maduell formula can be calculated as follows:

$$_{eq}(Kt/V)_{Mad} = [0.906 \times 1.23] - [0.26 \times 0.31] + 0.007 = 1.041$$

13.5.5 Original Rate Adjustment Method (Daugirdas-Schneditz Rate Equation)

The concept of using the rate of dialysis therapy to calculate $_{eq}(Kt/V)$ from $_{sp}(Kt/V)$ was first proposed by Daugirdas and Schneditz in 1995 (Daugirdas and Schneditz 1995; Daugirdas 1995). The mathematical relationship between the equilibrated and the single-pool Kt/V will vary depending upon the location of the angioaccess and the site from which the post-dialysis BUN sample is obtained. $_{sp}(Kt/V)$, calculated using an arterial post-dialysis BUN sample from an arteriovenous angioaccess ($_{art}Kt/V$), will be greater than that calculated from a mixed venous post-dialysis BUN, drawn through a venovenous angioaccess ($_{ven}Kt/V$). The equilibrated Kt/V ($_{eq}Kt/V$) can be compared with $_{sp}(Kt/V)$ by using the rate equation as follows (Daugirdas and Schneditz 1995):

$$_{eq}(Kt/V) = {}_{sp}(Kt/V) - \text{Rebound} \qquad (13.25)$$

The corresponding equilibrated Kt/V values are calculated by substituting the amount of urea rebound using Eq. (13.16) and Eq. (13.17) as follows:

For Arterial Access

$$_{eq}(Kt/V)_{rate.orig} = {}_{sp}(Kt/V) - \left(0.6 \times \frac{{}_{sp}(Kt/V)}{t} \right) + 0.03 \qquad (13.26)$$

For Venous Access

$$_{eq}(Kt/V)_{rate.orig} = {}_{sp}(Kt/V) - \left(0.47 \ ? \ \frac{{}_{sp}(Kt/V)}{t} \right) + 0.02 \qquad (13.27)$$

On average, the equilibrated Kt/V ($_{eq}Kt/V$) is 0.2 units smaller than the single-pool Kt/V, but as the discrepancy can be as much as 0.6 units (Daugirdas et al. 2004). Thus, a 4-hour treatment yielding a $_{sp}(Kt/V)$ of 1.3 is equivalent to a $_{eq}(Kt/V)$ of $1.3 - (0.6 \times 1.3/4) + 0.03$, or 1.14. The relationship between the single-pool and the $_{eq}(Kt/V)$ using either an arteriovenous or a venovenous access has been published as a nomogram by Daugirdas (1995) (see Fig. 13.6 and Fig. 13.7). For most patients, urea rebound is nearly complete 15 min after hemodialysis, but for a minority of patients, it may require up to 50 to 60 min. Therefore, the degree of rebound may be exaggerated in ESRD patients who are small-statured and during hemodialysis sessions that are complicated by intradialytic hypotension.

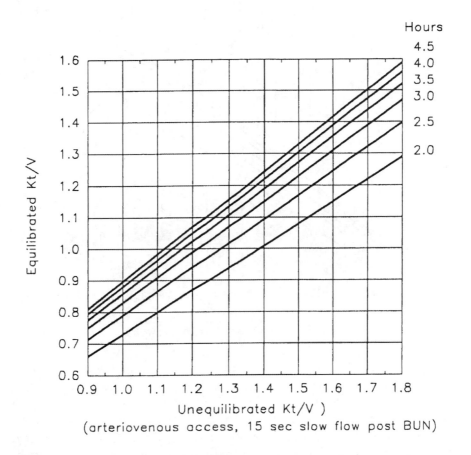

Fig. 13.6 Estimation of the $_{eq}(Kt/V)$ from the unequilibrated (single-pool) Kt/V for varying treatment times using an A-V access with the post-dialysis blood sample obtained from the arterial line 15 s after reducing the blood flow rate to about 50 mL/minute. [Adapted from Daugirdas JT (1995) Estimation of equilibrated Kt/V using the unequilibrated post dialysis BUN. Semin Dial.; 8(5): 283-284, with permission]

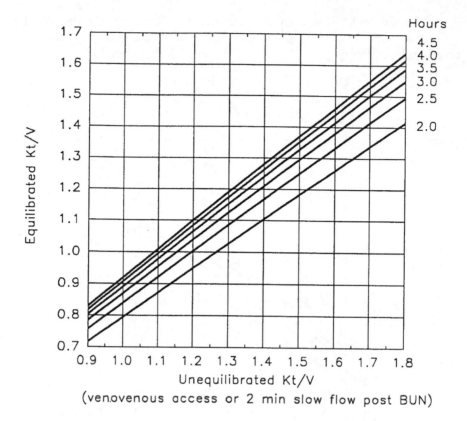

Fig. 13.7 Estimation of the $_{eq}(Kt/V)$ from the unequilibrated (single-pool) Kt/V for varying treatment times using a central vein access with the pos-dialysis blood sample obtained from the arterial line 15 s after reducing the blood flow rate Q_b to about 50 mL/minute. This nomogram can also be used for an A-V access when the post-dialysis blood sample is obtained from the arterial line 2 min after reducing Q_b to about 50 mL/min. [Adapted from Daugirdas JT (1995) Estimation of equilibrated Kt/V using the unequilibrated post dialysis BUN. Semin Dial.; 8(5): 283-284, with permission]

13.5.6 Modified Rate Equation: Results from the HEMO Study

Daugirdas et al (2004) developed a modified rate equation based on a large sample size of the HEMO trial to determine more precise values for coefficients in the prediction equations for rebound that might be appropri-ate for general application. They suggested that the rate of dialysis and the type of access are the prime determinants of the amount of post-dialysis urea rebound. The modified rate equations were evaluated first with

$_{sp}$(Kt/V) computed based on the pre-dialysis and the slow-flow post-dialysis BUN (denoted $_{sp}$(Kt/V)$_{20s}$) whether the analysis was based on the 20 s post-dialysis sample and again with $_{sp}$(Kt/V) computed from the pre-dialysis, and immediate full-flow post-dialysis BUN (denoted $_{sp}$(Kt/V)$_{0s}$) whether the analysis was based on the immediate 0-s post-dialysis sample. The modified rate equations are as follows:

With AV Access

▶ For single-pool Kt/V calculated based on 20 s post-dialysis samples:

$$_{eq}(Kt/V)_{rate.mod} = \,_{sp}(Kt/V) - \left(0.39 \times \frac{_{sp}(Kt/V)}{t} \right) \qquad (13.28)$$

▶ For single-pool Kt/V calculated based on immediate post-dialysis samples:

$$_{eq}(Kt/V)_{rate.mod} = \,_{sp}(Kt/V) - \left(0.46 \times \frac{_{sp}(Kt/V)}{t} \right) \qquad (13.29)$$

With venous Access

▶ For single-pool Kt/V calculated based on 20 s post-dialysis samples:

$$_{eq}(Kt/V)_{rate.mod} = \,_{sp}(Kt/V) - \left(0.22 \times \frac{_{sp}(Kt/V)}{t} \right) \qquad (13.30)$$

▶ For single-pool Kt/V calculated based on immediate post-dialysis samples:

$$_{eq}(Kt/V)_{rate.mod} = \,_{sp}(Kt/V) - \left(0.29 \times \frac{_{sp}(Kt/V)}{t} \right) \qquad (13.31)$$

According to the rate equations, substantial post-dialysis urea rebound can be anticipated when high-efficiency dialysis is delivered, particularly to a small patient, because then K/V will be high. The major advantage of the rate equation is that the $_{eq}$(Kt/V) can be predicted on the basis of a post-dialysis sample taken very soon after the end of dialysis avoiding the requirement of having to draw a post-dialysis BUN level 30–60 min after the completion of dialysis (Daugirdas et al. 2004).

13.5.7 Modified Tattersall Method Based on Modified Rate Equation

The estimate of time constant (B) in Tattersall's original description was 35 min (Tattersall et al. 1996b). In the study of Daugirdas et al (2004) data set, based on robust regression analyses, the modified Tattersall is as follows:

With AV Access

▸ For single-pool Kt/V calculated based on 20 s post-dialysis samples:

$$_{eq}(Kt/V)_{Tatt.mod} = sp(Kt/V) \times \left[\frac{t}{t+23.2}\right] \qquad (13.32)$$

▸ For single-pool Kt/V calculated based on immediate post-dialysis samples:

$$_{eq}(Kt/V)_{Tatt.mod} = sp(Kt/V) \times \left[\frac{t}{t+30.7}\right] \qquad (13.33)$$

With venous Access

▸ For single-pool Kt/V calculated based on 20 s post-dialysis samples:

$$_{eq}(Kt/V)_{Tatt.mod} = sp(Kt/V) \times \left[\frac{t}{t+13.9}\right] \qquad (13.34)$$

▸ For single-pool Kt/V calculated based on immediate post-dialysis samples:

$$_{eq}(Kt/V)_{Tatt.mod} = sp(Kt/V) \times \left[\frac{t}{t+18.5}\right] \qquad (13.35)$$

Example 13.8

Calculate the double pool Kt/V using the modified rate equation and the modified Tattersall equation if the delivered single pool Kt/V for a patient using venous access is 1.415 and the dialysis time is 210 min. The calculation of single pool Kt/V is based on 20 s post-dialysis sample technique.

Solution

The double pool Kt/V using the modified rate equation based on 20 s post-dialysis sample is calculated as:

$$_{eq}(Kt/V)_{rate.mod} = {_{sp}}(Kt/V) - \left(0.22 \times \frac{_{sp}(Kt/V)}{t} \right)$$

$$= 1.415 - \left(0.22 \times \frac{1.415}{3.5} \right) = 1.326$$

The double pool Kt/V using the modified Tattersall method is:

$$_{eq}(Kt/V)_{Tatt.mod} = sp(Kt/V) \times \left[\frac{t}{t+13.9} \right] = 1.415 \times \frac{210}{210+13.9} = 1.327$$

13.5.8 Leypoldt Formula

Leypoldt et al (2004) developed a new formula for estimating the equilibrated Kt/V based on empirical fitting of measured data. The Leypoldt equation has been shown to most closely predict actual rebound across a range of therapy rates and durations. The Leypoldt formula is as follows:

$$_{eq}(Kt/V) = \left(0.924 \times sp(Kt/V)\right) - \left(0.395 \times \frac{sp(Kt/V)}{t} \right) + 0.056 \quad (13.36)$$

Recognizing that some dialysis care teams may prefer to follow hemodialysis dosing using a double pool model for Kt/V, the HD Adequacy Work Group recommends that the minimum prescribed dose in a double pool model be considered to be 1.05 for patients dialyzing three times per week (NKF-K/DOQI 2001). Due to this variability of measuring Kt/V, DOQI guidelines recommended a target dose at least 15% higher than the listed minimum (1.4 for $_{sp}$(Kt/V) and 1.15 for $_{eq}$(Kt/V) (NKF-K/DOQI 2006).

13.6 REGIONAL BLOOD FLOW MODEL

The regional blood flow (RBF) model reported by Schneditz et al. in 1993 is alternative to the conventional double pool model, which can explain the solute rebound after hemodialysis (HD) (Schneditz et al. 1993, 1995; Schneditz and Daugirdas 1994). The basic concept is as follows. The distribution and clearance of a solute by the blood stream is related to the blood flow rate and diffusion through extravascular space. The clearance of highly diffusible solute such as urea is supposed to be flow limited rather than diffusion limited. Therefore the clearance of urea in the higher flow system is faster than that in lower flow system. In the RBF model, organ systems are divided into two groups according to a blood flow to water volume ratio. The organs that have a blood flow to water volume ratio of greater than 0.2/min are allocated to the high flow system and the other organ systems are allocated to the low flow system. The high flow system includes the kidneys, heart, brain, portal system, and lungs. The low flow system includes the muscles, bones, skin and fat. Based on physiologic data on organ perfusion and organ water content, organs allocated to the high flow system are supposed to contain 0.2 (volume fraction of high flow system: f_{VH}) (Schneditz et al. 1993, 1995; Schneditz and Daugirdas 1994) of total body water but to be perfused by 0.7 (flow fraction of high flow system: f_{QH}) (Schneditz et al. 1993) of the systemic blood flow. The high and low flow systems are perfused by parallel loops of the systemic circulation (see Fig. 13.8). Originally, f_{QH} was assumed as 0.7 based on the physiological data in reference 1. In the following reports f_{QH} was assumed as 0.8 (Schneditz and Daugirdas 1994) or as 0.85 (Schneditz et al.

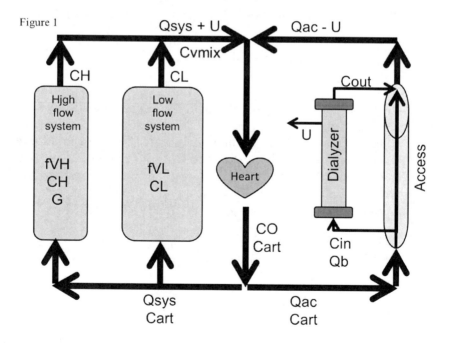

Fig. 13.8 A regional blood flow model with an arteriovenous fistula

1995). Which values is most appropriate for f_{QH} will be discussed later. In the RBF model, cardiac output (CO) is used for systemic blood flow (Q_{sys}) and access blood flow (Q_{ac}). The blood flow in high flow system is Q_{sys} multiplied by f_{QH} and that in low flow system is Q_{sys} multiplied by f_{QL}.

In the RBF model, solute in the high flow system is considered to be cleared faster than from the low flow system during a hemodialysis session. It will be simulated below. The disequilibrium of solutes between high and low flow systems is created during hemodialysis and causes the solute rebound after treatment.

According to Schneditz et al., blood flow distribution in hemodialysis patients is different from normal physiologic blood flow because renal blood flow is reduced or completely abolished due to end stage kidney disease. On the other hand, additional blood flow due to artificial arteriovenous fistula produces other regional blood flow and compensates for reduced renal blood flow in most cases.

13.6.1 Urea Kinetics in Variable Volume Regional Flow Model

Urea kinetic model, taking into account ultrafiltration and urea generation during a hemodialysis session will be explained in this section. In this model, the ratio of water volume of high flow system to that of low flow is assumed not to change during hemodialysis. Therefore, it is assumed that f_{QH} and f_{VH} are constant values during a hemodialysis session and the subsequent rebound phase as same as previous reports (Schneditz and Daugirdas 1994; Schneditz et al. 1995; Yamada et al. 2000). Total water volume (V) and water volume of each flow system (V_H, V_L) is expressed as follows.

$$V = V_0 - U \cdot t \tag{13.37}$$

$$V_H = (V_0 - U \cdot t) \cdot f_{VH} \tag{13.38}$$

$$V_L = (V_0 - U \cdot t) \cdot f_{VL} \tag{13.39}$$

where U refers to ultrafiltration rate. The urea generation is assumed to be restricted to the high flow system which includes the liver (Pedrini et al. 1988). The mass balance of urea in high flow system is expressed as follows:

$$\frac{d(V_H \cdot C_H)}{dt} = C_{art} \cdot Q_H - C_H \cdot (Q_H + U \cdot f_{VH}) + G \tag{13.40}$$

$$\frac{V_H \cdot dC_H}{dt} + \frac{C_H \cdot dV_H}{dt} = C_{art} \cdot Q_H - C_H \cdot (Q_H + U \cdot f_{VH}) + G \quad (13.41)$$

$$\frac{dV_H}{dt} = -U \cdot f_{VH} \quad (13.42)$$

Eq. (13.41) and Eq. (13.42) were combined and solved for dC_H/dt in Eq. (13.43)

$$\frac{dC_H}{dt} = \frac{1}{V_H} \cdot \left[Q_H \cdot (C_{art} - C_H) + G \right] \quad (13.43)$$

The mass balance of urea in low flow system is expressed as follows:

$$\frac{d(V_L \cdot C_L)}{dt} = C_{art} \cdot Q_L - C_L \cdot (Q_L + U \cdot f_{VL}) \quad (13.44)$$

$$\frac{V_L \cdot dC_L}{dt} + \frac{C_L \cdot dV_L}{dt} = C_{art} \cdot Q_L - C_L \cdot (Q_L + U \cdot f_{VL}) \quad (13.45)$$

$$\frac{dV_L}{dt} = -U \cdot f_{VL} \quad (13.46)$$

Eqs. (13.45) and (13.46) were combined and solved for dCL/dt in Eq. (13.47).

$$\frac{dC_L}{dt} = \frac{1}{V_L} \cdot \left[Q_L \cdot (C_{art} - C_L) \right] \quad (13.47)$$

When a central venous access is used, the blood entering the vascular access has the same composition as the mixed blood leaving the systemic tissue compartment. However, this assumption is not correct, when standard peripheral arteriovenous fistula is used as vascular access. The central venous flow and the blood flow from the peripheral access compose arterial blood flow. The composition of the blood entering the access during hemodialysis is same as that of arterial blood flow. As expected from Fig. 13.9, there are the following relation between Cart and C_{vmix}.

$$C_{art} \cdot (Q_{sys} + Q_{ac}) = C_{vmix} \cdot (Q_{sys} + U) + C_{art} \cdot (Q_{ac} - Q_b) + C_{out} \cdot (Q_b - U)$$
$$(13.48)$$

Urea clearance of a dialyzer is expressed as follows:

$$C_{in} \cdot K_d = C_{in} \cdot Q_b - C_{out} \cdot (Q_b - U) \quad (13.49)$$

When access recirculation can be ignored, C_{in} equals C_{art}.

Eq. (13.48) and Eq. (13.49) are combined to cancel C_{out} and solved for C_{art}.

$$C_{art} = C_{vmix} \cdot \left[\frac{Q_{sys} + U}{Q_{sys} + K_d} \right] \tag{13.50}$$

A term of a factor for cardiopulmonary recirculation in variable volume RBF model is defined.

$$f_{cp} = \left[\frac{Q_{sys} + U}{Q_{sys} + K_d} \right] \tag{13.51}$$

$$C_{art} = f_{cp} \cdot C_{vmix} \tag{13.52}$$

As U is inevitably lower than K_d, f_{cp} is less than 1. Therefore Cart is always lower than C_{vmix}. Because central venous blood stream is composed of blood flow from low and high flow system which include additional ultrafiltration rate, C_{vmix} is expressed as follows:

$$C_{vmix} = \frac{C_H \cdot (Q_H + Uf_{VH}) + C_L \cdot (Q_L + Uf_{VL})}{Q_{sys} + U} \tag{13.53}$$

Substitution C_{vmix} from Eq. (13.53) into Eq. (13.52)

$$C_{art} = f_{cp} \cdot \frac{C_H \cdot (Q_H + U \cdot f_{VH}) + C_L \cdot (Q_L + U \cdot f_{VL})}{Q_{sys} + U} \tag{13.54}$$

$$Q_H = Q_{sys} \cdot f_{QH} \tag{13.55}$$

$$Q_L = Q_{sys} \cdot f_{QL} \tag{13.56}$$

Substitution Q_H and Q_L from Eq. (13.55) and (13. 56) into Eq. (13.54)

$$C_{art} = f_{cp} \cdot \frac{C_H \cdot \left(Q_{sys} \cdot f_{QH} + U \cdot f_{VH} \right) + C_L \left(Q_{sys} \cdot f_{QL} + U \cdot f_{VL} \right)}{Q_{sys} + U} \tag{13.57}$$

Finally, the variable volume regional blood flow model is expressed following set of equations.

$$V_H = (V_o - U \cdot t) \cdot f_{VH} \qquad (13.38)$$

$$V_L = (V_o - U \cdot t) \cdot f_{VL} \qquad (13.39)$$

$$\frac{dC_H}{dt} = \frac{1}{V_H} \cdot \left[Q_H \cdot (C_{art} - C_H) + G \right] \qquad (13.43)$$

$$\frac{dC_L}{dt} = \frac{1}{V_L} \cdot \left[Q_L \cdot (C_{art} - C_L) \right] \qquad (13.47)$$

$$f_{cp} = \left[\frac{Q_{sys} + U}{Q_{sys} + K_d} \right] \qquad (13.51)$$

$$C_{art} = f_{cp} \cdot \frac{C_H \cdot (Q_{sys} \cdot f_{QH} + U \cdot f_{VH}) + C_L \cdot (Q_{sys} \cdot f_{QL} + U \cdot f_{VL})}{Q_{sys} + U} \qquad (13.57)$$

The time courses of C_{art}, C_H and C_L can be computed by numerical integration using the Runge-Kutta-Gill method. An example of macro in Excel for simulation is shown in APPENDIX C.

13.6.2 Simulation of Urea Concentration in a Dialysis Session and Post-Dialysis Rebound with Regional Blood Flow Model

For simulation, a patient with 60 kg of post-dialysis dry weight is assumed as a model case. The patient's initial total body water is 58% of dry weight plus 3L of total filtration volume ($V_0 = 60 \times 0.58 + 3$). Other parameters are $Q_{sys} = 5.5$ (L/min), UFR = 3/240 (L/min), $Q_b = 0.25$ (L/min), E = 0.2 and G = 0.224 (mmol/min) were assumed. The protein catabolic rate (PCR) corresponding to this G in the equilibrium state is about 70 g/day. The time course of urea in a dialysis session and post-dialysis rebound phase of this model patient is show in Fig. 13.9. Because there is a report (Yashiro et al. 2004) that agreement between simulation of urea rebound and real values was significantly improved by substituting 0.85 as f_{QH}, this value is adopted in this simulation.

Figure 2

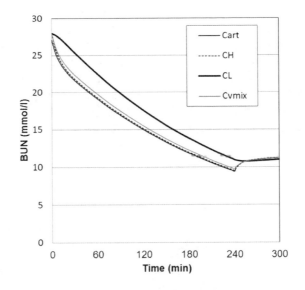

Fig. 13.9 The time course of urea in a dialysis session and post-dialysis rebound phase of a model patient

As shown in Fig. 13.9, C_{vmix} is close to C_H, because the major portion of blood flow in central vein system streams from high flow system. C_{art} is slightly lower than C_{vmix} due to cardiopulmonary recirculation. The difference in urea concentration between high and low flow systems at the end of a dialysis session causes post dialysis urea rebound.

In the rebound phase after the dialysis session, as the effect of cardiopulmonary recirculation disappears within 2 min (Schneditz et al. 1992b), f_{cp} can be assumed to equal 1 immediately after the dialysis session in simulation. It is also assumed that V_H and V_L were constant during the rebound phase. Therefore, the sharp increase in the arterial urea concentration will occur due to prompt disappearance of cardiopulmonary recirculation followed by gradual increase due to equilibrium between high and low flow systems.

13.6.3 Sensitivity of Post Dialysis Urea Rebound on Model Parameters

The effects of the fluctuation of f_{QH}, f_{VH}, and Q_{sys} on C_{art} in this model patient during 240 min of a dialysis session and 60 min of a following rebound phase are also indicated (see Fig. 13.10). The increase in f_{QH} and the decrease in f_{VH} and Q_{sys} caused the increase in C_{reb}, without significant impact on C_{end}. These results ascertained that RBF model can explain the tendency of increased post-dialysis urea rebound in the case of heart failure (George et al. 1996), whose Q_{sys} was thought to be suppressed.

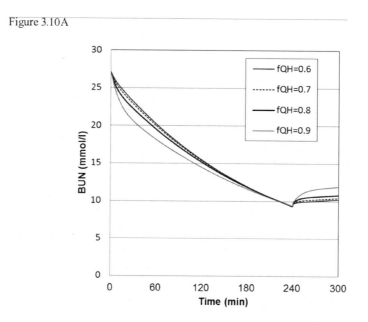

Fig. 13.10 The changes in the time course of urea nitrogen in arterial blood during the dialysis session and the rebound phase, accompanying the use of various values for flow fraction in high-flow system (f_{QH}) (A), volume fraction in high-flow fraction (f_{VH}) (B) and systemic blood flow (Q_{sys}) (C)

Figure 3.10B

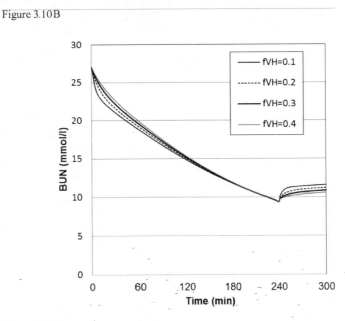

Figure 3.10C

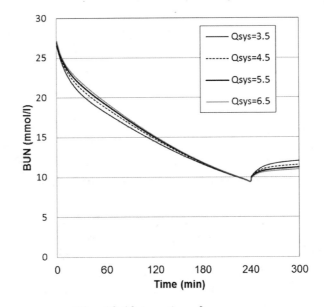

Fig. 13.10 (*continued*)

Kt/V with the following equation is also indicated in Fig. 13.11.

$$\frac{Kt}{V} = -\ln\left(R - 0.008 \times t\right) + \left(4 - 3.5 \times R\right) \times \frac{UF}{W} \qquad (13.58)$$

where R is C_{end}/C_0 or C_{reb}/C_0 and T is treatment time. Kt/V is called $_{sp}(Kt/V)$, when R is C_{end}/C_0 and $_{eq}(Kt/V)$, when R is C_{reb}/C_0 in this chapter.

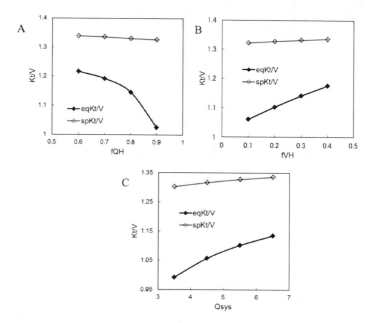

Fig. 13.11 The changes in $_{sp}(Kt/V)$ and $_{eq}(Kt/V)$ accompanying the use of various values for flow fraction in high-flow system (f_{QH}) (A), volume fraction in high-flow system (f_{VH}) (B) and systemic blood flow (Q_{sys}) (C).

The fluctuation of f_{QH}, f_{VH} and Q_{sys} doesn't significantly affect $_{sp}(Kt/V)$. However, $_{eq}(Kt/V)$ is significantly affected by these parameters fluctuations. The increase in f_{QH} and the decrease in f_{VH} and Q_{sys} causes a significant increase in C_{reb}, therefore significant reduction in Kt/V. The phenomenon that exercise in the late phase of a hemodialysis session increases urea clearance (Smye el al. 1998) may be explained by the increase in f_{VH}. Because skin and muscle which are included in low flow system at rest join the high flow system during exercise, f_{VH} increases. Since an increase in f_{VH} suppresses the urea rebound, in the removal of urea is increased. The advantage of the RBF model is that hemodynamics are physiologically linked to urea rebound.

13.6.4   Approach for Access Recirculation

The effect of access recirculation was not included in the above discussion. When significant amounts of access recirculation are present, C_{art} can't be assumed to equal C_{in}. In this situation, the following equations are valid as shown in Fig. 13.12.

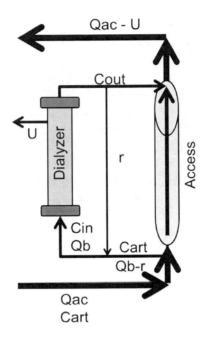

Fig. 13.12 An access blood flow and a recirculation flow

$$C_{art} \cdot K_d' = r \cdot C_{out} + C_{art} \cdot (Q_b - r) - C_{out} \cdot (Q_b - U) \quad (13.59)$$

$$C_{in} \cdot Q_b = C_{art} \cdot (Q_b - r) + r \cdot C_{out} \quad (13.60)$$

$$R_{ac} = \frac{r}{Q_b} \quad (13.61)$$

where K_d' is effective urea clearance taking access recirculation into consideration. Eq. (13.59), Eq. (13.60), Eq. (13.61) and Eq. (13.49) are combined and solved for K_d'.

$$K_d' = \frac{K_d \cdot (1 - R_{ac})}{\left[(1 - R_{ac}) \cdot \left(\dfrac{Q_b - K_d}{Q_b - U}\right)\right]} \tag{13.62}$$

When access recirculation can't be ignored, K_d' is substituted for K_d in simultaneous Eq. (13.43), (13.47), (13.51) and (13.57).

13.6.5 Estimation of Post Dialysis Urea Rebound with RBF Model in the Actual Patients

Having obtained informed consent, eight dialysis patients, dialyzed trice weekly, with negligible residual renal function were studied. Each patient had an ordinary arteriovenous fistula. The length of each dialysis session was 240 min. Blood samples were drawn before and end of a treatment. At the end of treatment, sampling from the arterial blood line was done without reduction of blood flow. To obtain urea rebound after hemodialysis, samples were drawn at 60 min after the end of dialysis (Pedrini et al. 1988). Blood samples were also drawn from the dialyzer venous line for the calculation of solute clearance (K_d; L/min). Total urea distribution volume at the start of dialysis session (V_0) was supposed to be 58% of post-dialysis body weight plus total filtration volume   (UFV). Urea generation rate was calculated as follows:

$$G = \frac{C_{0n} \cdot (0.58 \cdot BW + \Delta V) - C_{reb} \cdot (0.58 \cdot BW)}{\Delta t} \tag{13.63}$$

where C_{0n} is urea concentration at the start of next dialysis session, ΔV is water accumulation and Δt is period during two consecutive dialysis session. Q_{sys} was supposed to equal cardiac output (CO) minus 0.5 (L/min), as average access flow is assumed to be 0.5 L/min based on previous reports (Malovrh 1998). CO was approximated from the ultrasonic cardiogram according to the method of Teichholz (Teichholz et al. 1976). In Fig. 13.13, the curved lines indicate the simulation of post dialysis urea rebound by RBF model in the eight actual patients and the crosses indicate the actual rebound values at 60 min after the end of the session. Concentrations are expressed in the percentage of C_{end}. Ratio of estimated urea concentrations at the end of dialysis session to the real values were 99.9±4.5% and those at 60 min after dialysis session were 98.5±2.7%. These estimations can be improved by estimation of V_0 (Yashiro et al. 2004).

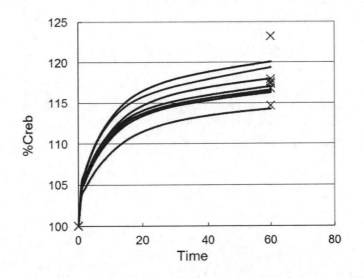

Fig. 13.13 The curved lines indicate the simulation of post dialysis urea rebound by the RBF model in the eight actual patients and the crosses indicate the actual rebound values at 60 min after the end of the treatment session. Concentrations are expressed in the percentage of C_{end}.

Example 13.9

Calculate urea concentration at the end of 240 min of dialysis and at 60 min after the treatment by variable volume RBF model with Runge-Kutta-Gill method if the pre-dialysis BUN is 105 mg/dl (37.5 mmol/L). The example of a macro for excel is shown in appendix.

For calculation, assume a patient with 60 kg of post-dialysis dry weight. The patient's initial total body water is 58% of dry weight plus 3L of total filtration volume ($V_0 = 60 \times 0.58 + 3$). Other parameters are $Q_{sys} = 5.5$ (L/min), U = 3/240 (L/min), $Q_b = 0.25$ (L/min), E = 0.2 and G = 0.224 (mmol/min). The protein catabolic rate (PCR) corresponding to this G in the equilibrium state is about 70 g/day. f_{QH} is 0.85 and f_{VH} is 0.2.

Solution

According to Eq. (13.35):

$$C_{in} \cdot K_d = C_{in} \cdot Q_b - C_{out} \cdot (Q_b - U)$$

Therefore,

$$K_d = Q_b - E \cdot (Q_b - U) = 0.25 - 0.2 \cdot (0.25 - 0.0125) = 0.2025$$

According to Eq. (13.37):

$$f_{cp} = \left[\frac{Q_{sys} + U}{Q_{sys} + K_d} \right] = 0.967$$

Thus,

At the end of dialysis session:

BUN = 34.5 mg/dL (12.3 mmol/L).

At 60 min after treatment (post-dialysis rebound):

BUN = 40.8 mg/dL (14.6 mmol/L)

13.7 CONCLUSION

In the conventional double pool model, the degree of the compartment effect is mainly determined by the intercompartmental mass transfer coefficient. In the RBF model, the compartment effect is dependent on variable hemodynamics. This variation depends on the variable perfusion of the low flow system, such as the vascular beds of the skin and the locomotors system. The flow of these organs is affected widely by the demands of perfusion of the important organs. The RBF model offers a hemodynamic explanation for the variability of the two pool effect and establishes a previously missing link between hemodynamics, solute removal, and efficiency of HD.

13.8 APPENDIX A

A-1 CALCULATION OF Kt/V WITH MATLAB

Program to get the Kt/V by Daugirda's formula-1995 using the Lowrie's method to calculate the monocompartimental one:

```
% Program to calculate the Kt/V by Daugirdas-1995
% using the monocompartimental Kt/V of Lowrie-1983
% Daugirdas-95: Kt/V = spKt/V - 0.6 x K/V + 0.03

home;
clear all;
clc;

%%%%%%%%% Data input %%%%%%%%%%

Cpre = input('Urea pre = ');
Cpost = input('Urea post = ');
K = input('K = ');
ts = input('Session time (in min) = ');
V = input('Volume = ');

%%%%%%%%% Calculations %%%%%%%%%%

spKtV = log (Cpre) - log (Cpost);
% Kt/V_daug95 = spKt/V - (0.6 x spKt/V / t) + 0.03. t en min
KTV = spKtV - (0.6 * spKtV / (ts/60)) + 0.03;


%%%%%%%%% Showing the results %%%%%%%%%%
disp(spKtV);
disp('The Kt/V calculated by Daugirdas-1995 is: ');
disp(KTV);

%%%%%%%%% FIN %%%%%%%%%%
```

A-2 Program to get the Kt/V by the Daugirdas formula of 1995 using the Daugirdas method to calculate the single pool Kt/V:

```
% Program to calculate the Kt/V by Daugirdas' formula of 1995
% using the 93 one to calcúlate the monocompartimental one
% Daugirdas-95: Kt/V = spKt/V - 0.6 x K/V + 0.03

home;
clear all;
clc;

%%%%%%%% Data input %%%%%%%%

Cpre = input('Urea pre = ');
Cpost = input('Urea post = ');
K = input('K = ');
ts = input('Session time (in min) ts = ');
V = input('Volume V = ');
UF = input('UF = ');
W = input('Post HD weight (Kg) = ');

%%%%%%%% Calculations %%%%%%%%

% Daugirdas-93 (7)  Kt/V = -ln (R - 0.008T) +(4 - 3.5R) x UF/W

R = Cpost / Cpre;
KTV93 = - log (R - 0.008 * (ts/60)) + (4 - 3.5 * R) * UF/W;

% Daugirdas-95: Kt/V = spKt/V - 0.6 x K/V + 0.03

KTV = KTV93 - 0.6 * KTV93 / (ts/60) + 0.03;

%%%%%%%% Showing results %%%%%%%%

disp('The Kt/V calculated by Daugirdas-1995 is: ');
disp(KTV);

%%%%%%%% FIN %%%%%%%%
```

APPENDIX B ABBREVIATIONS

BW (kg)	Body weight at the end of dialysis.
CO (L/min)	Cardiac output
CH (mmol/L)	Concentration of urea nitrogen in high flow system
CL (mmol/L)	Concentration of urea nitrogen in low flow system
Cart (mmol/L)	Concentration of urea nitrogen in arterial blood
Cvmix (mmol/L)	Concentration of urea nitrogen in mixed venous blood
C0 (mmol/L	Cart at the Start of dialysis
Cend (mmol/L)	Cart at the End of dialysis
Creb (mmol/L)	Cart at 60min After dialysis
C0n (mmol/L)	Cart at the Start of the next dialysis session
Cin (mmol/L)	Concentration of urea nitrogen In dialyzer arterial line
Cout (mmol/L)	Concentration of urea nitrogen in dialyzer venous line
E	Cout/Cin
fcp	A factor for cardiopulmonary recirculation
fQH	flow fraction of high flow system
fQL	flow fraction of low flow system, (1-Fqh)
fVH	Volume fraction of high flow system
fVL	Volume fraction of low flow system, (1-Fvh)
G (mmol/min)	Urea generation rate
Kd (L/min)	Urea clearance of a dialyzer
Kd'(L/min)	Modified urea Clearance of dialyzer taking access recirculation into consideration
spKt/V	Single pool Kt/V
eqKt/V	Equilibrated Kt/V
QH (L/min)	blood flow of high flow system
QL (L/min)	blood flow of low flow system
Qsys (L/min)	systemic blood flow
Qb (L/min)	dialyzer blood flow
Qac (L/min)	Access blood flow
r (L/min)	Recirculation blood flow
Rac	Access recirculation ratio
t (min)	Time from start of a dialysis session
Δt (min)	Time during two consecutive dialysis session minus 60 min
T (hr)	Treatment time

U (L/min)	Ultrafiltration rate
UFV (L)	Total ultrafiltration volume
V0	Total urea distribution volume at the start of a dialysis session
VH (L)	Urea distribution volume of high flow system
VL (L)	Urea distribution volume of low flow system
ΔV (L)	Body weight (volume) gain during Δt

APPENDIX C

Macro

```
Option Explicit

Public dc!(5), c#(5), c0!(5), tt!(10000), cc!(10000, 3)

Public nd, nn, dt, tl

Public Qsys, Qb, E, F, fQH, fVH, fQL, fVL, G, VH0, VL0, t
```

```
Public Sub MainRoutine()

    Datain

    nn = Int(tl / dt) + 2

    Runge

    Results

    DatainReb

    nn = Int(tl / dt) + 2

    Runge

    ResultsReb

End Sub
```

```
Public Sub Datain()

    Sheets("Sheet1").Select

    Qsys = Cells(12, 2)

    E = Cells(13, 2)

    F = Cells(14, 2)

    Qb = Cells(15, 2)

    G = Cells(16, 2)

    fQH = Cells(6, 2)
```

```
       fQL = Cells(7, 2)
       fVH = Cells(8, 2)
       fVL = Cells(9, 2)
       c0(1) = Cells(21, 2)
       c0(2) = Cells(18, 2)
       c0(3) = Cells(19, 2)
       tl = Cells(22, 2)
       nd = Cells(23, 2)
       dt = Cells(24, 2)
       VH0 = Cells(10, 2)
       VL0 = Cells(11, 2)
   End Sub
```

```
Public Sub Runge()
Dim i1%, j1%, t!, k#(3), r#(3), q#(3), sq
   sq = 0.7071068
   t = 0
   For i1 = 1 To nd
      q(i1) = 0
      c(i1) = c0(i1)
   Next i1
   For j1 = 1 To nn
      tt(j1) = t
      For i1 = 1 To nd
         cc(j1, i1) = c(i1)
      Next i1
      Derivative
      For i1 = 1 To nd
         k(i1) = dt * dc(i1)
         r(i1) = (k(i1) - 2 * q(i1)) / 2
         c(i1) = c(i1) + r(i1)
```

```
        q(i1) = q(i1) + 3 * r(i1) - k(i1) / 2
     Next i1
     Derivative
     For i1 = 1 To nd
        k(i1) = dt * dc(i1)
        r(i1) = (1 - sq) * (k(i1) - q(i1))
        c(i1) = c(i1) + r(i1)
        q(i1) = q(i1) + 3 * r(i1) - (1 - sq) * k(i1)
     Next i1
     Derivative
     For i1 = 1 To nd
        k(i1) = dt * dc(i1)
        r(i1) = (1 + sq) * (k(i1) - q(i1))
        c(i1) = c(i1) + r(i1)
        q(i1) = q(i1) + 3 * r(i1) - (1 + sq) * k(i1)
     Next i1
     Derivative
     For i1 = 1 To nd
        k(i1) = dt * dc(i1)
        r(i1) = (k(i1) - 2 * q(i1)) / 6
        c(i1) = c(i1) + r(i1)
        q(i1) = q(i1) + 3 * r(i1) - k(i1) / 2
     Next i1
     t = t + dt
  Next j1
End Sub
```

```
Public Sub Derivative()
    dc(1) = (1 / (Qsys + (1 - E) * Qb + E * F)) * (((Qsys * fQH + F * fVH) /
(VH0 - F * fVH * t)) * ((c(1) - c(2)) * Qsys * fQH + G) + ((Qsys * fQL + F *
fVL) / (VL0 - F * fVL * t)) * ((c(1) - c(3)) * Qsys * fQL))
```

```
dc(2) = (1 / (VH0 - F * fVH * t)) * ((c(1) - c(2)) * Qsys * fQH + G)
dc(3) = (1 / (VL0 - F * fVL * t)) * ((c(1) - c(3)) * Qsys * fQL)
End Sub
```

```
Public Sub Results()
Dim i
Sheets("Sheet1").Select
Range("e4:g52").ClearContents
For i = 1 To 49
Cells(3 + i, 5) = cc(1 + 50 * (i - 1), 1)
Cells(3 + i, 6) = cc(1 + 50 * (i - 1), 2)
Cells(3 + i, 7) = cc(1 + 50 * (i - 1), 3)
Next i
End Sub
```

```
Public Sub DatainReb()
Sheets("Sheet1").Select
    Qsys = Cells(34, 2)
    E = Cells(35, 2)
    F = Cells(36, 2)
    Qb = Cells(37, 2)
    G = Cells(38, 2)
    fQH = Cells(28, 2)
    fQL = Cells(29, 2)
    fVH = Cells(30, 2)
    fVL = Cells(31, 2)
    c0(1) = Cells(43, 2)
    c0(2) = Cells(40, 2)
    c0(3) = Cells(41, 2)
    tl = Cells(44, 2)
    nd = Cells(45, 2)
```

```
    dt = Cells(46, 2)
    VH0 = Cells(32, 2)
    VL0 = Cells(33, 2)
End Sub
```

```
Public Sub ResultsReb()
Dim i
Sheets("Sheet1").Select
Range("e53:g112").ClearContents
For i = 2 To 61
Cells(51 + i, 5) = cc(1 + 50 * (i - 1), 1)
Cells(51 + i, 6) = cc(1 + 50 * (i - 1), 2)
Cells(51 + i, 7) = cc(1 + 50 * (i - 1), 3)
Next i
End Sub
```

REEFERNCES

Abramson, F., Gibson, S., Barlee, V., Bosch, J.P.: Urea kinetic modeling at high urea clearances: Implications for clinical practice. Adv. Ren. Replace Ther. 1(1), 5–14 (1994)

Alloatti, S., Molino, A., Manes, M., Bosticardo, G.M.: Urea rebound and effectively delivered dialysis dose. Nephrol. Dial. Transplant. 13(6), 25–30 (1998)

Azar, A.T.: Adaptive Neuro Fuzzy system as a novel approach for predicting post-dialysis urea rebound. International Journal of Intelligent Systems Technologies and Applications (IJISTA) 10(3), 302–330 (2011)

Azar, A.T., Wahba, K.M.: Artificial Neural Network for Prediction of Equilibrated Dialysis Dose without Intradialytic Sample. Saudi J. Kidney Dis. Transpl. 22(4), 705–711 (2011)

Azar, A.T., Balas, V.E., Olariu, T.: Artificial Neural Network for Accurate Prediction of Post-Dialysis Urea Rebound (2010), doi:10.1109/SOFA.2010.5565606

Beige, J., Sharma, A.M., Distler, A., et al.: Monitoring dialysis efficacy by comparing delivered and predicted Kt/V. Nephrol. Dial. Transplant. 14(3), 683–687 (1999)

Bhaskaran, S., Tobe, S., Saiphoo, C., et al.: Blood urea levels 30 minutes before the end of dialysis are equivalent to equilibrated blood urea. ASAIO J. 43(5), M759–M762 (1997)

Brahm, J.: Urea permeability of human red cells. J. Gen. Physiol. 82(1), 1–23 (1983)

Burgelman, M., Vanholder, R., Fostier, H., Ringoir, S.: Estimation of parameters in a two-pool urea kinetic model for hemodialysis. Med. Engl. Phys. 19(1), 69–76 (1997)

Canaud, B., Bosc, J.Y., Cabrol, L., et al.: Urea as a marker of adequacy in hemodialysis: lesson from in vivo urea dynamics monitoring. Kidney Int. suppl. 76, S28–S40 (2000)

Canaud, B., Bosc, J.Y., Leblanc, M., et al.: A simple and accurate method to determine equilibrated post-dialysis urea concentration. Kidney Int. 51(6), 2000–2005 (1997)

Cappello, A., Avanzolini, G., Chiari, L.: Estimation of parameters in a two-pool urea kinetic model for hemodialysis. Med. Eng. Phys. 20(4), 315–318 (1998)

Castro, M.C.M., Romao Jr., J.E., Marcondes, M.: Measurement of blood urea concentration during hemodialysis is not an accurate method to determine equilibrated post-dialysis urea concentration. Nephrol. Dial. Transplant. 16(9), 1814–1817 (2001)

Chithat, T., Tungsanga, K., Eiam-Ong, S.: Accuracy of using 30-minute post-dialysis BUN to determine equilibrated Kt/V. J. Med. Assoc. Thai. 89(suppl. 2), 54–64 (2006)

Daugirdas, J.T., Blake, P.G., Ing, T.S. (eds.): Handbook of Dialysis, 4th edn. Lippincott, Williams and Wilkins, Philadelphia (2007)

Daugirdas, J.T., Greene, T., Depner, T.A., et al.: Factors that Affect Post-dialysis Rebound in Serum Urea Concentration, Including the Rate of Dialysis: Results from the HEMO Study. J. Am. Soc. Nephrol. 15(1), 194–203 (2004)

Daugirdas, J.T., Greene, T., Depner, T.A., et al.: Relationship between apparent (single-pool) and true (double-pool) urea distribution volume. Kidney Int. 56(5), 1928–1933 (1999)

Daugirdas, J.T., Depner, T.A., Gotch, F.A., et al.: Comparison of methods to predict equilibrated Kt/V in the HEMO Pilot Study. Kidney Int. 52(5), 1395–1405 (1997)

Daugirdas, J.T., Schneditz, D., Leehey, D.J.: Effect of access recirculation on the modeled urea distribution volume. Am. J. Kidney Dis. 27(4), 512–518 (1996a)

Daugirdas, J.T., Burke, M.S., Balter, P., et al.: Screening for extreme post-dialysis urea rebound using the Smye method: patients with access recirculation identified when a slow flow method is not used to draw the postdialysis blood. Am. J. Kidney Dis. 28(5), 727–731 (1996b)

Daugirdas, J.T., Schneditz, D.: Overestimation of hemodialysis dose depends on dialysis efficiency by regional blood flow but not by conventional two pool urea kinetic analysis. ASAIO J. 41(3), M719–M724 (1995)

Daugirdas, J.T.: Estimation of equilibrated Kt/V using the unequilibrated post dialysis BUN. Semin. Dial. 8(5), 283–284 (1995)

Daugirdas, J.T.: Second generation logarithmic estimates of single-pool variable volume Kt/V: an analysis of error. J. Am. Soc. Nephrol. 4(5), 1205–1213 (1993)

Dedrick, R.L., Bischoff, K.B.: Pharmacokinetics in applications of the artificial kidney. In: Chem. Eng. Prog. Symp. Ser., vol. 64, pp. 32–44 (1968)

Dedrick, R.L., Gabelnick, H.L., Bischoff, K.B.: Kinetics of urea distribution. In: Proc. Ann. Conf. Eng. Med. Biol., vol. 10, 36.1 (1968)

Depner, T.A., Rizwan, S., Cheer, A.Y., et al.: High venous urea concentrations in the opposite arm: A consequence of hemodialysis-induced compartment disequilibrium. ASAIO J. 37(3), 141–143 (1991)

Depner, T.A.: Multicompartment models. In: Depner, T.A. (ed.) Prescribing Hemodialysis: A Guide to Urea Modeling, pp. 91–126. Kluwer Academic, Dordrecht (1991)

Duchesne, R., Klein, J.D., Velotta, J.B., et al.: UT-A urea transporter protein in heart: Increased abundance during uremia, hypertension, and heart failure. Circ. Res. 89(2), 139–145 (2001)

Evans, J.H., Smye, S.W., Brocklebank, J.T.: Mathematical modelling of haemodialysis in children. Pediatr. Nephrol. 6(4), 349–353 (1992)

Fernandez, E.A., Valtuille, R., Willshaw, P., Perazzo, C.A.: Using Artificial Intelligence to Predict the Equilibrated Post-dialysis Blood Urea Concentration. Blood Purif. 19(3), 271–285 (2001)

Flanigan, M.J., Fangman, J., Lim, V.S.: Quantitating hemodialysis: A comparison of three kinetic models. Am. J. Kidney Dis. 17(3), 295–302 (1991)

Garred, L.J., Canaud, B., Bosc, J.Y., Tetta, C.: Urea rebound and delivered Kt/V determination with a continuous urea sensor. Nephrol. Dial. Transplant. 12(3), 535–542 (1997)

George, T.O., Priester-Coary, A., Dunea, G., et al.: Cardiac output and urea kinetics in dialysis patients: Evidence supporting the regional blood flow model. Kidney Int. 50(4), 1273–1277 (1996)

Goldstein, S.L., Brewer, E.D.: Logarithmic extrapolation of a 15- minute postdialysis BUN to predict equilibrated BUN and calculate double-pool Kt/V in the pediatric hemodialysis population. Am. J. Kidney Dis. 36(1), 98–104 (2000)

Gotch, F.A., Keen, M.L.: Kinetic modeling in hemodialysis. In: Nissenson, A.R., Fine, R.N. (eds.) Clinical Dialysis, 4th edn., pp. 153–202. McGrraw-Hill, New York (2005)

Grandi, F., Avanzolini, G., Cappello, A.: Analytic solution of the variable-volume double-pool urea kinetics model applied to parameter estimation in hemodialysis. Comput. Biol. Med. 25(6), 505–518 (1995)

Guh, J., Yang, C., Yang, J., Chen, L., Lai, Y.: Prediction of equilibrated postdialysis BUN by an artificial neural network in high-efficiency hemodialysis. Am. J. Kidney Dis. 31(4), 638–646 (1998)

Goldau, R.: Clinical Evaluation of Novel Methods to Determine Dialysis Parameters Using Conductivity Cells. Ph. D. Würzburg University (2002)

Heineken, F.G., Evans, M.C., Keen, M.L., Gotch, F.A.: Intercompartmental fluid shifts in hemodialysis patients. Biotechnol. Progr. 3(2), 69–73 (1987)

Jean, G., Chazot, C., Charra, B., et al.: Is post-dialysis urea rebound significant with long slow hemodialysis? Blood Purif. 16(4), 187–196 (1998)

Jean, G., Charra, B., Chazot, C., Laurent, G.: Quest for post-dialysis urea rebound-equilibrated Kt/V with only intradialytic urea samples. Kidney Int. 56(3), 1149–1153 (1999)

Kaufman, A.M., Schneditz, D., Smye, S., et al.: Solute disequilibrium and multicompartment modeling. Adv. Ren. Replace Ther. 2(4), 319–329 (1995)

Kooman, J.P., van der Sande, F.M., Leunissen, K.M.: Kt/V: Finding the Tree within the Woods. Nephrol. Dial. Transplant. 16(9), 1749–1752 (2001)

Leblanc, M., Charbonneau, R., Lalumiere, G., et al.: Postdialysis Urea Rebound: Determinants and Influence on Dialysis Delivery in Chronic Hemodialysis Patients. Am. J. Kidney Dis. 27(2), 253–261 (1996)

Leypoldt, J.K., Jaber, B.L., Zimmerman, D.L.: Predicting treatment dose for novel therapies using urea standard Kt/V. Semin. Dial. 17(2), 142–145 (2004)

Maduell, F., Garcia-Valdecasas, J., Garcia, H., et al.: Urea reduction ratio considering urea rebound. Nephron 78(2), 143–147 (1998)

Maduell, F., Garcia-Valdecasas, J., Garcia, H., et al.: Validation of different methods to calculate KtV considering postdialysis rebound. Nephrol. Dial. Transplant. 12(9), 1928–1933 (1997)

Malovrh, M.: Non-invasive evaluation of vessels by duplex sonography prior to construction of arteriovenous fistula for haemodialysis. Nephrol. Dial. Transplant. 13(1), 125–129 (1998)

Matthews, D.E., Downey, R.S.: Measurement of urea kinetics in humans: a validation of stable isotope tracer methods. Am. J. Physiol. 246(6 Pt 1), E519–E527 (1984)

Metry, G.S., Attman, P.O., Lönnroth, P., et al.: Urea kinetics during hemodialysis measured by microdialysis–a novel technique. Kidney Int. 44(3), 622–629 (1993)

NKF-K/DOQI: Clinical Practice Guidelines and Clinical Practice Recommendations, Updates: Hemodialysis Adequacy, Peritoneal Dialysis Adequacy, Vascular Access. Am. J. Kidney Dis. 48(suppl. 1), S28–S58 (2006)

NKF-K/DOQI: Clinical practice guidelines for hemodialysis adequacy: Update. Am. J. Kidney. Dis. 37(1 suppl. 1), S7–S64 (2001)

Pedrini, L.A., Zereik, S., Rasmy, S.: Causes, kinetics and clinical implications of post-hemodialysis urea rebound. Kidney Int. 34(6), 817–824 (1988)

Pflederer, B.R., Torrey, C., Priester-Coary, A., Lau, A.H., Daugirdas, J.T.: Estimating equilibrated Kt/V from an intradialytic sample: effects of access and cardiopulmonary recirculations. Kidney Int. 48(3), 832–837 (1995)

Renkin, E.M.: Effects of blood flow on diffusion kinetics in isolated, perfused hindlegs of cats; a double circulation hypothesis. Am. J. Physiol. 183(1), 125–136 (1955)

Ronco, C., Brendolan, A., Crepaldi, C., et al.: Ultrafiltrations-rates and dialyse hypotension. Dialyse J. 40, 8–15 (1992)

Sargent, J.A., Gotch, F.A.: Principles and biophysics of dialysis. In: Maher, J.F. (ed.) Replacement of Renal Function by Dialysis, 3rd edn., pp. 87–143. Kluwer Academic, Dordrecht (1989)

Schneditz, D., Platzer, D., Daugirdas, J.T.: A diffusion-adjusted regional blood flow model to predict solute kinetics during haemodialysis. Nephrol. Dial. Transplant. 24(7), 2218–2224 (2009)

Schneditz, D., Daugirdas, J.T.: Compartment effects in hemodialysis. Semin. Dial. 14(4), 271–277 (2001)

Schneditz, D., Fariyike, B., Osheroff, R., Levin, N.W.: Is intercompartmental urea clearance during hemodialysis a perfusion term? A comparison of two pool urea kinetic models. J. Am. Soc. Nephrol. 6(5), 1360–1370 (1995)

Schneditz, D., Daugirdas, J.T.: Formal analytical solution to a regional blood flow and diffusion based urea kinetic model. ASAIO J. 40(3), M667–M673 (1994)

Schneditz, D., VanStone, J., Daugirdas, J.T.: A regional blood circulation alternative to in-series two compartment urea kinetic modeling. ASAIO J. 39(3), M573–M577 (1993)

Schneditz, D., Roob, J., Oswald, M., et al.: Nature and rate of vascular refilling during hemodialysis and ultrafiltration. Kidney Int. 42(6), 1425–1433 (1992a)

Schneditz, D., Kaufman, A.M., Polaschegg, H.D., et al.: Cardiopulmonary recirculation during hemodialysis. Kidney Int. 42(6), 1450–1456 (1992b)

Sharma, A., Espinosa, P., Bell, L., et al.: Multicompartment Urea Kinetics In Well-Dialyzed Children. Kidney Int. 58(5), 2138–2146 (2000)

Sharma, A.K.: Reassessing hemodialysis adequacy in children: The case for more. Pediatr. Nephrol. 16(4), 383–390 (2001)

Sherman, R.A., Kapoian, T.: Recirculation, urea disequilibrium, and dialysis efficiency: Peripheral arteriovenous versus central venovenous vascular access. Am. J. Kidney Dis. 29(4), 479–489 (1997)

Smith, C.P.: Mammalian urea transporters. Exp. Physiol. 94(2), 180–185 (2009)

Smye, S.W., Tattersall, J.E., Will, E.J.: Modeling the postdialysis rebound: the reconciliation of current formulas. ASAIO J. 45(6), 562–567 (1999)

Smye, S.W., Lindley, E.J., Will, E.J.: Simulating the effect of exercise on urea clearance in hemodialysis. J. Am. Soc. Nephrol. 9(1), 128–132 (1998)

Smye, S.W., Will, E.J.: A mathematical analysis of a two-compartment model of urea kinetics. Phys. Med. Biol. 40(12), 2005–2014 (1995)

Smye, S.W., Dunderdale, E., Brownridge, G., Will, E.: Estimation of treatment dose in high-efficiency haemodialysis. Nephron 67(1), 24–29 (1994)

Smye, S.W., Evans, J.H., Will, E., Brocklebank, J.T.: Paediatric haemodialysis: Estimation of treatment efficiency in the presence of urea rebound. Clin. Phys. Physiol. Meas. 13(1), 51–62 (1992)

Spiegel, D.M., Baker, P.L., Babcock, S., et al.: Hemodialysis urea rebound: the effect of increasing dialysis efficiency. Am. J. Kidney Dis. 25(1), 26–29 (1995)

Star, R., Hootkins, J., Thompson, J., et al.: Variability and stability of two pool urea mass transfer coefficient. J. Am. Soc. Nephrol. 3, 395A (1992)

Tattersall, J., Farrington, K., Bowser, M., et al.: Underdialysis caused by reliance on single pool urea kinetic modeling. J. Am. Soc. Nephrol. 3, 398 (1996a)

Tattersall, J.E., DeTakats, D., Chamney, P., et al.: The post-haemodialysis rebound: predicting and quantifying its effect on KtV. Kidney Int. 50(6), 2094–2102 (1996b)

Tattersall, J.E., Chamney, P., Aldridge, C., Greenwood, R.N.: Recirculation and the post-dialysis rebound. Nephrol. Dial. Transplant. 11(suppl. 2), 75–80 (1996c)

Teichholz, L.E., Kreulen, T., Herman, M.V., et al.: Problems in echocardiographic volume determinations: echocardiographic-angiographic correlations in the presence of absence of asynergy. Am. J. Cardiol. 37(1), 7–11 (1976)

Timmer, R.T., Klein, J.D., Bagnasco, S.M., et al.: Localization of the urea transporter UT-B protein in human and rat erythrocytes and tissues. Am. J. Physiol. Cell Physiol. 281(4), C1318–C1325 (2001)

Yamada, T., Hiraga, S., Akiba, T., et al.: Analysis of Urea Nitrogen and Creatinine Kinetics in Hemodialysis: Comparison of a Variable-Volume Two-Compartment Model with a Regional Blood Flow Model and Investigation of a Appropriate Solute Kinetics Model for Clinical Application. Blood Purif. 18(1), 18–29 (2000)

Yashiro, M., Watanabe, H., Muso, E.: Simulation of post-dialysis urea rebound using regional flow model. Clin. Exp. Nephrol. 8(2), 139–145 (2004)

Vanholder, R., Burgelman, M., De Smet, R., et al.: Two-Pool versus Single-Pool Models in the Determination of Urea Kinetic Parameters. Blood Purif. 14(6), 437–450 (1996)

Wagner, L., Klein, J.D., Sands, J.M., Baylis, C.: Urea transporters are distributed in endothelial cells and mediate inhibition of L-arginine transport. Am. J. Physiol. Renal. Physiol. 283(3), F578–F582 (2002)

Zhao, D., Sonawane, N.D., Levin, M.H., Yang, B.: Comparative transport efficiencies of urea analogues through urea transporter UT-B. Biochim. Biophys. Acta 1768(7), 1815–1821 (2007)

ESSAY QUESTIONS

1. Differentiate between single pool and double pool urea kinetic models.
2. Describe the concept of urea rebound
3. Write a matlab program to calculate Kt/V by Daugirdas' formula (1995) using the Daugirdas' method to calculate the monocompartimental one.
4. List the main methods for calculating equilibrated dialysis dose.
5. What is the main advantage of the rate equation for calculating urea rebound and $_{eq}(Kt/V)$?
6. Explain the regional blood flow model and the mechanism producing urea rebound after treatment.
7. Explain cardiopulmonary recirculation.
8. List the simultaneous equations expressing RBF model.
9. In the conventional double pool model, the degree of the compartment effect mainly determined intercompartmental mass coefficients. Indicate the factors that affect the degree of the compartment effect in the RBF model and explain how they affect equilibrated Kt/V.
10. Exercise in the late phase of a hemodialysis session is known to increase urea clearance. Explain this mechanism of this phenomenon based on RBF model

MULTIPLE CHOICE QUESTIONS

Choose the best answer

1. If the pre-dialysis BUN is 133 mg/dL; intradialytic urea concentration after 120 min of hemodialysis is 70 mg/dL; post-dialysis urea concentration is 45 mg/dL The time of dialysis is 240 min. the equilibrated post-dialysis urea concentration using Smye method is...
   A. 52 mg/dL
   B. 53 mg/dL
   C. 55 mg/dL
   D. 58 mg/dL

2. Using the same patient's data as in question 1, the percentage of urea rebound using the Smye method is...
   A. 18.2%
   B. 19.5%
   C. 25.6%
   D. 22.22%

3. The urea rebound process takes about ... to equilibrate 95% of an initial urea gradient over the cell membrane.
   A. 30 min
   B. 60 min
   C. 50 min
   D. 20 min

4. In relation to urea kinetic modeling...
   A. The 1-pool model consistently underestimates urea removal, and the 2-pool model slightly overestimates urea removal.
   B. The 1-pool model consistently overestimates urea removal, and the 2-pool model slightly underestimates urea removal.
   C. Both models underestimate urea removal.
   D. Both models overestimate urea removal.

5. If the pre-dialysis BUN is 125 mg/dL; post-dialysis urea concentration is 42 mg/dL and the equilibrated urea concentration after 30 min of dialysis is 48 mg/dL. The ratio of single pool to double pool urea distribution volume is...
   A. 0.95
   B. 0.92
   C. 1.00
   D. 0.98

6. The time constant for Tattersall's original formula is...
   A. 18.5 min
   B. 23.2 min
   C. 30.7 min
   D. 35 min

7. If the delivered single pool Kt/V value is 1.501 and the dialysis time is 240 min, then the rate of dialysis is...
   A. 0.31
   B. 0.38
   C. 0.33
   D. 0.32

8. If the delivered single pool Kt/V value is 1.274 and the dialysis time is 180 min, then $_{eq}$(Kt/V) using the Leypoldt formula is...
   A. 0.953
   B. 1.023
   C. 0.856
   D. 1.095

9. The delivered single pool Kt/V for a patient using an arterial access is 1.348 and the dialysis time is 210 min. The calculation of single pool Kt/V is based on immediate 0 s post-dialysis sample technique. The double pool Kt/V using modified rate equation is…
  A. 1.15
  B. 1.12
  C. 1.17
  D. 1.08

10. How large is the minimum eKt/V recommended by DOQI guidelines for a schedule of three hemodialysis sessions per week?
  A. $_{eq}(Kt/V) = 0.9$
  B. $_{eq}(Kt/V) = 1.2$
  C. $_{eq}(Kt/V) = 1.1$
  D. $_{eq}(Kt/V) = 1.3$

11. Due to the variability in measuring Kt/V, which are the target values recommended by DOQI guidelines for $_{eq}(Kt/V)$?
  a) $_{eq}(Kt/V) = 1.05$
  b) $_{eq}(Kt/V) = 1.15$
  c) $_{eq}(Kt/V) = 1.05$
  d) $_{eq}(Kt/V) = 1.15$

12. The flow fraction to the high flow system in regional flow model is usually assumed as…
  A. 0.8
  B. 0.6
  C. 0.4
  D. 0.2
  E. 0.1

13. The factor that doesn't affect cardiopulmonary recirculation is…
  A. Q_{sys}
  B. Q_b
  C. Q_{ac}
  D. U
  E. K_d

14. Which concentration of urea is the highest during hemodialysis?
    A. C_{art}
    B. C_{vmix}
    C. C_H
    D. C_L
    E. C_{out}

15. The increase of … augments the rebound of urea after treatment.
    A. f_{QH}
    B. f_{QL}
    C. f_{VH}
    D. f_{VL}
    E. Q_{sys}

16. The organ included in low flow system is…
    A. Kidneys
    B. Skin
    C. Lungs
    D. Heart
    E. Brain

17. The cut off value for specific perfusion to divide organs between high and low flow system is…
    A. 0.1 /min
    B. 0.2 /min
    C. 0.3 /min
    D. 0.4 /min
    E. 0.5 /min

18. Select the variable not affecting modified urea clearance of dialyzer
    A. Kd'
    B. R_{ac}
    C. K_d
    D. Q_b
    E. U
    F. Q_{sys}

19. How long does it take to dissipate effects caused by cardiopulmonary recirculation?
   - A. 2sec
   - B. 20sec
   - C. 2min
   - D. 20min
   - E. 2hr

20. The nearest concentration to C_{art} during hemodialysis is…
   - A. C_H
   - B. C_L
   - C. C_{out}
   - D. C_{vmix}

21. When…increases, the hemodialysis efficiency decreases.
   - A. f_{QH}
   - B. f_{QL}
   - C. f_{VH}
   - D. f_{VL}
   - E. Q_{sys}

Chapter 14

Applications of Bioimpedance to End Stage Renal Disease (ESRD)

Laura M. Roa, David Naranjo, Javier Reina-Tosina, Alfonso Lara,
José A. Milán, Miguel A. Estudillo, J. Sergio Oliva

CHAPTER OUTLINES

- Introduction
- History of bioimpedance
- Physical principles of bioimpedance
- Bioimpedance instrumentation basics
- Bioimpedance measurement techniques
- Nephrology applications
- Commercial devices
- Case studies
- Conclusion

CHAPTER OBJECTIVES

Provide the reader with knowledge to:

- Understand the physical principles of bioimpedance.
- Estimate body composition from bioimpedance measurements.
- Know how to apply different bioimpedance analysis techniques to improve the nutritional and hydration status of dialysis patients.

KEY TERMS

- Bioimpedance.
- Bioelectrical impedance analysis.
- Body composition.
- Overhydration.
- Bioimpedance spectroscopy.

ABSTRACT

This chapter develops a thorough review of the methods and techniques used for the analysis of body composition of renal patients based on bioimpedance measurements. The work ranges from the physical principles, to bioelectric models of human body, instrumentation, configurations in the position of electrodes, equations to calculate body composition, bioimpedance nephrological applications and clinical analysis of results. This text provides a multidisciplinary approach that will allow the reader to understand and comprehend this kind of technology, so it can be used both by engineers as a basis for the development of bioimpedance medical devices, and by medical staff to apply the bioimpedance analysis techniques in a better control and management of patients with ESRD.

A.T. Azar (Ed.): Modeling and Control of Dialysis Systems, SCI 404, pp. 689–769.
springerlink.com © Springer-Verlag Berlin Heidelberg 2013

14.1 INTRODUCTION

The body is a multicompartmental system, where each compartment is a whole space separated from the others by a membrane; hence, strictly speaking, every cell should be considered as a compartment itself. It is clear that the infinite complexity that this issue entails makes the modeling of such multicompartmental system unfeasible. Regarding the fact that the concentration of ions dissolved in water is different inside and outside the cells, in a first instance, a two-compartment model of the human body composed by the intracellular fluid and extracellular fluid could be set (Kyle et al. 2004a) (Gibney et al. 2005), where the word "fluid" refers to merging water plus the solutes dissolved in it (sodium, potassium, magnesium, chlorides and bicarbonates, etc.). The boundary between the two media is the cell membrane. Using a two-compartment model supposes a closer and more accurate estimation of parameters than the monocompartment one.

The intracellular environment includes all the fluids that are within the cell membrane and it is the place where the body metabolic processes take place. This medium is commonly referred to as Intra-Cellular Water (ICW), because the volume it occupies could be identified with the water that it contains. The extracellular environment is outside the cell membrane and is usually referred to as Extra-Cellular Water (ECW). The ECW amount of water in healthy adults is usually between 13 and 21 liters (Wabel et al. 2009). Unlike the intracellular environment, the extracellular environment can be divided, from the structural and functional standpoints, in the following submedia (Callaghan et al. 2003): plasma, interstitial and lymphatic fluids, dense connective tissue, cartilage (70% water), bone (6.6% water) and transcellular fluids. The overall content of water in the human body consists of the sum of ICW and ECW which is often referred to as Total Body Water (TBW).

Due to the high hydraulic permeability of the cell membrane, water moves freely between the intracellular and extracellular media (Charra 2007). Sodium is the passive motor of these water movements from a point where there is a higher concentration of water to a lower one in order to equalize the concentrations. This keeps an equal osmolarity in all body fluids compartments. As the sodium concentration inside the cells is usually kept constant, the sodium content in the body determines the volume of ECW. An increase in the amount of sodium represents an increase of osmolarity, and it stimulates the thirst and reduces the urine volume (antidiuresis). A further intake of water would increase the ECW. This ECW overload unleashes the excess of water and sodium excretion through urine so as to restore the normal levels within a few hours. A decrease in water intake also increases the osmolarity, and it stimulates the thirst and antidiuresis. Normally, sodium (usually salt-based) and water intakes are balanced by the excretion of urine, keeping constant the volume of ECW.

As water distribution is not uniform throughout the human body, it can be seen as a biocompartmental model composed by fat mass (FM) and another compartment called fat free mass (FFM) (Kyle et al. 2004a). FM represents the lipid mass of the body, which does not include any amount of water, while FFM is anything that is not fat (see Fig 14.1).

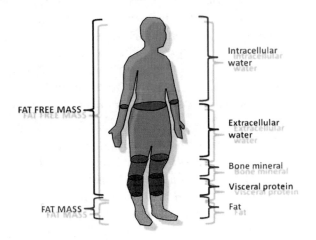

Fig. 14.1 Compartmental model of the human body

It is possible to calculate TBW by means of the FFM, because in healthy individuals it represents a 73.2% average of water (Eisenkolbl et al. 2001), which is its principal component. However, this fraction does not remain constant during life span. FFM is a broad term that includes lean body mass (LBM) and bone mass (Earthman et al. 2007) (Coupaye et al. 2007). The LBM compartment can be divided between extracellular mass (ECM) and body cell mass (BCM). The ECW and the structural bone matrix are the components that make up the ECM. The ICW is included in the BCM. In fact, ICW measurements are used as an approach to BCM.

Uremic patients treated with both hemodialysis and peritoneal dialysis show alterations in the metabolism of water with continuous variations in hydration status (Charra 2007), which are difficult to understand. The relative distribution of ECW and ICW in such patients is different compared to a healthy population and the increase or decrease in water and sodium is often accompanied by metabolic abnormalities associated with edema (overhydration) (Wabel et al. 2008). In such circumstances, after a dialysis session it is quite common for patients to have a significant fluid excess or to be in an undesirable state of dehydration, which can cause or aggravate any cardiovascular disease (Wabel et al. 2009). In addition, these patients typically show a reduction in fat mass and FFM (Basaleem et al. 2004).

If fluid excess is not removed, long-term consequences can be severe. Hypervolemia is considered a predisposing factor for the development of hypertension in patients on dialysis, and other conditions such as pulmonary edema, peripheral edema, left ventricular hypertrophy, heart failure and other cardiovascular sequelae (Wizemann et al. 2009). Cardiovascular disease is the leading cause of death in the general population and in patients with End Stage Renal Disease (ESRD), and the mortality rate of patients with ESRD is 10 to 20 times higher than the general population (Naiman et al. 2009). On the other hand, removing too much fluid is also dangerous because the patient ends suffering from hypotension, which is also associated with increased mortality in hemodialysis patients (Wabel et al. 2008).

In this sense, in renal patients treated by hemodialysis it is very important to assess the amount of excess fluid to determine how much should be removed through ultrafiltration to achieve a desired state of normohydration (Woodrow et al. 1996; Pastan and Gassensmith 1992). It is also important to know how to distribute the losses of fluids between the ECW and ICW compartments, because sometimes patients suffer alterations in the distribution of liquids, especially in obese individuals or patients with weight loss (Jaffrin and Morel 2008). In addition, BCM is an important indicator of the nutritional status of the patient and a decrease in its value is often associated with poor prognosis (Kyle et al. 2004a). However, estimating the size of this compartment is difficult due to its complexity, which includes both non-fat cells and the aqueous compartment of adipocytes. In overhydrated patients, although an accurate estimate of the FFM could be made, a major malnutrition may be masqueraded due to an expansion of the ECW. Summarizing, knowledge of body fluid volumes and other body compartments such as BCM and fat mass is essential for the description of the hydration status in renal patients.

The reference methods for the measurement of body fluid volumes are based on solutions of radio-isotopes (Jaffrin and Morel 2008), which are freely distributed to all cell compartments without any barrier (Watson et al. 1980). In studies with humans, TBW is usually estimated with solutions of deuterium oxide, tritium or antipyrine. ECW can be measured with solutions that contain radioactive isotopes of sodium or non-radioactive tracer bromide (Wabel et al. 2009). ICW can be found by means of the radioactive isotope of potassium, which is included in the corporal potassium (Jaffrin and Morel 2008). ICW could also be obtained by subtracting ECW from TBW.

Generically, the methods based on solutions involve an initial sample of blood or urine, followed by the intake of an isotope or tracer (may be several for many estimations). After several hours to establish the steady state, a final sample of blood or urine is taken. The volume (ECW or TBW) can be calculated taking into account that $C_1 V_1 = C_2 V_2$ (Earthman et al. 2007), where C_1 is the initial concentration of the isotope in the solution volume (V_1) and C_2 is the final concentration of the isotope or tracer in the urine or blood, so that the body water volume corresponds to V_2.

Although the methods of multiple solutions provide precise measurements of body compartments and are considered as reference methods in the determination of fluid volumes, they are not ideal methods for the clinical application for several reasons (Earthman et al. 2007; Jaffrin and Morel 2008; Moissl et al. 2006): they are expensive because they require the use of mass spectrometers and technical expertise; they are time-consuming procedures; they involve the administration of radioactive isotopes or tracers; they are invasive procedures when using blood samples; they require the availability of the patient for many hours; it takes at least 2-3 weeks for the tracer to be completely eliminated from the body in order to apply the measurement technique again, so these techniques cannot be used to measure changes in volume in a short period of time. For all these reasons, solution methods are not the right choice for the estimation of fluid compartments and BCM in the routine clinical practice.

To avoid these problems, many authors have proposed equations based on anthropometric measurements for a quick estimate of TBW, like the correlation of Watson et al (1980) or Hume and Weyers (Fenech et al. 2001). However, as these correlations were established using data from healthy subjects, they should not be applied to people with disorders in their body composition, such as patients on dialysis. The dry weight reached at the end of dialysis is considered the patient's ideal weight, so the correlation equations should be applied using the dry weight obtained for the estimation of the volume of TBW. However, if a personalization that takes into account individual physiological characteristics such as muscle or adipose tissue is not considered, the anthropometric relationships can lead to significant errors in the estimation of TBW, which give rise to an inadequate hemodialysis.

All these factors have made bioimpedance methods to be one of the most used techniques to estimate body composition because they have not the restrictions of solution methods and provide more accurate estimations than the anthropometric methods (Moissl et al. 2006). Thanks to bioimpedance techniques, it is possible to obtain an accurate estimation of body fluids and body composition in both normal and disease states. Besides, it also identifies protein/lean reserves (FFM) and fat reserves (FM). It is capable of assessing changes in hydration, which are important in hemodialysis to avoid complications related to fluid overload, and allows an adjustment of dry weight to provide the best possible treatment.

Bioimpedance measurements also have many practical advantages that have led to their rapid development (Earthman et al. 2007; Jaffrin and Morel 2008; Ellis et al. 1999). The instrumentation is portable, relatively inexpensive, and the measurements can be quickly performed with minimal operator training. Bioimpedance methods require little maintenance, and they are safe and easy to perform. It is a noninvasive technique, which requires only the positioning of electrodes on the body. The results are obtained immediately, and the measurement can be repeated as often as desired, with a large inter-observer reproducibility. The level of participation of the subjects under examination is relatively low, and it requires them neither the intake of bad-tasted solutions, nor taking blood samples nor a too long time of rest as required for the dissolution methods for the balance of oral tracers (3-4 hours).

After years of research in bioimpedance analysis with dialysis patients, this technique has significantly increased its clinical use (Kyle et al. 2004b). The provided estimates of ECW and ICW have been validated through dissolution methods, which are considered the gold standard (Kotanko et al. 2008). In this context, the objective of this chapter is to perform a detailed introduction to bioimpedance analysis techniques applied to kidney patients. After this introductory section an historical review of impedance applications in medicine will be carried out. In a later section, the basic physical principles of bioimpedance measures will be outlined and, afterwards, the details of the instrumentation will be explained. The chapter will continue with the presentation of the different methods of bioimpedance analysis to estimate body composition. Later, some of the most important uses and applications of bioimpedance in nephrology will be exposed. A section will also feature some of the commercial solutions currently available and others used in the literature. Finally, three case studies that highlight the clinical utility of bioimpedance measurements will be presented.

14.2 HISTORY OF BIOIMPEDANCE

The earliest findings into the bioelectricity phenomenon date from 1787 when L. Galvani (Galvani 1791) discovered that a frog muscle was twitched when it was struck by a spark. According to these experiments, Galvani formulated the theory of animal electricity, which was refuted by Alessandro Volta. In 1820, Hans Cristian Oersted found a relationship between electricity and magnetism, leading to the invention of the galvanometer. These first devices were not appropriate to measure bioelectric signals since they were not sensitive enough and they were not able to detect the fast current changes from muscles and nerves. Thanks to the development of more sensitive galvanometers (Nobili 1825), the existence of endogenous currents and charges in living tissue was subsequently demonstrated. In 1843, Carlo Matteucci measured the electric current from heart muscles (Matteucci 1842). DuBois-Reymond studied these phenomena in detail and introduced the action potential term in order to designate the electrical current changes during muscle contraction (Du Bois-Reymond 1848). Koelliker y Müller became the first to observe the action potentials from myocardiocyteal muscle cells. In 1901, Willem Einthoven introduced a new high-sensitive string galvanometer to record the heart potentials (Einthoven 1901). Five years later, Einthoven published a detailed paper (Einthoven 1906) that depicted the major clinical applications of electrocardiogram, thereby laying the foundations for the development of the ECG analysis, which is still the most important medical examination procedure in hospitals worldwide.

Hermann Müller found the capacitive properties of tissue and anisotropy of muscle conductivity in 1870. In addition to his famous equations, James Clerk Maxwell calculated the resistance of a homogeneous suspension of uniform spheres as a function of the volume concentration of the spheres. In fact, this mathematical model for cell suspensions and tissues is still used today. Since 1871, researchers have worked to get a better insight of the electrical properties of tissue, both healthy and damaged as well as before and after death, setting up their properties as a function of frequency.

The implementation of bioimpedance measurements started in 1930, when Atzler and Lehman realized that flow changes from thoracic cavity as a result of the pumping of the blood through the heart, also produced changes in the thoracic impedance (Atzler and Lehmann 1931). The bioimpedance measurement technique is based on injecting a very low AC current into the human body or living tissue, below the threshold of perception. The electric current produces a drop in voltage, which increases with a higher electrical impedance of the tissue. Fenning measured rat breathing by using a similar method in 1937 (Fenning 1937), where the animal's body was modeled as a variable capacitor whose capacitance depended on the respiratory movements. In 1940, Rósa applied this technique in order to detect the heart and blood vessels movements. In 1949, Whitehorn and Perl calculated the blood volume pumped through the heart with similar techniques.

Holzer et al. became the first to use an alternating signal to avoid the problems related to electrode polarization in bioimpedance measurements (Éninya and Ondzuls 1962). They were able to detect the changes of the heart flow by using a device called rheograph. The fluctuations in the blood flow caused very weak alterations in the conductivity, around 1%, thus bioimpedance measurements only detected changes in blood flow when the signal was amplified enough without interferences. Therefore, they included an electronic amplifier and a Wheatstone bridge into the detector in order to increase its sensitivity. Nyboer et al. found a high correlation between the thoracic impedance variation and the volume changes related to breathing, which were recorded by means of a spirometer (Nyboer 1950). Their studies led to the foundations for impedance plethysmography. A plethysmograph based on impedance contains a sinusoidal voltage source that is transformed into current by using a converter. The current flows through the body segment that is being studied by means of two electrodes (current electrodes). The voltage generated in the current path is measured with another pair of electrodes (voltage electrodes). Therefore, the amplitude of the voltage signal is proportional to the impedance of the body segment. Bioimpedance can be modified both by the volume changes caused by breathing movements and by pulsatile changes of blood flow in the thorax. Impedance variations due to flood movements have a different frequency than impedance changes caused by breathing movements, thereby a mathematical algorithm can be developed to remove them and only calculate the volume changes related to breathing. The first device for hemodynamic parameters monitoring was developed in 1966, in collaboration with the Apollo program, leading to the progress of impedance cardiography for the estimation of the systolic volume. The resistivity of cardiac muscle is greater than that of the blood, and therefore the impedance variations are mainly due to the movement of the blood, decreasing with the filling of the heart chambers and increasing with emptying. This is the basic of impedance cardiography, which has also been used for the estimation of the cardiac output for decades by means of Kubicek equation (Kubiczek et al. 1966).

Thereafter, bioimpedance has been applied in the development of new diagnostic tools and medical devices. In 1978, Webster and Henderson tried to reproduce the technique of X-ray tomography, but using low frequency electric signals (Henderson and Webster 1978). However, the bases of what today is understood by electrical impedance tomography were not developed until the 80s at the English University of Sheffield (Holder 2004). Images related to the distribution of the impedances within the body were obtained by measuring the electrical potentials on the body surface (see Fig.14.2). The impedance varies depending on tissue physiological state, so it has been used to monitor the viability of the organs (Edd 2006), to know the skin hydration or diagnose skin diseases (Aberg et al. 2003), and even as a non-invasive method to measure blood glucose levels (Amaral and Wolf 2007; Tura et al. 2007). Bioimpedance has also been used as a tool for cell measurements at clinical laboratories (coulter counter, hematocrit measures and monitoring of cell cultures) (Piacentini et al. 2008; Zheng et al. 2007; Trebbels et al. 2009; Dziong et al. 2007). Furthermore, it is still applied in diagnostic equipment related to volume changes (impedance plethysmography, impedance cardiography, impedance pneumograph, etc.) (Wang et al. 2008; Pandey and Pandey 2007).

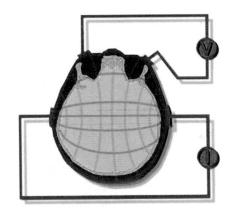

Fig. 14.2 Scheme of electrical potentials measurement in the human body

Nevertheless, one of the major bioimpedance applications is the study of body composition, very useful in several clinical areas (nephrology, nutrition, obstetrics, gastroenterology, postoperative follow-up, patients with HIV, deficit of growth hormone, obesity, or in critical-care). In 1963, Tomasset carried out the first estimations of water content of the whole body from impedance measurements using a fixed frequency AC current

(Baumgartner 1996). In order to increase the sensitivity of the devices, Nyboer and Hoffer et al. proposed a scheme of four electrodes, which is the most used today (Hoffer et al. 1969). The first equations for the estimation of body fluid volumes were based on linear regressions defined from height^2/resistance at 50 kHz. The regression parameters differed depending on the population group with which they were obtained (Kyle et al. 2004a). Subsequent equations included other components to improve the accuracy of the estimations, such as weight, age, gender, ethnicity or anthropometric measurements of trunk and/or limbs.

However, these methods are based on correlations and linear regression techniques; thus, they can only be used for the population group for which they were obtained, thereby showing wrong results in patients with irregular hydration states. Tomasset became the first to use the Cole-Cole model in order to differentiate between the extracellular water and the body water (Thommasset 1963). To do this, he chose two frequencies, 1 kHz and 100 kHz. As the electric resistance is related to the fluid volume that the current crosses, the extracellular water can be estimated at low frequencies and the total body water at high frequencies by using linear regression approaches. In 1992, the impedance spectroscopy technique was introduced (Matthie et al. 1992). This tecnique uses Cole model (Cole 1972) and Hanai's mixture theory in order to estimate the extracellular water and the body water, avoiding the population imbalances obtained by linear regression approaches. Since then, bioimpedance measurements have been broadly used to quantify body composition, estimate fluid volume and locate mass anatomy (muscles, fat, water) in certain parts of the body.

14.3 PHYSICAL PRINCIPLES OF BIOIMPEDANCE

The impedance (Z) is described as the opposition of a conductor to the flow of an alternating current (Grimnes and Martinsen 2000). It is defined as the ratio between a voltage and the electrical current that produces that voltage (Z = V/I) (see Fig. 14.3). This property depends on the frequency and the characteristics of the medium through which current flows.

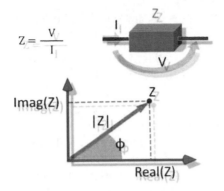

Fig. 14.3 Graphical representation of the impedance

Generically, the impedance is considered as a complex number consisting of the sum of a real part called resistance (R) and an imaginary part called reactance (X_C), both expressed in units of ohms. The parameter j is the imaginary unit, such that $j^2 = -1$.

$$Z = R + j \cdot X_C \qquad (14.1)$$

To show its features, in many cases we can find the value of the impedance plotted in vector form on a plane where the horizontal axis corresponds to the resistance and the vertical axis corresponds to the reactance. As we shall see in later sections, sometimes it is useful to express the impedance in polar coordinates, i.e. by specifying the module (|Z|) and phase (φ) of the impedance vector, whose values can be obtained from R and of X_C by the following equations:

$$|Z| = \sqrt{R^2 + X_C^2} \qquad (14.2)$$

$$\varphi = \tan^{-1}\left(\frac{R}{X_C} \right) \qquad (14.3)$$

When the impedance is related to a biological tissue, this property is also called bioimpedance (Grimnes and Martinsen 2000). The bioelectrical impedance in this case is evaluated through electrodes placed in different positions on the biological tissue or body section to be measured, by measuring the voltage response to a small excitation current. R is described as the opposition of the conductor to the flow of direct and alternating electrical current (DC and AC) and is equal to the inverse of the conductance (Buchholz et al. 2004). The other component, X_C, is inversely proportional to the capacitance and can be defined as the opposition to the passage of an alternating current.

There is an inseparable relationship between electricity and chemistry both in tissues and in cells. It is not possible to understand what is happening in a tissue during electrical current flow without considering the electrolytic theory. In a simple in vitro model, as a vessel containing an aqueous solution, the electrical current is carried by ions dissolved in a solution. Conductivity, or the amount of electricity that can be conducted, is directly proportional to the concentration of ions in the solution. Therefore, the resistance of the solution will increase if the concentration of ions is decreased (Buchholz et al. 2004). Other factors that increase the resistance are an augment in the viscosity of the solution, an increase in the concentration of non-conductive material, an enlargement of the distance between the electrodes (electrical path length), and a decrease of the cross-sectional area of the container. Factors such as temperature and elemental composition of ions also influence the resistance. Bioimpedance and its frequency dependence differ considerably between different tissues and cell suspensions. There are also significant changes in their electrical properties when cells or tissues pass from a physiological state to another, e.g. alive to dead, dry to hydrated or from normal to pathological.

The analysis by means of bioelectrical impedance is based on the principle that biological tissues behave as conductors of electric current and/or dielectric (insulator) depending on their composition (Piccoli 2002a). As the conductivity is directly proportional to the concentration of ions (electrolytes) present in fluids, electrolyte solutions of body fluids (blood, lymph, etc.) and all soft tissues (in particular non fatty tissues as muscles) are optimal electric conductors. Bone is not so easily crossed by electric currents and behaves as a poor conductor (insulator). In the adipose tissue, the current may flow through the interstitial electrolyte solutions and adipocytes, with the exception of the lipid droplets, which are hydrophobic and consequently do not conduct current. Therefore, bioimpedance can be considered as a measure of the ionic electrical conduction through soft tissue.

In order to simplify the study of bioimpedance, the human body can be conceptualized as a constant diameter cylinder whose length is the height (Kyle et al. 2004a). The resistance (R) of a homogeneous conductive material is proportional to its length and inversely proportional to its cross-sectional area (A) and conductivity (σ) of that material. According to the cylindrical model, the impedance of the human body would depend on the specific conductivity of the non-lipid tissue, its section and its length according to the following expression:

$$R = \frac{L}{\sigma A} \qquad (14.4)$$

There is another property related to the flow of electric current in materials, in addition to resistance or conductance: the permittivity. Permittivity is a physical property that is related to the material's ability to transmit an electric field (Gabriel et al. 1996a). In general, in dielectric materials, a decrease of permittivity with frequency is observed, due to the absorption of electromagnetic energy by the same materials. The largest energy losses are caused by the relaxation effects associated with molecular dipoles of the medium. At low frequencies, the field changes slowly enough to allow the dipoles to reach equilibrium before the field has reversed its polarity. For frequencies at which the orientations of the dipoles cannot follow the applied field due to the viscosity of the medium, a temporary delay is produced in the response of the medium and absorption of field energy, which is dissipated as heat.

Biological tissues also show dispersion effects as a result of the interaction of electromagnetic radiation with cellular and molecular components. The main dielectric characteristics of tissues as a function of frequency are well known and have already been presented by Foster and Schwan in 1989, showing that the dielectric spectrum of tissues is characterized by tree major dispersion regions where permittivity is decreased as the frequency increases (Gabriel et al. 1996a):

- α dispersion: low frequency in the range of 10 Hz up to 10 kHz, due particularly to the phenomena of ionic diffusion in the cell membrane.
- β dispersion: at intermediate frequencies (between 10 kHz and 100 MHz), it is associated with the polarization of cell membranes, but also contribute to polarization of proteins and other organic macromolecules.
- γ dispersion: about gigahertz, is mainly due to dipolar polarization of water molecules.

Each of these dispersion or relaxation regions (Lorenzo et al. 1997) (see Fig. 14.4) is a manifestation of a polarization mechanism characterized by a time constant (τ), which, in a first-order approximation gives the following expression for the relative complex permittivity (ε^{*}) as a function of angular frequency ($\omega = 2\pi\cdot$frequency):

$$\varepsilon^* = \varepsilon_\infty + \frac{\varepsilon_s - \varepsilon_\infty}{1 + j\omega\tau} \tag{14.5}$$

This is the well-known Debye expression (Gabriel et al. 1996b), where ε_∞ is the permittivity at infinite frequency and ε_s is the permittivity at zero frequency. The magnitude of the dispersion is described as $\Delta\varepsilon = \varepsilon_s - \varepsilon_\infty$. Hurt proposed in 1985 modeling the dielectric spectrum of tissues as the sum of five dispersions plus a conductivity term in which σ is the static ionic conductivity of the tissue and ε_0 is the permittivity in free space (Gabriel et al. 1996b):

$$\varepsilon^* = \varepsilon_\infty + \sum_{n=1}^{5} \frac{\Delta\varepsilon_n}{1 + j\omega\tau_n} + \frac{\sigma}{j\omega\varepsilon_0} \tag{14.6}$$

However, the complexity of both the structure and composition of biological materials is such that each dispersion region should be extended by introducing distribution parameters as defined in the Cole-Cole model for dispersions, with a tuning parameter $0 < a \le 1$,

$$\varepsilon^*(\omega) = \varepsilon_\infty + \frac{\Delta\varepsilon}{1 + (i\omega\tau)^a} \tag{14.7}$$

Finally, global tissue model would consist of the sum of the individual dispersions. As mentioned above, the β dispersion is in the range of low frequencies and is caused by cell membranes, whose behavior is similar to a capacitor. These capacitive effects occur when regions of high conductivity, such as ECW and ICW, are separated by regions of low conductivity, the cell membranes in this case, behaving then the regions of high conductivity as the plates of a capacitor (Buchholz et al. 2004).

Biological tissue consists of cells, which are separated by ECW and whose inner part is composed of ICW. At a frequency of 0 kHz (direct current), the "biological plates" can be charged, but no conduction current passes through the membrane capacitor. Thus, at very low frequencies, there will be minimal conduction through the cells due to the high impedance of the cell membrane (a capacitor at a low frequency has a very high impedance), and the conduction process is governed mainly by the properties of ECW, which are resistive in greater proportion due to the concentration

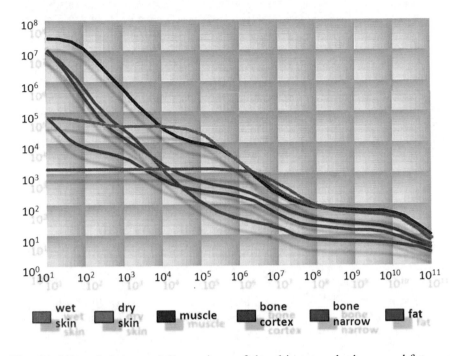

Fig. 14.4 Permittivity and dispersions of the skin, muscle, bone and fat as a function of frequency

of ions (see Fig.14.5). Current will flow in this case through the ECW around the cells, which will increase the electrical length of the path. The virtual increment in the length of the current path also increases the resistance of the medium. As the frequency of alternating current is progressively augmented, the capacitance of the membrane will be charged and uncharged, reducing the impedance of the membrane and allowing a small penetration of the current in the ICW compartment. This increases the area of cross section through which current flows and decreases the effective length of the current path. Thus, the impedance of the medium will reduce as the frequency augments, since the amount of conductor volume is increased. At high frequencies (> 5 MHz) the rate of loading and unloading of the membrane is such that the capacitive effect can be considered negligible (the capacity of the membrane is short-circuited) and current flows directly through the ICW and ECW compartments depending on the relative conductivity of these media. The impedance is almost exclusively composed of its term R (when frequency is high), which is also lower due to the higher effective area of the conductor.

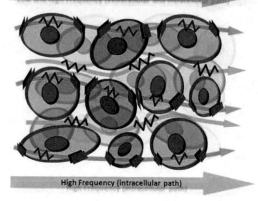

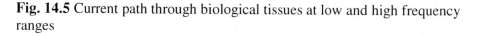

Fig. 14.5 Current path through biological tissues at low and high frequency ranges

The simplest model of this complex situation represents the current path into two parallel branches, one through extracellular fluids and another through the intracellular fluid (Cornish et al. 1993). The extracellular path is considered purely resistive while the intracellular path includes the capacitive effects in the cell membrane, so that the magnitude of the impedance of intracellular path is dependent on frequency. To model this behavior many electrical circuits have been used. Modeling is essential because it is the only way to independently analyze the individual components of a heterogeneous material system. In some models, the resistors and capacitors are in series, in others they are in parallel, but there are more complex configurations (Kyle et al. 2004a). The circuit used in a standard way to represent in vivo biological tissues is formed by a resistor to define the extracellular path of the current (R_e) placed in parallel with the second arm of the circuit that represents the path of intracellular current, which is a capacitance and a resistance (R_i) arranged in series (see Fig.14.6).

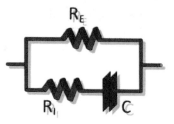

Fig. 14.6 Circuit model of a biological tissue

The relationship between the capacitances and resistances are interesting because they reproduce the different electrical properties of tissues which may be affected in different ways by disease, nutritional status and hydration status (Kyle et al. 2004a). The resistance is directly related to the fluids, while the reactance, which derives from the properties of the cell membrane, may be related to nutritional status. The impedance of a resistor is R and the impedance of a capacitor is $1/(j\omega C)$, and thus the impedance of the circuit in Fig. 14.6 corresponds to the following expression:

$$Z = \frac{R_e \left(R_i + \dfrac{1}{j\omega C} \right)}{R_e + R_i + \dfrac{1}{j\omega C}} \tag{14.8}$$

Multiplying the numerator and denominator by $j\omega(R_e+R_i)$ and rearranging the terms, the impedance can be expressed in terms of R_0 (resistance at zero frequency) and R_∞ (resistance at infinite frequency) as follows (Cornish et al. 1993):

$$Z = R_\infty + \frac{R_0 - R_\infty}{1 + j\omega\tau} \tag{14.9}$$

Where R_∞ is the parallel of the extracellular and intracellular resistances (R_e,R_i) and R_0 is equivalent to extracellular resistance (R_e),

$$R_\infty = \frac{R_i R_e}{R_i + R_e} , \quad R_0 = R_e \tag{14.10}$$

and τ represents the time constant of the circuit, which describes the dispersion due to the capacitive component, producing a dependence of the impedance as a function of frequency. For the circuit in Fig.14.6, the time constant has the following value:

$$\tau = \left(R_e + R_i \right)C \tag{14.11}$$

Separating the real and imaginary parts, the following expressions can be derived for the resistance (R) and reactance (X_c):

$$R = R_\infty + \frac{R_0 - R_\infty}{1 + \omega^2\tau^2} \tag{14.12}$$

$$X_C = -\frac{\omega\tau(R_0 - R_\infty)}{1 + \omega^2\tau^2} \tag{14.13}$$

Adding R^2 y X_C^2 and rearranging terms to eliminate the parameter $\omega\tau$, yields:

$$R^2 + X_C^2 - R(R_0 + R_\infty) + R_0 R_\infty = 0 \tag{14.14}$$

Which, in a representation of R in the x-axis and X_C in the y-axis, is the equation of a circle (Cornish et al. 1993) with center point in $((R_0+R_\infty)/2$, and radius $(R_0-R_\infty)/2$. The maximum of the reactance X_C corresponds to the value of ω for which the derivative of the reactance with respect to ω is equal to zero. This value of ω is called the characteristic angular frequency (ω_C), which in this case corresponds to the following expression:

$$\omega_C = \frac{1}{\tau} \tag{14.15}$$

To identify the parameters of the circuit model, an impedance diagram called Cole-Cole plot is typically used (De Lorenzo et al. 1999), which is a graphical representation of the resistance vs. the reactance depicted as in Fig. 14.7 (note that the reactance axis is negated for convenience). If we represent the impedance of the circuit model for each of the frequencies from zero to infinity, it is obtained a circular impedance curve whose shape is the result of electrical and structural characteristics of the tissue. At DC, capacitors act as insulators and all the current passes through the extracellular fluid. The zero-frequency impedance is completely resistive (R_0), standing on the real axis, and with the same value as R_e. If the circuit is excited with an electrical current at infinite frequency, the capacitor would act as a perfect conductor and the current would pass through both resistances, R_i and R_e, arranged in parallel, resulting in a completely resistive impedance (R_∞). As the frequency increases, the position of the impedance moves counter clock-wise along the semicircle from R_0 to R_∞.

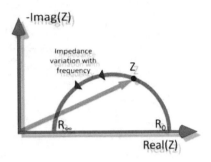

Fig. 14.7 Cole-Cole plot

The consequence of the capacitive behavior of cell membranes is that the extracellular resistance (R_e) should be measured at very low frequency (below 1 kHz) and the resistance of intracellular and extracellular media as a whole (R_∞) should be measured at very high frequency (above 5 MHz) (Jaffrin and Morel 2008). However, the application of DC or currents at very high frequency using electrodes placed on the skin is not allowed for practical reasons, so bioimpedance meters are limited in their application in the range from 5 kHz to 1 MHz. In this situation, R_e and R_∞ must be calculated by extrapolating the impedance for frequencies zero and infinity, respectively. This extrapolation can be easily made by observing the impedance semicircle in the Cole-Cole plane. R_0 corresponds to the intersection point farthest from the center of the impedance semicircle with the real axis, and R_∞ corresponds to the other point of intersection of the curve. The determination of R_0 and R_∞ is the first step in estimating body volume based on bioimpedance measurements.

In 1928, Cole found that the impedance measurements of biological materials had a circular shape, but its center was located below the axis of resistance (Cornish et al. 1993). The cause of this effect comes from the fact that cell membranes are not perfect capacitors and the great differences between tissue types and sizes of cells in biological organisms cause a distribution of the time constants. This behavior can be seen as the superposition of multiple dispersion effects of membranes, each one with different time constants, as shown in Fig. 14.8.

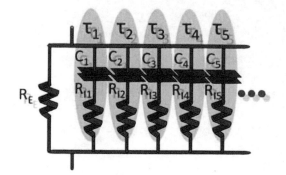

Fig. 14.8 Distribution of time constants

In 1941, Cole and Cole showed that, when there is a distribution of the time constants, the complex impedance can be represented by the following expression:

$$Z = R_\infty + \frac{R_0 - R_\infty}{1 + (j\omega\tau)^{(1-\alpha)}} \qquad (14.16)$$

where α $(0 \leq \alpha \leq 1)$ is a characteristic parameter of the distribution of relaxation frequencies due to the different structures in a heterogeneous material, and $\theta = (\pi/2)\,\alpha$ is the angle at which the center of the circle moves below the real axis, as it is shown in Fig. 14.9.

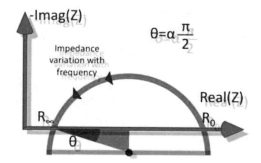

Fig. 14.9 Center displacement of the semicircle of impedance

An equivalent circuital for this impedance was proposed by Salter (1979) which is known as Salter's circuit model, which introduces a nonlinearity in the impedance of the membrane as shown in Fig. 14.10.

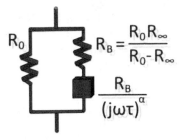

Fig. 14.10 Salter's circuit model

Finally, the Cole-Cole model was extended to introduce a time delay invariant with frequency (Td), which is due to many causes (De Lorenzo et al. 1995). This new component is modeled by a phase lag that increases linearly with frequency as shown in the following equation:

$$Z = \left(R_\infty + \frac{R_O - R_\infty}{1 + (j\omega\tau)^{(1-\alpha)}} \right) e^{-j\omega T_d} \qquad (14.17)$$

14.4 BIOIMPEDANCE INSTRUMENTATION BASICS

Bioimpedance measurement systems are based on injecting an oscillating signal at a certain frequency (usually an electric current) in the body under test and the measurement of the signal (usually voltage) that occurs as a result of the injection. According to Ohm's Law, the quotient between the voltage and current provides the impedance measurement of the body section. It is easier to build a current injector using current technology than a current detector with the same features and benefits. This is the reason why most applications developed by bioelectrical impedance analysis are performed by exciting the tissue with an alternating current and measuring the potential difference that it causes between the end points of the section under test. Moreover, given the interest in obtaining the impedance behavior as a function of frequency, many of impedance analyzers are capable of generating currents and measurement voltages at multiple frequencies, what implies an increase in the complexity of the instrumentation.

Since bioimpedance analyzers inject an electrical current inside the human body, they must comply strictly with the national and international security regulations, avoiding any interference with pacemakers or other biomedical equipments (Piccoli 2002a). Furthermore, to avoid any possible adverse effects in the health of exposed individuals as well as any interference with the user biological signals, electromagnetic exposures from the devices must be within the safety limits set by the international and national laws (ICNIRP 1998, 2009). For this reason, commercial devices typically inject a current density lower than 1 mA/cm^2.

In a system of biological impedance measurement, one of the most critical parts is the electrodes. Their function is to provide an electrochemical interface between the tissue and the electronic measurement subsystem, both for current injection and voltage detection. The electrodes are indispensable, but the dispersion in the impedance values that they present, the introduced noise, fluctuations and contact problems make them one of the most variable parameters, that can become a serious problem. The electrode-skin contact consists of a metal electrode, an electrolytic gel (usually containing Cl⁻) and human skin (see Fig.14.11). One of the most common types is Ag-AgCl electrodes with an electrolyte containing Cl⁻ (Webster 2009). Its popularity is mainly due to two major advantages. The first is that it generates very little noise, less than 10 uV. The second is that they are virtually impossible to be polarized, so that the current flows freely through the electrode union. A polarizable electrode would behave like a capacitor and current would not ease through the electrode union.

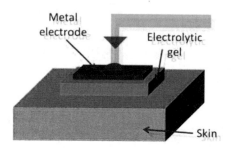

Fig. 14.11 Elements that constitute an electrode

For many applications, the electrode interface can be modeled as a source of offset voltage with in-series impedance (Webster 2009) (see Fig.14.12). The offset voltage is due to the double layer potential between the electrode and the electrolyte, and between the electrolyte and the skin. The impedance consists of a parallel RC circuit (R_d and C_d) in series with a resistance (R_s). R_d represents the conduction currents resulting from the double layer of ionic charge on the electrode-electrolyte interface. C_d represents the displacement currents. Resistance R_s is associated with the losses due to conduction in the electrolyte. The range of impedances can be from hundreds of ohms to several megaohms, depending on the frequency of the electrical signal that is flowing.

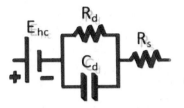

Fig. 14.12 Circuit model of an electrode

Once the current has been injected into the human body, bioimpedance measurements can be performed in two different configurations, depending on the number of electrodes, giving rise to two possibilities in measurement systems: 2 electrodes and 4 electrodes (Neves and Souza 2001). In the first case, the current is injected through two electrodes and the voltage is measured from the same 2 electrodes. The impedance is then determined by dividing the measured voltage over the injected current. However, the most common methods for measuring bioimpedance use the configuration of four electrodes, in which an alternating current of very low intensity (imperceptible to the subject) is passed through the electrodes further away (distal). The voltage drop along the section of the body is measured using the voltage sensing electrodes (proximal), placed a short distance from the distal electrodes (see Fig. 14.13). The impedance is then determined by dividing the voltage measured at the proximal electrodes over the current injected through the distal electrodes. In the configuration of two electrodes,

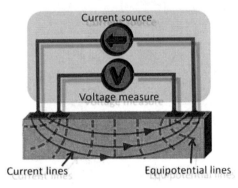

Fig. 14.13 Scheme of a four electrodes system

the impedance between the skin and the electrode is in series with the impedance of the body, and thus it is not easy to separate the two impedances to derive the correct value of the bioimpedance.

In a configuration of four electrodes, the impedance input of a pre-amplifier, which measures the voltage difference in the proximal electrodes, is typically much larger than the impedance of the electrodes (Neves and Souza 2001). Thus, the impedance of the electrodes can be neglected in the bioimpedance analysis, because the voltage across the electrodes is much lower than that observed at the pre-amplifier input.

There are two basic techniques for measuring the impedance of biological tissues: the method of the impedances bridge and the phase detection method (Songer 2001), although other alternatives have also been proposed based on the response to pulses (Min et al. 2004) or white noise (Kennedy 2006), as opposed to sinusoidal current excitation. Both the impedance bridge method and the phase detection method can be used either in a configuration of two electrodes or with four electrodes, although for both techniques it is recommended the tetrapolar configuration.

In the impedance bridge method, the biological tissue or body section is situated in an impedance bridge as shown in Fig.14.14. Biological impedance is represented by Z_B. The impedances Z_2 and Z_3 are known and the impedance of Z_1 is modified automatically until no current flows through M, which occurs when the terminals of M have the same voltage. Z_B can then be calculated by using the following equation:

$$Z_B = \frac{Z_3 Z_1}{Z_2}$$
(14.18)

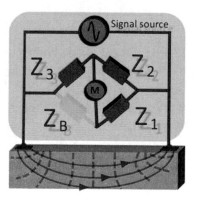

Fig. 14.14 The impedance bridge method

The phase detection method has many advantages over the impedance bridge method, such as its greater accuracy in the entire frequency range, speed and simplicity. For these reasons, the phase detection method has become the most widely used in bioimpedance measurement systems. Fig. 14.15 shows the basic structure of a bioelectrical impedance meter based on phase detection method for a configuration of four electrodes. As the input impedance of the instrumentation amplifier is very high, no current flows virtually by the sensing electrode, so that the tissue impedance measurements are not affected by the electrode contact impedance, which can be neglected compared to the impedance of the tissue.

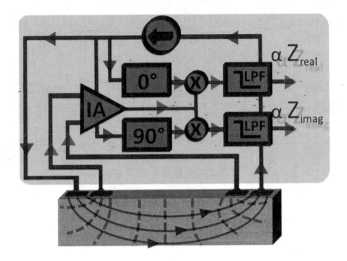

Fig. 14.15 Phase detection method

The basic principle of this approach is based on two coherent demodulations of the input voltage signal (Yang and Wang 2005) (see Fig. 14.15). The voltage between the electrodes as a function of time can be represented as $V_{IN}(t) = Z \cdot I \cdot \sin(\omega_0 t + \theta)$ where I is the amplitude of the current source, which is known, Z is the module and θ is the phase of the biompedance. At the output of the instrumentation amplifier, voltage can be represented as $V(t) = V \cdot \sin(\omega_0 t + \theta)$ and according to the trigonometric relations, also as $V(t) = V \cdot \cos(\theta) \cdot \sin(\omega_0 t) + V \cdot \sin(\theta) \cdot \cos(\omega_0 t)$. The value of V can be determined through an analog to digital converter (ADC). The signal $V(t)$ is then divided into two lines, and multiplied in one of these lines with a signal in phase with the original reference signal, represented as U·sin ($\omega_0 t$) and a quadrature signal with the signal original reference in the other line, which is represented as U·cos ($\omega_0 t$). The signals from each of the lines are demodulated through a low pass filter, so that DC components obtained at the output of the demodulators are proportional to the functions $\cos(\theta)$ and $\sin(\theta)$ respectively. Thus, these signals are proportional to the resistive and reactive impedance, respectively, since the real part of impedance is proportional to V·$\cos(\theta)$/I and the imaginary part of impedance is proportional to V·$\sin(\theta)$/I. Their values are also obtained through analog-to-digital conversion for subsequent processing.

One might add that these bioimpedance analyzers do not measure body composition directly. Instead, the real and imaginary parts (or the module and phase) of the measured impedance during the analysis are then processed and mathematical models are used to obtain one or more components related to body composition. These methods will be studied in detail in the next section.

14.5 BIOIMPEDANCE MEASUREMENT TECHNIQUES

In a typical application of bioimpedance, a current is injected into the user through a pair of electrodes called distal electrodes, one placed on the hand over the third metacarpophalangeal joint, and another on the foot over the third metatarsophalangeal joint (Chamney et al. 2002). A pair of additional electrodes, called proximal electrodes, are located one on the wrist (over the carpus) and another on the ankle (tibio-tarsal) to measure the potential difference between them as it is shown in the global lateral configuration of Fig. 14.16. To avoid interference between different sections of the body and obtain accurate enough impedance values, it is recommended that measurements are carried out with the body in supine position, remaining at rest for several minutes before the measurements to establish an equilibrium in the body fluids, with legs apart about 45° one from the other and arms away 30° from the body.

It is possible to obtain measurements of other body segments through variants of the global lateral configuration, as proposed by Patterson in (Patterson 1989) and represented in Fig. 14.16. Thus, keeping the location of the current injector electrodes and the voltage detector electrodes on hands and feet, changing their configuration it is possible to measure the impedance along the two arms, one arm, trunk, left leg or right leg.

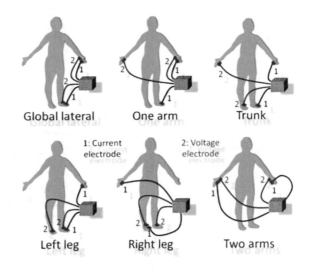

Fig. 14.16 Different configurations in the position of electrodes for segmental analysis

As shown above, once the values of impedance of the body section are known in magnitude and phase it is possible to derive the resistance values of the extracellular compartment (R_E) and the intracellular compartment (R_I). These resistances depend on the volume of fluids and tissue composition of the respective compartments. The values of ECW and ICW can then be derived by combining these resistances with the resistivity constant of the tissues. From the estimation of these volumes it is possible to determine other parameters of body composition. Some equations are purely empirical, while others are based on models of the electrochemical conductance of the tissues. The following subsections outline the different approaches that have been applied to measurements of body water and compartmental composition based on bioimpedance measurements at one or multiple frequencies.

14.5.1 Single Frequency Bioimpedance Analysis (SFBIA)

As explained in section 14.3, if the human body is modeled as a cylinder with uniform cross section and as an isotropic conductor with conductivity σ, the value of its resistance can be obtained by the following expression:

$$R = \frac{\text{Height}}{\sigma \text{Area}} = \frac{\text{Length}^2}{\sigma \, \text{Volume}} \tag{14.19}$$

From Eq. (14.19), Hoffer et al. derived the basic model of electrical bio-impedance, which is widely used today (Buchholz 2004).

$$\text{Volume} = \frac{\text{Length}^2}{\sigma R} \tag{14.20}$$

Although the body is not a uniform cylinder and its conductivity is not constant, an empirical relationship can be established between the ratio ($Length^2/R$) and the water volume, which contains electrolytes that can conduct electrical current through the body (Kyle et al. 2004a). In applications of body composition height is commonly used rather than length. These approaches based on empirical relationships with impedance values obtained at a single frequency are generically referred to as Single Frequency Bioelectrical Impedance Analysis (SFBIA). These empirical equations are usually based on measurements at 50 kHz, with surface electrodes placed on the hand and foot. The frequency of 50 kHz is considered as the standard frequency for bioimpedance measurements (Cornish et al. 1993). At this frequency, current passes through the extracellular and intracellular fluids, although the proportion of current that flows through the two compartments varies from one tissue to another. Many authors suggest that the frequency of 5 kHz is the best for ECW estimations using relationships as $Height^2/R_{5kHz}$, since at these frequencies the current passes predominantly through the extracellular fluid; however, to calculate TBW the optimal frequency is 100 kHz (Cornish et al. 1993). In this sense, the intermediate frequency of 50 kHz is considered adequate for the estimation of both TBW and ECW. The different SFBIA methods are generally based on linearizations obtained by regression lines that are specific for a given population with similar anthropometric characteristics. These expressions relate the parameter $Height^2/R$ with water volumes obtained by dissolution methods, resulting expressions of the following fashion (Buchholz et al. 2004):

$$\text{TBW}(L) = A\frac{\text{Height}^2}{R} + B \tag{14.21}$$

Where A corresponds with the slope and B the intercept of the population group regression line according to weight, age and sometimes sex. The X_C term is usually ignored because it represents a negligible impedance at 50 kHz ($< 4\%$). Table 14.1 shows some of the empirical relationships proposed in the literature for the estimation of TBW (Kyle et al. 2004a) (Jaffrin and Morel 2008).

Table 14.1 Examples of SFBIA equations for TBW estimation

TBW (liters) Equations
$0.5561 \times Height(cm)^2/R_{50kHz}$ (ohm) $+ 0.0955 \times Weight(kg) + 1.726$ For Men and women, obese and non-obese   (Kushner et al. 1986)
$0.446 \times Height(cm)^2/R_{50kHz}$ (ohm) $+ 0.126 \times Weight (kg) + 5.82$ For Women and men, surgical patients   (Hannan et al. 1994)
Women: $6.53 + 0.3674 \times Height(cm)^2/Z_{50kHz}$ (ohm) $+ 0.1753 \times$ Weight (kg) $- 0.11 \times Age$ (years)   Men: TBW(Women) + 2.83   For Men and women, 7-83 years, large   (Deurenberg et al. 1991)   variation body composition
Men: $1.02 + 0.449\ Height(cm)^2/R_{50kHz}$ (ohm) $+ 0.176\ Weight(kg)$ Women: $3.747 + 0.45\ Height(cm)^2/R_{50kHz}$ (ohm) $+ 0.113\ Weight(kg)$ For Healthy subjects,12-94 years   (Sun et al. 2003)

The same regression procedure has been also used for the estimation of ECW. Table 14.2 contains two of the equations proposed by different authors. There are anthropometric regression equations for ICW calculations as well (Table 14.3), although once TBW and ECW are known, the value of ICW can be obtained since TBW=ECW+ICW. FFM can also be obtained from TBW assuming that FFM is hydrated in a 73.2% rate (TBW=0.732·FFM), as proposed in numerous studies, although population approaches have also been made by regression techniques (Table 14.4). In order to calculate body fat, anthropometric estimations based on measurements of bioimpedance have been proposed as well (Table 14.5).

Table 14.2 Examples of SFBIA equations for ECW estimation

ECW (liters) Equations
$0.0119 \times Height\ (cm)^2/X_{50kHz}$(ohm) $+ 0.123 \times Height\ (cm)^2/R_{50kHz}$ (ohm) $+ 6.15$ For Heterogeneous group of surgical   (Hannan et al. 1995)   patients (women and men)
Men: $-5.22 + 0.2 \times Height(cm)^2/R_{50kHz}$ (ohm) $+ 0.005 \times Height(cm)^2/X_{50kHz}$ (ohm) $+ 0.08 \times Weight (kg) + 1.9$ Women: ECW (Men) + 1.86   For Men and woman, healthy subjects,   (Sergi et al. 1994)   chronic heart failure, chronic renal failure

Table 14.3 Example of SFBIA equation for ICW estimation

ICW (liters) Equations
Women: $9.182 + 20.285 \times$ Height $(cm)^2/|Z|_{5kHz}$ (ohm) $+ 7.114$ (Phase angle)
Men: ICW(Women) $+ 2.113$
For Elderly (60-80 years)   (Dittmar and Reber 2002)

Table 14.4 Examples of SFBIA equations for FFM estimation

FFM (kg) Equations
Women: $-4.104 + 0.518 \times$ Height$(cm)^2/R_{50kHz}$ (ohm) $+ 0.231 \times$ Weight(kg) $+ 0.13 \times X_{C50kHz}$
Men: FFM (Women) $+ 4.229$
For Healthy adults (18-94 years)   (Kyle et al. 2001)
Women: $-12.44 + 0.34 \times$ Height$(cm)^2/R_{50kHz}$ (ohm) $+ 0.1534 \times$ Height (cm) $+ 0.273 \times$ Weight(kg) $- 0.127 \times$ Age (years)
Men: FFM (Women) $+ 4.56$
For Healthy adults (>16 years)   (Deurenberg et al. 1991)

Table 14.5 Example of SFBIA equation for % body fat estimation

Body Fat (% of the Weight) Equations
Women: $14.94 - 0.079 \times$ Height $(cm)^2/R_{50kHz}$ (ohm) $+ 0.818 \times$ Weight (kg) $- 0.231 \times$ Height (cm) $+ 0.077 \times$ Age (years)
Men: Body Fat (Men) $- 0.064 \times$ Weight (kg)
For Healthy subjects (35-65 years)   (Heitmann et al. 1990a, b)

14.5.2 Multi Frequency Bioimpedance Analysis (MFBIA)

Some studies have suggested that the frequency of 50 kHz may not be ideal to estimate body composition (Buchholz et al. 2004). However, at 50 kHz, the path of the electrical current is mainly extracellular, with some unknown penetration into the intracellular compartment. Although it is the resistance of body fluids and not the capacitance what is related to the water volume, both resistance and capacitance of the tissues affect the values of the measured resistance and reactance. Therefore, the capacitive effects of the measured values cannot be excluded. This led many researchers to reconsider which frequencies were the most suitable to detect and differentiate between ECW and TBW.

According to this approach, impedance measurements at low frequency, such as 1 or 5 kHz, can be used to estimate ECW because penetration of currents in ICW is negligible at such low frequencies. The resistance measured at low frequency can be interpreted as the extracellular resistance ($R_0=R_E$). At higher frequencies, like 100, 500 or 1,000 kHz, current passes through the cell membrane and impedance measurements can be used to estimate TBW, considering that the current penetrates almost completely into the cell (Earthman et al. 2007). The measured resistance at high frequency can be interpreted as the total resistance (R_∞, which is the shunt resistance of the intra and extracellular paths).

Multi Frequency Bioelectrical Impedance Analysis (MFBIA) was used for the first time by Tomasset, who proposed the use of impedance values measured at two different frequencies: one at a very low frequency (normally 1 or 5 kHz) and another at a very high frequency (usually 50, 100, 200, 500 kHz or 1 MHz). These impedances at different frequencies are applied to empirical models of linear regression to estimate TBW y el ECW. Intracellular water volume is usually calculated as the difference between TBW and ECW. Table 14.6 shows two examples of MFBIA equations proposed by different authors for the body composition analysis (Kyle et al. 2004a).

Table 14.6 Examples of MFBIA equations for ECW and TBW estimations.

ECW (liters) Equations
$5.75 + 0.01 \times \text{Height (cm)}^2/X_{C50kHz}$ (ohm) $+ 0.165 \times \text{Height (cm)}^2/R_{5kHz}$ (ohm)
For Surgical patients   (Hannan et al. 1994)
TBW (liters)
$23.1898 + 0.0154 \times (\text{Body volume}/Z_{1kHz}) + 0.3315 \times (\text{Body volume}/Z_{1kHz})(Z_{1kHz} - Z_{100kHz})/(Z_{1kHz} \, Z_{100kHz})$
For Obese woman   (De Lorenzo et al. 1999)

14.5.3 Bioimpedance Spectroscopy (BIS)

The Bioimpedance Spectroscopy method (BIS) is based on bioimpedance measurements at multiple frequencies and in the correspondence of the measured values with the parameters of Cole-Cole model (Moissl et al. 2006). This method has more solid theoretical foundations than SFBIA and MFBIA, due to the incorporation of the physical principles that derive from bioimpedance measurements. As MFBIA, the determination of body fluid volumes is based on the fact that low-frequency electric current does not penetrate cell membranes, so it flows only within the ECW compartment, while high-frequency current flows through both the ECW and ICW compartments. Therefore, the resistance at low and high frequencies are related to ECW and TBW, respectively. Thus, the main current path at low frequencies is the ECW and at high frequencies is the TBW.

14.5.3.1 BIS Based on the Cole-Cole Model

When the resistance and reactance of each of the frequencies generated by the impedance analyzer are graphically represented, the result is a locus with a semicircular shape (Cornish et al. 1993). Due to technical and safety reasons, bioimpedance meters using surface electrodes are usually limited in its application to the frequency range from 5 kHz to 1 MHz, so that the resistance of ECW (R_e) and TBW (R_∞) must be calculated by extrapolation to zero and infinite frequency, respectively (Buchholz et al. 2004) (see Fig. 14.17). A processing algorithm calculates the curve that best fits the shape of the impedance.

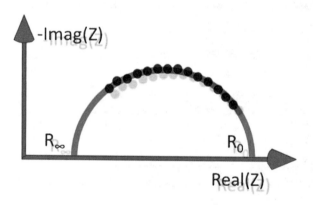

Fig. 14.17 Extrapolation of the curve that best fits the shape of the impedance

The point of intersection of the curve farthest from the center of the diagram corresponds to the impedance at zero frequency and is equivalent to the resistance of extracellular fluid (R_{ECW}). The point of intersection of the curve with the horizontal axis closer to the infinite frequency is equivalent to the resistance of TBW (R_{TBW}). At infinite frequency the circuit model can be seen as the parallel between R_{ECW} and R_{ICW}, whose value corresponds to R_{TBW}, so the value of R_{ICW} can be derived from the other two:

$$R_{ECW} = R_0; \quad R_{TBW} = R_\infty; \quad R_{ICW} = \frac{R_{TBW}R_{ECW}}{R_{ECW} - R_{TBW}} \quad (14.22)$$

R_{ECW} and R_{ICW} values are estimated by means of regression to ECW and TBW values obtained by dissolution techniques to produce Cole-Cole linear equations as shown in Table 14.7 (Kyle et al. 2004a):

Table 14.7 Examples of regressed BIS equations for ECW and ECW estimations

ECW (liters)
-3.511 + 0.351 × Height $(cm)^2/R_{ECW}$ (ohm) + 0.05 × Weight (kg)   For Healthy (obese and non-obese)   (Cox-Reijven et al. 2000)
ICW (liters)
12.2 + 0.37065 × Height $(cm)^2/R_{ICW}$ (ohm) + 0.105 × Weight (kg) – 0.132 × age (years)   For Healthy men (23-53 years)   (De Lorenzo et al. 1995)

14.5.3.2 BIS Based on Hanai Mixture Theory

The major drawback of the methods of analysis based on equations of the type Volume = K_1*Height$^2/R + K_2$, with K_1 and K_2 parameters obtained empirically, is that these equations can be applied only to populations for which they were defined not be adequate for altered states of hydration or body composition (Moissl et al. 2006). If these equations are applied to populations different than the specifically used for their production, or with different hydration, different proportions of fat mass or other anatomical geometries, significant errors arise from the assumption of a constant resistivity and geometry. For this reason, the multifrequency model of Cole-Cole was extended with the application of the Hanai mixture theory to in-vivo systems. Mixture theory describes the effect that a concentration of a non-conductive material produces in the effective resistivity of surrounding conductive tissue. According to this theory, the effective conductivity of the material would be modified according to the following expression, where c is the non-conductive fraction of the volume (Lorenzo et al. 1997):

$$\rho ef = \frac{\rho}{(1-c)^{\frac{3}{2}}} \quad (14.23)$$

By applying the mixtures theory of Hanai, the human body is considered as a superposition of a conductive medium (water, electrolytes, soft
tissue, etc.) and a non-conductive (bone, fat, air, etc.). If the human body is
modeled as a cylinder of resistivity ρ ($\rho = 1 / \sigma$), the resistance value can
be expressed as:

$$R = \rho \frac{\text{Height}}{\text{Area}} = \rho \frac{\text{Height}^2}{\text{Volume}} \qquad (14.24)$$

A correction factor K_B is applied to this equation to adjust the cylindrical geometry to the human body form.

$$R = K_B \rho \frac{\text{Height}^2}{\text{Volume}} \qquad (14.25)$$

In Van Loan et al (1993), the value 4.3 is proposed for K_B for a model
consisting of five cylinders (trunk and extremities) from statistical anatomical measurements in adults. This geometric correction and Hanai mixture
theory can be used to predict in a more direct way the ECW and ICW volumes from values and R_{ECW} y R_{ICW}. These modifications improve the
Cole-Cole model by introducing the effects of non-conductive substances
in body water, eliminating the apparent population specificity found in the
regression equations and improving its sensitivity to changes in body hydration status. Furthermore, no assumptions as 73.2% of hydration of FFM
or a uniform distribution of ICW and ECW are done, which may not be
right in disease states such as severe diarrhea or patients on dialysis.

14.5.3.2.1 Determination of the ECW

For a zero frequency, all the current passes through the outer of cells, so
that the variable c in the expression of Hanai takes the value (Jaffrin and
Morel 2008):

$$c = \frac{\text{Total Volume} - \text{Extracellular Volume}}{\text{Total Volume}} \qquad (14.26)$$

If we refer to ρ_{ECW} as the resistivity of the medium at zero frequency
(ECW), the effective resistivity according to the Hanai mixture theory is:

$$\rho_{\text{ECWef}} = \rho_{\text{ECW}} \left(\frac{\text{Total Volume}}{\text{Extracellular Volume}} \right) \qquad (14.27)$$

The value of resistance in this case corresponds to the extracellular resistance (R_{ECW}) and replacing the value of the previous resistivity in the equation the following expression is obtained:

$$R_{ECW} = \frac{\text{Total Volume}^{\frac{1}{2}} \rho_{ECW}}{\text{Extracellular Volume}^{\frac{3}{2}}} K_B \text{Height}^2 \qquad (14.28)$$

If the total volume is replaced by the ratio $Weight/Density_{Body}$, where $Weight$ is body weight and $Density_{Body}$ is the body density, then the ECW volume can be expressed as:

$$\text{Extracellular Volume} = \text{ECW} = K_{ECW}\left(\frac{\text{Height}^2 \text{Weight}^{\frac{1}{2}}}{R_{ECW}}\right)^{\frac{2}{3}} \qquad (14.29)$$

With the extracellular volume expressed in liters, the height in centimeters, body density in kg/l and the resistivity in ohm * cm, K_{ECW} takes the following expression (the scale factor of 10^{-2} is introduced to correct the result with the units above):

$$K_{ECW} = 10^{-2}\left(\frac{K_B \rho_{ECW}}{\text{Density}_{Body}^{\frac{1}{2}}}\right)^{\frac{2}{3}} \qquad (14.30)$$

Comparing the results with ECW values obtained by the technique of bromide solution, the authors of (Van Loan et al. 1993) proposed a K_{ECW} value equal to 0.306 for men and 0.316 for women. Body density value equal to 1.05 Kg/l and K_B equal to 4 were considered. These values are also used in the equations shown below.

14.5.3.2.2 Determination of the TWB

TBW can also be calculated by using the same method as for ECW (Jaffrin and Morel 2008). Therefore the volume of TBW was considered as an electrically homogeneous fluid on the macroscopic scale. Thus, for an infinite frequency, there would be an expression similar to Eq. (14.29), but for TBW and the resistivity at infinite frequency:

$$TBW = K_\infty \left(\frac{Height^2 Weight}{R_\infty} \right)^{2/3}$$
(14.31)

K_∞ takes the following expression:

$$K_\infty = 10^{-2} \left(\frac{Height^2 Weight}{R_\infty} \right)^{2/3}$$
(14.32)

A resistivity of 104.3 ohm cm for men and 100.5 ohm cm for women were found comparing the TBW estimated by this technique with the volumes obtained in a healthy population with the reference methods (Jaffrin and Morel 2008). The average error in the estimates with respect to the reference method was 0.79 liters, and applying the method in patients on hemodialysis was possible to estimate the ultrafiltration volume with an error of 9%.

14.5.3.2.3 A Modification of the Method (Two Conductive Fluid in the Equation of Hanai)

To provide a better approach, it would be necessary to consider separately the paths of intracellular and extracellular current, which have different resistivities (Jaffrin and Morel 2008; Moissl et al. 2006). From the Hanai mixtures equation for two conductive fluids, Matthie (Matthie 2005) obtained the following expression for the resistivity at infinite frequency whereas a conductive fluid is the ECW and the other is the ICW:

$$\rho_\infty = \rho_{TBW} = (\rho_{ICW} - \rho_{ECW}) \left(\frac{R_{TBW}}{R_{ECW}} \right)^{2/3}$$
(14.33)

From this value of resistivity and considering that the TBW is the sum of ICW and ECW the following expressions of volume could be obtained:

$$ECW = \left(\frac{K_b \rho_{ECW}}{D_b^{1/2}} \right)^{2/3} \left(\frac{Height^2 Weight^{1/2}}{R_{ECW}} \right)^{2/3}$$
(14.34)

$$ICW = ECW \left(\left(\frac{\rho_{TBW} R_{ECW}}{\rho_{ECW} R_{TBW}} \right)^{2/3} - 1 \right)$$
(14.35)

This method is implemented in the Xitron Hydra 4200 multi-frequency bioimpedance meter of Xitron Technologies with values: ρ_{ICW}=273.9 ohm cm and ρ_{ECW}=40.5 ohm cm for men and ρ_{ICW}=264.9 ohm cm and ρ_{ECW}=39.0 ohm cm for women.

14.5.3.2.4 Modification of the Method BIS (Adapted to Body Mass Index)

The previous method shows systematic errors in the difference between estimated fluid volumes and reference values for subjects with extreme values of body mass index (BMI). To correct these differences, Moissl et al proposed a modification of the BIS method based on Hanai mixture theory (Moissl et al. 2006), but adapting the parameters of the equations in terms of BMI to take into account the personal morphology of the subject, and in particular, the proportion of fatty tissues. This method is based on the equations for calculating ECW and ICW already seen:

$$ECW = K_{ECW} \left(\frac{Height^2 Weight^{1/2}}{R_O} \right)^{2/3} \tag{14.36}$$

$$ICW = K_{ICW} \left(\frac{Height^2 Weight^{1/2}}{R_I} \right)^{2/3} \tag{14.37}$$

But with K_{ECW} and K_{ICW} as a function of the *BMI*:

$$K_{ECW} = \frac{a}{BMI} + b; \quad K_{ICW} = \frac{C}{BMI} + d \tag{14.38}$$

From a population of 120 healthy subjects and 32 renal patients, the following values were obtained for the parameters: a = 0.188, b = 0.2883, c = 5.8758, d = 0.4194, comparing to the reference values obtained using methods of solution of bromide. Results showed fewer errors in the determination of the ICW and TBW compared with other BIS methods in both healthy population and renal patients.

14.5.4 Segmental Bioelectrical Impedance Analysis

In the clinical setting, the analysis by bioimpedance is normally based on a hand-foot tetrapolar configuration modeling the human body as a cylindrical conductor of constant cross section (Nescolarde et al. 2008). This hypothesis fails because it ignores differential aspects as the proportion of fat, hydration or different anatomical forms. Due to this, many authors have proposed localized bioimpedance analysis on well-defined body segments to minimize modeling errors (Kyle et al. 2004a). It would be reasonable to think that segmental measurements on arms, legs and trunk can reduce electrical modeling errors against measurements of the whole body, as a cylindrical model provides a closer approximation for one segment than for the entire body.

Many researchers prefer to see the human body as a structure consisting of five cylinders (two arms, two legs and trunk) with different areas for cross sections, which are connected by an in-series configuration (Buchholz et al. 2004). Since the resistance is inversely proportional to the cross-sectional area, the resistance of the whole body mainly depends on the resistance of the extremities, which have lower cross-sections than the trunk. Thus, total volume of ECW and ICW is calculated as the sum of segmental volumes obtained from localized bioimpedance measurements. From the total volumes of ECW and ICW, the value of TBW be could derived (Zhu et al. 2006).

$$ECW = 2\left(ECW_{ARM} + ECW_{LEG}\right) + EGM_{TRUNK} \qquad (14.39)$$

$$ICW = 2\left(ICW_{ARM} + ICW_{LEG}\right) + ICW_{TRUNK} \qquad (14.40)$$

$$TBW = ECW + ICW \qquad (14.41)$$

Some studies assume that the resistivity of the segments is constant; however, it has been proven that the use of specific resistivity for each of the segments improves the estimation of fluid volumes in hemodialysis patients. Since total volumes of ECW and ICW estimated by segmental bioimpedance do not include fluids in hands, feet, head and neck, due to the location of the electrodes, final results should be corrected to add the fractions of hydration of each of them (Zhu et al. 2006).

14.5.5 Bioelectrical Impedance Vector Analysis (BIVA)

The method of Bioelectrical Impedance Vector Analysis (BIVA) was developed by Piccoli et al. as a technique for body composition estimate independently of the body weight and anthropometric characteristics of the user (Piccoli et al. 1994). BIVA allows a direct assessment of the patient from bioimpedance measurements, not depending on equations or models.

In addition, direct analysis of bioimpedance measurements avoids errors due to regression approaches or model limitations (Piccoli et al. 2002b). The BIVA method is based on measurements of the complex electrical impedance, usually at 50 kHz, between the right hand and the right foot (if it is possible this configuration). The components of the impedance vector, i.e., resistance R and reactance X_C (in absolute value), are normalized by the subject's height (R/height y X_C/height) and represented in a plot with R/height in the x-axis and X_C/height in the y-axis (Nescolarde et al. 2004). Due to the correlations between R and X_C an ellipsoidal shape is established for the distribution of impedances of the different subjects on the plane R-X_C, which is known as R-Xc graph.

If R/Height and X_C/Height are considered as two variables of normal (gaussian) bivariate distribution and impedance values corresponding to a healthy population are taken as a reference, three reference percentiles or tolerance ellipses (50%, 75% and 95%) can be established. These ellipses are gender specific, representing the zone where the normal impedance values are distributed. They indicate the probability interval within which a specific proportion of a population will fall with a fixed probability of 100%. From the impedance values of a reference population it is possible to calculate the lengths of the semiaxis of the tolerance ellipses (L_1 and L_2) and theirs slopes (b_1 y b_2) using the following equations (Piccoli et al. 1994):

$$K = \frac{F_a(n+1)}{n(n-2)}$$

$$L_1, L_2 = \sqrt{K}\sqrt{(n-1)\left(s_x^2 + s_y^2\right) + \sqrt{\left[(n-1)\left(s_x^2 + s_y^2\right)\right]^2 \pm 4(n-1)^2\left(1-r^2\right)s_x^2 s_y^2}}$$

$$b_1 = \frac{\left(s_y^2 - s_x^2\right)}{2rs_x s_y} + \sqrt{1 + \left[\frac{\left(s_y^2 - s_x^2\right)}{2rs_x s_y}\right]^2}, \qquad b_2 = \frac{-1}{b_1}$$

$$\text{inclination} = \tan^{-1}(b_i), i = 1, 2$$

$$(14.42)$$

With s_x and s_y denoting the sample standard deviations in each of the axes, r for the correlation coefficient, α for the level of probability ($\alpha=0.05$, 0.25, and 0.50 for 95%, 75%, and 50% tolerance ellipses, respectively), and F_α for the value of the Snedecor's F with 2 and n-2 degrees of freedom and a probability α.

Piccoli established in (Piccoli et al. 1994) reference ellipses in a study of a healthy Italian population. Since then, numerous reference ellipses have been proposed for different population groups in order to provide more accurate results, as the shape, position and orientation of the ellipses vary by race, age and body size. In Table 14.8 it is shown as an example the parameters of the ellipses for the Italian population presented in (Piccoli et al. 1994) and other proposed later for different population groups (Espinosa-Cuevas 2007; Piccoli et al. 2002b).

Table 14.8 Examples of regressed BIS equations for ECW and ECW estimations

	CENTER			MAJOR AXIS				MINOR AXIS		
	R/H	X/H	I_1 (°)	Semiaxis L1			I_2 (°)	Semiaxis L2		
				95%	75%	50%		95%	75%	50%
Italian population										
Men	298.6	30.8	69.3	187	127	89	-20.7	89	61	43
Women	371.9	34.4	69.27	199	135	95	-20.73	105	71	50
U.S. population, non-Hispanic, Caucasian										
Men	277.2	38.1	68.68	161	110	77	-21.32	62	42	30
Women	372.9	46.9	64.58	189	129	91	-25.42	79	54	38
U.S. population, non-Hispanic, Afro-American										
Men	282.9	41.4	68.42	183	124	88	-21.58	67	45	32
Women	372.5	50.6	65.88	218	148	104	-24.12	75	51	36
U.S. population, Hispanic, Mexican										
Men	293.1	42.2	68.22	175	119	84	-21.78	66	45	31
Women	390.6	51.1	66.04	212	144	102	-23.96	79	54	38
Mexican population										
Men	308.7	39.8	65.86	168	114	81	-24.14	72	49	35
Women	398.2	44.3	69.44	185	125	89	-20.56	101	68	48

Using the parameters of Table 14.8, the following equations can be used to represent the tolerance ellipses in an R-X_C graph. Varying the parameter t from 0 to 360°, the different values of 'X' and 'Y' can then be obtained.

$$X = L_1 \cos(I_1)\cos(t) - L_2 \sin(t) + \text{Centro}(R / \text{Height}) \quad (14.43)$$

$$Y = L_1 \sin(I_1)\cos(t) + L_2 \cos(I_1)\sin(t) + \text{Centro}(X_c / \text{Height}) \quad (14.44)$$

In BIVA method, the impedance vector of a new subject, normalized by his/her height, is confronted graphically (R-X_C graph) with the reference tolerance ellipses of 50%, 75% and 95% of healthy individuals of the same gender (see Fig. 14.18). Bioimpedance vectors that fall outside of the 75%

tolerance ellipse indicate abnormal physiological states and their location on the graph can be interpreted as follows (Piccoli et al. 2002b):

- *Variations along the direction of the major axis:* The upper pole of the ellipse of tolerance of 75% represents the dehydration threshold, while the lower pole of the same ellipse represents the overhydration threshold (edema). A shift along the major axis of the ellipse at any point in the R-X_C plane in the direction that increases the impedance indicates a dehydration of the body. A displacement in the direction that decreases the impedance means that the body has acquired a greater proportion of water. Hemodialysis patients are considered under an ideal situation if the variations of impedance vector are always within the 75% tolerance ellipse.

- *Variations along the direction of the minor axis:* A shift along the minor axis of the ellipse at any point in the R-X_C plane in the sense that decreases the phase angle indicates a smaller amount of soft tissue or cells. Depending also of the hydration status, they may be malnourished or cachectic (overhydration) or anorexic (dehydration). A displacement in the sense that the phase angle increases means a greater amount of soft tissue or cells. Depending of the hydration status, individuals may be obese (overhydration) or athletes (dehydration).

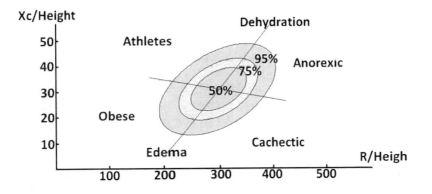

Fig. 14.18 R-X_C graph

The BIVA technique thus provides a direct method for the analysis of hydration and nutritional status of the subjects under study, being useful for both healthy subjects (Piccoli et al. 1996) and people with altered hydration status like hemodialysis patients, in intensive care units or during weight loss diets (Piccoli et al. 2002b).

14.6 NEPHROLOGY APPLICATIONS

From the review of published studies, five areas could be identified for the clinical application of bioimpedance in dialysis: identification of the dry weight, improvement of cardiovascular management, monitoring of fluid transfer during ultrafiltration, estimate of urea distribution volume in the calculation of Kt/V and nutritional assessment.

14.6.1 Identification of the Dry Weight

Hydration status is the most important predictor of mortality in hemodialysis patients after diabetes (Wabel et al. 2009). There is a high correlation between mortality and overhydration in hemodialysis patients due to the high risk of pulmonary and cardiovascular problems (Nescolarde et al. 2004). This fact has led to establish the concept of dry weight as a key factor for the adjustment of the dialysis treatment. In hemodialysis, the patient's weight reached at the end of a session, in which the maximum amount of fluid is removed without inducing hypotension during the absence of anti-hypertensive, is defined as dry weight and is conventionally considered as a therapeutic target (Charra 2007).

If the patients are not dialyzed up to their optimal weight, these can be in a permanent state of hydration, which can induce the development of hypertension and cardiovascular problems (Wabel et al. 2008; Machek et al. 2008). On the other hand, if a patient desires a final goal weight after several sessions of dialysis and there is an increase in his/her lean mass and fat due to a better nutrition, patient's dehydration will progressively be increased unleashing dialysis intolerance (Piccoli 2002a). The search of the dry weight of the patient is likely to produce episodes of hypotension leading to unpleasant effects such as dizziness, fatigue and muscle cramps (Kotanko et al. 2008).

The relative lack of precision in the clinical estimation of dry weight has led to the proposal of numerous non-clinical methods based on measurements of bioelectrical impedance for estimation of the dry weight and the hydration status of dialysis patients (Charra 2007). In this regard, many proposals have been developed based on measurements of the whole-body (hand-to-ankle) or segmental bioimpedance to estimate ECW, ICW and TBW (Kotanko et al. 2008). Dry weight estimates based on the ratio of

ICW to ECW, ECW to TBW, or the ratio of ECW and body weight have also been made.

It would also seem reasonable to use the BIS technique for the estimation of dry weight, as it provides more accurate measurements of body volume. However, as the errors in the estimates of ECW and ICW are around ± 1 L and > ± 1.5 L, respectively, the BIS technique may lead to significant errors in the estimation of dry weight (Kotanko et al. 2008). This lack of precision in measurements can be caused by an inadequate human body composition model. Most authors suggest a model divided into fat tissue and not fat tissue (FFM), and they also assume that fat mass is not hydrated and the water content in the FFM is 73.2%. However, numerous factors can affect the hydration proportions in these tissues, making very difficult to estimate the excess of fluid. Besides, the quantification of the dry weight is only possible once the benchmark of hydration has been established. To this end, (Chamney et al. 2007) proposed a new body composition model based on three compartments, which is consistent with the previous one that divides the body into fat mass and FFM, which has been modified to facilitate the quantification of excess fluids due to pathological causes (see Fig. 14.19).

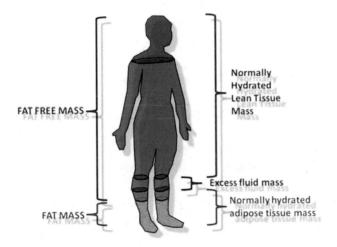

Fig. 14.19 Body composition model for quantification of excess fluids

In this model the fluid excess is a sub-compartment of the FFM, so that this model is divided into "normally hydrated lean tissue" mass ($M_{NH\ LT}$) and excess fluid mass (M_{ExF}). The fat tissue is referred to as "normally hydrated adipose tissue" mass (M_{NH_AT}) that includes the proportion of water associated with the adipose tissue, which is also included in the FFM in traditional models. If an excess of fluid happens, it can be located in the adipose tissue or the soft tissue (edema), or being part of a separate compartment (ascites).

The authors concluded a series of relationships between different body compartments of the model by means of normal hydration values of healthy subjects. These relations can be used both to establish the state of hydration and to estimate the nutritional status of patients (Chamney et al. 2007). In order to estimate mass excess fluid they propose the following equation:

$$M_{EXF} = 1.136 \cdot ECW - 0.430 * ICW - 0.114 \cdot Weight \qquad (14.45)$$

The normally hydrated lean tissue mass can be approximated as:

$$M_{NH\_LT} = 2.725 \cdot ICW + 0.191 \cdot M_{EXF} - 0.191 \cdot Weight \qquad (14.46)$$

The normally hydrated adipose tissue is calculated as follows:

$$M_{NH\_AT} = Weight - M_{EXF} - M_{NH\_LT} \qquad (14.47)$$

And, considering a constant rate of hydration, the fat mass corresponds to:

$$M_{FAT} = 0.752 \cdot M_{NH\_AT} \qquad (14.48)$$

This model makes possible to obtain more accurate estimates of dry weight and excess fluids. Experimental results have shown maximum errors in excess fluid of up to 0.5 kg (Wabel et al. 2009) adjusted the hydration status of patients at a hemodialysis center for a year using this model. The normohydration objective was to obtain the excess fluid volume lower than 2.5 liters before the dialysis sessions, maintaining when possible an overhydration between -1.1 and 1.1 liters at the end of the session. They gradually adjusted the treatment to achieve the hydration objectives, which was achieved in a period between 1 and 5 months, depending on the particular patient case. The results showed an improvement in the hypertension control, allowing a reduction in the anti-hypertensive medication, and also avoiding the occurrence of adverse events during dialysis. It also improved the quality of life of patients recovering their appetite and the possibility of developing a normal life.

14.6.2 Improvement of Cardiovascular Management

Since 1960 it is known that hypertension in dialysis patients can be controlled through a strict ultrafiltration (Charra 2007). In fact, through a combination of long-term hemodialysis and low sodium diet it was possible to normalize blood pressure in the 90% of hemodialysis patients during the first decade of application. The sodium in the human body controls the volume of extracellular water. In patients with advanced renal failure, sodium balance becomes positive and the extracellular water volume expands. This leads to hypertension, causing vascular changes that have severe consequences. Over the years, dialysis sessions were generally shortened by increasing the sodium output. Thus, the importance of a low sodium diet was gradually forgetting, resulting in a progressive loss of blood pressure control. Hypertension and fluid overload are considered as triggers of left ventricular hypertrophy which affects in large proportion to the population in hemodialysis programs (Wabel et al. 2008). Numerous studies have shown that left ventricular hypertrophy is associated with a significant proportion of deaths in hemodialysis patients. The HEMO study found that nearly 70% of chronic patients undergoing hemodialysis in the United States had hypertension despite taking anti-hypertensive medication (Rocco et al. 2001). If anti-hypertensive medication is partially effective in controlling blood pressure, it is likely to decrease the sensitivity of blood pressure as a marker of fluid overload, so that the dry weight may be underestimated. In addition, hypertension can be caused by other factors different to the fluid excess.

Low blood pressure is also associated with an increased risk of death in patients in hemodialysis and peritoneal dialysis because there is an increment in cardiovascular risk when the systolic pressure is less than 110 mm Hg (Wabel et al. 2008). The high correlation between low systolic blood pressure and the increment in mortality is associated with a higher rate of heart failure as a result of a continuous hypertension. A constant descend in blood pressure over months also increases the mortality risk (Wabel et al., 2009). A 10% of hemodialysis patients have low blood pressure and excess fluid, so that the patient remains in a state of continuous overhydration as they are not adequately treated (Wabel et al., 2008).

Bioimpedance has been used in numerous studies to provide better control of blood pressure in hemodialysis patients, because of its usefulness as a marker for estimation of dry weight (Zhou et al. 2010; Passauer et al. 2009) and fluid excess (Chamney 2007). With the aim of improving the efficiency of cardiovascular management, in Wabel et al. (2008) proposed a graphical method that can help the medical staff to estimate the level of necessary intervention to control blood pressure and hydration status was presented. This method, called hydration reference graph, is based on a two-dimensional chart which represents the excess of fluid in the horizontal axis and systolic blood pressure in the vertical one. This graph allows a quick identification and interpretation of the patient state through their situation on different regions. It also allows the comparison of patients with respect to the healthy population or other groups of patients. The hydration reference graph is composed of the following regions (see Fig. 14.20):

Region N: Patients who are in the region *N* have a hydration status and blood pressure comparable to those of the healthy population. Patients who have an excess of fluid greater than 1.1 L are considered to be overhydrated, while those with a value lower than -1.1 L are considered to be dehydrated. Patients with blood pressure above 140 mm Hg are considered to be hypertensive, while those below 100 mm Hg are considered hypotensive.

Region Dx: Patients in pre-dialysis have a higher excess fluid than the healthy population. Establishing a new frontier for the excess fluid at 2.5 L, below which the pre-dialysis patients normally are. It is also increased the threshold from which a hypertension is considered, above 150 mm Hg.

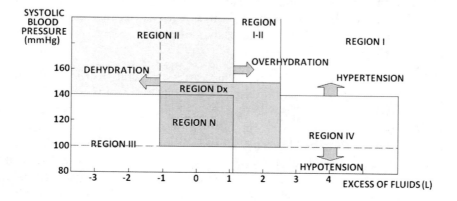

Fig. 14.20 Systolic blood pressure versus overhydration

Region I: This region represents patients with an excess of fluid greater than 2.5 L and a systolic blood pressure above 140 mm Hg. Hypertension in these patients may be related to fluid excess.

Region I–II: This region represents patients with fluid excess between 1.1 and 2.5 L, and systolic blood pressure above 150 mm Hg.

Region II: This region represents patients with a normal state of hydration but systolic blood pressure above 150 mm Hg. Patients in this region are hypertensive, but it is unlikely that excess fluid is the cause.

Region III: In which the patients are dehydrated with normal or low systolic blood pressure (below 140 mm Hg).

Region IV: Patients in this region reflect a serious fluid excess fluid, over 2.5 L, which is not reflected in systolic blood pressure as it is below 140 mm Hg.

The strategies for achieving a state of normotension are based on fluid reduction, the administration of anti-hypertensive drugs or a combination of both. The hydration reference graph provides a quick way to distinguish if a state of hypertension is caused by a fluid excess or, in contrast, it is caused by other factors, although it should not be used as a clinical diagnosis, but as a support tool. It can also help to prevent an excessive removal of fluids in dehydrated patients who have high blood pressure.

14.6.3 Fluid Transfer Monitoring During Ultrafiltration

During hemodialysis treatment, plasma water is removed by ultrafiltration and replaced by water from other compartments of the body, especially from interstitial fluids. These fluids transfer mechanisms during hemodialysis are complex and difficult to address. A deeper understanding of these changes is essential to improve the treatment efficacy, control the blood pressure, reduce complications and determine if the target weight of the patient has been reached (Jaffrin et al. 2002). In this regard, numerous studies have associated the measurements of bioimpedance and their variations with the changes during the dialysis treatment. The results of (Shulman et al. 2001) showed that bioimpedance measurements were consistent with the changes in weight and hematocrit levels during therapy.

The removal of fluid by ultrafiltration produces an increase in the value of the bioimpedance (Al-Surkhi et al. 2007). Also, a significant reduction in TBW and ECW is produced. However, variations in ICW are not the same in all the patients, what indicates that in some patients the removed water proceeds from the extracellular compartment in a greater proportion. These changes were also observed in the parameters of the Cole-Cole model during hemodialysis sessions, with increments in the values of R_0 and R_∞, and greater variations in R_0. Instead, R_{ICW} can both increase and decrease. The characteristic frequency, which is an indicator of cell size, decreases during hemodialysis session, while the α parameter increases.

Ultrafiltration causes a blood volume reduction, but central blood volume, which is formed by the volume of blood in the lungs, the heart and great vessels, must be preserved (Shulman et al. 2001). Then, a series of compensatory physiological mechanisms are activated, as an increase in stroke volume, tachycardia, peripheral vasoconstriction, release of vasoactive hormones or increase of venous return (Prakash et al. 2002). These mechanisms can be damaged in patients treated by dialysis, especially in diabetic patients, with vascular problems or elderly people, which can show episodes of hypotension during hemodialysis and other associated symptoms, such as muscle cramps, dizziness and fatigue. Intradialytic hypotension is a fairly common complication that often requires the infusion of hyperosmotic fluids (with dextrose or sodium), the interruption of ultrafiltration, changes in posture, and even the administration of vasoactive drugs. Some authors have associated it with a higher mortality rate (Charra 2007).

As a result of the compensation mechanisms of the human body, volume changes are more dynamic in the ECW of the legs than those in the trunk, which may explain the frequency of leg cramps during and after hemodialysis (Zhou et al. 2010). For this reason, segmental bioimpedance measurements are more accurate than measurements made over the whole body (Shulman et al. 2001) to estimate the volume of ultrafiltration that will be removed from a patient, the distribution of ECW and ICW or their changes during hemodialysis.

With estimations based on bioimpedance measurements, a continuous and accurate monitoring of changes in body fluids could be made, which could help in the determination of the volume and the best ultrafiltration rate in each time (Medrano et al. 2010). Thus, a closed loop control could be established to minimize the occurrence of hypotension episodes, but maintaining the final objective of dry weight. In addition, bioimpedance measurements can also serve as predictors of the occurrence of adverse events. In (Swatowski et al. 2004), it was reported a greater increase in thoracic impedance during episodes of intradialytic hypotension despite that the ultrafiltration rate was kept constant. Furthermore, a hop was observed in the thoracic impedance value at the beginning of an atrial arrhythmia. These results highlight the usefulness of bioelectrical impedance to predict and attend possible complications during hemodialysis treatment, before their symptoms appear.

14.6.4 Urea Distribution Estimate in Kt/V Calculation

Urea kinetic modeling and the Kt/V index are commonly used in hemodialysis treatments (Wuepper et al. 2003). Kinetic modeling aims to estimate the value of the amount of dialysis provided to a patient through the Kt/V, which is the key parameter to quantify and manage the dialysis dose. This parameter is defined as the ratio of the dialyzer clearance liquid (K) multiplied by the duration of dialysis (t) over the urea distribution volume (V).

The K parameter can be calculated by using the dialyzer mass transfer coefficient and the blood pump flow, which are characteristic parameters of the machine, and finally adjusting it to the hematocrit and the recirculation. The dialysis time is an adjustable parameter and the volume of urea distribution (V) is considered equivalent to the total body water (TBW) (Lowrie and Teehan 1983). Currently, hemodialysis machines allow the real time monitoring of clearance without the need of blood samples. The medical staff usually estimated TBW from anthropometric formulas in order to obtain the Kt/V. These indirect measurements use body weight and other parameters such as age and sex to estimate the volume of urea distribution. However, the volumes estimated this way are significantly higher than the urea distribution volume determined by urea kinetic modeling through blood samples (Dumler 2004). In order to provide a better estimate of Kt/V many authors have proposed bioimpedance to calculate the Volume of Distribution of Urea (Wuepper et al. 2003). In Lindley et al (2009) there is a comparison among the TBW volumes obtained from various anthropometric formulas and the bioimpedance measurements obtained from the volume of urea distribution by means of urea kinetic modeling in a single compartment. The results showed that the volume obtained using bioimpedance was the best approximation for the volume of urea distribution. The correspondence between the parameter Kt/V through bioimpedance measurements and the one obtained from blood samples has also been demonstrated. However, in some patients there is a small but systematic difference, around 5%. This error can be caused by differences in body composition that are not assumed by the bioimpedance model or can be caused from other errors introduced by the calculation of Kt/V through blood samples. However, these authors recommend the use of the bioimpedance as a method for determining the volume, whenever possible, and otherwise use Watson's formula confirming the results from blood samples.

14.6.5   Nutritional Assessment

Malnutrition is a serious health problem that affects between 40 and 50% of patients with chronic renal failure (Basaleem et al. 2004). It is associated with an increased morbidity and mortality of patients (Edefonti et al. 2006), an increase of the infection risk, a poor injury healing, a loss of muscle mass, a decreased quality of life of patients and an increase in the instability of the blood pressure (Stolarczyk et al. 1994). The kidneys, in addition to the role of removing organic waste, are also busy keeping the hormone nutrients and water levels, and play an important role in the generation of energy, maintaining the blood pressure and regenerating the bone mass, so that kidneys dysfunction has a direct impact on the nutritional status of the patient. Besides, many other causes can also affect these patients: dietary restrictions, loss of nutrients through ultrafiltration, the presence of uremic toxins, catabolic effects of dialysis, gastrointestinal disorders, chronic infections, post-dialytic fatigue, etc.

These issues suggest that it is appropriate to periodically assess the nutritional status of renal patients for a better management of nutrients that properly maintain the different functionalities of the body. The Body Mass Index (BMI = weight (kg) / height (m)^2) provides an estimate of the nutritional status discriminating between extremely obese, obese, normal, thin or very thin subjects (WHO 2010). The weight loss may be indicative of possible malnutrition; however, in other cases, this malnutrition can be masked if there is an accumulation of fluid in the body (edema) while the cell mass decreases (Earthman et al. 2007).

In order to avoid this, there have been many proposals based on bioimpedance measurements so as to provide simple, precise and effective tools to be incorporated in the dialysis routine for the assessment of the nutritional status of patients. Many studies link this nutritional status with the BCM value, which is directly related to the ICW. Others link the nutritional status with the ICW/ECW ratio (Fein et al. 2008). Nevertheless, the most accurate studied are those that provide measurements of muscle mass and fat mass (Chamney 2007; Kaysen et al. 2005) proposed a model for estimating muscle mass from ICW values obtained by the BIS method, which proved to be as accurate as the estimates obtained from the total body potassium. The BIVA method has also been proposed as a method to find the nutritional status, even in altered states of hydration, since it avoids errors caused by the assumption of a constant hydration of soft tissues (Piccoli et al. 2002b).

14.7 COMMERCIAL DEVICES

The first commercial bioimpedance instruments designed to analyze body composition date from 1981, when *RJL Systems* (USA) introduced the legendary *BIA-101*, which is the bioimpedance analysis device most referred in the literature (Rjlsystems 2011). This device was the result of collaboration with the Italian company *Akern*, which was responsible for introducing it in Europe (Akern 2011). Since then, *RJL Systems* and *Akern* have continued working together on the development of new products related to the bioimpedance analysis. Some *BIA-101* analyzers are still in use after more than 20 years because of the consistency and reliability of its measurements and the solidness of its basic specifications based on the injection of a small current at 50 kHz. These specifications have been maintained in current RJL bioelectrical impedance (*Quantum II, X, III, IV*) and Akern (modern *BIA-101*, *BIA-101 Anniversary*, *EFG*) analyzers systems. Several models of body composition analyzers from different manufacturers appeared in the 90s, either for *MFBIA* analysis at 50 kHz (*Valhalla Scientific Inc.*) (Valhalla 2011) or for ITBFS analysis (*BODYSTAT* Limited, Isle of Man) (Bodystat 2011) or for BIS analysis (*Xitron*) (Ellis 1999). Non-commercial impedance analyzers have also been developed in academic research laboratories. UniQuest Limited, which is the technology transfer company of the University of Queensland (Australia), marketed the *SFB3 SEAC* multifrequency bioimpedance analyzer, which has been used in many subsequent researches (Earthman et al. 2007). This device was an early version of the BIS SFB7 analyzer marketed by *Impedimed* (Impedimed 2011).

In 1994 there were more than 30 bioimpedance manufacturers worldwide. This led the National Institute of Health in the United States to assess the validity and interpretation of data obtained through bioelectrical impedance analysis to estimate body composition in the Technology Assessment Conference Statement of 1994 (NIH 1994). The conference discussed in detail the variety of bioimpedance instrumentation and studied the applicability of this technique in both healthy subjects and patients. A deep review of the state of knowledge and technological development of bioelectrical impedance to date was developed. This review ended in a set of recommendations for its application use (measurement standardization, safety, clinical use limitations, range of validity, etc.).

Since then, commercial devices have been used in numerous areas related to the monitoring of body composition (sports performance, clinical assessment, weight reduction, biomedical research). In the United States, *Xitron Technologies Inc.* became the leading manufacturer of MFBIA / BIS devices. Their first model, the *Xitron 4000B*, has been used in numerous studies since 1990 (Earthman et al. 2007), and was later replaced by the *Hydra 4200* model (Jaffrin and Morel 2008). This device performs a BIS analysis in the frequency range between 5 and 1000 kHz to calculate ECW and ICW volumes using the Cole-Cole model, the Hanai theory of mixed conductivity and the resistivity from De Lorenzo et al (1997). Recently, *Fresenius Medical Care* (Germany), the most important distribution company of dialysis products in the world, bought the license for the technology developed by *Xitron* for the manufacture of the *Body Composition Monitor* (Fresenius 2011). This device, in addition to providing measurements of ECW, ICW, TBW, FFM and fat mass, estimates the excess of fluid, which is a parameter that can be helpful to medical staff for the prescription of hemodialysis treatments. In 2007, *Impedimed* acquired *Xitron Technologies Inc.*, which has stopped manufacturing the *Hydra* device (Xitron 2011). Fresenius holds the license of *Xitron* technology to implement devices for patients with renal failure, although *Impedimed* is the one who manufactures them. The *Xitron* technology license for other applications (like vascular insufficiency, loss of muscle mass, hydration monitoring, lymphedema, etc.) remains being an *Impedimed* property. Table 14.9 shows a summary of commercial bioimpedance analyzers along with their main features, some of them currently available and others used in the literature.

Table 14.9 Commercial devices for bioimpedance analysis

Analyzer	Manufacturer	Frequencies	Current	Measures
BIA 101	Akern	SFBIA, 50 KHz	800 uA	TBW, ECW, ICW, FFM, FAT, BCM, impedance
BIA 101 Anniversary	Akern	SFBIA, 50 KHz	300 uA	TBW, ECW, ICW, FFM, FAT, BCM, impedance
EFG	Akern	SFBIA, BIVA, 50 KHz	330 uA	TBW, ECW, ICW, FFM, FAT, BCM, impedance
Body Comp MF	Akern	MFBIA, 5, 50 and 100 kHz	300 uA	TBW, ECW/ICW, FFM, FAT, BCM, impedances
QUANTUM II, X, III, IV	RJL Systems	SFBIA, 50 KHz	425 uA	Impedance
BF-906, BF-907	Maltron Interntional Ltd.	SFBIA, 50 KHz	700 uA	FAT, FFT, TBW, Impedance

Table 14.9 (*continued*)

BIOSCAN 916	Maltron Interntional Ltd.	SFBIA, 50 KHz	700 uA	FAT, FFT, TBW, ECW, ICW, Impedance
BIOSCAN 920	Maltron Interntional Ltd.	MFBIA, 5, 50 and 100, 200 kHz	800 uA	FAT, FFT, TBW, ECW, ICW, Impedance
SFB7	Impedimed	BIS, 256 frequencies between 4 KHz and 1 MHz	200 uA	TBW, ECW, ICW, FFM, FAT, Impedance
DF50	Impedimed	SFBIA, 50 KHz		TBW, ECW, ICW, FFM, FAT, Impedance
Hydra 4200	XitronTechnologies	BIS, 50 frequencies between 5 KHz and 1 MHz	50–700μA	TBW, ECW, ICW, FFM, FAT, Impedance
4000B	Xitron Technologies	BIS, 50 frequencies between 5 KHz and 1 MHz	800 uA	IMPEDANCES
BCMU	Fresenius Medical Care	BIS, 50 frequencies between 5 KHz and 1 MHz		TBW, ECW, ICW, FFM, FAT, Impedances Fluid Excess
1500MDD	Bodystat http://www.bodystat.com	MFBIA, 5, 50 KHz		TBW, FFM, FAT, Impedances
Quadscan 4000	Bodystat	MFBIA, 5, 50, 100 and 200 KHz		ECW, ICW, TBW, FFM, FAT, Impedances AT 50 KHz
ZOE - Fluid Status Monitor	Noninvasive Medical Technologies, Inc.	Segmental SFBIA (thoracic), 100 KHz	2 mA	Resistance

Table 14.9 (*continued*)

S331S	Tanita	SFBIA, 50 KHz	90 uA	TBW, FFM, FAT, Resistance
BC-418, TBF-310	Tanita	SFBIA, 50 KHz	500 uA	TBW, FFM, FAT, Resistance
MC-180	Tanita	MFBIA, 5 frequencies between 1 KHz and 500 KHz		TBW, ECW, ICW, FFM, FAT, Resistances
SEAC SFB3	Uniquest	486 frequencies,4 to 1024 kHz	100 uA	Impedances
MODEL 1260A	Solartron Analytical	Up to 32 MHz	6-600 uA	Impedances
MP150 + EBI100C	Biopac	12.5, 25, 50, 100 KHz	400 uA	Impedances
Bioscan Spectrum	Biológica Tecnología Médica S.L.,	MFBIA, 20 frequencies, 1-300 KHz		Impedances
BCS-1, 2, 3	Valhalla Scientific Inc.	SFBIA, 50 KHz	500 uA	TBW, FFM, FAT, Resistance

14.8 CASE STUDIES

Five case studies of patients undergoing hemodialysis are described below in order to show the applicability and usefulness of bioimpedance as an aid in the treatment of patients with terminal renal failure. For this sake, biomedical variables obtained by using the body composition evolution by means of bioelectrical impedance spectroscopy (Body Composition Monitor from Fresenius Medical Care) (Fresenius 2011) are shown. These variables allow a direct estimate of the hydration and nutritional status of patients that often remain hidden for the medical staff.

14.8.1 Case Study I

This case presents the biomedical parameters obtained of a 167 cm tall, 63 years old and 80 kg male at the end of a hemodialysis session through bioimpedance analysis. Fig. 14.21 shows the impedance values obtained at 50 analyzer operation frequencies (from 5 kHz to 1MHz). Using an error minimization algorithm the device calculates Cole-Cole modified model parameters that best fits the impedance values. Parameters in the figure show the value of these variables.

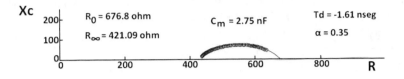

Fig. 14.21 Impedance values versus modified Cole-Cole model in Case Study I

The bioimpedance analyzer estimated the following values for body composition variables using the BIS technique (see Table 14.10), which are defined according to the model described in (Chamney 2007).

Table 14.10 Body composition in Case Study I

TBW	38.2 L	Lean Tissue Mass	46.9 Kg
ICW	22.7 L	Fat Mass	26.3 Kg
ECW	15.5 L	Adipose Tissue Mass	35.8 Kg
Overhydration	-3.2 L	Body Cell Mass	27.4 Kg

These values correspond to a FFM of 53.7 kg and fat mass of 26.3 kg for the two-compartment model described in the second paragraph of this chapter. Patient's systolic and diastolic blood pressures were 132 mmHg and 69 mmHg, respectively. According to the reference graph of hydration described in (Wabel et al. 2008) the patient is in the region III, and shows a major water shortage that would be advisable to be reduced up to values such as those proposed in (Wabel et al. 2008) so as to avoid the occurrence of adverse events during dialysis, and improve patient's quality of life (see Fig. 14.22)

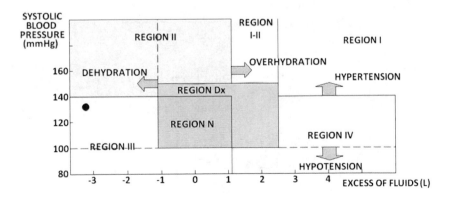

Fig. 14.22 Systolic blood pressure versus overhydration in Case Study I

This dehydration is also evident if we develop a vector analysis using the reference ellipses defined in (Piccoli et al. 2002b). The value of the impedance at 50 kHz normalized by the height of these tolerance ellipses has been represented in Fig. 14.23. The shift in the positive direction of the axis of the ellipse is indicative of a state of dehydration, while the displacement in the direction of the minor axis indicates that the patient's nutritional status is adequate, although having little overweight.

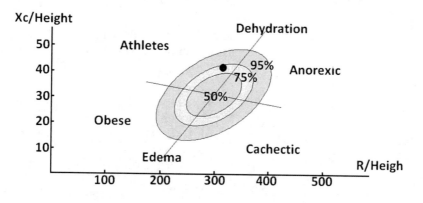

Fig. 14.23 BIVA analysis in Case Study I

According to the classification of the World Health Organization (WHO 2010), if the Body Mass Index (BMI) is used to assess the nutritional status, the patient is in the pre-obesity stage (BMI = 28.7) (see Fig. 14.24) and it is recommended to lose weight (Colombo et al. 2008) (BMI > 25). We can confirm that the patient is significantly overweight (Hoeger and

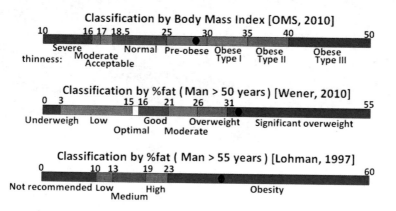

Fig. 14.24 Nutritional classification of the patient in Case Study I by BMI and %FAT

Hoeger 2010; Lohman et al. 1997) using the fat percentage obtained by bioimpedance analysis (% fat = 32.9% relative). Colombo et al (2008) stated that the patient is at high risk of metabolic syndrome (male, FAT relative > 21.9%), being highly recommended to lose weight (male, 60-79 years, FAT relative > 31%).

Fat Mass Index (FMI), which is obtained by dividing the fat mass in kilograms by the square of height in meters, is also used to provide a more accurate assessment utilizing independently the fat content of the subject. According to (Coin et al. 2008; Kyle et al. 2003, 2004c) and (Schutz et al. 2002), the patient has a significant excess of fat (IMF = 9.43 kg/m2), and is therefore highly recommended to lose weight (Colombo et al. 2008) (Males, IMF > 8.3 kg/m^2) (see Fig. 14.25).

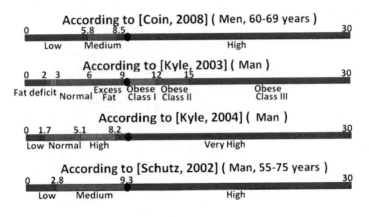

Fig. 14.25 Nutritional classification of the patient in Case Study I by FMI

The Index of Fat-Free Mass (FFMI), which is obtained by dividing the fat-free mass in kilograms by the square of height in meters, is very useful to assess the muscle condition of the patient. According to (Coin et al. 2008; Kyle et al. 2003; Kyle et al. 2004c; Schutz et al. 2002), the patient has a very suitable FFM value for his/her age and sex (see Fig. 14.26).

14.8.2 Case Study II

This case corresponds to a woman of 158 cm tall, 29 years old and 50 kg. The following variables of body composition (see Table 14.11) were obtained by mean the commercial bioimpedance analyzer (Fresenius 2011), derived according to the model described in (Chamney 2007):

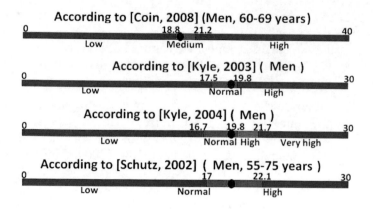

Fig. 14.26 Nutritional classification of the patient by FFMI

Table 14.11 Body composition in Case Study II

TBW	22.5 L	Lean Tissue Mass	18.7 Kg
ICW	10.2 L	Fat Mass	20.5 Kg
ECW	12.3 L	Adipose Tissue Mass	27.9 Kg
Overhydration	3.4 L	Body Cell Mass	8 Kg

These values are consistent with a FFM of 29.5 kg and fat mass of 20.5 kg. Patient's systolic blood pressure was 120 mm Hg and diastolic 60 mm Hg. According to the reference graph of hydration described in (Wabel et al. 2008) the patient is in the region number IV (see Fig. 14.27), which corresponds to a serious fluid excess fluid is not reflected in blood pressure because it is below 140 mm Hg. In this case, it would be advisable to rule out possible heart damage.

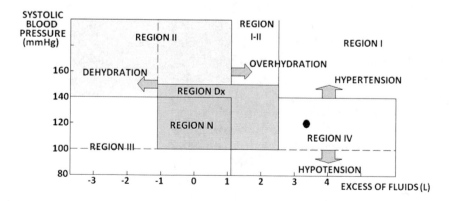

Fig. 14.27 Systolic blood pressure versus overhydration in Case Study II

Fig. 14.28 shows the value of the impedance at 50 kHz normalized by height for BIVA analysis on tolerance ellipses. The shift in the negative direction of the major axis of the ellipses indicates a significant fluid excess, out of the tolerance ellipses, confirming the results shown in the figure above. In addition, the position of the bioimpedance warns about a possible situation of malnutrition of the patient, although the BMI is within the normal range (BMI=20) according to the WHO classification (WHO 2010).

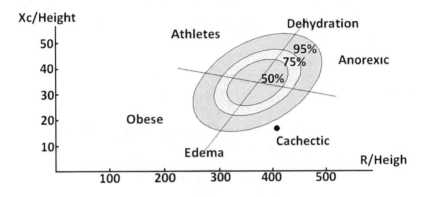

Fig. 14.28 BIVA analysis in Case Study II

If the fat percentage obtained by bioimpedance analysis is used (% relative fat= 42.4%) for a nutritional classification, a significant overweight of the patient is observed (Hoeger and Hoeger 2010; Lohman et al. 1997). According to Colombo et al. (2008), the patient is in serious risk of metabolic syndrome (Woman, % relative fat > 37.2%), being highly recommended weight loss (Woman, 20-39 years, % relative fat >39%) (see Fig. 14.29).

However, the FMI obtained by the analysis of bioimpedance measures (FMI=8.21 Kg/m^2) not confirm this excess of fat in the patient (Coin et al. 2008; Kyle et al. 2003, 2004c; Schutz et al. 2002), since the obtained value obtained is at the limit of normality, although it would be advisable to reduce it (Colombo et al., 2008) (Woman, FMI >8.2 Kg/m^2) (see Fig. 14.30).

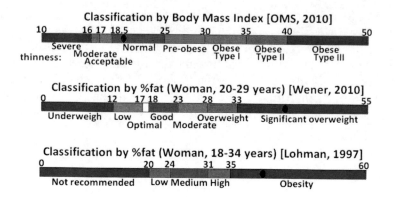

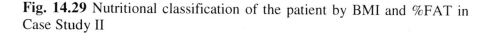

Fig. 14.29 Nutritional classification of the patient by BMI and %FAT in Case Study II

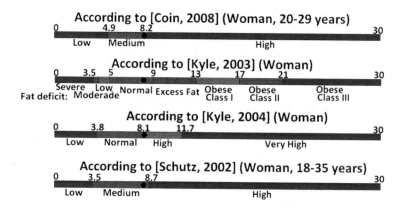

Fig. 14.30 Nutritional classification on the patient by FMI in Case Study II

The FFMI in this case really provides an important information about the patient's nutritional status since its value is below the recommended range for their age and sex (FFMI=8.21 Kg/m^2) according to the classification proposed in (Kyle et al. 2004c, 2003; Schutz et al. 2002; Coin et al. 2008), showing a clear lack of muscle mass (see Fig. 14.31).

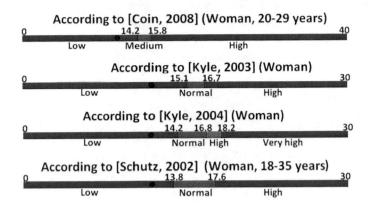

Fig. **14.31** Nutritional classification of the patient by FFMI in Case Study II

14.8.3 Case Study III

This case study shows the evolution of bioimpedance values of a male patient of 171 cm tall, 73 years old and 79.2 kg of weight before a hemodialysis session. The following figure shows the impedance values obtained for the 50 frequencies of operation of the BIS analyzer (Fresenius 2011) before the start of hemodialysis, together with those obtained at the end of the session for an ultrafiltration volume of 1.7 liters. Figure 14.32 shows the values for the parameters of Cole-Cole model that best approximates the obtained impedances.

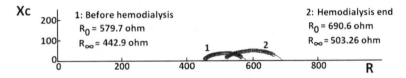

Fig. **14.32** Evolution of impedance values versus modified Cole-Cole model in Case Study III

Figure 14.32 shows an increase in the values of the impedances, which was expected after the removal of 1.7 liters of fluid by ultrafiltration. From the parameters of Cole-Cole model, bio-impedance analyzer derived the following volumes of fluids (see Table. 14.12).

Table 14.12 Fluids volumes evolution in Case Study III

Before hemodialysis session		After hemodialysis session	
TBW	34.5 L	TBW	32.6 L
ICW	16.8 L	ICW	17 L
ECW	17.7 L	ECW	15.6 L
Overhydration	1.7 L	Overhydration	1.7 L

On the other hand, patient's blood pressure was taken before and after hemodialysis. The table shows the pressure values obtained (see Table 14.13).

Table 14.13 Blood pressure evolution in Case Study III

Before hemodialysis session		After hemodialysis session	
Systolic blood pressure	140 mm Hg	Systolic blood pressure	166 mm Hg
Diastolic blood pressure	80 mm Hg	Diastolic blood pressure	90 mm Hg

According to the hydration reference graph described in (Wabel et al. 2008), the patient at the start of hemodialysis was in the region Dx (see Fig. 14.33), with an excess of fluid comparable to the pre-dialysis population. His blood pressure was high, although within the normal range for this fluid excess. At the end of the hemodialysis session the patient was within the region II, having reduced the fluid excess to values of hydration within normal limits. However, systolic blood pressure increased significantly. This hypertension, therefore, is unlikely to be associated with fluid excess, and may be associated with a vascular cause.

BIVA representation of the bioimpedance on the population tolerance ellipses population corroborates the evolution of the patient from an initial state of overhydration to a final state of hydration within normal limits (see Fig. 14.34). In addition, the position of bioimpedance values shows signs of a possible nutritional deficiency in the patient.

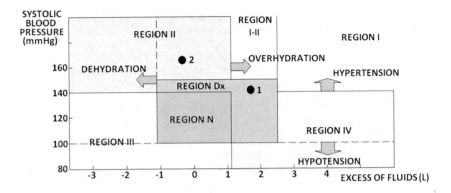

Fig. 14.33 Evolution of systolic blood pressure versus overhydration in Case Study III (1: Before Hemodialysis; 2: Hemodialysis end)

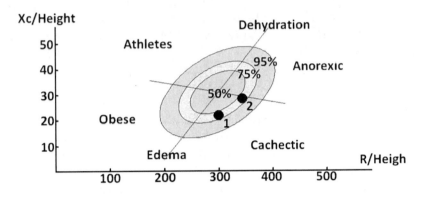

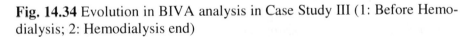

Fig. 14.34 Evolution in BIVA analysis in Case Study III (1: Before Hemodialysis; 2: Hemodialysis end)

14.9 CONCLUSION

Uremic patients treated with both hemodialysis and peritoneal dialysis show alterations in the metabolism of water with continuous variations in hydration status. After a dialysis session, it is quite common for patients to have a significant fluid excess or to be in an undesirable state of dehydration, which can cause or aggravate any cardiovascular disease. In this sense, in renal patients treated by hemodialysis it is very important to assess the amount of excess fluid to determine how much should be removed through ultrafiltration to achieve a desired state of normohydration. Bioimpedance methods are one of the most used techniques to estimate body composition because they have not the restrictions of solution methods and provide more accurate estimations than the anthropometric methods.

The most common methods for measuring bioimpedance use the configuration of four electrodes instead of two, with two electrodes to inject current and two electrodes for voltage measurement, because this configuration allows neglecting the effects of electrodes on bioelectrical impedance measurements. On the other hand, there are two basic techniques for measuring the impedance of biological tissues: the method of the impedances bridge and the phase detection method. However, the phase detection method has become the most widely used in bioimpedance measurement systems because it has many advantages over the impedance bridge method, such as its greater accuracy in the entire frequency range, speed and simplicity.

Thanks to bioimpedance analysis techniques, it is possible to obtain an accurate estimation of body fluids and body composition and hydration status in both normal and disease states. Besides, it also identifies protein/lean reserves (FFM) and fat reserves (FM). SFBIA technique is generally performed at a frequency of 50 kHz. At this frequency the current passes through both the intracellular and extracellular fluid and consequently total body water (TBW) may be calculated. But shifts in intracellular fluid cannot be easily detected due to the current passes through both intra and extracellular compartments. In addition, SF-BIA relies on regression approximations which have been determined from healthy individuals, so are not suitable for all subjects. As the frequency of 50 kHz may not be ideal to estimate body composition, many researchers have reconsidered which frequencies are the most suitable to detect and differentiate between ECW, ICW and TBW. To make this, MFBIA technique has been proposed, which involves taking impedance measurements at low and high frequencies. However, these impedances are applied to empirical models of linear regression to estimate TBW and ECW, and they must be applied only in populations for which they were defined, and they are not adequate for altered states of hydration or body composition. BIS takes measurements at greater number of frequencies and uses mathematical modeling to estimate the resistance at zero and infinite frequencies. These values are utilized through Hanai mixture theory to derive fat-free mass and fat mass. This technique improves the Cole-Cole model by introducing the effects of non-conductive substances in body water, eliminating the apparent population specificity found in the regression equations and improving its sensitivity to changes in body hydration status. Experimental results have shown that the BIS method can be as accurate as the dissolution reference methods when measurement conditions are under control.

The use of bioimpedance devices as a support tool in dialysis is widely proved. BIA helps Nephrologists providing them with patient's hydration status. Hydration status is the most important predictor of mortality in hemodialysis patients after diabetes. If the patients are not dialyzed up to their optimal weight, these can be in a permanent state of hydration, which can induce the development of hypertension and cardiovascular problems. On the other hand, if in a patient the goal weight is obtained after several sessions of dialysis and there is an increase in his/her lean or fat mass due to a better nutrition, patient's dehydration will progressively be increased unleashing dialysis intolerance and unpleasant effects such as dizziness, fatigue and muscle cramps. Bioimpedance analysis also facilitates an assessment of the patient's nutritional status, another major problem in hemodialysis patients. This parameter directly affects the morbidity and mortality of patients and it is fundamental to carry out an estimate of their life expectancy. Bioimpedance also allows an early detection of disturbances in the patient's health status, thus helping to prevent complications. During dialysis session the doctor may operate in real time, avoiding complications by intervention even before it occurs, simply observing the results of bioimpedance measures and acting on-line accordingly. Bioimpedance can be used too to estimate urea distribution volume, thus helping nephrologists in prescribing adequate dialysis dose. Finally, it is a tool for customizing the health care because it provides information about the particular state of the patient, which is used to individualize treatments taking into account such data.

Furthermore, bioimpedance measurements also have many practical advantages that have led to their rapid development: they have not the restrictions of solution methods and provide more accurate estimations than the anthropometric methods; the instrumentation is portable, relatively inexpensive, and the measurements are noninvasive, easy to obtain, quick to get with minimal operator training, consistent, reproducible, safe, harmless and non-uncomfortable.

REFERENCES

Aberg, P., Nicancer, I., Ollmar, S.: Minimally invasive electrical impedance spectroscopy of skin exemplified by skin cancer assessments. In: Proceedings of the 25th Annual International Conference of the IEEE Engineering in Medicine and Biology Society, vol. 4, pp. 3211–3214 (2003)

Akern web site (2011), http://www.akern.com/ (accessed August 2011)

Al-Surkhi, O.I., Riu, P.J., Vazquez, F.F., et al.: Monitoring Cole-Cole Parameters During Haemodialysis (HD). In: Proceedings of the 29th Annual International Conference of the IEEE EMBS, pp. 2238–2241 (2007)

Amaral, C.E.F., Wolf, B.: Effects of glucose in blood and skin impedance spectroscopy. In: AFRICON (2007), doi:10.1109

Atzler, E., Lehmann, G.: Über ein Neues Verfahren zur Darstellung der Herztätigkeit (Dielektrographie). Arbeitsphysiol. 6, 636–680 (1931)

Basaleem, H.O., Alwan, S.M., Ahmed, A.A., et al.: Assessment of the Nutritional Status of End-Stage Renal Disease Patients on Maintenance Hemodialysis. Saudi J. Kidney Dis. Transplant. 15(4), 455–462 (2004)

Baumgartner, R.N., Heymsfield, S.B., Lichtman, S., et al.: Body composition in elderly people: effect of criterion estimates on predictive equations. Am. J. Clin. Nutr. 53(6), 1345–1353 (1991)

Bodystat web site, http://www.bodystat.com/ (accessed August 2011)

Buchholz, A.C., Bartok, C., Schoeller, D.A.: The Validity of Bioelectrical Impedance Models in Clinical Populations. Nutr. Clin. Pract. 19(5), 433–446 (2004)

Callaghan, J.J., Rosenberq, A.G., Rubash, H.E.: The adult knee, 2nd edn. Lippincott Williams & Wilkins (2003)

Chamney, P.W., Krämer, M., Rode, C., et al.: A new technique for establishing dry weight in hemodialysis patients via whole body bioimpedance. Kidney Int. 61(6), 2250–2258 (2002)

Chamney, P.W., Wabel, P., Moissl, U.M., et al.: A whole-body model to distinguish excess fluid from the hydration of major body tissues. Am. J. Clin. Nutr. 85(1), 80–89 (2007)

Charra, B.: Fluid balance, dry weight, and blood pressure in dialysis. Hemodial. Int. 11(1), 21–31 (2007)

Coin, A., Sergi, G., Minicuci, N., et al.: Fat-free mass and fat mass reference values by dual-energy X-ray absorptiometry (DEXA) in a 20–80 year-old Italian population. Clin. Nutr. 27(1), 87–94 (2008)

Cole, K.S.: Membranes, ions and impulses: a chapter of classical biophysics. Univ. of California Press, Berkeley (1972)

Colombo, O., Villani, S., Pinelli, G., et al.: To treat or not to treat: comparison of different criteria used to determine whether weight loss is to be recommended. Nutr. J. 7, 5 (2008)

Cornish, B.H., Thomas, B.J., Ward, L.C.: Improved prediction of extracellular and total body water using impedance loci generated by multiple frequency bioelectrical impedance analysis. Phys. Med. Biol. 38(3), 337–346 (1993)

Coupaye, M., Bouillot, J.L., Poitou, C., et al.: Is Lean Body Mass Decreased after Obesity Treatment by Adjustable Gastric Banding? Obes. Surg. 17(4), 427–433 (2007)

Cox-Reijven, P.L., Soeters, P.B.: Validation of bio-impedance spectroscopy: effects of degree of obesity and ways of calculating volumes from measured resistance values. Int. J. Obesity Rel. Metab. Disord. 24(3), 271–280 (2000)

De Lorenzo, A., Candeloro, N., Andreoli, A., et al.: Determination of intracellular water by multifrequency bioelectrical impedance. Ann. Nutr. Metab. 39(3), 177–184 (1995)

De Lorenzo, A., Andreoli, A., Matthie, J., et al.: Predicting body cell mass with bioimpedance by using theoretical methods: a technological review. J. Appl. Physiol. 82(5), 1542–1558 (1997)

De Lorenzo, A., Sorge, R.P., Candeloro, C., et al.: New insights into body composition assessment in obese women. Can. J. Physiol. Pharmacol. 77(1), 17–21 (1999)

Deurenberg, P., van der Kooy, K., Leenen, R., et al.: Sex and age specific prediction formulas for estimating body composition from bioelectrical impedance: a cross-validation study. Int. J. Obes. 15(1), 17–25 (1991)

Dittmar, M., Reber, H.: Evaluation of different methods for assessing intracellular fluid in healthy older people: a cross-validation study. J. Am. Geriatr. Soc. 50(1), 104–110 (2002)

Du Bois-Reymond, E.: Untersuchungen über thierische Elektricität. Reimer Verlag (1848)

Dumler, F.: Best Method for Estimating Urea Volume of Distribution: Comparison of Single Pool Variable Volume Kinetic Modeling Measurements with Bioimpedance and Anthropometric Methods. ASAIO J. 50(3), 237–241 (2004)

Dziong, D., Bagnaninchi, P.O., Kearney, R.E., et al.: Nondestructive Online In Vitro Monitoring of Pre-Osteoblast Cell Proliferation Within Microporous Polymer Scaffolds. IEEE Trans. Nanobioscience 6(3), 249–258 (2007)

Earthman, C., Traughber, D., Dobratz, J., et al.: Bioimpedance Spectroscopy for Clinical Assessment of Fluid Distribution and Body Cell Mass. Nutr. Clin. Pract. 22(4), 389–405 (2007)

Edd, J.F., Rubinsky, B.: Assessment of the Viability of Transplant Organs with 3D Electrical Impedance Tomography. In: 27th Conf. Proc. IEEE Eng. Med. Biol. Soc., vol. 3, pp. 2644–2647 (2006)

Edefonti, A., Paglialonga, F., Picca, M., et al.: A prospective multicentre study of the nutritional status in children on chronic peritoneal dialysis. Nephrol. Dial. Transplant. 21(7), 1946–1951 (2006)

Einthoven, W.: Un nouveau galvanometer. Arch. Néerland Sci. Exactes Naturelles 6, 625–633 (1901)

Einthoven, W.: Le telecardiogramme. Arch. Int. Physiol. 4, 132–164 (1906)

Eisenkolbl, J., Kartasurya, M., Widhalm, K.: Underestimation of percentage fat mass measured by bioelectrical impedance analysis compared to dual energy X-ray absorptiometry method in obese children. Eur. J. Clin. Nutr. 55(6), 423–429 (2001)

Ellis, K.J., Shypailo, R.J., Wong, W.W.: Measurement of body water by multifrequency bioelectrical impedance spectroscopy in a multiethnic pediatric population. Am. J. Clin. Nutr. 71(6), 1618 (1999)

Espinosa-Cuevas, M.A., Hivas-Rodripuez, L., Gonzalez-Medina, E.C., et al.: Vectores de impedancia en población mexicana. Rev. Invest. Clin. 59(1), 15–24 (2007)

Éninya, G.I., Ondzuls, P.A.: A portable rheograph for clinical studies. Biull. Eksp. Biol. Med. 52, 105–107 (1961)

Fein, P., Chattopadhyay, J., Paluch, M.M., et al.: Enrollment Fluid Status Is Independently Associated with Long-Term Survival of Peritoneal Dialysis Patients. Adv. Perit. Dial. 24, 79–83 (2008)

Fenech, M., Maasrani, M., Jaffrin, M.Y.: Fluid volumes determination by impedance spectroscopy and hematocrit monitoring: application to pediatric hemodialysis. Artif. Organs 25(2), 89–98 (2001)

Fenning, C.: A new method of recording physiologic activities–I: Recording respiration in small animals. J. Lab. Elin. Med. 22, 1279–1280 (1937)

Fresenius web site, http://www.bcm-fresenius.com/ (accessed August 2011)

Gabriel, C., Gabriel, S., Corthout, E.: The dielectric properties of biological tissues: I. Literature survey. Phys. Med. Biol. 41(11), 2231–2249 (1996a)

Gabriel, S., Lau, R.W., Gabriel, C.: The dielectric properties of biological tissues: III. Parametric models for the dielectric spectrum of tissues. Phys. Med. Biol. 41(11), 2271–2293 (1996b)

Galvani, A.L.: De viribus electricitatis in motu musculari commentarius. De Boloniensi Scient. Et art. Instituto Etque Academia Commentarii 7, 363 (1791)

Gibney, M.J., Elia, M., Ljungqvist, O., et al.: Clinical Nutrition. The Nutrition Society Textbook. Blackwell Science (2005)

Grimnes, S., Martinsen, O.G.: Bioimpedance and Bioelectricity Basics. Academic Press, San Diego (2000)

Hannan, W.J., Cowen, S.J., Fearson, K.C.H., et al.: Evaluation of multi-frequency bioimpedance analysis for the assessment of extracellular and total body water in surgical patients. Clin. Sci. (Lond.) 86(4), 479–485 (1994)

Hannan, W.J., Cowen, S.J., Plester, C.E., et al.: Comparison of bio-impedance spectroscopy and multifrequency bio-impedance analysis for the assessment of extracellular and total body water in surgical patients. Clin. Sci. 89(5), 651–658 (1995)

Heitmann, B.L.: Prediction of body water and fat in adult Danes from measurement of electrical impedance: A validation study. Int. J. Obes. 14(9), 789–802 (1990a)

Heitmann, B.L.: Evaluation of body fat estimated from body mass index, skinfolds and impedance: A comparative study. Eur. J. Clin. Nutr. 44(11), 831–837 (1990b)

Henderson, R.P., Webster, J.G.: An Impedance Camera for Spatially Specific Measurements of the Thorax. IEEE Trans. Biomed. Eng. 25(3), 250–254 (1978)

Hoeger, W.K., Hoeger, S.A.: Principles and Labs for Fitness and Wellness. Cengage Learning. Wadsworth, USA (2010)

Hoffer, E.C., Meador, C.K., Simpson, D.C.: Correlation of whole-body impedance with total body water volume. J. Appl. Physiol. 27(4), 531–534 (1969)

Holder, D.S.: Electrical Impedance Tomography: Methods, History and Applications. Institute of Physics Publishing (2004)

ICNIRP: International Commission on Non-Ionizing Radiation Protection, Guidelines for Limiting Exposure to Time-Varying Electric, Magnetic, and Electromagnetic Fields up to 300 GHz. Health Phys. 74(4), 494–522 (1998)

ICNIRP: International Commission on Non-Ionizing Radiation Protection, ICNIRP Statement on the Guidelines for limiting exposure to time-varying electric, magnetic and electromagetic fields (up to 300 GHz). Health Phys. 97(3), 257–258 (2009)

Impedimed web site, http://www.impedimed.com/ (accessed August 2011)

Jaffrin, M.Y., Fenech, M., de Fremont, J.F., et al.: Continuous Monitoring of Plasma, Interstitial, and Intracellular Fluid Volumes in Dialyzed Patients by Bioimpedance and Hematocrit Measurements. ASAIO J. 48(3), 326–333 (2002)

Jaffrin, M.Y., Morel, H.: Body fluid volumes measurements by impedance: A review of bioimpedance spectroscopy (BIS) and bioimpedance analysis (BIA) methods. Med. Eng. Phys. 30(10), 1257–1269 (2008)

Kaysen, G.A., Zhu, F., Sarkar, S., et al.: Estimation of total-body and limb muscle mass in hemodialysis patients by using multifrequency bioimpedance spectroscopy. Am. J. Clin. Nutr. 82(5), 988–995 (2005)

Kennedy, J.: Multifrequency Bioimpedance Determination. US Patent 2006/0004300 A1 (2006)

Kotanko, P., Levin, N.W., Zhu, F.: Current state of bioimpedance technologies in dialysis. Nephrol. Dial. Transplant. 23(3), 808–812 (2008)

Kushner, R.F., Schoeller, D.A.: Estimation of total body water by bioelectrical impedance analysis. Am. J. Clin. Nutr. 44(3), 417–424 (1986)

Kyle, U.G., Genton, L., Karsegard, L., et al.: Single prediction equation for bioelectrical impedance analysis in adults aged 20–94 years. Nutrition 17(3), 248–253 (2001)

Kyle, U.G., Nicod, L., Raguso, C., et al.: Prevalence of low fat-free mass index and high and very high body fat mass index following lung transplantation. Acta Diabetol. 40(suppl. 1), S258–S260 (2003)

Kyle, U.G., Bosaeus, I., Antonio, D.D., et al.: Bioelectrical impedance analysis—part I: review of principles and methods. Clinical Nutrition 23, 1226–1243 (2004a)

Kyle, U.G., Bosaeus, I., De Lorenzo, A.D., et al.: Bioelectrical impedance analysis—part II: utilization in clinical practice. Clin. Nutr. 23(6), 1430–1453 (2004b)

Kyle, U.G., Morabia, A., Schutz, Y., et al.: Sedentarism Affects Body Fat Mass Index and Fat-Free Mass Index in Adults Aged 18 to 98 Years. Nutrition 20(30), 255–260 (2004c)

Kubiczek, W.G., Karnegis, J.N., Patterson, R.P., et al.: Development and evaluation of an impedance cardiac output system. Aerospace Med. 37(12), 1208–1212 (1966)

Lindley, E.J., Chamney, P.W., Wuepper, A., et al.: A comparison of methods for determining urea distribution volume for routine use in on-line monitoring of haemodialysis adequacy. Nephrol. Dial. Transplant. 24(1), 211–216 (2009)

Lohman, T.G., Houtkooper, L.B., Going, S.B.: Body fat measurement goes hi-tech: not all are created equal. ACSM's Health Fitness J. 1, 30–35 (1997)

Lorenzo, A., Andreoli, A., Matthie, J., et al.: Predicting body cell mass with bioimpedance by using theoretical methods: a technological review. J. Appl. Physiol. 82(5), 1542–1558 (1997)

Lowrie, E.G., Teehan, B.P.: Principles of prescribing dialysis therapy: Implementing recommendation from the National Co-operative Dialysis Study. Kidney Int. 23(13), S113–S122 (1983)

Machek, P., Jirka, T., Moissl, U., et al.: Optimal fluid status assessed with bioimpedance spectroscopy reduces IMES and hospitalisation in hemodialysis patients. NDT Plus 1(2), ii322–ii322 (2008)

Matteucci, L.: Sur un phénomène physiologique produit par les muscles en conctraction. Ann. Chim. Et. Phys. 6, 339 (1842)

Matthie, J.R., Withers, P.O., Van Loan, M.D., Mayclin, P.L.: Development of commercial complex bio-impedance spectroscopic system for determining intracellular and extracellular water volumes. In: Proc. of the 8th Int. Conf. on Electrical Bio-Impedance, pp. 203–205 (1992)

Matthie, J.R.: Second generation mixture theory equation for estimating intracellular water using bioimpedance spectroscopy. J. Appl. Physiol. 99(2), 780–781 (2005)

Medrano, G., Eitner, F., Floege, J.Ü., et al.: A Novel Bioimpedance Technique to Monitor Fluid Volume State During Hemodialysis Treatment. ASAIO J. 56(3), 215–220 (2010)

Min, M.M., Kink, A., Land, R., et al.: Modification of Pulse Wave Signals in Electrical Bioimpedance Analyzers for Implantable Medical Devices. In: Proceedings of the 26th Annual International Conference of the IEEE EMBS, San Francisco, vol. 3, pp. 2263–2266 (2004)

Moissl, U.M., Wabel, P., Chamney, P.W., et al.: Body fluid volume determination via body composition spectroscopy in health and disease. Physiol. Meas. 27(9), 921–933 (2006)

Naiman, N., Cheung, A.K., Goldfarb-Rumyantzev, A.S.: Familiality of cardiovascular mortality in end-stage renal disease patients. Am. J. Nephrol. 29(3), 237–243 (2009)

Nescolarde, L., Piccoli, A., Román, A., et al.: Bioelectrical impedance vector analysis in haemodialysis patients: relation between oedema and mortality. Physiol. Meas. 25(5), 1271–1280 (2004)

Nescolarde, L., Doñate, T., Piccoli, A., et al.: Comparison of segmental with whole-body impedance measurements in peritoneal dialysis patients. Med. Eng. Phys. 30(7), 817–824 (2008)

Neves, C.E.B., Souza, M.N.: A Comparison Between Impedance Measufled by a Commercial Analyzer and Your Value Adjusted by a Theoretical Model in Body Composition Evaluation. In: Proceedings of the 23rd Annual EMBS International Conference, vol. 4, pp. 3388–3391 (2001)

NIH: National Institutes of Health, Bioelectrical Impedance Analysis in Body Composition Measurement. In: Technology Assessment Conference Statement, vol. (11-12), pp. 749–762 (1994)

Nyboer, J.: Electrical Impedance Plethysmography: A Physical and Physiologic Approach to Peripheral Vascular Study. Circulation 2(6), 811–821 (1950)

Nobili, L.: Ueber einen neuen Galvanometer. J. Chem. und Physik. 45, 249–254 (1825)

Pandey, V.K., Pandey, P.C.: Wavelet Based Cancellation of Respiratory Artifacts in Impedance Cardiography. In: 15th Int. Conf. on Digital Signal Processing, pp. 191–194 (2007)

Passauer, J., Petrov, H., Schleser, A., et al.: Evaluation of clinical dry weight assessment in haemodialysis patients using bioimpedance spectroscopy: a cross-sectional study. Nephrol. Dial. Transplant. 25(2), 545–551 (2009)

Pastan, S., Gassensmith, C.: Total body water measured by bioelectrical impedance in patients after hemodialysis: comparison with urea kinetics. ASAIO J. 38(3), M186–M189 (1992)

Patterson, R.: Body fluid determinations using multiple impedance measurements. IEEE Eng. Med. Biol. Soc. Mag. 8(1), 16–18 (1989)

Piacentini, N., Demarchi, D., Civera, P., et al.: Blood cell counting by means of impedance measurements in a microsystem device. In: 30th Conf. Proc. IEEE Eng. Med. Biol. Soc., pp. 4824–4827 (2008)

Piccoli, A., Rossi, B., Pillon, L., et al.: A new method for monitoring body fluid variation by bioimpedance analysis: The RXc graph. Kidney Int. 46(2), 534–539 (1994)

Piccoli, A., Piazza, P., Noventa, D., et al.: A new method for monitoring hydration at high altitude by bioimpedance analysis. Med. Sci. Sports Exerc. 28(12), 1517 (1996)

Piccoli, A., Nescolarde, L.D., Rosell, J.: Análisis convencional y vectorial de bioimpedancia en la práctica clínica. Nefrología 12(3), 228–238 (2002a)

Piccoli, A., Pillon, L., Dumler, F.: Impedance Vector Distribution by Sex, Race, Body Mass Index, and Age in the United States: Standard Reference Intervals as Bivariate Z Scores. Nutrition 18(2), 153–167 (2002b)

Prakash, S., Reddan, D., Heidenheim, A.P., et al.: Central, Peripheral, and Other Blood Volume Changes During Hemodialysis. ASAIO J. 48(4), 379–382 (2002)

Rjlsystems (2011), http://www.rjlsystems.com/ (accessed August 2011)

Rocco, M.V., Yan, G., Heyka, R.J., et al.: Risk factors for hypertension in chronic hemodialysis patients: baseline data from the HEMO study. Am. J. Nephrol. 21(4), 280–288 (2001)

Salter, D.C.: Quantifying skin disease and healing in vivo using electrical impedance measurements. In: Rolfe, P. (ed.) Non-invasive Physiological Measurements, vol. 1, pp. 21–68. Academic Press, London (1979)

Schutz, Y., Kyle, U.U.G., Pichard, C.: Fat-free mass index and fat mass index percentiles in Caucasians aged 18 – 98 y. Int. J. Obes. Relat. Metab. Disord. 26(7), 953–960 (2002)

Sergi, G., Bussolotto, M., Perini, P., et al.: Accuracy of bioelectrical impedance analysis in estimation of extracellular spaces in healthy subjects and in fluid retention. Ann. Nutr. Metab. 38(3), 158–165 (1994)

Shulman, T., Heidenheim, A.P., Kianfar, C., et al.: Preserving Central Blood Volume: Changes in Body Fluid Compartments During Hemodialysis. ASAIO J. 47(6), 615–618 (2001)

Songer, J.: Tissue Ischemia Monitoring Using Impedance Spectroscopy: Clinical Evaluation. M.Sc. Worcester Polytechnic Institute (2001)

Stolarczyk, L.M., Heyward, V.H., Hicks, V.L., et al.: Predictive accuracy of bioelectrical impedance in estimating body composition of Native American women. Am. J. Clin. Nutr. 59(5), 964–970 (1994)

Sun, S.S., Chumlea, W.C., Heymsfield, S.B., et al.: Development of bioelectrical impedance analysis prediction equations for body composition with the use of a multicomponent model for use in epidemiologic surveys. Am. J. Clin. Nutr. 77(2), 331–340 (2003)

Swatowski, A., Wizemann, V., Zaluska, W., et al.: Thoracic Impedance Measurements During Orthostatic Change Test and During Hemodialysis in Hemodialyzed Patients. ASAIO J. 50(6), 581–585 (2004)

Thommasset, A.: Bio-electrical properties of tissue impedance measurements. Lyon Med. 209, 1325–1352 (1963)

Trebbels, D., Hradetzky, D., Zengerle, R., et al.: Capacitive on-line hematocrit sensor design based on impedance spectroscopy for use in hemodialysis machines. In: Conf. Proc. IEEE Eng. Med. Biol. Soc., pp. 1208–1211 (2009)

Tura, A., Maran, A., Pacini, G.: Non-invasive glucose monitoring: Assessment of technologies and devices according to quantitative criteria. Diabetes Res. Clin. Pract. 77(1), 16–40 (2007)

Valhalla web site, http://www.valhallascientific.com/ (accessed August 2011)

Van Loan, M.D., Withers, P., Matthie, J., et al.: Use of bioimpedance spectroscopy to determine extracellular fluid, intracellular fluid, total body water and fat-free mass. In: Ellis, K.J., Eastman, J.D. (eds.) Human Body Composition: in Vivo Methods, Models and Assessment, vol. 60, pp. 67–70. Plenum, New York (1993)

Wabel, P., Moissl, U., Chamney, P., et al.: Towards improved cardiovascular management: the necessity of combining blood pressure and fluid overload. Nephrol. Dial. Transplant. 23, 2965–2971 (2008)

Wabel, P., Chamney, P., Moissl, U., et al.: Importance of Whole-Body Bioimpedance Spectroscopy for the Management of Fluid Balance. Blood Purif. 27(1), 75–80 (2009)

Wang, J.J., Hu, W.C., Kao, T., et al.: On Measuring the Changes in Stroke Volume from a Peripheral Artery by Means of Electrical Impedance Plethysmography. In: The 2nd International Conference on Bioinformatics and Biomedical Engineering, ICBBE 2008, Shanghai, May 16-18, pp. 1409–1412 (2008)

Watson, P.E., Watson, I.D., Batt, R.D.: Total body water volumes for adult males and females estimated from simple anthropometric measurements. Am. J. Clin. Nutr. 33(1), 27–39 (1980)

Webster, J.G.: Medical Instrumentation: Application and Design, 4th edn. John Wiley & Sons, New York (2009)

WHO web site, http://www.who.int/en/ (accessed December 2010)

Wizemann, V., Wabel, P., Chamney, P., et al.: The mortality risk of overhydration in haemodialysis patients. Nephrol. Dial. Transplant. 24(5), 1574–1579 (2009)

Woodrow, G., Oldroyd, B., Turney, J.H., et al.: Measurement of total body water by bioelectrical impedance in chronic renal failure. Eur. J. of Clin. Nutr. 50(10), 676–681 (1996)

Wuepper, A., Tattersall, J., Kraemer, M.: Determination of urea distribution volume for Kt/V assessed by conductivity monitoring. Kidney Int. 64(6), 2262–2271 (2003)

Xitron web site, http://www.xitrontech.com/ (accessed August 2011)

Yang, Y., Wang, J.: Tetrapolar Method for Complex Bioimpedance Measurement: Theoretical Analysis and Circuit Realization. In: Proc. of the 2005 IEEE Engineering in Medicine and Biology: 27th Annual Conference, Shanghai, vol. 6, pp. 6605–6607 (2005)

Zheng, S., Nandra, M.S., Chong, Y.T.: Human Blood Cell Sensing with Platinum Black Electroplated Impedance Sensor. In: 2nd IEEE International Conference on Nano/Micro Engineered and Molecular Systems, NEMS 2007, January 16-19, pp. 520–523 (2007)

Zhou, Y.L., Liu, J., Sun, F.: Calf bioimpedance ratio improves dry weight assessment and blood pressure control in hemodialysis patients. Am. J. Nephrol. 32(2), 109–116 (2010)

Zhu, F., Kuhlmann, M.K., Kaysen, G.A.: Segment-specific resistivity improves body fluid volume estimates from bioimpedance spectroscopy in hemodialysis patients. J. Appl. Physiol. 100(2), 717–724 (2006)

ESSAY QUESTIONS

1. Briefly describe the most widely used compartmental model of the human body.
2. List some of the advantages provided by bioimpedance measurements in order to establish the body composition compared with other estimation techniques.
3. Describe the frequency behavior of the human body under the injection of electric currents.
4. Which are the advantages of the configuration of four electrodes for bioimpedance measurements compared to two-electrode configuration?
5. In which nephrology applications can bioimpedance meters be useful?
6. Calculate the TBW of the patient whose data are shown below using the Watson equation (Fenech et al. 2001).

	Sex	Age (years)	Height (m)	Weight (kg)	TBW-BIS (liters)
Patient	woman	38	1.56	69.9	30.1

7. Use the SFBIA approximation of Deurenberg et al (1991) for TBW estimation in patient of question 6, considering the impedance values shown in the following table for hand-foot tetrapolar configuration. From the TBW values, estimate the amount of FFM.

	R (50 KHz) ohm	X (50 KHz) ohm
Patient	522.99	45.85

8. Graphically, approximate the parameters of Cole-Cole model (R_{ECW}, R_{ICW}, $C_{membrane}$ and α) from bioelectrical impedance values associated with the following frequencies:

Frequency	R (ohm)	X_C (ohm)	Frequency	R (ohm)	X_C (ohm)
5 kHz	719.8	30.8	54 kHz	635.6	57.6
7 kHz	712.1	36.6	67 kHz	626.6	56.5
9 kHz	705.8	41.2	83 kHz	617.9	54.8
13 kHz	694.8	47.9	128 kHz	601.7	50.4
15 kHz	689.8	50.0	159 kHz	594.4	47.7
23 kHz	672.8	55.4	245 kHz	581.2	42.0
28 kHz	664.4	57.0	304 kHz	575.5	38.8

35 kHz	654.5	58.0	378 kHz	570.2	35.7
39 kHz	649.8	58.1	582 kHz	561.4	29.0
43 kHz	645.5	58.2	723 kHz	557.7	25.3
50 kHz	639.0	57.8	1000 kHz	553.7	18.9

9. Make the estimation of TBW in the patient of question 6 by using the BIS technique based on the body mass index (Moissl et al. 2006). Assume the following values for R_0 and R_∞.

	R_0 (ohm)	R_∞ (ohm)
Patient	616.7	442.74

10. Estimate the mass excess fluid and the fat mass for hypothetical patients by using the relationships of Chamney et al. (Chamney et al. 2007) in order to establish the state of hydration and to estimate their nutritional status. The following table shows the parameters of the patients needed for the calculations.

	Weight (kg)	ECW (liters)	ICW (liters)
Patient 1	71	15.5	17
Patient 2	73.5	14.6	14.8
Patient 3	57.3	10.7	13.8

MULTIPLE CHOICE QUESTIONS

Choose the best answer

1. The circuit used in a standard way to represent in vivo biological tissues is composed by:
   A. A shunt circuit composed by a resistor to define the intracellular path of the current and by a resistor and a capacitor in series representing the path of extracellular current.
   B. A shunt circuit composed by a capacitor to define the extracellular path of the current and by a resistor and a capacitor in series representing the path of intracellular current.
   C. A shunt circuit composed by a resistor to define the extracellular path of the current and by a resistor and a capacitor in series representing the path of intracellular current.
   D. A shunt circuit composed by a capacitor to define the intracellular path of the current and by a resistor and a capacitor in series representing the path of extracellular current.

2. To avoid any possible adverse health effects in exposed individuals as well as any interference with the user biological signals, bioimpedance commercial devices typically inject a current:
  A. Lower than 1 mA/cm^2.
  B. Lower than 1 μA/cm^2.
  C. Lower than 10 μA/cm^2.
  D. No matter the size of the electrode while the current is lower than 10 mA.

3. In what position could the electrodes of a bioelectrical impedance analyzer be fixed to measure the impedance of the trunk?
  A. Current injection electrodes on the hand and foot, and sensing electrodes on the wrist and ankle, all in the extremities of the same side.
  B. Current injection electrodes on the hand and foot of the limbs on one side, and sensing electrodes on the wrist and ankle on the opposite side.
  C. Current injection electrodes on the hand and foot of the limbs on one side, and sensing electrodes placed one on each ankle.
  D. Current injection electrodes fixed one on each hand, and sensing electrodes fixed one on each wrist.

4. What frequency is considered as the standard for bioimpedance measurements?
  A. 50 kHz.
  B. 5 kHz.
  C. 100 kHz.
  D. 20 kHz and 100 kHz.

5. In BIVA analysis, a change in the direction of the major axis of tolerance ellipses from the center to the upper pole of the tolerance ellipse of 50% represents:
  A. Unfavorable evolution to malnutrition.
  B. Unfavorable evolution to obesity.
  C. Unfavorable evolution to overhydration.
  D. Unfavorable evolution to dehydration.

6. Using the SFBIA approximation of Sergi et al. (Sergi et al. 1994) to estimate ECW, what would the ECW volume be of a hypothetical male patient of height 158 cm that presents a global lateral impedance value at 50 kHz with resistance equal to 459.8 ohms and reactance in absolute value equal to 26.1 ohms?

A. 5.16 liters
B. 9.67 liters
C. 10.42 liters
D. 18.46 liters

7. Using the SFBIA approximation of Kyle et al. (Kyle et al. 2001) for FFM estimation, calculate the proportion of FFM of a hypothetical female patient of height 156 cm and weight 55.8 kg that presents a global lateral impedance value at 50 kHz with resistance equal to 675.3 ohms and reactance in absolute value equal to 40.5 ohms:
A. 23.12 Kg
B. 32.72 Kg
C. 34.01 Kg
D. 42.53 Kg

8. With the BIS approximation based on the Cole-Cole model of De Lorenzo et al. (De Lorenzo et al. 1995) for ICW estimation, obtain the ICW volume of a hypothetical male patient of height 167 cm, weight 81.4 kg and 63 years old that presents a R_{ICW} resistance equivalent to 1014.9 ohms:
A. 14.97 liters.
B. 16.63 liters.
C. 20.51 liters.
D. 22.62 liters.

9. Using the BIS approximation based on Hanai mixture theory of Van Loan et al. (Van Loan et al. 1993), what would the ECW volume be of a hypothetical female patient of height 161 cm and weight 64.1 kg that presents a R_{ECW} resistance equivalent to 796.5 ohms?
A. 12.89 liters.
B. 14.71 liters.
C. 18.93 liters.
D. 21.56 liters.

10. Using the modification of BIS approximation based on Hanai mixture theory described by Moissl et al. (Moissl et al. 2006), calculate the ICW volume of a hypothetical patient of height 161 cm and weight 75.4 kg that presents a R_{ICW} resistance equivalent to 1311.3 ohms:
A. 15.62 liters.
B. 17.87 liters.
C. 19.19 liters.
D. 21.23 liters.

11. Using the BIVA method from the graph of Case Study II, perform an assessment of hydration and nutritional status of a hypothetical woman of height 155 cm that presents a global lateral impedance value at 50 kHz with resistance equal to 310 ohms and reactance in absolute value equal to 23 ohms:
   A. Normal nutritional status, normal hydration.
   B. Normal nutritional status, dehydrated.
   C. Malnourished, dehydrated.
   D. Obese, overhydrated.

12. Using the BIVA method from the graph of Case Study I, perform an assessment of hydration and nutritional status of a hypothetical man of height 169 cm that presents a global lateral impedance value at 50 kHz with resistance equal to 760 ohms and reactance in absolute value equal to 84 ohms:
   A. Normal nutritional status, normal hydration.
   B. Normal nutritional status, dehydrated.
   C. Malnourished, dehydrated.
   D. Obese, overhydrated.

13. Using the BIVA method from the graph of Case Study II, perform an assessment of hydration and nutritional status of a hypothetical woman of height 153 cm that presents a global lateral impedance value at 50 kHz with resistance equal to 535 ohms and reactance in absolute value equal to 53 ohms:
   A. Normal nutritional status, normal hydration.
   B. Normal nutritional status, dehydrated.
   C. Malnourished, dehydrated.
   D. Obese, overhydrated.

14. According to the reference graph of hydration presented by Wabel et al (2008), realize an assessment of the status of a patient that presents an fluid excess of 2 liters and a systolic blood pressure of 140 mmHg.
   A. Patient with hydration status and blood pressure comparable to healthy population.
   B. Patient with hydration status and blood pressure comparable to pre-dialysis population.
   C. Patient overhydrated but with a blood pressure within normal levels.
   D. Overhydrated and hypertensive patient.

15. According to the reference graph of hydration described by Wabel et al (2008), realize an assessment of the status of a patient that presents an fluid excess of 0.9 liters and a systolic blood pressure of 135 mmHg.
   A. Patient with hydration status and blood pressure comparable to healthy population.
   B. Patient with hydration status and blood pressure comparable to pre-dialysis population.
   C. Patient overhydrated but with a blood pressure within normal levels.
   D. Overhydrated and hypertensive patient.

16. In relation to the fluid control in dialysis patients, which situation is considered undesirable?
   A. An excess of fluid is dangerous, as it may be a predisposing factor for the development of hypertension or left ventricular hypertrophy. However, it is recommended that the patient is somewhat dehydrated.
   B. Removing too much fluid is dangerous because the patient ends suffering from hypotension, which is also associated with increased mortality in hemodialysis patients.
   C. An excess of fluid is dangerous, the patient ends suffering from hypotension, which is also associated with increased mortality in hemodialysis patients.
   D. Removing too much fluid is dangerous, as it may be a predisposing factor for the development of hypertension or left ventricular hypertrophy.

17. In hemodialysis, which is the definition of patient dry weight?
   A. The patient's weight at the beginning of an hemodialysis session.
   B. The patient's weight reached at the end of an hemodialysis session.
   C. The patient's weight reached at the end of an hemodialysis session, in which the maximum amount of fluid is removed without inducing hypotension.
   D. The patient's weight at the beginning of an hemodialysis session, in which the minimum amount of fluid is removed without inducing hypertension.

18. Regarding the dielectric properties of tissues, which of the following options is correct?
   A. The permittivity of tissues increases with frequency.
   B. β dispersion is associated with the polarization of cell membranes.
   C. β dispersion occurs at low frequencies in the range of 10 Hz up to 10 kHz.
   D. γ dispersion occurs about in the range of gigahertzs, and it is mainly due to dipolar polarization of water molecules.

19. Regarding the resistance values of the human body circuit model:
   A. The extracellular resistance is measured at a very high frequency (above 5 MHz).
   B. To measure the resistance at zero frequency (R_0), a direct current (DC) is applied.
   C. The application of DC or currents at a very high frequency using electrodes placed on the skin is not allowed.
   D. Bioimpedance meters are normally limited in their application to the range of 5 kHz up to 10 MHz.

20. What is the recommended position for bioimpedance measurements to determine body composition?
   A. It is recommended that measurements are carried out with the body in vertical position, with legs apart about 45° one from the other and arms 30° away from the body.
   B. It is recommended that measurements are carried out with the body in vertical position, with hands and feet close to the body.
   C. It is recommended that measurements are carried out with the body in supine position, with legs apart about 45° one from the other and arms 30° away from the body.
   D. It is recommended that measurements are carried out with the body in supine position, with hands and feet close to the body.

Author Index

Printed by Publishers' Graphics LLC
BT20130108.19.20.135